Sears's
Anatomy and Physiology for Nurses

Sears's Anatomy and Physiology for Nurses

As per INC Syllabus

Seventh Edition

Indira CK MBBS MD
Associate Professor
Government Medical College
Konni, Kerala, India

Mini Vasudevan MBBS MD
Additional Professor
Government Medical College
Thrissur, Kerala, India

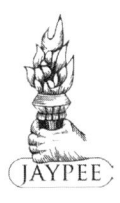

The Health Sciences Publisher
New Delhi | London | Panama

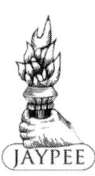 **Jaypee Brothers Medical Publishers (P) Ltd**

Headquarters
Jaypee Brothers Medical Publishers (P) Ltd
4838/24, Ansari Road, Daryaganj
New Delhi 110 002, India
Phone: +91-11-43574357
Fax: +91-11-43574314
Email: jaypee@jaypeebrothers.com

Overseas Offices

J.P. Medical Ltd
83 Victoria Street, London
SW1H 0HW (UK)
Phone: +44 20 3170 8910
Fax: +44 (0)20 3008 6180
Email: info@jpmedpub.com

Jaypee-Highlights Medical Publishers Inc
City of Knowledge, Bld. 235, 2nd Floor, Clayton
Panama City, Panama
Phone: +1 507-301-0496
Fax: +1 507-301-0499
Email: cservice@jphmedical.com

Jaypee Brothers Medical Publishers (P) Ltd
17/1-B Babar Road, Block-B, Shaymali
Mohammadpur, Dhaka-1207
Bangladesh
Mobile: +08801912003485
Email: jaypeedhaka@gmail.com

Jaypee Brothers Medical Publishers (P) Ltd
Bhotahity, Kathmandu
Nepal
Phone: +977-9741283608
Email: kathmandu@jaypeebrothers.com

Website: www.jaypeebrothers.com
Website: www.jaypeedigital.com

© 2018, Jaypee Brothers Medical Publishers

The views and opinions expressed in this book are solely those of the original contributor(s)/author(s) and do not necessarily represent those of editor(s) of the book.

All rights reserved. No part of this publication may be reproduced, stored or transmitted in any form or by any means, electronic, mechanical, photocopying, recording or otherwise, without the prior permission in writing of the publishers.

All brand names and product names used in this book are trade names, service marks, trademarks or registered trademarks of their respective owners. The publisher is not associated with any product or vendor mentioned in this book.

Medical knowledge and practice change constantly. This book is designed to provide accurate, authoritative information about the subject matter in question. However, readers are advised to check the most current information available on procedures included and check information from the manufacturer of each product to be administered, to verify the recommended dose, formula, method and duration of administration, adverse effects and contraindications. It is the responsibility of the practitioner to take all appropriate safety precautions. Neither the publisher nor the author(s)/editor(s) assume any liability for any injury and/or damage to persons or property arising from or related to use of material in this book.

This book is sold on the understanding that the publisher is not engaged in providing professional medical services. If such advice or services are required, the services of a competent medical professional should be sought.

Every effort has been made where necessary to contact holders of copyright to obtain permission to reproduce copyright material. If any have been inadvertently overlooked, the publisher will be pleased to make the necessary arrangements at the first opportunity. The **CD/DVD-ROM** (if any) provided in the sealed envelope with this book is complimentary and free of cost. **Not meant for sale.**

Inquiries for bulk sales may be solicited at: jaypee@jaypeebrothers.com

Sears's Anatomy and Physiology for Nurses

Sixth Edition: **1985 (Publisher: Edward Arnold ELBS)**

Seventh Edition: **2018**

ISBN: 978-93-86261-55-7

Printed at Sanat Printers

Dedicated to
Our families and colleagues

Preface to the Seventh Edition

This seventh edition has been revised with a view to include the facts of Anatomy and Physiology which should be known to the graduates in Nursing Schools. It includes understanding the basics of Human Anatomy and Physiology in such a way that—when assisting a doctor or left alone to deal with an emergency, the students should be able to realize the purpose of studying the subject. All that are to be known to a Nursing student regarding Anatomy and Physiology are explained with simple diagrams and notes so that the student can easily correlate to clinical aspects as well. Though not all, contents are modified in such a way that students will find it easy learning of Anatomy and Physiology. Diagrams are included to make learning this subject interesting.

In this edition, it is our goal to find new ways to help instructors teach more easily and effectively and students to learn pleasantly. This can be a unique solution to study Anatomy and Physiology in a concise manner for the nursing students.

Indira CK
Mini Vasudevan

Acknowledgments

We are indebted to Mr Rajee Reghunath (Principal) Amala Nursing College, Thrissur, Kerala, India for extending help towards writing the book. Also we are grately thankful to all the faculties of Government Nursing College, Thrissur, especially Lata CR (Principal) and her supporting staff. Special thanks to Ms Sreedevi CR for her motivation in editing the book. The authors sincerely thanks Dr Amar Jayanthi (Professor), Government Medical College, Idukki and Dr Arunkumar KG for the helping hands.

The authors sincerely thanks the faculties of Physiology Department, Government Medical College, Thrissur for their whole-hearted cooperation.

The authors also thanks their family members for their constant inspiration extended in writing this book.

Sincere thanks to Jaypee Brothers Medical Publishers (P) Ltd, New Delhi for the encouragement given to us to bring this book.

INC Syllabus

FIRST YEAR BSc NURSING ANATOMY

Placement: First Year
Time: Theory: 60 Hours

Course Description: The course is designed to enable students to acquire knowledge of the normal structure of various human body systems and understand the alterations in anatomical structures in disease and apply this in practice of nursing. Course content is divided into 3 categories: **must know, desirable to know and nice to know,** which is indicated as must know (***), desirable to know (**) and nice to know (*). 60% of questions for the examination should be from must know portions of content, 40% may be from desirable to know portions of content. Nice to know content may be discussed in the class but avoid questions from this part for university examination.

Unit	Time (hrs)	Learning Objectives	Content	Teaching Learning Activities	Assessment Methods	Chapter
I	3	Describe the anatomical terms, organization of human body and structure of cell, tissues, membranes and glands	Introduction to anatomical terms organization of the human body *** Human cell structure, tissues–definition, types, characteristics, classification, location, functions and formation, membranes and glands, classification and structure ** Organelle-structure and functions * Cell junctions	Lecture, discussion, explain using charts, microscopic slides, skeleton and torso	Short answer questions, objective Type	1, 2
II	5	Describe the structure of bones and joints	The Skeletal System *** Bones–types, structure, bone formation and growth, bones of limbs (description of bones), Joints–classification and major Joints-hip, shoulder, structure ** Knee joint, elbow joint Ossification-types, vertebra, ribs, sternum, bony pelvis, fetal skull * Wrist, carpometacarpal, tibiofibular, radioulnar joints, mention rickets, malignancies of bone	Lecture, discussion, explain using charts, skeleton, loose bones and joints	Structured essay, short answer questions, objective type	4, 5, 6

Unit	Time (hrs)	Learning Objectives	Content	Teaching Learning Activities	Assessment Methods	Chapter
III	3	Describe the structure of muscles	The muscular system *** Types and structure of muscles, gluteal muscles, thigh muscles and deltoid *** Structure of muscle in detail. Actions of various individual and groups of muscles * Myasthenia Gravis	Lecture, discussion, explain using charts, models and films Demonstrate muscular movements	Short answer questions, objective type	4, 7
IV	8	Describe the structure of nervous system	The nervous system *** Structure of neurons, meninges, CNS, ANS, parts of brain, spinal cord, cranial nerves, spinal nerves, peripheral nerves, auxillary, sciatic, femoral, radial, important cutaneous nerves ** Difference in function of sympathetic and parasympathetic, blood supply of cerebrum autonomic nervous system ventricles of brain * Structure of spinal cord, cerebrum, cerebellum hydrocephalus	Lecture, discussion, explain using models, charts, slides, specimens	Structured essay questions, short answer questions, objective type	17
V	4	Explain the structure of sensory organs	The sensory organs *** Structure of skin, eye-layers, ear, nose, tongue ** Muscles of eyeball, middle ear * Common sensory dysfunction	Lecture, discussion, explain using models, charts, slides, specimens	Short answer questions, objective type	15
VI	7	Describe the structure of circulatory and lymphatic system	Circulatory and lymphatic system *** Heart-layers chambers- features, blood supply, structure of blood vessels Arterial and venous system, Circulation: systemic pulmonary, coronary, lymph- atic system, lymphatic tissues: - Thymus gland - Lymph nodes - Spleen tonsil ** Major arteries of limbs, head and neck, thorax, abdomen and pelvis veins usually used for IV injections * Conducting system of heart, sites of portosystemic anastomosis, microscopic structure of lymphoid organs IHD, myocardial infarction, tonsillectomy splenomegaly	Lecture, discussion, explain using models, charts, slides, specimens	Structured essay questions, short answer questions, objective type	10, 11

Unit	Time (hrs)	Learning Objectives	Content	Teaching Learning Activities	Assessment Methods	Chapter
VII	5	Describe the structure of respiratory system	The respiratory system *** Trachea, bronchi, lungs, pleura Muscles of respiration: intercostal and diaphragm ** Bronchopulmonary segments * Investigations for lung diseases-pneumonia, pleural effusion, pneumothorax, site for pleural, lung function tests	Lecture, discussions, explain using models, torso, charts, slides, specimens	Short answer questions, objective type	8
VIII	7	Describe the structure of digestive system	The digestive system *** Parts of alimentary tract-esophagus extent, constrictions stomach, pancreas, liver, cecum, appendix, large intestine, rectum and anal canal in detail, blood supply accessory organs of digestion ** Structure of stomach, intestines, liver, pancreas * Liver function tests, investigations-barium studies hernias	Lecture, discussion, explain using models, torso, charts, slides, specimens	Structural essay questions, short answer questions, objective types	12
IX	6	Describe the structure of excretory system	The excretory system *** Structure of organs of urinary system: Kidney, ureter, urinary bladder, urethra- male, female ** Structure of nephron * Microscopic structure of kidney, ureter, urinary bladder, investigations of the renal system, catheterization	Lecture, discussion, explain using models, torso, charts, slides, specimens	Short answer questions, objective type	16
X	5	Describe the structure of endocrine system	The endocrine system *** Parts of pituitary, pancreas, thyroid, parathyroid, and adrenal glands, thymus ** Diseases caused by hyper and hypofunctions of organs * Microscopic structure of organs	Lecture, discussion, explain using models, torso, charts, slides, specimens	Short answer questions, objective type	14

Unit	Time (hrs)	Learning Objectives	Content	Teaching Learning Activities	Assessment Methods	Chapter
XI	5	Describe the structure of reproductive system	The reproductive system including breast *** Female reproductive organs- uterus, tubes, vagina Male reproductive organs-testis, mammary gland ** Prostate, vas deferens, ovary investigations of reproductive system * Microscopic structure of organs, common causes of infertility and their treatment	Lecture, discussion, explain using models, torso, charts, slides, specimens	Short answer questions, objective type	19

REFERENCES

- Dr Sreedevi P, Fundamental Aspects of Anatomy, 1st edn.
- Ashalatha PR, Textbook of Anatomy and Physiology for Nurses, Jaypee Brothers, New Delhi.
- Chaurasia BD, Human Anatomy Vol I, II and III, CBS Publishers, Delhi-32.
- Williams et al., Gray's Anatomy-39th edn., Churchil Livingstone, New York.
- Tortora and Grabowski, Principles of Anatomy and Physiology, 8th edn. Harper Collins.
- Kimber and Grey, Textbook of Anatomy and Physiology, CV Moshy Co., St Louis.
- Millard et al. Human Anatomy and Physiology, WB Saunders Company Philadelphia.
- Bajpai RN, Human Histology, Jaypee Brothers Medical Publishers, New Delhi.
- Singh Inderbir, Essentials of Anatomy, 2nd edn. Jaypee Brothers.

PHYSIOLOGY

Placement: First Year
Time: Theory: 60 Hours

Course Description: The course is designed to enable the students to acquire knowledge of the normal physiology of various human body systems and understand the alterations in physiology in diseases and apply this in practice of nursing.

Course content is divided into 3 categories: **must know, desirable to know and nice to know,** which is indicated as must know (***), desirable to know (**) and nice to know (*). 60% of questions for the examination should be from must know portions of content, 40% may be from desirable portions of content. Nice to know content may be discussed in the class but avoid questions from this part for university examination.

Unit	Time (hrs)	Learning Objectives	Content	Teaching Learning Activities	Assessment Methods	Chapter
I	3	Describe the physiology of cell, tissues, membranes and glands	General and cell physiology *** Membranes and glands-functions Concept of ECF and ICF homeostasis ** Intravenous fluid therapy-basic principles only * Tissue-formation, repair, alterations in disease	Lecture, discussion	Short answer questions, objective type	2
II	2	Describe the bone formation and growth and movements of skeletal system	Skeletal system * Bone formation and growth Bones-functions and movements of bones of axial and appendicular skeleton, bone healing, joints and joint movement, alterations in disease, applications and implications in nursing	Lecture, discussion, explain using charts, models and films, demonstration of joint movements	Short answer questions, objective type	5
III	5	Describe the muscle movements and tone and demonstrate muscle contraction and tone	Muscular system (nerve and muscle) *** Nerve: Stimulus–impulse definitions and mechanism, Membrane potentials briefly, functions of neurons and neurolgia, physiology of muscle contraction, comparative study of skeletal, cardiac and smooth muscle. Neuromuscular transmission ** Alterations in disease, mention myasthenia gravis and dystrophies * Muscle movements	Lecture, discussion, explain using charts, models slides, specimen and films, demonstration of muscle movements, tone and contraction	Short answer questions, objective type	7

Unit	Time (hrs)	Learning Objectives	Content	Teaching Learning Activities	Assessment Methods	Chapter
IV	8	Describe the physiology of nerve stimulus, reflexes, brain, cranial and spinal nerves, demonstrate reflex action and stimulus	Nervous system *** Organization: Brain, spinal cord, cranial and spinal nerves. Autonomic nervous system, ascending and descending tracts ascending tracts. Pain: Somatic, visceral, and referred, cerebrospinal fluid-composition, circulation and function. Synapse: Properties, functions reflex arc, reflex action and reflexes. Function of thalamus, hypothalamus, basal ganglia, cerebellum-functions. ** Mention muscle tone levels and maintenance of posture. Parkinsonism, spinal cord injury, hemiplegia, paraplegia, lumbar puncture, raised ICT, stroke, alterations in disease sleep and disturbances * Autonomic learning and biofeedback	Lecture, discussion, explain using charts, models slides, and films. Demonstrate nerve stimulus, reflex action, reflexes	Structured essay, short answer questions, objective type	17
V	8	Describe the physiology of blood and functions of heart, demonstrate blood cell count, coagulation grouping, Hb: BP and Pulse monitoring	Circulatory system blood *** Functions, composition, [formed elements: RBC, WBC platelets] Blood groups, blood coagulation, hemoglobin: estimation blood transfusion, reactions lymph ** Jaundice, leukocytosis, leukemia, polycythemia, anemia * Structure, synthesis and breakdown of hemoglobin: Variation of molecules, Immunity, formation of T cells and B cells, types of immune response, antigens, antibodies, cytokines. Circulation: Circulation-principles, functions of heart, conduction, cardiac cycle, BP and Pulse: control, factors influencing ** BP, hypertension, circulatory shock, cardiac failure ECG Alterations in disease, applications and implications in nursing	Lecture, discussion, explain using charts, films demonstration of blood cell count, coagulation, grouping, hemoglobin estimation, heart conduction system, measurement of pulse, BP	Structured essay, Short answer questions, objective type	3, 9, 10

INC Syllabus

Unit	Time (hrs)	Learning Objectives	Content	Teaching Learning Activities	Assessment Methods	Chapter
VI	6	Describe the physiology and mechanisms of respiration, demonstrates spirometry	The respiratory system *** Functions of respiratory organs, volumes, pulmonary ventilation, mechanics of ventilation, gaseous exchange in lungs, carriage of oxygen and carbon dioxide, exchange of gases in tissues ** Alterations in disease-hypoxia, asphyxia, artificial respiration, periodic breathing, cyanosis, O_2 therapy, O_2 toxicity, regulation of respiration	Lecture, discussion, explain using charts, films, demonstration of spirometry	Structured essay, short answer questions, objective type	8
VII	6	Describe the physiology of digestive system, demonstrates BMR	The digestive system *** Functions of organs of digestive tract, movements of alimentary tract Digestion in mouth, stomach, small intestines, large intestines, absorption of food Functions of liver, gallbladder and pancreas, vomiting and diarrhea ** Jaundice * Metabolism of carbohydrates, protein and fat (in biochemistry)	Lecture, discussion, explain using charts, films	Structured essay, short answer questions objective type	12
VIII	6	Describe the physiology of excretory system	Excretory system *** Functions of kidneys, composition of urine, mechanism of urine formation, filtration, reabsorption, secretion urinary bladder ** Alterations in disease-impaired renal function, dialysis * Role of kidney in fluid and acid base balance *** Functions of skin, regulation of body temperature	Lecture, discussion, explain using charts, films	Structured essay, short answer questions, objective type	16
IX	3	Describe the physiology of sensory organs	Special senses (sensory organs) *** Vision audition olfaction taste ** Errors of refraction, glaucoma, color blindness, deafness	Lecture, discussion, explain using charts, films, demonstration of BMR	Short answer questions, objective type	18

Unit	Time (hrs)	Learning Objectives	Content	Teaching Learning Activities	Assessment Methods	Chapter
X	5	Describe the physiology of endocrine glands	Endocrine system *** Functions of pituitary, thyroid, parathyroid, pancreas, suprarenal, placenta and ovaries and testes ** (Briefly about common diseases) * Pineal body, thymus	Lecture, discussion, explain using charts, films, demonstration of BMR	Short answer questions, objective type	14
XI	8	Describe the physiology of male and female reproductive system	Reproductive system *** Functions of female reproductive organs, functions of breast, menstrual cycle, ovulation, pregnancy tests ** Physiological principles underlying contraception * Reproduction of cells- DNA, mitosis, meiosis, spermatogenesis, oogenesis, introduction to embryology *** Functions of male reproductive organs	Lecture, discussion, explain using charts, films, models, specimens	Structured essay, short answer questions, objective type	19

REFERENCES

- Choudhary, Concise Medical Physiology
- Jain AK, Textbook of Physiology for Nurses
- Ashalatha PR, Textbook of Anatomy and Physiology for Nurses, Jaypee Brothers, New Delhi
- Khurana I (2006) Textbook of Medical Physiology, New Delhi, Elsevier
- Guyton AC and Hall JE (2006), Medical Physiology, Philadelphia, Guyton and Hall
- Review of Medical Physiology, Ganong 23rd edn.

Contents

1. **Introduction** — 1
2. **Cells and Tissues** — 7
   - Cell *7* • Cellular Organization *7* • General and Cell Physiology *11*
   - Body Fluids and Intravenous Fluid Therapy *16* • Tissues *17*
   - Epithelium *18* • Connective Tissue *19* • Cartilage *20* • Bone *21*
   - Muscular Tissue *23* • Nerve *24* • Properties of Neurons *25*
   - Action Potential *26*
3. **Immunity** — 28
   - Innate Immunity *28* • Acquired Immunity *30*
4. **The Body as a Whole** — 33
   - The Skull *34* • The Thorax *34* • The Abdomen *35*
   - Systems of the Body *36*
5. **The Skeleton** — 37
   - Development of Bone *39* • Growth of Bones *39*
   - Practical Considerations *40* • The Skeleton as a Whole *40*
   - Types of Bone *40* • The Human Skeleton *42* • Bones of the Shoulder Girdle and Upper Limb *43* • Bones of the Pelvic Girdle *49* • The Bones of the Lower Limb *52* • The Skull *56* • The Vertebral Column *69*
   - Bones of the Thorax *75*
6. **Joints or Articulations** — 79
   - Joints of Upper Limb *80* • Joints of Pelvic Girdle and Lower Limb *83*
   - Vessels and Nerves *84*
7. **Physiology of Muscle Contraction** — 89
   - Skeletal Muscle *89* • Sarcomere *89* • Sarcolemma *90* • Properties of Skeletal Muscle *91* • Mechanism of Muscle Contraction *92*
   - Cardiac Muscle *94* • Smooth Muscle *95* • Neuromuscular Transmission *96*
   - Skeletal Muscles *97* • Principal Groups of Muscles *99*
8. **Respiratory System** — 110
   - Nasal Cavity *110* • Pharynx *112* • Larynx *113* • Pleura and Lungs *115*
   - Respiratory Movements *116* • Voice Production *118* • Physiology of Respiration *119* • Histology of Terminal Bronchiole *120* • Functions of Lungs *122* • Measurement of Pulmonary Ventilation *123* • Spirogram *124*

- Changes Occurring in Lungs *128* • Regulation of Respiration *129*
- Chemical Regulation *131* • Hypoxia *133* • Asphyxia *134*
- Disorders of Respiration *135* • Artificial Respiration *135*

9. **The Blood (Hemopoietic System)**   137
   - Composition and Functions of Blood *137* • Formed Elements *139* • Variations in Size, Shape, and Structure of RBC *140*
   - Anemia *144* • Erythropoiesis *146* • Eosinophil *152* • Leukopenia *154*
   - Blood Group *161*

10. **Circulatory System**   166
    - Heart and Great Vessels *167* • Cardiovascular Physiology *170* • Heart *170* • ECG *175* • Vascular System *188* • Poiseuille's Law *188* • Nervous Control of the Heartbeat *189* • The Blood Pressure *190* • Cardiac Failure *194* • Shock *195* • Regional Circulations *196* • Cereberal Circulation *197* • Brain Metabolism and Oxygen Requirements *198* • Cutaneous Circulation *198*

11. **The Mononuclear Phagocytic and Lymphoid Systems**   200
    - The Lymphoid System *200*

12. **The Digestive System**   207
    - Salivary Glands *208* • Stomach *208* • Duodenum *210* • Jejunum *210*
    - Ileum *210* • Cecum *211* • The Accessory Organs of Digestion *215*
    - Physiological Anatomy *222* • Ingestion of Food *222* • Acid Secretion *226*
    - Regulation of Pancreatic Secretion *229* • Jaundice *232*
    - Digestion and Absorption of Food *235*

13. **Metabolism and Nutrition**   238
    - Basal Metabolic Rate *239* • Vitamins *246* • Water *248* • Fiber *248*
    - Nutrition *248* • Control of Food Intake *249*

14. **The Endocrine System**   251
    - Classification of Hormones *252* • Pituitary Gland *253* • Anterior Pituitary Hormones *253* • Growth Hormone *256* • Somatomedins or Insulin Like Growth Factors *257* • Pituitary Insufficiency in Humans *259*
    - Panhypopituitarism in the Adult *259* • Pituitary Hyperfunction *259*
    - Posterior Pituitary *261* • The Thyroid Gland *264* • The Thyroid *265*
    - Antithyroid Drugs *269* • Calcium Metabolism *271* • Phosphorus Metabolism *272* • The Parathyroid Glands *273* • Abnormalities *274*
    - The Pineal Gland *275* • The Sex Glands or Gonads *275* • The Suprarenal Glands *275* • Adrenal Cortex *278* • Actions of Glucocorticoids *279*
    - Hormones of Adrenal Medulla *281* • Pheochromocytoma *283*
    - The Pancreas *283* • The Endocrine Pancreas *284* • Insulin *284*
    - Applied Physiology *286* • Diabetes Mellitus *286* • Glucagon *287*
    - Somatostatin *288* • Pancreatic Polypeptide (PP) *288*

15.	**The Skin and Regulation of Body Temperature**	289
	• The Skin *289* • Functions of the Skin *294* • Regulation of Body Temperature *294*	
16.	**Excretory System**	298
	• The Kidneys *298* • Structure *299* • Blood Supply *301* • Functions of Kidneys *301* • Functional Anatomy *304* • Tubular Function *305* • Aquaporins *311* • Water Intoxication *311* • Tubular Secretion *311* • Hypokalemia *312* • Concentration and Dilution of Urine *313* • Role of Urea *316* • Acidification of Urine *316* • Diuretics *317* • Urinary Bladder *317* • Micturition Reflex *318*	
17.	**The Nervous System**	320
	• Nervous System *320* • The Meninges *321* • Cerebrospinal Fluid *322* • CSF Composition *323* • The Spinal Cord *324* • Structure of Spinal Cord *326* • The Spinal Nerves *327* • Sensation and the Sensory Path *331* • Neurotransmitters *332* • The Cranial Nerves *333* • Pain *338* • The Brain *343* • Cerebrum *344* • Motor System *345* • Functional Areas of Cerebral Cortex *347* • Thalamus *349* • Hypothalamus *350* • Internal Capsule *350* • Ventricles *350* • Hydrocephalus *352* • Blood Brain Barrier *352* • The Brainstem *354* • Reticular Formation *354* • Cerebellum *355* • Basal Ganglia *356* • Movement and the Motor Path *359* • Synapse *361* • Synaptic Transmission *363* • Reflexes *366* • Receptors *372*	
18.	**The Sense Organs**	375
	• Sensation in the Skin *375* • The Sense of Smell *376* • The Sense of Taste *376* • The Sense of Hearing *377* • The Sense of Sight—Vision *382*	
19.	**Reproductive System**	391
	• Sex Organs *391* • Male Reproductive System *392* • Female Reproductive System *398* • The Female Climacteric and Menopause *404* • The Breasts (Mammary Glands) *404* • Functions of the Breast *405* • Pregnancy *406*	
20.	**Ageing**	413
	• Changes due to Ageing *413* • The Special Senses *415* • Temperature Regulation *415* • Thirst *416* • Pain *416* • Resistance to Infection *416* • The Relevance of Ageing to Clinical Medicine *416*	

Weights and Measures   417

SI Units   418

Index   419

CHAPTER 1

Introduction

Life is, perhaps, the most mysterious fact in the Universe and it is not unreasonable that humans have devoted much study to this phenomenon. One of the results of their labors is the science of biology. In its broad sense, this subject embraces all living matter, both animal and vegetable, in all its forms, both visible and microscopic.

The study of the simplest forms of life contributes to the better understanding of those which have attained a more complicated and advanced degree of development in the scale of nature.

From the earliest concepts of the subject, careful study and the application of logical thinking, backed by evidence supported by ever-growing scientific techniques, has provided an enormous amount of knowledge. Much of this knowledge is so advanced and so specialized that it can only be appreciated by the few and even they would be the first to admit that such knowledge is incomplete and always capable of further expansion.

Human biology may be studied as a pure science. On the other hand, for doctors, nurses and many other workers it is the practical application of this knowledge to the understanding of disease and the general well-being of the human race that is of greatest importance.

In order to attain the necessary understanding, some familiarity with science in general is essential and, in order to apply it to full advantage, there must be further appreciation of the workings of the human mind and the development of one of the greatest of human attributes, namely sympathy.

To return to the basic aspects of human biology, this has numerous subdivisions which include anatomy, physiology and biochemistry. However, 'the divisions of the sciences are like the branches of a tree that join in one trunk' (Francis Bacon) and they are, therefore, more or less closely related to one another.

Anatomy is the study of the parts of the body, their form, position and relationship to each other.

This knowledge has been obtained by careful dissection and further expanded by the detailed study of the structure of the various tissues under the microscope (Histology).

A greater understanding of the subject has been obtained by studying the anatomy of other members of the animal kingdom (comparative anatomy), development from conception to birth (embryology), and a general consideration of evolution.

In recent years it has been increasingly possible to gain knowledge of the internal anatomy of the living subject by means of non-invasive imaging techniques.

Ultrasonography uses the echoes of ultrasound waves to build up a picture of the contents of the abdomen in which a fetus or any abnormal masses may be studied (Fig. 1.1).

Echocardiography uses the same principles to obtain structural and

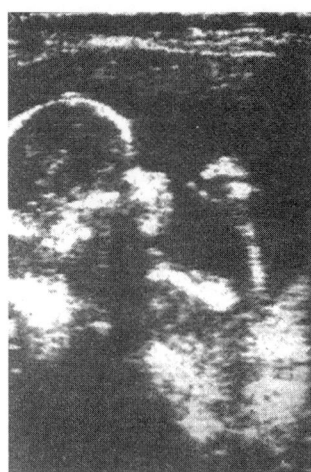

Fig. 1.1: Ultrasound image of a fetus in the womb (*in utero*) with hand to mouth

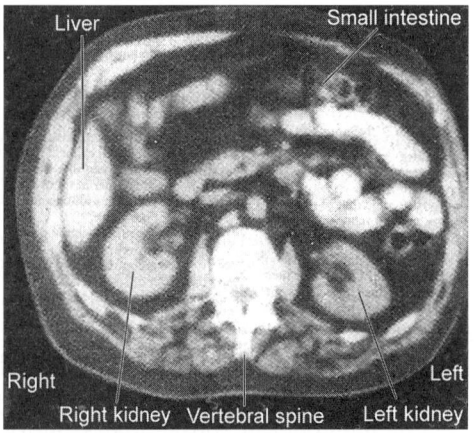

Fig. 1.2: CT scan at the level of the kidneys

functional information about the heart. With this technique, the opening and closing of the valves and the wall-motion may be seen and measured.

Computerized tomography (CT scanning) (Fig. 1.2) produces sharp clear images of normal and abnormal structures by distinguishing between their relative densities. Cross sections of the head and trunk may be studied at any level. The anatomical display may be helpful in teaching but is primarily used for diagnostic purposes. Abscesses, cysts and tumors may be detected and the exact anatomical position for a needle biopsy determined. Similarly, the investigation may be helpful in planning radiotherapy.

Nuclear magnetic resonance (NMR) is the latest major non-invasive imaging technique to be developed but its availability is currently limited by its cost.

Many techniques are available for the study of physiology and its alteration by disease. The electroencephalogram (EEG) is a well-known example of one which is non-invasive. It provides information on brain function and dysfunction and this method of investigation is frequently complementary to a CT scan.

Physiology is the study of the functions of the body as a whole and of the individual structures and organs contained therein. Some of this is reasonably simple; some involves complicated chemical, physical and electrical details.

Every living structure, whether it be animal or vegetable, is derived, so far as we know, from another living structure. It has the power of growth and reproduction, and its life is dependent upon its ability to absorb non-living material which it builds up into the framework of its own body.

Before considering living matter, it is necessary to go back a step further and ascertain the nature of the chemical substances of which it is composed, and which are, therefore, found in the human body as a whole.

Broadly speaking, there are two types of matter—elements and compounds. The latter may be divided into inorganic and organic.

An element is a substance which contains only one kind of matter. The following are the most important elements found in the human body—carbon, hydrogen, nitrogen, oxygen, sulfur, phosphorus, chlorine, iodine, sodium, potassium, magnesium, calcium and iron.

Of these, oxygen and nitrogen commonly occur in their uncombined natural state. The others are found combined with one another in the form of compounds.

A chemical compound is a combination of two or more elements in fixed proportions forming an entirely new substance in which the individual elements apparently lose their identity, thereby differing from a simple mixture. Every part of a compound has exactly the same composition and properties as every other part.

Inorganic compounds are relatively simple combinations of the elements found especially in non-living matter such as minerals, water and salts.

The essential feature of organic compounds is the presence of the element carbon, usually combined with hydrogen and oxygen. In addition, nitrogen and other elements may also be included and form compounds of a highly complicated nature which are found especially in living matter.

The main organic compounds found in the body are carbohydrates, fats and proteins.

All three of these contain carbon, hydrogen and oxygen but proteins also contain nitrogen and other elements.

Going back one stage further in the structure of matter, and in order to understand some of the principles which must be considered in physiology, it is necessary to have some knowledge of the atomic theory which was propounded by Dalton nearly one hundred and eighty years ago. This has been the basis of chemical science ever since.

Stated simply, this implies the following:
- The basis of all matter is the atom.
- If further subdivided, an atom consists of protons, neutrons and electrons. The protons and electrons each carry a unit charge of electricity. That of the former is positive and that of the latter negative. The neutrons, as their name implies, are electrically inactive (Fig. 1.3).

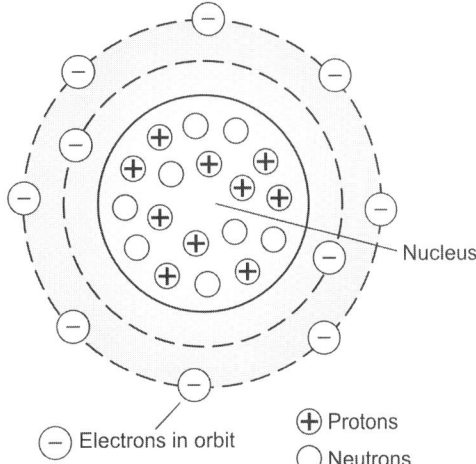

Fig. 1.3: Diagram of an atom with ten positive protons in the nucleus and ten negative electrons in orbit

- Every atom consists of a central particle or nucleus around which constantly revolve in their own orbit one, a few or many smaller electrons. On an astronomical scale these are rather like planets revolving around the sun.
- The nucleus consists of a compressed mass of protons and neutrons. Because of the protons, it is positively charged with electricity. In order to render the atom as a whole electrically neutral, it has an appropriate number of circulating negative electrons.
- For example, the atom of hydrogen carries one electron; that of carbon, six; nitrogen, seven; oxygen, eight; sodium, eleven; chlorine, seventeen, and so on.
- Under ordinary circumstances the atoms of each element (except for its radioactive isotopes) are stable. In 1919 Rutherford succeeded in splitting the atom and his work led, step by step, to the modern science of nuclear physics.
- The atoms of most elements have the property of combining with atoms of other elements to form the molecules of new compounds.

- This power can best be visualized by imagining that the atom of each element has one or more hooks or bonds which can link up with a similar hook or hooks of another atom or atoms, e.g. hydrogen, sodium and chlorine have one hook; oxygen, calcium and sulfur, two; nitrogen, three; carbon, four; and so on.

  Thus, one atom of sodium can combine with one atom of chlorine to form one molecule of the compound, sodium chloride or common salt. Using standard chemical symbols this might be expressed thus:

  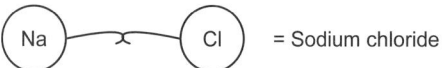

  and one atom of oxygen can combine with two of hydrogen:

  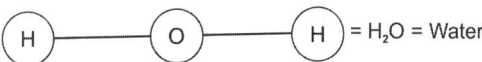

  Nitrogen having three 'hooks' can link up with three atoms of hydrogen to make a molecule of the compound ammonia.

  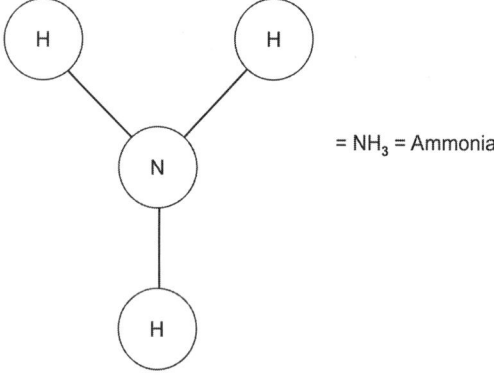

- In other words, the atoms of elements, by union with those of other elements, form the molecules of chemical compounds which have the combined mass of the individual elements which compose them. Therefore in scientific terms an atom is said to have its own atomic weight and a compound its molecular weight.

The atomic weight of an element is the average weight of an atom of that element in relation to the weight of an atom of hydrogen, which is taken as 1, e.g. carbon, 12; iron, 56; lead, 207.

Because the nucleus of some elements does not always have the same number of neutrons but still has the identical number of protons and electrons, there is a slight variation in the weights of individual atoms of a particular element. Those atoms which vary in weight from the standard are called isotopes. Many of these are unstable and are radioactive, discharging their nuclei (alpha particles) at high velocity.

Such radioactive isotopes introduced into the body can be detected and traced by a Geiger counter. Thus radioactive iodine given to an individual may be traced to the thyroid gland. In larger doses radioactive isotopes, for example radium, may be used to destroy the abnormal cells which occur in cancer.

The following table lists the elements present in the body and their respective symbols.

Carbon (C)	Chlorine (Cl)
Hydrogen (H)	Iodine (I)
Nitrogen (N)	Sodium (Na)
Oxygen (O)	Potassium (K)
Sulfur (S)	Magnesium (Mg)
Phosphorus (P)	Calcium (Ca)
	Iron (Fe)

Many other elements are present in only minute amounts and are known as trace elements. Some of these are essential to life; examples are cobalt, copper, manganese, molybdenum and

possibly selenium. Chromium may protect arteries from atherosclerosis. Some trace elements serve no useful purpose in the body but are contaminants.
- Returning to the example of sodium chloride, it will be recalled that the atom of sodium has eleven electrons and that of chlorine seventeen. In effecting the combination to form compound there is a rearrangement of the electrons in such a way that the sodium atoms become positively charged with electricity and the chlorine atoms become negatively charged. Such electrically charged atoms are called **ions**.
- When such compounds are dissolved in water some, but not all, of the molecules of the compound become *ionized* into their individual electrically charged atoms. Some of these atoms will carry a positive charge and the others a negative charge. In the case of sodium chloride, the sodium ions are positive (+) and the chlorine ions negative (−).

Atoms in this state of ionization, because they carry an electric charge, are referred to as electrolytes, and the solution containing them, an electrolyte solution. It is in this form that many salts, circulate in the water contained in the blood and tissue fluids of the body.
- Another aspect of this subject is the 'acid/alkaline' reaction of body fluids. The hydrogen ions (H^+) have a positive charge and are acid, while the hydroxyl ions (OH^-) are negative and cause alkalinity. If the H^+ ions and the OH^- ions are equally balanced the reaction of the fluid will be neutral:

$H^+ + OH^- = H_2O$ (or water which is neutral)

For practical purposes a scale has been devised and numbered from 1 to 14. The central figure of 7 is taken to represent neutrality and the hydrogen ion concentration is indicated by the symbol pH (Fig. 1.4).

Fluids having a pH of 1 to 7 are acid and those with a pH exceeding 7 are alkaline.

It must be understood that this is a scale only used to measure very small degrees of acidity and alkalinity. For example, the pH of the blood is kept constant at 7.4, i.e. very slightly alkaline but never acid. That of urine is usually slightly acid with a pH of 5 to 6.

One of the most important functions of the various salts present in the body is to keep the pH of the blood constant and

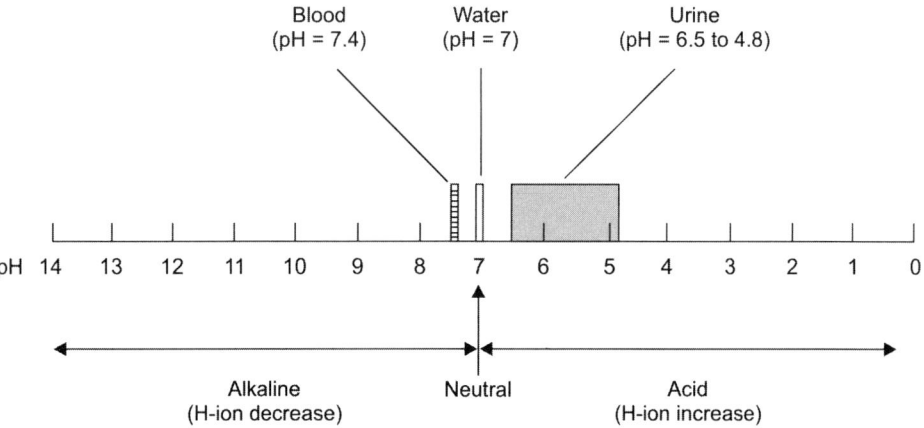

Fig. 1.4: Diagram illustrating hydrogen ion concentration (pH) in the body

there is a continuous interchange of various positive and negative ions in the tissues to maintain this equilibrium. Any excess of acid hydrogen ions is excreted in the urine by the kidney cells.

On the other hand, one of the most important end products of carbohydrate and fat metabolism is carbon dioxide (CO_2). When this is dissolved in water it forms a weak acid (carbonic acid):

$$CO_2 + H_2O \rightleftharpoons H_2CO_3 \rightleftharpoons H^+ + HCO_3$$

carbon dioxide — water — carbonic acid — hydrogen ion — bicarbonate ion

This, when ionized, also liberates acid H^+ in considerable quantity which would tend to lower the pH of the blood towards the neutral figure of 7. However, the respiratory center in the medulla of the brain is particularly sensitive to any change in the pH of the blood and immediately causes an increase in the rate and depth of breathing which is maintained until the excess of carbon dioxide (and at the same time the excess of hydrogen ions in the blood) is removed.

There are also certain salts together with the blood plasma which themselves are neutral but which have the power of reacting with hydrogen ions without becoming acid. These are called buffer substances which also help to maintain the pH of the blood at a constant level.

CHAPTER 2

Cells and Tissues

■ CELL

The shapes of mammalian cells vary widely depending on their interactions with each other, their extracellular environment and internal structure. Their surfaces are often highly folded for absorptive and transport functions.

Most cells are between 5–50 micrometer in diameter, lymphocytes 6 micrometer, RBC 7.5 micrometer, columnar epithelial cells 20 micrometer tall and 10 micrometer wide. Megakaryocytes in bone marrow are 200 micrometer (Fig. 2.1).

■ CELLULAR ORGANIZATION

Each cell is contained within limiting plasma membrane which encloses cytoplasm. All cells except mature RBC contain nucleus that is surrounded by nuclear membrane. The nucleus contain chromosomes, the

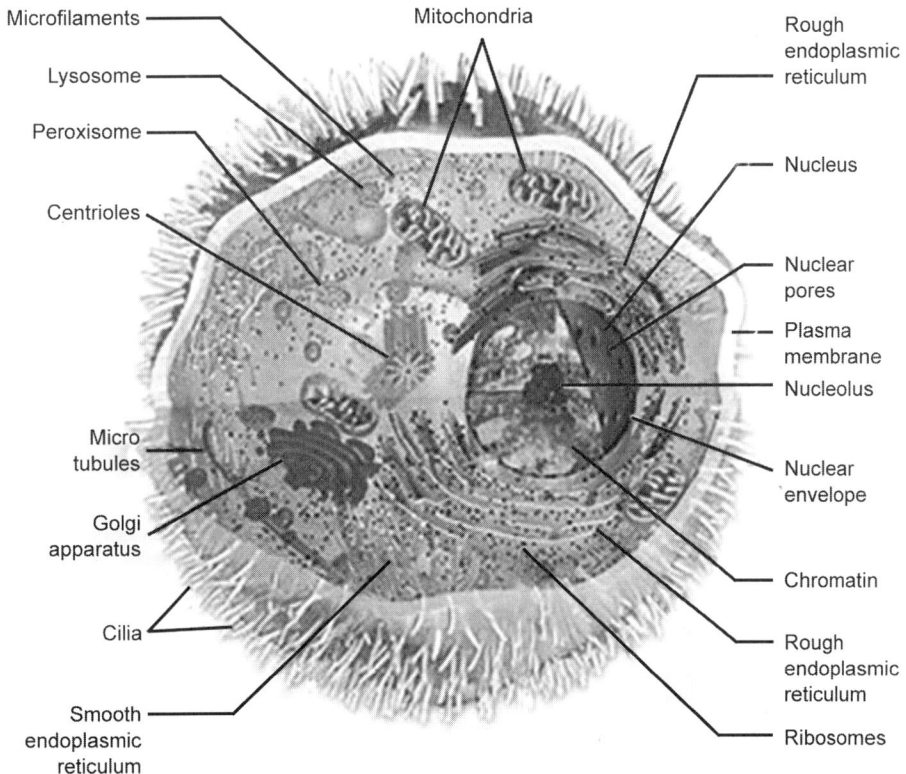

Fig. 2.1: Anatomy of the animal cell

nucleolus and membrane bound structures such as rough endoplasmic reticulum, Golgi apparatus, lysosomes, peroxisomes, mitochondria and vesicles for transport, secretion and storage of cellular component. Structures like ribosomes, filamentous protein are seen in cytosolic compartment. The cytoskeleton determine the shape of cell.

Cytoplasm

It is highly concentrated with 200 mg/mL of protein. It has extremely low levels of Ca^{++}, high K^+, low Na^+ in cytoplasm. Key organizer of the cytoplasm is the cytoskeleton. This is composed of actin and myosin.

Endoplasmic Reticulum (Fig. 2.2)

It is a membrane lined channel within cytoplasm. Channels include cisternae (flattened sac) tubules and vesicles. The membranes divide the cytoplasm into two major compartments, the intra membranous compartment and the extra membranous cytosol which is made of enzymes carbohydrates and small proteins. Channel system is divided into rough endoplasmic reticulum (granular endoplasmic reticulum) and smooth endoplasmic reticulum (agranular endoplasmic reticulum) which lacks ribosomes. Vesicles are budded off from the rough endoplasmic reticulum for transport to Golgi apparatus as a part of protein targeting mechanism.

Smooth Endoplasmic Reticulum

It is associated with carbohydrate metabolism, and many other metabolic processes including detoxification and synthesis of lipids, cholesterol and other steroids.

Ribosomes (Fig. 2.3)

The ribosomes catalyze the synthesis of proteins from amino acids. Large number of proteins are applied to the surface of the subunits cores of RNA. Subunits are separated into coefficients like 40S and 60S. A typical cell contains millions of ribosomes. They may be solitary or may be in groups attached to mRNA.

40S subunit is the site of attachment and translation of mRNA. 60S subunit is responsible for the release of the new protein. Protein synthesis on ribosomes may be suppressed by a class of RNA molecule known as small interfering RNA (si RNA) or silencing RNA.

Golgi Apparatus (Golgi Complex) (Fig. 2.4)

It is a distinct cytoplasmic region near the nucleus. Proteins synthesized in rough endoplasmic reticulum undergo post-translational modification and are targeted to cell surface for secretion and storage.

Golgi apparatus is a membranous organelle consisting of a stack of several membranous cisternae surrounding its

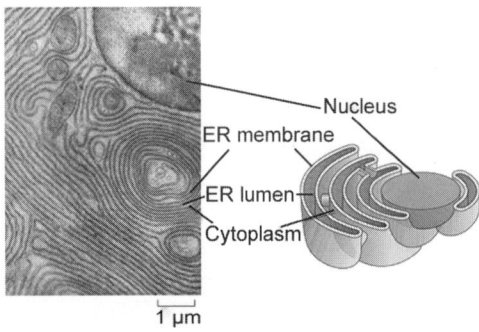

Fig. 2.2: Endoplasmic reticulum

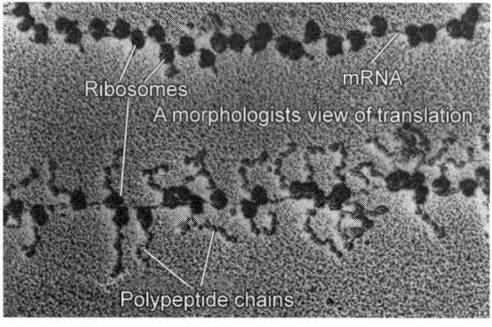

Fig. 2.3: Ribosomes

Cells and Tissues

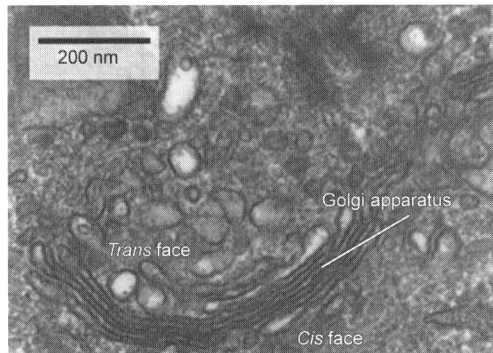

Fig. 2.4: Golgi apparatus

surface. In addition to cisternae there are cis-Golgi and trans-Golgi network.

Endosomes, Lysosomes, Proteosomes, Peroxisomes: Endosome system of vesicles originates in small endocytic vesicles or larger phagosomes. Endocytic system is linked to second series of membranous structures the lysosomes. Lysosomes contain acid hydrolases which degrade exogenous materials and intracellular damaged organelles.

Tay-Sachs disease, Hurlers disease are due to defective lysosomal enzymes caused by gene mutation.

Mitochondria (Fig. 2.5)

They are membrane bound organelle. They are the principal source of chemical energy in most cells, site of TCA cycle electron transport where complex organic molecules are oxidized to CO_2 and H_2O.

The various enzymes of TCA cycle are located in mitochondrial matrix and some in inner mitochondrial membrane. Mitochondria usually appear as round or elliptical bodies, lined by outer and inner unit membrane separated by inter-membranous space.

Cytoskeleton

It is a system of filamentous intercellular protein of different shape and size that form a complex interconnected network. It provides mechanical support for projections from cell surface such as microvilli and cilia and anchors them to cytoplasm. The major filamentous structures found in non-muscle cells are microfilaments, microtubules, intermediate filaments. Intermediate filaments include keratin and genetic abnormalities in keratin cause skin diseases like epidermolysis bullosa (Fig. 2.6).

Cell Surface Projections

These are structures which project from surface of different types of cells. These

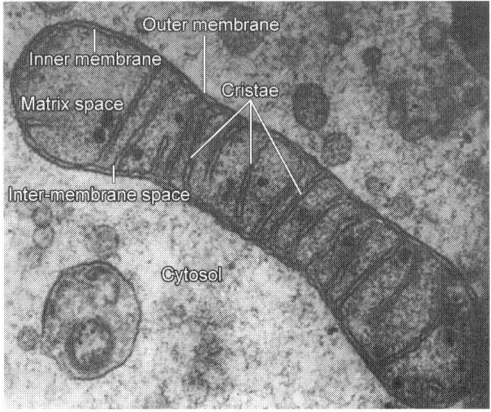

Fig. 2.5: Mitochondria

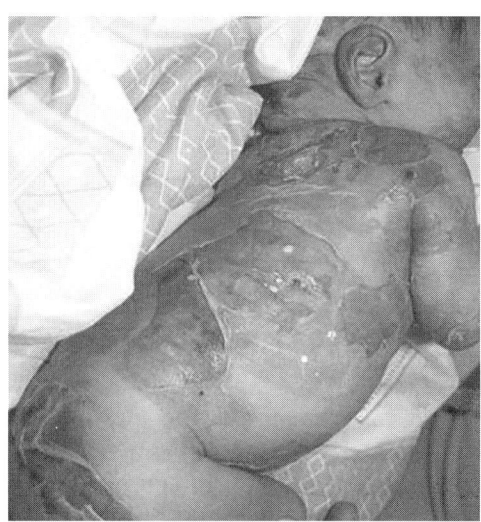

Fig. 2.6: Epidermolysis bullosa

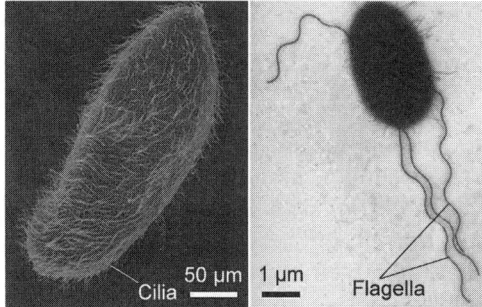

Fig. 2.7: Cilia and flagella

projections permit movement of cell (flagella) or of fluids across apical cell surface (cilia) or increase surface area for absorption (microvilli) (Fig. 2.7).

Chromosomes

The work of Gregor Mendel in 1885 on garden pea can be considered as the discovery of genes. The term 'Gene' was first coined by Danish, botanist in 1909. Within nucleus of cell, there are several thread like structures known as chromosomes (chroma-color, soma body). In 1903, Sutton and Boveri proposed that chromosomes carry hereditary factors or genes. Chromosome number being 46, loss or gain of chromosomes or genes may result in chromosome disorder which can run in family. Watson and Crick discovered the structure of DNA in 1953. DNA can be regarded as the basic template that provides a blueprint for formation and maintenance of an organism. DNA is packaged into chromosomes made up of tightly coiled long chains of genes. Chromosomes are the factors that distinguish one species from another and that enable transmission of genetic information. Somatic cell division in mitosis provides means of ensuring that each daughter cell retains its own genetic complement and meiosis enables each mature ovum and sperm to contain a unique single set of parental gene. The study of chromosomes and cell division is referred to as cytogenetics. Chromosome number in human is 46 and maleness is determined by 'Y' chromosome.

Human Chromosome (Fig. 2.8)

Morphology: During cell division, each chromosome consists of 2 identical strands known as chromatids which are the result of DNA replication. These sister chromatids are joined at primary constriction known as centromere (Fig. 2.9). Centromere consists of several hundred kilobases of repetitive DNA. Each centromere divides chromosome to short arm (p arm) and long arm (q arm). Tip of chromosome is known as telomere. Telomeres seal the ends of chromosomes and maintain structural integrity. Telomeres consist of tandem repeats of TTA.

Morphologically, chromosomes are classified according to position of centro-

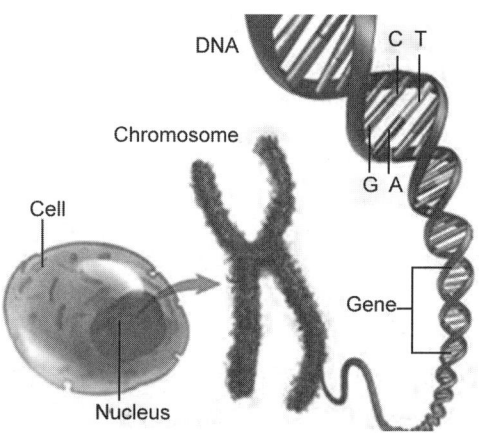

Fig. 2.8: Human chromosome

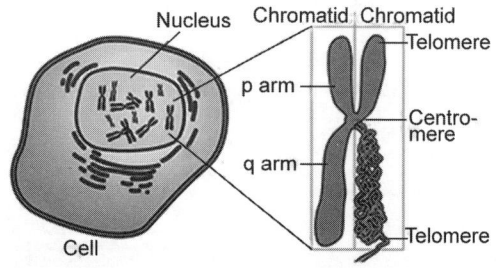

Fig. 2.9: Structure of chromosome

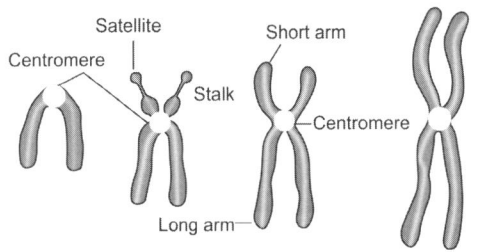

Fig. 2.10: Morphology of chromosomes

meres: Metacentric—centrally placed, submetacentric—intermediate position, acrocentric—terminally placed (Fig. 2.10).

Acrocentric has stalk like appendages called satellites.

In human cells, nucleus contains 46 chromosomes, 22 pairs of autosomes and a pair of sex chromosomes, XX in females and XY in males.

Members of a pair of chromosomes are called homologs. Somatic cells have diploid number (46) of chromosomes whereas gametes have haploid number (23). X and Y are known as sex chromosomes.

Y chromosomes are smaller than X chromosomes and carry a few genes, mostly SRY gene (testis determining factor).

Chromosome analysis: Chromosome analysis is done by karyotyping and chromosome constitution is called karyotype (Fig. 2.11).

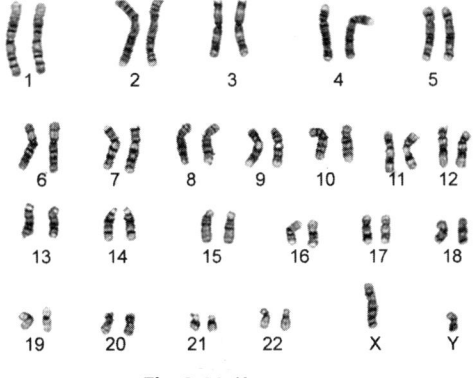

Fig. 2.11: Karyotype

Chromosome banding: Several staining methods can be utilized to identify individual chromosomes.

G-Banding (Giemsa): Chromosome denatured with trypsin and stained with Giemsa which gives each chromosome a characteristic pattern of dark and light bands.

Other banding techniques are Q-banding, R-banding, C-banding, high resolution banding.

Chromosomal Abnormalities

Numerical abnormalities: Involve the loss or gain of one or more chromosomes referred to as aneuploidy. Loss of single chromosome results in monosomy and presence of extra chromosome is trisomy. Trisomy 21 is called Down syndrome. Polyploidy contain multiples of the haploid number of chromosomes such as 69-triploidy, 92-tetraploidy.

Structural abnormalities: Structural chromosome rearrangements result from chromosome breakage with subsequent reunion in a different configuration. Chromosome rearrangement may be balanced or unbalanced resulting in serious clinical effects in children.

■ GENERAL AND CELL PHYSIOLOGY

The cell is the smallest structural and functional unit of the body. The human body contains about 100 trillion cells. Typical cell as seen by the light microscope, consists of three basic components.
- Cell membrane
- Cytoplasm
- Nucleus

Cell membrane (Fig. 2.12): Cell membrane or the plasma membrane is the protective sheath enveloping the cell body. It separates the contents of cell from the external environment and controls exchange of

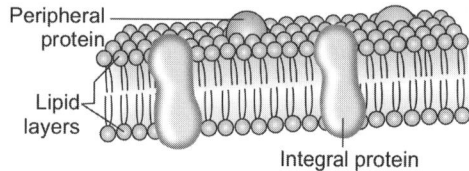

Fig. 2.12: Cell membrane-structure

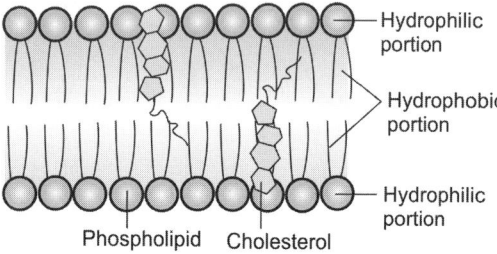

Fig. 2.13: Lipid bilayer

materials between the fluid outside the cell (extracellular fluid) and the fluid inside the cell (intracellular fluid). A detailed knowledge of its structure is essential for the understanding of cell functions.

Symbol of angstrom: Electron microscopy has shown that cell membrane or plasma membrane has a trilayer structure having a total thickness of 7–10 nm (70–100Å) and is known as unit membrane. The three layers consist of two electron-dense layers separated by an electron lucent layer (clear zone). Biochemically the cell membrane is composed of a complex mixture of lipids (40%), proteins (55%) and carbohydrates (5%).

Fluid mosaic model of membrane structure: In 1972, Singer and Nicholson put forward the fluid mosaic model of membrane structure which is presently most accepted. According to this model, phospholipid bilayer is the basic continuous structure forming the cell membrane. The phospholipids are present in fluid form. This fluidity makes the membrane quite flexible and thus allows the cells to undergo considerable changes in the shape without disruption of structural integrity. The protein molecules are present as a discontinuous mosaic of globular proteins which float about in the fluid, the phospholipid bilayer forming a fluid mosaic pattern.

Arrangement of Different Molecules in Cell Membrane

Lipid bilayer (Fig. 2.13): Each lipid molecule in the lipid bilayer of the cell membrane primarily consists of phospholipids, cholesterol and glycolipids. The lipid molecule is pin shape and consists of a head and a tail end. Head end or globular end of the molecule is positively charged and quite soluble in water (i.e. polar or hydrophilic). The tail end consists of two chains of fatty acids or steroid radical of cholesterol. It is insoluble in water (nonpolar or hydrophobic). These lipid molecules are arranged as bilayer in such a way that their nonpolar hydrophobic tail ends are directed towards the center of the membrane where as their polar hydrophilic head ends are directed outwards on either side of the membrane. In this way head ends of the molecules face the aqueous phases, i.e. extracellular fluid on outer side and the intracellular fluid (cytoplasm) on inner side.

Functional significance of the lipid bilayer: The lipid bilayer of the cell membrane makes it a semipermeable membrane which constitutes the major barrier for the water soluble molecules like electrolytes, urea, and glucose. On the other hand, fat soluble substances like oxygen fatty acids and alcohol can pass through the membrane with ease.

Arrangement of proteins in the cell membrane: Most protein molecules float about in the phospholipid bilayer forming a fluid mosaic pattern.

The two types of proteins are:
- Lipoproteins
- Glycoproteins

Proteins in the Cell Membrane

- *Peripheral protein:* Present peripheral to the lipid bilayer both inside and outside to it.
  - *Intrinsic proteins:* Proteins located in the inner surface of lipid bilayer and serve as enzymes.
  - *Extrinsic or surface proteins:* Proteins located on the outer surface of the lipid bilayer. Some of these proteins serve as cell adhesion molecules that anchor cells to neighboring cells and to the basal lamina.
- *Integral proteins or transmembrane proteins:* These are the proteins which extend into the lipid bilayer. They serve as:
  - Channel proteins
  - Carrier proteins
  - Receptor proteins
  - Antigens pumps.

Arrangements of Carbohydrates in the Cell Membrane

The carbohydrates are attached either to the proteins (glycoproteins) or the lipids (glycolipids). Throughout the surface of cell membrane, carbohydrate molecules form a loose covering called glycocalyx.

Functions of Cell Membrane Carbohydrates

Being negatively charged the carbohydrate molecules of the cell membrane do not allow the negatively charged particles to move out of the cell. The glycocalyx helps in tight fixation of the cells with one another. Some of the carbohydrate molecules serve as receptors.

Cytoplasm

Cytoplasm is an aqueous substance (cytosol) containing a variety of cell organelles and other structures. The structures dispersed in the cytoplasm can be grouped into three.
1. *Organelles:* They are the permanent components of the cells which are bounded by limiting membrane and contain enzymes, hence participate in the cellular metabolic activity. These include:
   - Mitochondria
   - Endoplasmic reticulum
   - Golgi apparatus
   - Ribosomes
   - Lysosomes
   - Peroxisomes
   - Centrosome
2. *Cytoplasmic inclusions:* Lipid droplets, glycogen, proteins are secretary granules. Melanin pigment is seen in the cells of epidermis, retina and basal ganglia.
3. *Cytoskeleton:*
   - Microtubules
   - Intermediate filaments
   - Microfilaments.

Molecular Motors

They help in the movement of different proteins, organelles and other cell parts (their cargo) to all parts of the cell. These can be divided into two types:
1. Microtubule based molecular motors, which produce motion along microtubules.
   a. Conventional kinesins
   b. Dyneins
2. Actin-based molecular motors, e.g. myosin. This is a motor that produces motion along the actin.

Nucleus

Nucleus is present in all the eukaryotic cells. It controls all the activities in the cell including reproduction. Nucleus consists of:
- Nuclear membrane
- Nucleoplasm
- Nucleolus.

Intercellular Junctions (Fig. 2.14)

The cell membranes of the neighboring cells are connected with one another through

14 Anatomy and Physiology for Nurses

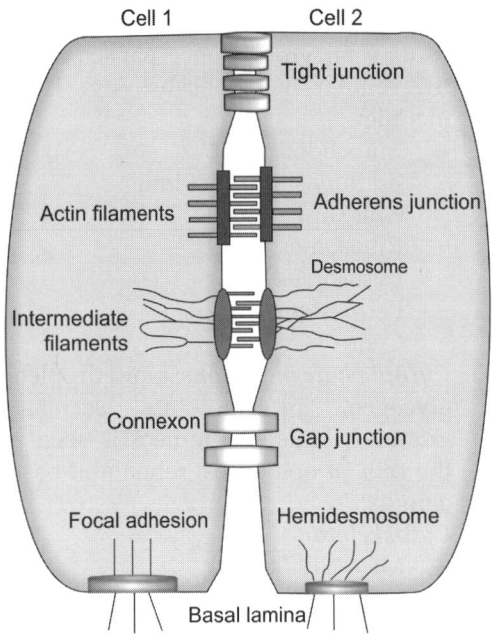

Fig. 2.14: Intercellular junctions

the intercellular junctions or junctional complexes. These are of three types:
1. Tight junctions
2. Adherens junctions—desmosome and hemidesmosome
3. Gap junction.

Cell Adhesion Molecules (CAMs)

These are the prominent parts of the intercellular connections by which the cells are attached to the basal lamina and to each other.
- Integrins
- Adhesion molecules of IgG subfamily
- Cadherins
- Selectins

Functions of Cell Membrane
- First function of cell membrane is to establish, maintain and vary in a controlled fashion, the concentration

Tissues			Functions/locations
1. Epithelium	Squamous	Simple	Linings of organs (e.g. endothelium of heart)
		Stratified	Coverings (e.g. skin)
		Transitional	Linings of organs (e.g. bladder)
	Columnar	Glandular	Secretion (e.g. gastric juices)
			Absorption (e.g. walls of intestine)
		Ciliated	Movement of mucus (e.g. respiratory system)
2. Connective tissue	Fibrous	White	Supporting (e.g. ligaments)
			Protecting—outer coverings of organs (e.g. kidneys)
		Yellow elastic	In walls of arteries and bronchi of lungs
	Areolar		Packing and supporting (e.g. under skin)
	Adipose	Fat	Protection around organs (e.g. eyes, kidneys)
		Brown fat	Protection (e.g. thermogenesis)
	Cartilage	Hyaline	Protection (e.g. covering articular surfaces)
		Fibrocartilage	Supporting (e.g. intervertebral discs)
		Elastic	Supporting (e.g. epiglottis, pinna of ear)
	Bone	Compact	Support and protection (i.e. hard surface of bone)
		Cancellous	Provides lightness with strength (i.e. spongy bone); also contains red bone marrow
	Blood	Red cells	Carriage of oxygen and carbon dioxide
		White cells	Protection of body from infection
		Platelets	Coagulation of blood
3. Muscle	Voluntary (striated)		Power of movement (i.e. muscles attached to skeleton)
	Involuntary (plain)		Present in internal organs (e.g. colon)
	Cardiac		Specialized muscle of heart
4. Nerves	Nerve cells (neurons)		Generation of impulses
			Transmission of impulses
	Neuroglia		Support for nerve cells

of electrolyte, non-electrolytes or water between two separate aqueous compartments the ICF and ECF.
- It maintains the membrane potential, i.e. potential difference between inside and outside of membrane.
- Membranes are a site of signal transduction.
- They serve as surfaces favoring certain molecular interations.

Transport Across Cell Membranes
- Diffusion
  - Simple diffusion
  - Facilitated diffusion
- Osmosis
- Movement through ion channels
- Active transport
  - Primary active transport
  - Secondary active transport
- Endocytosis
- Exocytosis

Diffusion

Diffusion is the process by which a gas or a substance in solution expands because of the motion of its particles to fill all of the available volume. Diffusion through the cell membrane is divided into two subgroups.
1. Simple diffusion
2. Facilitated diffusion

Simple Diffusion
- Through interstices of lipid bilayer if the diffusing substance is lipid soluble, e.g. O_2, N_2, CO_2, alcohol.
- Through coating channels in some transport proteins.

Types of Channels
- Open
- Gated
  - Voltage gated
    - Na^+ channels
    - K^+ channels
  - Ligand gated
    - ACh channels

Facilitated Diffusion (Fig. 2.15)
It is also called carrier mediated diffusion. Proteins act as carriers that bind ions and other molecules and then change their configuration moving the bound molecule from one side of the membrane to the other. No energy is required for the process. This takes place, along the concentration gradient or electrical gradient. The difference from diffusion through open channels is the rate of diffusion approached a maximum called V max as the concentration of substance increases, e.g. glucose transport by glucose transporter which move glucose from ECF to the cytoplasm of the cell down concentration gradient.

Osmosis
The diffusion of solvent molecule into a region in which there is a higher concentration of the solute to which the membrane is impermeable is called osmosis.

Active Transport
When a cell membrane move molecules or ions uphill against a concentration gradient (or uphill against an electrical or pressure gradient) the process is called active transport, e.g. Na^+, K^+, Ca^{++}, Fe^{++}, H^+, it, I^-, urate sugers, amino acids.

Primary Active Transport
In this, energy is derived directly from the breakdown of ATP or some other high energy phosphate compound.

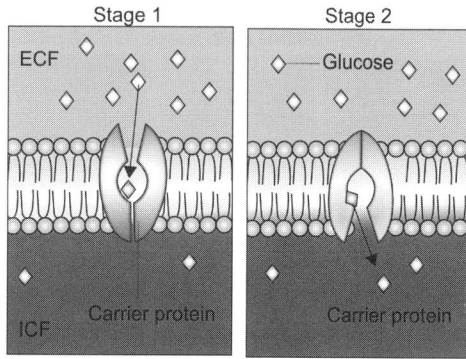

Fig. 2.15: Facilitated diffusion

For example, Na$^+$, K$^+$, ATPase pump, catalyzes the hydrolysis of ATP to ADP and uses the energy to extrude 3 Na$^+$, from the cell and take 2 K$^+$, into the cell, for each mole of ATP hydrolyzed.

Primary active transport of Ca^{++} (muscle).

Primary active transport of H$^+$ (gastric glands of stomach, late distal tubules of kidney).

Secondary Active Transport

- Co-transport → SGLT, intestine, renal tubules
- Counter-transport → Na$^+$, H$^+$, counter transport in proximal kidney tubules (Fig. 2.16).

Exocytosis

Proteins that are secreted by cells move from the ER to GA and from trans-Golgi, they are extruded into secretary granules or vesicles. The granules or vesicles move to the cell membrane. Their membrane then fuses with the cell membrane and area of fusion breakdown. This leaves the contents outside and the cell membrane intact. This extrusion process is called exocytosis. It requires Ca^{++} and energy along with docking proteins.

Endocytosis

Cell eating or phagocytosis is the process by which bacteria, dead tissue or other bits of material are engulfed by cells such as PML of blood.

Cell drinking or pinocytosis is the process with the difference that the substance ingested as in solution.

■ BODY FLUIDS AND INTRAVENOUS FLUID THERAPY

Body Fluids

Distribution of Total Body Water

i. 7% of BW - Mineral
ii. 15% - Fat
iii. 18% - Protein
iv. 60% - Water (TBW)

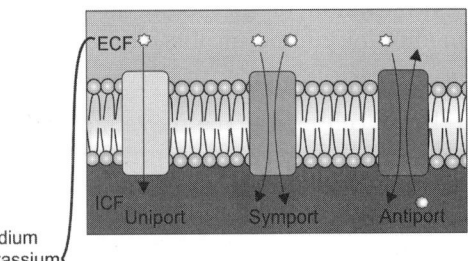
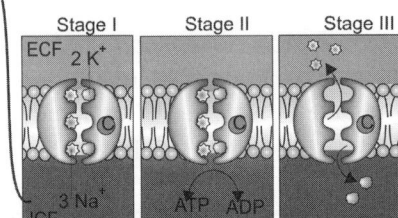
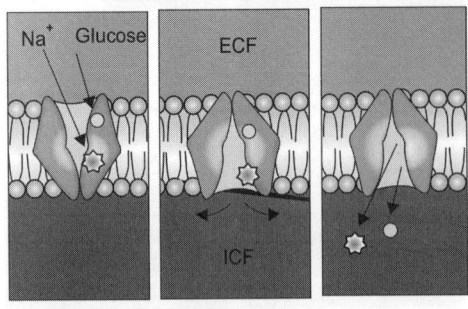

Fig. 2.16: Sodium glucose cotransport

TBW Comp	Volume (L)	% Body Weight	Body Water
TBW	42	60	100
ECF	14	20	33 (1/3rd^{TBW})
ICF	28	40	67 (2/3rd)

ECF Comp	Volume (L)	% Body Weight	% Body Water
Plasma (25%)	3.5	4-5	8
(Interstitial + Trancellular F) 75% of ECF (include lymph)	10.5	15	25

10 Ionic Composition of Body Fluids (mEq/L of H$_2$O)

Cells and Tissues

10n	ECF	ICF
Cation		
+ve Na⁺	145	12
K⁺	5	155
Mg^{++}	2	15
Others	2	2
Total cation	154	184
Anions		
-ve c/-	110	8
HCO_3^-	27	8
PO_4^{3-}	2	90
Proteins	15	60
Others	-	18
Total anions	154	184
Total 10	308	368

Sum of anions in ECF = sum of cations in ECF. Na^+, Ca^{2+}, Cl^-, HCO_3^- are largely extracellular K^+, Mg^{2+}, organic PO_4^{3} and proteins mainly present in ICF.

Only exchangeable solutes are osmotically active.

pH refers to negative logarithm of (H^+) counteraction.
Refers to negative log. Of the (H^+)
Blood pH – 7.4 (6.9–7.7)

Compatable with life
The cell membrane seperates the ICF from ECF.

Cause of difference is the Logic Composition of ICF and ECF
i. Resting cell membrane is impermeable or moderately permeable to Na^+
ii. Resting cell memb is freely permeable to K^+ and Cl^- (50-100 times)
iii. Cell membrane is impermeable to most intracellular anions such as protein and organic PO_4^- ions.

RMP (steady potential)
Inside –ve to exterior
-10 mv (RBC)
-100 mv (ske. muscle cell)

Cause
1. Difference in ionic composition of ECF and ICF
2. $Na^+ K^+$ pump.

Intravenous Fluid Therapy

Fluid loss may also be replaced by a solution containing low molecular weight dextran.

Normal saline (9% saline) ⎫
5% dextrose ⎬ Less efficient as volume Expanders. Avoid risk of blood products
Ringer lactate solution ⎭

Water Balance

	Volume (mL)			Volume (mL)	
Intake	Cold	Hot		Cold	Hot
Drinks	1600	2400	Urine	1500	1000
Food	1000	1000	Sweat	100	1500
Oxidation	200	200	Skin	500	500
			Airway	400	300
			Feces	300	300
Total	2800	3600		2800	3600

Obligatory urine volume 500 mL
Insensible perspiration 200 mL
Insensible loss in expired air 200 mL
3 mechanism – aldosterone
- ADH
- Osmoreceptors in Hypothalamus → Thirst
- ANF

TISSUES

The cells of the human body differ in appearance according to the particular type of tissue to which they belong, and the specialized functions which these tissues perform.

The following are the principal kinds of tissues found in the body. Each consists of individual types of cells which can be seen and recognized under a microscope.

EPITHELIUM

Epithelium is a tissue composed of cells generally arranged to form a membrane or lining, covering either an internal or external body surface.

Simple squamous epithelium (also known as pavement epithelium) consists of a single layer of flattened cells. It is found in the alveoli of the lungs, lining the interior of the heart and blood vessels, and the lymphatic vessels (Fig. 2.17). It forms a smooth, flat membrane, which is lined up by an internal surface is sometimes called endothelium

Stratified squamous epithelium is composed of similar cells arranged in layers. The surface cells are flattened like the simple variety, but the deeper ones are rounded (Fig. 2.18).

The epidermis of the skin consists of stratified epithelium, the outer layers of which become hard and horny because they contain a substance called **keratin.** Stratified epithelium is also found in the mouth, pharynx, esophagus, vagina and part of the urethra. Its structure is specially adapted to the wear and tear experienced by body surfaces. The superficial layers are constantly being shed and replaced by growth from the deeper layers.

Transitional epithelium is composed of cells which provide a watertight surface, but are also capable of expansion. It is found by lining parts of the urinary tract, where it is able to withstand the action of urine with which it is in constant contact.

Columnar epithelium consists of cylindrical-shaped cells, one layer thick, and is found in the secretory glands of the body, such as the salivary glands and the breasts (Fig. 2.19). The stomach and intestines are also lined with columnar epithelium, where some of the cells are responsible for the absorption of fluids and foodstuffs, whilst others secrete a thick, sticky, protective substance called mucus.

Ciliated columnar epithelium is a special form of columnar epithelium (Fig. 2.20).

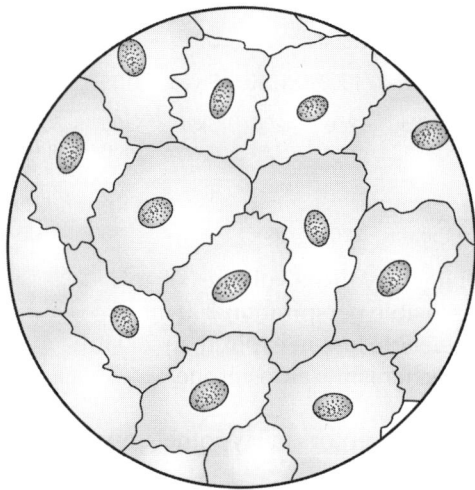

Fig. 2.17: Simple squamous epithelium

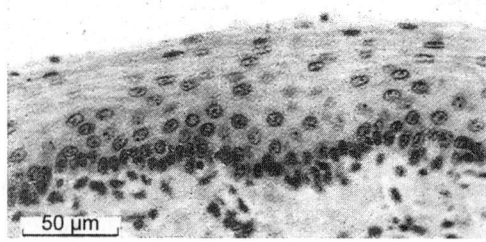

Fig. 2.18: Stratified squamous epithelium from the pharynx

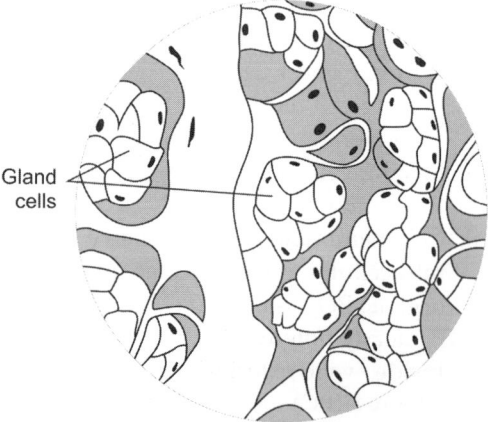

Fig. 2.19: Glandular epithelium from a salivary gland (submandibular gland)

Cells and Tissues

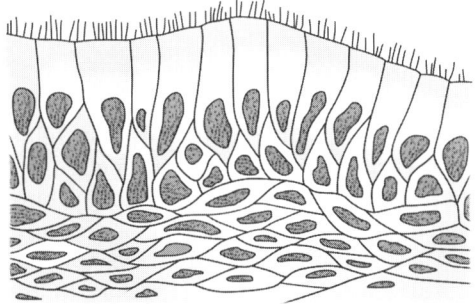

Fig. 2.20: Ciliated columnar epithelium from the trachea

The free surface of each cell is surmounted by fine hair-like processes or cilia. The cilia bend rapidly to one side and then straighten again; this whipping movement sweeps onwards in one direction any substance or fluid in contact with the surface of the cell. Ciliated epithelium is found in the respiratory system, and lines the nasal cavities, the trachea and bronchi. The movement of the cilia conveys mucus, dust, etc. from the deeper parts of the lungs towards the exterior. It is also found in the Fallopian (uterine) tubes, where it assists the ovum on its passage to the uterus.

■ CONNECTIVE TISSUE
Irregular Connective Tissue

Irregular connective tissue is further subdivided to loose, dense, adipose tissue.

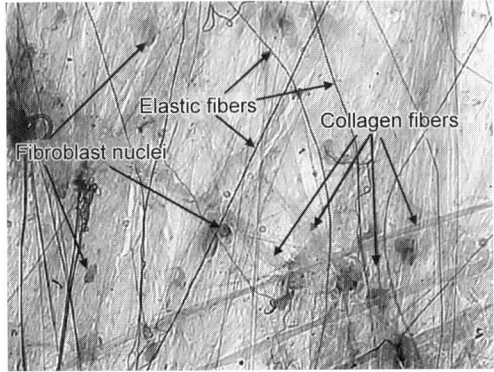

Fig. 2.21: Loose areolar connective tissue

Loose (Areolar) Connective Tissue (Fig. 2.21)

Extensively distributed and its function is to bind parts together allowing considerable movement to take place because of its elasticity. It forms subcutaneous tissue in regions devoid of fat like eyelids, scrotum. It is also found between muscles, nerves and vessels. Loose connective tissue has collagen and elastic fibers.

Dense Irregular Connective Tissue (Fig. 2.22)

It gives protection to unsheathed organs and found in regions susceptible to mechanical stress. Thick bundles of collagen fibers seen which have considerable strength, e.g. sclera of eye, capsule of glands, periosteum, perichondrium.

Adipose Tissue (Fig. 2.23)

It consists of adipocytes and it is divided into lobules by stronger fibrous septa containing blood vessels. Fat cells in lobules are compressed and hence polygonal.

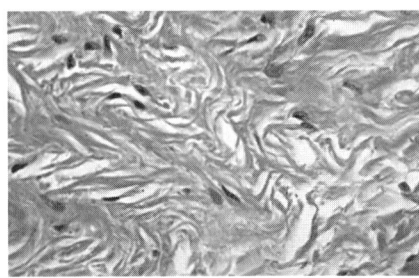

Fig. 2.22: Dense irregular connective tissue

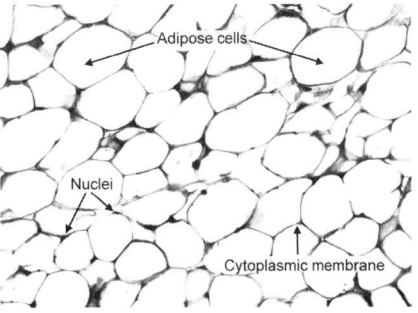

Fig. 2.23: Adipose tissue

Regular Connective Tissue

Regular connective tissue includes highly fibrous tissue which are regularly oriented to form sheaths and aponeuroses. Fibroblasts secrete the fibers. Fibroblasts in external surface are active and repair damage. Connective tissues are predominantly collagenous. Elastic components may occur.

Mucoid Tissue (Fig. 2.24)

This is fetal or embryonic connective tissue. It exists in jelly of Wharton in umbilical cord. Matrix contains fine mesh work of collagen fibers with nucleated cells having branching process.

■ CARTILAGE

In skeletal tissue, cartilage and bone essentially specialized connective tissue. It is covered by fibrous perichondrium except at synovial surfaces.

Structure of Cartilage

Cartilage is a type of stiff load bearing connective tissue. It is covered by fibrous perichondrium except at synovial surfaces.

Cartilage matrix: This contains chondroblasts and chondrocytes. There is hyaline cartilage (hyalos means glass), white fibrocartilage (with much collagen) and yellow elastic cartilage (with an elastin network).

Cartilage cells: These cells occupy small lacunae in matrix. Young cells (chondroblasts) are smaller and often flat, possessing surface projections (filopodia). Mature cartilage cells lose ability to divide. These mature cells are called chondrocytes. They have round nucleus and possess nucleoli. Cytoplasm is filled with granular endoplasmic reticulum, Golgi complex and mitochondria.

Intercellular matrix: Composed of collagen and elastin fibers. Ground substance is a firm gel, rich in carbohydrates which are predominantly acidic.

Proteoglycan of cartilage: They consist of branched carbohydrates called glycosaminoglycan (GAG).

Varieties of Cartilage

Cartilage may be hyaline cartilage, white fibrocartilage, yellow elastic cartilage, cellular cartilage.

Hyaline cartilage: It is glassy, homogenous, bluish in appearance, firm in consistency and possess elasticity (Fig. 2.25). Costal cartilage, nasal cartilage, most laryngeal cartilage, most articular cartilage are hyaline. Cells are flat towards perichondrium and seen in groups of two or more (cell nests).

Matrix is typically basophilic and metachromatic.

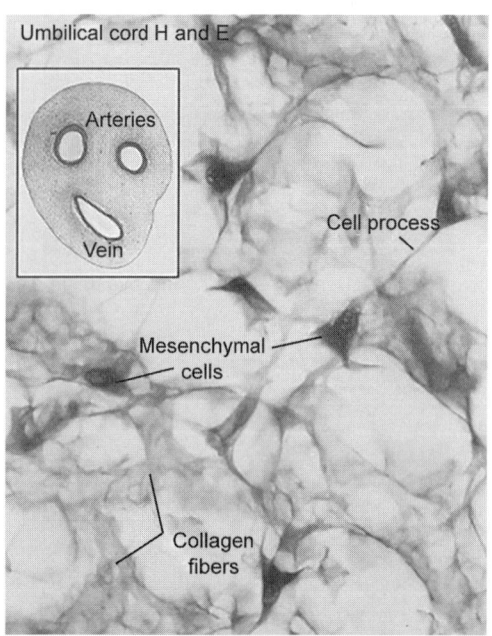

Fig. 2.24: Mucoid tissue

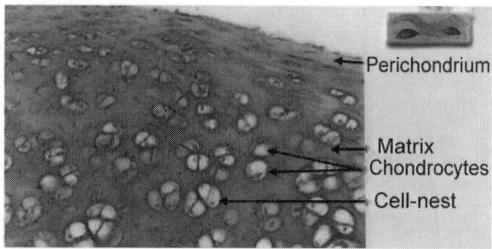

Fig. 2.25: Hyaline cartilage

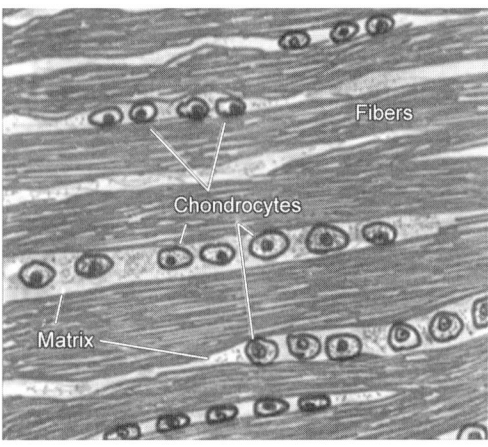

Fig. 2.26: Fibrocartilage

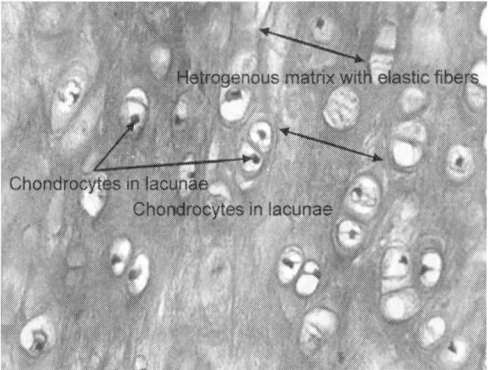

Fig. 2.27: Elastic cartilage

White fibrocartilage: Is dense white fibrous tissue with fibroblasts and group of chondrocytes (Fig. 2.26). White fibrocartilage has great tensile strength with elasticity and resist pressure. Type 1 collagen form matrix.

Yellow elastic cartilage: Occurs in external ear, epiglottis, corniculate cartilage (Fig. 2.27). It contains chondrocytes and matrix of yellow elastic fibers. Most sites in which yellow elastic fibers occur have vibrational functions like laryngeal sound wave production.

Growth of Cartilage

Cartilage is formed from embryonic mesenchyme. Mesenchymal cells proliferate and become tightly packed, foreshadowing subsequent cartilage. Cells soon begin to secrete matrix composed of type 2 collagen filaments, type 9 collagen core protein. Continued secretion of matrix separate cells and hyaline cartilage becomes recognizable.

■ BONE

Bone is highly vascular, constantly mineralized connective tissue. It is remarkable for its hardness and regenerative capacity. Bone consists of cells, intercellular matrix and osteocytes are embedded in its matrix. Matrix is composed of mainly collagen fibers, calcium, phosphate. There are vascular canals within bone providing cells with its metabolic support. Cells include osteoclasts which remove bone and osteoblasts which deposit bone. Bone has collagen framework oriented as coarse bundles (woven bone) when young, and as parallel sheets in mature condition (lamellar bone). Collagen fibers and matrix form cylinders (osteons) arranged concentrically around blood vessels. Outer surface of bone is lined by periosteum. Developmentally bone may form by direct transformation of condensed mesenchyme (intramembranous) or be preceded by cartilage model which bone later replaces (endochondral bone).

Macroscopic Structure of Bone

It has either dense texture like ivory (compact bone) or has large cavities with bars and plates (spongy bone or cancellous bone). Compact bone is related to cortex and spongy bone lies in the interior. Compact bone provides strength whereas cancellous bone supports bone marrow. Bone forms a reservoir for metabolic calcium and phosphate.

Microscopy

Cells of bone consists of number of types (Fig. 2.28):

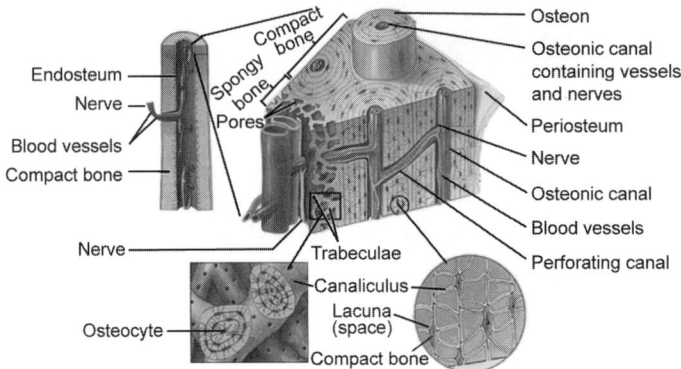

Fig. 2.28: Microscopy of bone

- Osteoprogenitor stromal cells which give rise to various bone cells
- Osteoblasts which lay down bone
- Osteocytes within bone
- Osteoclasts which erode it

Osteocytes are derived from osteoblasts and are caught in matrix, retain contact with each other. They are ellipsoid in shape and fine processes emerge from cell body.

Microscopy of Cells of Bone

Osteoprogenitor cells: Resemble young fibroblasts and are mesenchymal origin. They are responsible for synthesis, deposition, mineralization of bone matrix. Some cells get embedded in bone matrix and become osteocytes. The cells have oval nucleus and extensive granular endoplasmic reticulum, numerous secretory vesicles and Golgi complex. The cells play an indirect role in hormone regulation of bone resorption.

Osteocytes

Bone lining cells: These are flattened epithelium like cells. They are in contact with each other and neighboring osteocytes. They play an active role in regulating differentiation of osteoprogenitor cells.

Osteoclasts: These are large polymorphous cells with variable number of oval, closely packed nuclei (15–20). They are found where there is active removal of bone and lie in close contact with bone surface in pits termed resorption bays or lacunae of Howship.

Functionally, osteoclasts are responsible for the removal of bone. They cause demineralization by proton release. They also degrade collagen.

Microscopy of bone matrix: Ground substance consists of collagen fibers arranged in parallel arrays. It has inorganic mineral salts, collagen, non-collagenous protein. Collagen is type 1 and the fibers of collagen are synthesized by osteoblasts.

Microscopic Organization of Bone

Two different types of organization:
1. Woven bone
2. Lamellar bone

In woven bone, collagen fibers are irregularly arranged. It is formed by active osteoblasts.

Lamellar bone: Seen in all adult skeleton.

In compact bone, collagen fibers arranged in layers and embedded in it are osteocytes. They form layers called lamellae. When arranged in concentric cylinders around neurovascular channel (Haversian canal), they form basic unit called Haversian system or osteon (Fig. 2.29).

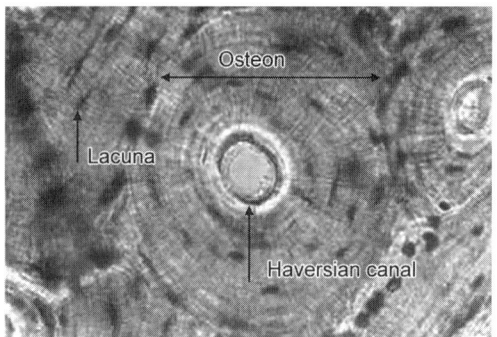

Fig. 2.29: Osteon

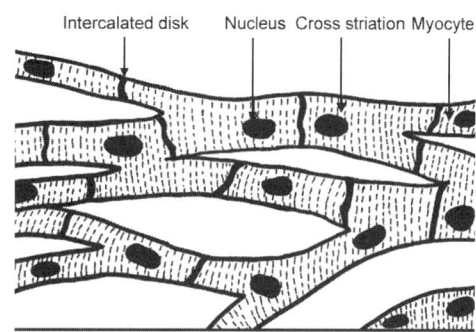

Fig. 2.31: Cardiac muscle

MUSCULAR TISSUE

Muscle cells are known as myocytes. Myocytes differentiate to skeletal, cardiac and smooth muscle. Skeletal and cardiac muscle are referred to as striated muscle because myosin and actin filaments are organized to give cross striated appearance.

Skeletal muscle: Has parallel bundles of long multinucleated fiber (Fig. 2.30).

Light microscopy of skeletal muscle: Muscle fibers are long cylindrical structures and transverse striations are produced due to sarcomeres. Multiple nuclei are flattened and situated at periphery of fibers.

Cardiac muscle (Fig. 2.31): Consists of branching network of individual cells. Compared to skeletal muscle, cardiac muscle is less powerful. Skeletal muscle power is (100 watts/kg) and cardiac 3–5 watts per kg. In cardiac muscle, spaces are occupied by blood vessels and mitochondria for continuous supply of energy. Cardiac muscle contraction is not under hormonal or ANS control. Sarcomeres in muscle are arranged across fibers and produce fine cross-striations. Cardiac muscle cells are up to 100 micron long. Each cells has large nucleus, occasionally two, occupying central part of cell. Cells are branched at their ends and the branches of adjacent cells are tightly associated and anastomotic fibers. Electron microscopy show junction binding cells together called intercalated disc. Thus the fibers of cardiac muscle are not single cells as they are in skeletal muscle. Fine connective tissue found between cardiac muscle fiber. A linear arrangement of cardiac muscle fiber seen in papillary muscle of heart. Ventricles of heart are composed of spiralling fibers running in different direction. Cross striations of cardiac muscle is less conspicuous because it is embedded in abundant sarcoplasm.

Smooth muscle (Fig. 2.32): The cytoplasm has smooth unstriated appearance from which the name implies. It is also called nonstriated muscle. Myocytes of smooth muscle are smaller than striated muscle. Length of cells range from 50 micron to 500 micron in uterus. Cells are spindle shaped and tapering towards ends with single nucleus situated in the middle of cell.

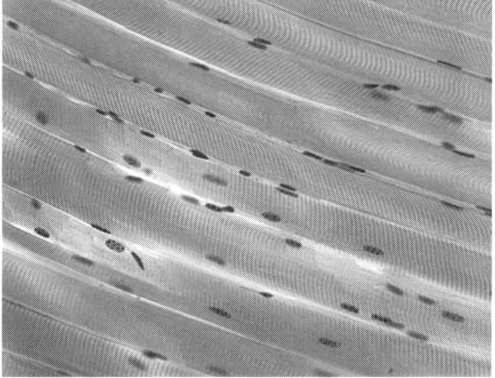

Fig. 2.30: Skeletal muscle

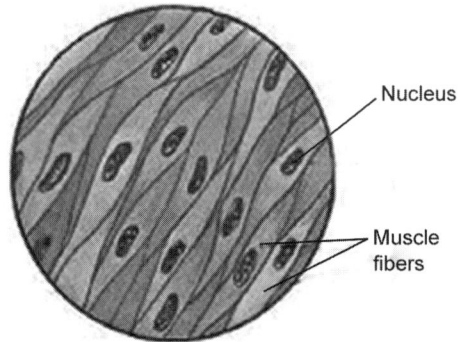

Fig. 2.32: Smooth muscle

Smooth muscle cells are typically found in walls of tubular structures and hollow viscera (blood vessels and bronchial tree). Smooth muscle has the capacity for self-renewal following damage.

Myoepithelial Cells

Found in association with number of secretory glands like salivary, lacrimal, sweat, mammary gland.

■ NERVE

Human central nervous system contains about 10^{11} (100 billion) neurons. It also contains 10–50 times this number of glial cells.

Morphology

The neuron consists of a body (Soma, Perikaryon) and 2 types of processes the dendrites and axon.

Types of Neurons
- *Unipolar:* Those with axon and dentrite arise by a common stem, e.g. dorsal root ganglion cells.
- *Bipolar:* Axon and dentrite spring from opposite portions of soma. Olfactory or auditory nerve.
- *Multipolar:* From different portions of soma spinal motor neuron.

Within grey matter the axons are enclosed only by the plasma membrane. Upon leaving the grey matter they acquire a sheath of cupid materials called myelin. These myelin sheaths are associated with somatic nerves of large diameter (>1 µm) which conduct faster than smaller unmyelinated nerve fibers. Schwann cells spiralling concentrically around the axons forms the myelin sheath. Outer layer of myelin contains flattened nuclei of Schwann cells called neurilemma. Myelinated neuron appear as if constricted at regular intervals due to absence of myelin at these points called nodes of Ranvier. Neurilemma is absent in CNS and optic nerves.

It is replaced by glial cells which form sheaths. Glia are of three types asterocytes, oligo dendrocytes and microglia.

The neurilemma in the region of node of Ranvier become highly permeable to sodium and potassium ions compared to myelin sheath. So conduction of impulse is leaping from node to node (called saltatory conduction) rather than a continuous process.

The cell body (Fig. 2.33): It can be of various sizes and forms, stellate, round, pyramidal, fusiform, etc. The cytoplasm contains 1) Neurofibrils 2) Nissl bodies 3) Golgi apparatus, 4) Mitochondria, 5) Ribosomes, 6) Endoplasmic reticulum. Mitochondria found along the entire length of axon and contains all the enzymes required for respiration of cell. Nucleus contain 1 or 2 nuclei, but no centrosome, absence of centrosome indicates the nerve cell has lost its power of division. Dendrite is the receptive process of the neuron. Axon is discharging process. In peripheral sensory nerves, the dendrites are comparable in length with an axon.

Synapse: The contact of the axon terminal of one nerve cell with the body, dendritic process, or sometimes the axon of another is called synapse.

Afferents: Carry impulse to CNS.

Efferents: Carry impulse from CNS to periphery.

A mixed nerve contains both types of fibers.

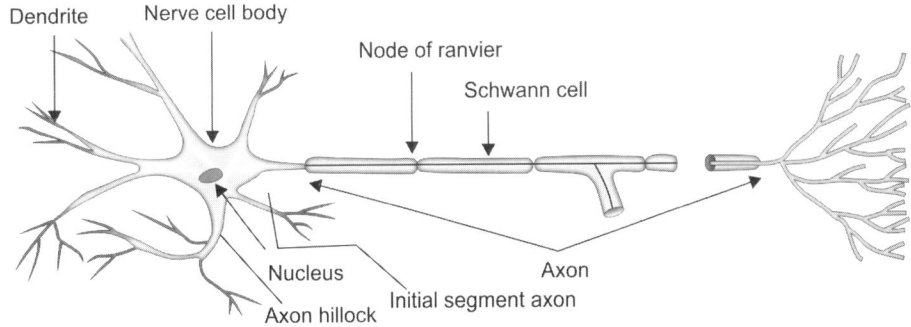

Fig. 2.33: Structure of neuron

Functions of Myelin

- Increase velocity of conduction.
- Reduce energy expenditure for nerve conduction.
- Myelin acts as an insulator so prevents cross stimulation of adjacent axons.

■ PROPERTIES OF NEURONS

- Conductivity
- Excitability

Excitability: It means the events leading to the generation of action potentials.

Conduction: It refers to the propagation of AP which proceeds away from the site of excitation.

Stimulus: It is a sudden change in the environment of a living organism which causes it to react in the case of nerve to set up an impulse: (1) electrical, (2) thermal, (3) mechanical or chemical.

Resting Membrane Potential and its Ionic Basis

There is a potential difference across the membrane of most cells with the inside of the cells negative relative to be exterior. This is resting membrane potential and is written with a minus sign signifying that the inside is negative relative to exterior. Its magnitude varies from tissues to tissues ranging from –9 to –100 mv. In neurons it is –70 mv.

Origin of Normal Resting Membrane Potential (RMP)

The RMP is developed by mainly by two factors:
a. Diffusion of ions along concentration and electrical gradient
b. Pumps

A large concentration gradient exists for Na^+ and K^+ across the resting nerve membranes. The gradients are:

Outside	Inside
Na^+ – 142 meq/L	Na^+ – 10 meq/L
K^+ – 4 meq/L	K^+ – 140 meq/L
Cl – 125 mmol/L	Cl – 9 mmol/L

1. *Diffusion of K^+ ions through membrane:* Concentration gradient for K^+ facilitates its movement out of the cell via K^+ channels. But its electrical gradient is directed inward. At equilibrium—the tendency of K^+ to move out of the cell is balanced by its tendency to move into the cell. At equilibrium there is a slight excess of cations (+ve) on the outside and slight excess of anions (–ve) on the inside. If K^+ were the only factor causing RMP. RMP inside the fiber would be –94 mv.)
   $(\log \frac{140}{24} \times 61.5 = \log 35 \times 61.5)$

2. *Diffusion of Na^+ through nerve membrane:* There is a slight permeability of nerve membrane to Na^+ ions and

minute diffusion of Na⁺ ions occur through leak channels from outside to inside. The calculated Nernst potential for Na⁺ is +60 mv inside the membrane.

The membrane is highly permeable to K⁺ but only slightly permeable to Na⁺ (permeability of K⁺ is about 100 times as great as to Na⁺) therefore diffusion of K⁺ contributes far more to membrane potential than does diffusion of Na⁺. Therefore by using Goldman equation the value comes nearer to the K⁺ potential.

Chloride ions are in electrochemical equilibrium with the RMP. They diffuse freely through the membrane potential at rest.

3. *Contribution of Na⁺ K⁺ pump:* The measured RMP of a nerve is not in accordance with the calculated E_K or E_{Na}. So if only passive electrical and chemical forces were acting across the membrane, the cell would gradually gain Na⁺ or lose K⁺, but intracellular Na⁺ and K⁺ concentration remain constant because of Na⁺ K⁺ pump.

There is continuous pumping of 3 Na⁺ to the outside for each 2 K⁺ pumped to the inside of the membrane. So there is a continuous loss of the positive charges from inside the membrane which create an additional degree of negativity on the inside of the membrane and make an additional contribution to the RMP (electrogenic pump).

Measurement of the Membrane Potential

Measured from squid (Loligo) especially in the neck region. One electrode inserted into body of axon other outside the cell and connecting to voltmeter.

■ ACTION POTENTIAL

Action potential is propagated disturbances produced due to changes in the conduction of ions across the cell membrane that are produced by alternations in ion channels (Fig. 2.34).

If the axon is stimulated and a conducted impulse occurs, a characteristic series of potential changes known as AP is observed as the impulse passes the external electrode.

When the stimulus is applied, there is a brief irregular deflection of the baseline,

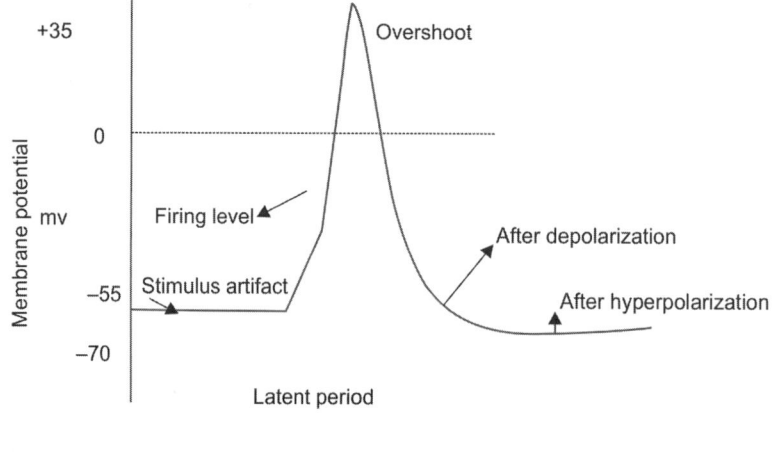

Fig. 2.34: Action potential in a neuron

which is called stimulus artifact. This is due to current leakage from the stimulating electrodes to recording electrodes. It indicates the point at which stimulus is applied.

Latent period is the isoelectric interval that ends with the start of the action potential. LP is directly proportional to distance between stimulating and recording electrode. Inversely proportional to the speed of conduction.

Firing level or threshold, after initial 15 mV of depolarization, the rate of depolarization, increases, then the tracing reaches and overshoots zero potential line to +35 mV.

Then it reverses and repolarization falls rapidly to resting level till 70% repolarization to complete.

Sharp rise and rapid fall—spike potential slower fall at the end of repolarization—after depolarization.

After reaching resting level, tracing overshoots slightly in hyperpolarizing direction to form a small propagated hyperpolarization.

Ionic Basis of AP

Resting stage: RMP before the AP occurs— 70 mV

Depolarization stage: Increase in sodium permeability and tremendous numbers of Na^+ ions flow to the interior of the axon. During depolarization membrane potential overshoots beyond zero level and become positive.

Repolarization: Within a few 10,000th of a second after the membrane become highly permeable to sodium ions, sodium channels opens more than normal. Rapid diffusion of K^+ ions to exterior reestablishes negativity inside. This is called repolarization. In addition to the $Na^+ K^+$ leak channels, the two voltage gated sodium and potassium channels are necessary for causing both depolarization and repolarization of membrane.

Functions of Neuroglia

Microglia: Phagocytic (increase in inflammation)

Asterocytes: Related to blood vessels synapses, support, transport mechanism inflammatory and reparative reactions and isolation of neuronal elements.

Olegodentroglia: Formation of myelin layer within CNS.

Different Types of AP

1. Monophasic AP
2. Biphasic AP
3. Spike potential — Nerve filter / Skeletal muscle
4. *Plateau type AP:* Cardiac muscle cell
5. *Rhythmic type AP:* Heart in SA nodes, AV node, conducting system, smooth muscle, neurons of CNS.
6. *Compound AP:* Action potential with multiple peak, a property of mixed nerve.

CHAPTER 3

Immunity

The body has a variety of defenses against microbial invaders. Some of these immune mechanisms are innate and are present from birth; they are non-specific in that they counteract a wide variety of infective agents. In contrast, acquired immune mechanisms are specific, each being directed against a particular microorganism.

■ INNATE IMMUNITY

There are major differences between species, and between strains within species, in susceptibility to infection. A dog, for example, stands no risk whatever of catching a cold from its master. Lesser determinants of innate immunity are individual genetic factors, age, sex, nutritional status and hormonal balance.

The intact skin, and particularly its outer horny layer, affords an effective mechanical barrier to the entry of microorganisms into the body. The mucous membranes, not having a horny layer, afford less protection but have mechanical mechanisms of their own. For example, the mucosa of the respiratory tract traps particles in its moisture and they are swept upwards, by the hair-like processes or cilia (performing mechanical cleansing), to reach the oropharynx, from which they are swallowed or expectorated. Unfortunately the cilia may be disabled by a variety of agents, including viruses which infect the respiratory tract. In the gastrointestinal tract, a layer of mucus traps organisms and peristaltic movement prevents stagnation and bacterial overgrowth. A high flow rate of secretions, as in the urinary and biliary tracts, discourages bacterial proliferation; such regions are usually sterile but may become infected if flow is impeded, by calculi or by prostatic obstruction of the bladder neck, for example. Temperature is also a factor in the innate immunity of an animal to some infective agents. Whilst warm blooded animals are susceptible to tuberculosis, for example, cold-blooded animals are immune because the tubercle bacillus is temperature dependent.

Chemical factors also protect against infection. Among these, the fatty acids on the surface of the skin have an antiseptic action. These are present in the secretions of the sebaceous glands and are also produced by Proprionobacterium acnes, which is a member of the normal microflora of the skin. The normal microflora also provides protection from pathogens in other ways. Large numbers of microorganisms live in a close harmonious relationship with humans and are known as commensals. The acidity of sweat (pH 5.5) also has a microbiocidal effect.

Lysozyme, an enzyme secreted by macrophages, is found in large quantities in human tears and helps to prevent bacterial conjunctivitis. It is found in relatively high concentration in most tissue fluids and in polymorphonuclear leukocytes, although it is nor synthesized by these cells. Lysozyme disables or destroys many Gram-positive bacteria by chemically attacking their cell walls, breaking them up, a process known as lysis. The macrophages then remove damaged cells and bacteria from the tissues. Macrophages are large cells which are derived from the bone marrow but are distributed widely throughout the body and congregate at the site of an inflammatory response.

In the course of infection and inflammation, a variety of basic polypeptides released from damaged cells have a destructive effect on certain bacteria. The levels of a number of other 'acute phase' substances are increased in the blood in the inflammatory response but the roles of many of them are unclear.

A major defense mechanism is provided by a complex group of proteins, all of large molecular size, collectively known as complement. They form a series of enzymes which can be activated directly by some bacteria and indirectly, with the help of antibody, in other cases. Activated products of the complement system help in the first-line host defence against microorganisms, destroying them by lysis, and they mediate inflammatory changes. Complement can also lyse red cells (hemolysis) and indeed much of our knowledge of the complement system comes from studies of immune hemolysis.

The complement system is a triggered enzyme cascade system in which circulating inactive forms (proenzymes) are converted into active forms by their predecessors in the cascade. The complement system can be activated in two ways, known as the classical pathway and the alternate pathway. Tile classical pathway is typically initiated by complexes of antibody and antigen whereas the alternate pathway can be activated in the absence of antibody. Three stages are involved in the activation of the system, namely the recognition stage, the activation stage and the membrane attack stage.

The components of the complement system are known by their numbers, C1 to C9 and, of these components, C3 is the most abundant. The main sources of complement components are the intestinal epithelium, the macrophages, the liver and the spleen.

When attacked by a virus, many cells rapidly respond by producing interferon. This is a family of proteins which block the replication (multiplication) of viruses, both in the cells which produce the interferon and in other cells. Expressed simply, it interferes with the synthesis of new virus by the cells of the host. Interferons have two important actions:
(a) They alter the properties of the cell membrane against accessibility by viruses; and
(b) They activate cellular genes to produce intracellular enzymes which interact with double-stranded RNA to inhibit protein synthesis in the virus.

Because of their protective properties, lysozyme and interferons have been described as 'natural antibiotics.' They provide rapid protection against invaders, lysozyme against bacteria and interferon against viruses.

Phagocytes

Certain cells in the body have the power of engulfing bacteria and other foreign materials. They are known as phagocytic cells and are of two types, the circulating polymorphonuclear leukocytes of the blood and the mononuclear phagocytic cells known as macrophages. The latter are distributed throughout the body and are themselves of two kinds, namely those which circulate in the blood (monocytes) and those which are fixed in the tissues (e.g. histiocytes in the connective tissues). These actively phagocytic cells are collectively referred to as the mononuclear phagocytic system. The phagocytes either digest the material which they engulf or store it out of harm's way so that it can no longer act as an irritant. They quickly clear the blood of bacteria and other particulate matter.

The macrophages form an important link between the innate and acquired immune systems. They pass on to the lymphoid cells some of the antigens, or their products, but at the same time retain some of them so that the lymphoid cells are not overwhelmed.

The normal function of phagocytes depends upon their ability to *recognize, bind* and *ingest* microorganisms and other particles. This is, in part, non-specific but, in addition, bacteria coated with antibody and complement adhere to the phagocyte because the phagocyte cell membrane has receptors for a part of the antibody molecule and a component of the complement system. Antibodies can greatly enhance the phagocytosis and even the intracellular digestion of bacteria. An antibody which coats the surface of a bacterium or other particle (antigen), and makes it more susceptible to phagocytosis, is known as an opsonizing antibody or opsonin. IgM antibodies are particularly effective opsonizing agents. Clearly, the complement also acts as an opsonic in this situation.

Generally, polymorph nuclear neutrophils are more effective than monocytes or macrophages in the rapid killing of bacteria. However, macrophages are more versatile than neutrophils and are essential for the elimination of various chronic infusive agents.

Immunity refers to resistance exhibited by the host towards injury caused by microorganism, or its products.

Immune response is reaction of body against foreign antigen.

Antigen is a substance which when introduced into the body can generate immune response, and is usually a protein. The antibody formed reacts specifically and in an observable manner. Antigenicity depends on the presence of an antigenic determinant or epitope on the surface of the antigen, represented by a small area on the surface of antigen.

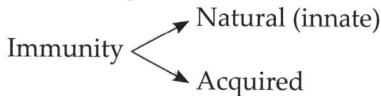

Natural immunity refers to resistance to infection which an individual possess because of his genetic and constitutional make up. It does not require prior exposure to antigen, or immunization, e.g. phagocytosis of bacteria by neutrophil.

■ ACQUIRED IMMUNITY

It is the resistance an individual acquire during life can be active or passive.

Active immunity is the resistance developed by an individual as a result of antigenic stimulation. It involves active functioning of the immune system.

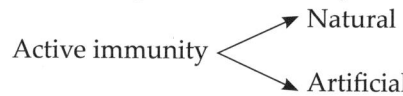

Natural: Infections produce natural active immunity.
Artificial: Vaccines provide artificial active immunity.

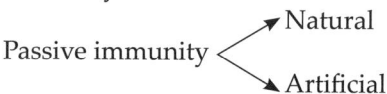

Passive immunity: Body's immune system plays no role in its development.
Natural passive immunity: From mother to fetus through placenta or breast milk.
Artificial passive immunity: Introducing preformed antibody.

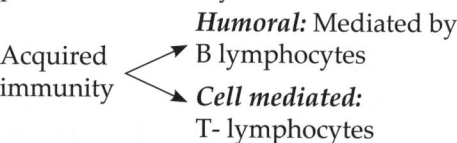

Humoral Immunity

Mediated by circulating antibodies which are carried by globulin fraction of plasma proteins produced by plasma cells derived from lymphocytes.

In early neonatal life committed stem cells give rise to pre-B lymphocytes which mature in red bone marrow (RBM). They escape from RBM enter the peripheral lymphoid tissue like lymph node—peyer's patch, tonsil, white pulp of spleen and circulate back and forth between circulation and peripheral lymphoid organs. B lymphocytes produce 5 classes of immunoglobulins (Ig) (Fig. 3.1):
1. IgG
2. IgA
3. IgM
4. IgD
5. IgE

Complement System

Consisting of several enzymes also interact with immune system.

Cellular Immunity

Mediated by sensitized T lymphocytes constitute major defense against infection by viruses, fungi, and few intracellular bacteria, e.g. tubercle bacillus also defense against malignant tumors. Cells of both these systems interact in many ways.

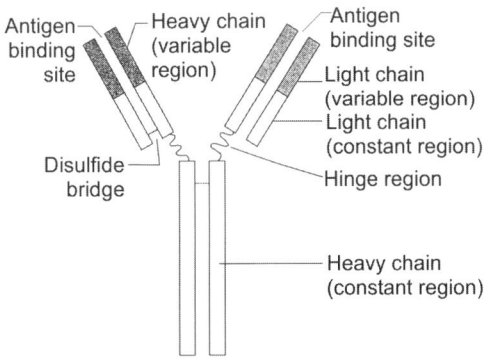

Fig. 3.1: An immunoglobulin molecule

Development of Immune System

In the thymus the lymphocytes proliferate and develop extreme diversity for reacting against specific antigens. This proliferation in the thymus is not dependent on antigenic stimulus. In the thymus lymphocytes are educated so that they become capable of mounting cell mediated immune response against appropriate antigens. They acquire surface receptors and become immunologically competent cells. These cells have antigen recognition sites on their surface which enables each cell to recognize only one antigen specifically. T lymphocytes are also taught not to react against proteins or other antigens that are present on bodies own tissues. These cells migrate to peripheral lymphoid tissue, spleen lymph node etc. They circulate through blood, lymph node and tissues so that they can reach any site immediately following introductions of antigen into any part of body. These cells are capable of:
- Recognizing antigens
- Storage of immunological memory
- Immune response to specific antigens

T cells can be classified to:
- Helper T cells
- Suppressor T cells
- Memory T cells
- Cytotoxic T cells

Helper T cells

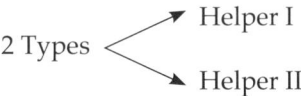

Helper I: Recreates interleukin 2, interferone and is involved in cell mediated immunity.
Helper II: Secretes interleukin 4, 5 and interact with B lymphocytes in bringing about humoral immunity.

Suppressor T Cells

Inhibit antibody production by B cells and immune response of cytotoxic T cells. Thus they regulate the activities of other cells.

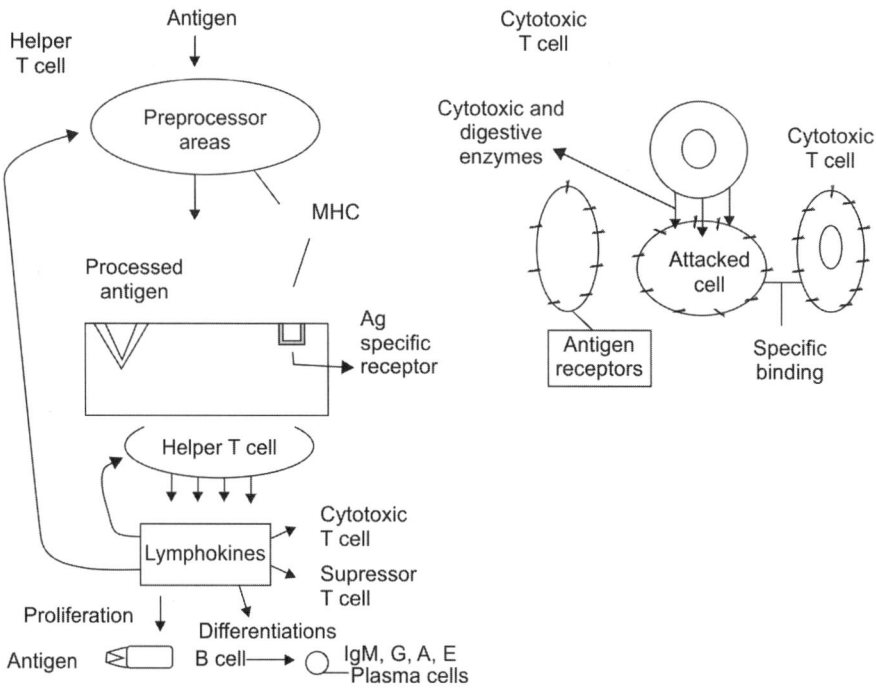

Fig. 3.2: Mechanism of action of helper T cells, cytotoxic T cell mediated lysis

It prevent them from causing excessive immune reaction damaging to the tissues.

Helper and Suppressor T cells together are called regulatory cells. Normal balance between helper and suppressor is registered for normal immune response.

T cells can be differentiated into subsets depending on presence of certain antigenic determinants on the surface. Most cytotoxic T cells have a CD_8 antigenic determinant (Fig. 3.2).

Antigenic determinant in helper T cell is CD_4 antigen.

Memory Cells

When stimulated, both B cell and T cell undergo clonal selection and proliferation so that the antigen is eliminated. After elimination of antigen lymphocytes of this particular clone die, but a few lymphocytes of this clone survive with in the lymph node in a dorment state. Memory cells can be either B or T memeory cell. Memory cells retain the memory of the particular antigen. If a second attack by same antigen occurs, memory cells begin to proliferate and lymphocytes of that particular clone are released with in few days.

Cytotoxic T Cell

Individed accurate and pinpoint destruction of the antigen together with the macrophage which have engulfed the antigen occurs with the help of cytotoxic T cells.

CHAPTER 4

The Body as a Whole

All the various cells and tissues which have been described from the basis of the separate systems of the body. A system may be defined as a group of structures or organs which carry out an essential fundamental function of the individual. Although, to some extent, each system works and can be considered on its own, the functions of the various systems are very closely connected and are dependent on each other. For example, the bones, joints, ligaments and muscles are all concerned with the function of movement which in turn is controlled by the activity of the nervous system. The vitality of the nervous system is dependent on an adequate circulation of blood and a supply of oxygen which enters the blood via the respiratory system.

It is essential to be familiar with certain terms used in anatomical description. The body is considered in the upright or erect position with the palms of the hands facing to the front and the toes pointing forwards. The following terms are then applied:

Anterior (ventral)	Towards the front of the body or limbs
Posterior (dorsal)	Towards the back of the body or limbs
Median	In the middle
Medial	The side nearest the mid-line of the body
Lateral	The side farthest away from the mid-line
Superior	Above any point referred to
Inferior	Below any point referred to
Plantar	Belonging to the sole of the foot
Palmar	Belonging to the palm of the hand

The terms internal and external should only be used to describe the relationship to the inner and outer surfaces of the body and not as alternatives to medial and lateral (Fig. 4.1).

In describing the limbs, the upper part nearest the trunk is called the proximal part; the lower portion farthest away from the trunk is called the distal part. The proximal part is the more central and the distal part is the more peripheral.

The terms for common movements are:

Flexion	A bending at a joint so that two connected parts are approximated together
Extension	A straightening out from a position of flexion
Abduction	A drawing away from the median axis of the body
Adduction	A bringing towards the median line of the body

The body as a whole is built up around the bony framework of the skeleton and consists of three main parts:
- The head and neck
- The trunk
  - The chest or thorax
  - The abdomen and pelvis
- The limbs
  - The upper limbs
  - The lower limbs.

The head is separated into two parts, the cranium or brain case and the face. The trunk is divided into the thorax or chest and the abdomen or belly. There are two pairs of limbs, the upper and lower, each divided into parts which roughly correspond.

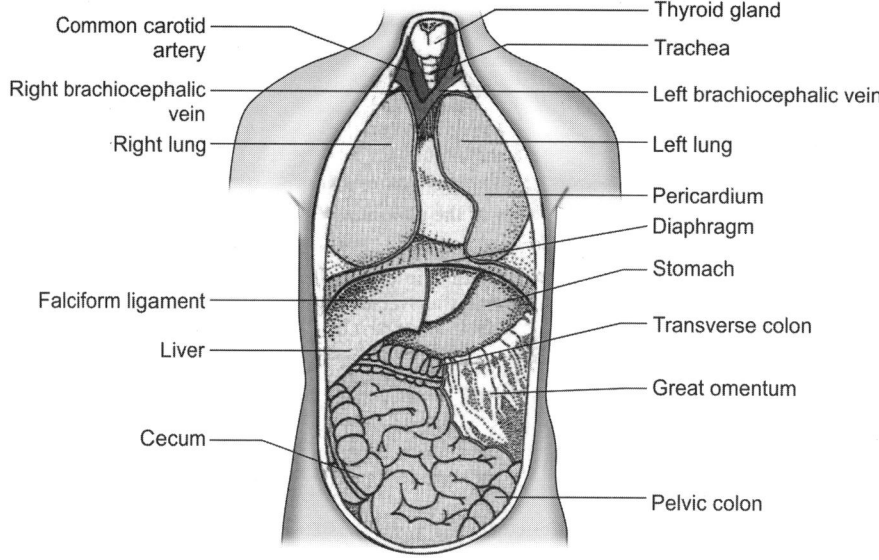

Fig. 4.1: The viscera of the body from the front

Upper limbs:	Upper arm, elbow, forearm, wrist, hand, fingers
Lower limbs:	Thigh, knee, leg, ankle, foot, toes

The fingers and toes are referred to as digits, the bony parts of which, separated by joints are called phalanges.

Covering the bones and giving rise to the general contour of the body are numerous muscles. Blood vessels and nerves traverse all parts of the human frame.

The chief organs of the body are contained in special cavities:
- The brain in the cavity of the skull (cranium)
- The lungs and heart in the cavity of the thorax
- The digestive organs in the abdominal cavity.

It is of importance to know the boundaries of these cavities and the structures which they contain. All those mentioned will be referred to later, but are included now for purposes of classification.

■ THE SKULL

This consists of the cranium which protects the brain and the eyes, and the mandible or lower jaw which is hinged to it. The movements of the mandible are essential for the chewing of food and for the production of speech.

■ THE THORAX

This important cavity is situated in the upper part of the trunk and its walls consist of a bony framework supporting various muscles.

Boundaries of the thorax (Fig. 4.2)

Anterior: The sternum, costal cartilages and front ends of the ribs

Posterior: The thoracic or dorsal part of the vertebral column or backbone, consisting of twelve individual vertebrae and the intervertebral discs of cartilage between them

Lateral: The twelve ribs and the intercostal muscles

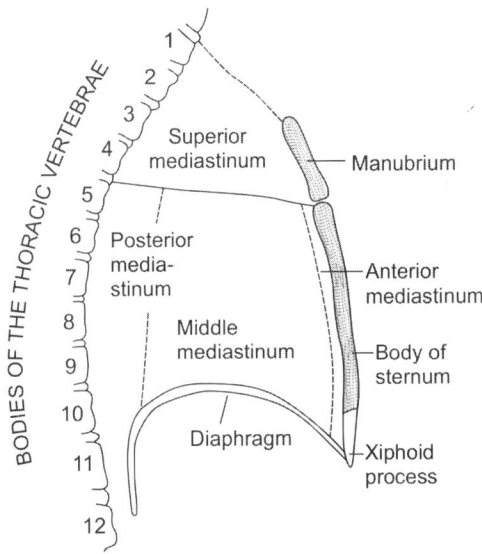

Fig. 4.2: Section of the thorax, showing the divisions of the mediastinum

Superior: The root of the neck with its muscles and blood vessels

Inferior: The diaphragm—a large dome-shaped muscular structure, separating the cavity of the thorax from that of the abdomen, through which pass the esophagus, aorta and inferior vena cava.

Contents of the Thorax

- The lungs occupy the greater part of the thoracic cavity except for a central portion behind the sternum which extends backwards to the vertebral column and is known as the mediastinum
- The heart is situated in the mediastinum in the central part of the thoracic cavity and is enclosed in a fibrous bag or sac known as the pericardium.
- The trachea or windpipe enters the thorax through its upper opening from the neck and passes down in the posterior part of the mediastinum until it divides into the two main bronchi at the level of the fourth thoracic (dorsal) vertebra. A bronchus passes to each lung.
- The esophagus or gullet also enters the superior opening of the thorax from the neck where it commences as a continuation of the pharynx. The esophagus lies just in front of and to the left of the vertebral column and behind the trachea. It leaves the thorax by passing through an opening in the diaphragm and enters the abdominal cavity where it immediately joins the stomach.

Other structures in the thorax include the thymus gland, the phrenic and vague nerves, the aorta, some important veins (the superior vena cava and inferior vena cava), the thoracic duct and lymphatic glands.

■ THE ABDOMEN

The abdominal cavity is the largest cavity in the body. It is described in two parts, the abdomen proper and the pelvic cavity. The latter is directly continuous with the rest of the abdomen but is situated in the space bounded by the sacrum behind, the ischium on each side and the pubic bones in front.

Boundaries of the Abdominal Cavity

Anterior: The muscles of the abdominal wall (the rectus, internal and external oblique and transverses on each side)

Posterior: The lumbar part of the vertebral column in the mid-line and the psoas, quadratus lumborum and iliacus muscles on either side

Superior: The diaphragm

Inferior: The abdominal cavity is continuous with the superior opening of the pelvic cavity

Contents of the Abdominal Cavity

- The stomach and intestines
- The liver, gallbladder and spleen

- The pancreas, kidneys and suprarenal glands. The abdominal aorta and inferior vena cava. All of these structures lie outside the peritoneum and are situated on the posterior wall of the cavity.

Boundaries of the Pelvic Cavity

Anterior: The pubic bones and syphilis pubis
Posterior: The sacrum
Lateral: The ischium on each side
Superior: The pelvis is continuous with the abdominal cavity
Inferior: The muscles of the pelvic floor (elevator any, etc.). Through the pelvic floor pass the lower part of the bowel (rectum) in the hollow formed by the sacrum behind, the urethra and, in the female, the vagina towards the front.

Contents of the Pelvic Cavity

- The lower part of the large intestine (the sigmoid or pelvic colon and the rectum)
- The bladder
- The female organs of reproduction (uterus, ovaries and Fallopian tubes).
- Some loops of small intestine may also be present in the pelvis.

■ SYSTEMS OF THE BODY

As a matter of convenience the various systems of the body are generally described separately but it must be remembered that functionally they are all closely related and interwoven. The major systems are:
- The locomotor system (bones, muscles and joints)
- The nervous system (central and peripheral, somatic and autonomic)
- The skin and organs of special sense (sight, hearing, smell and taste)
- The cardiovascular system (heart, blood vessels and lymphatics)
- The blood (the hemopoietic system) The respiratory system
- The digestive system
- The endocrine system (ductless glands) The urinary system
- The reproductive system.

Anatomically there is a close relationship between the urinary and reproductive systems. Hence they are frequently described together under the heading 'The Urogenital System'.

The nervous system receives and utilizes information from the sense organs and controls voluntary and involuntary (reflex) movements of muscles. The higher centers regulate thought, memory and social behavior. The cardiovascular or circulatory system enables nutrients to be conveyed to and waste products removed from all parts of the body by means of the blood. The respiratory system provides for the intake of oxygen and discharge of carbon dioxide. The digestive system provides for the intake and breakdown of food into relatively simple chemical compounds suitable for absorption. The ductless glands influence metabolism, growth and reproduction. The urinary system removes waste products circulating in the blood and helps to keep its chemical and physical properties constant.

It should be noted that there is a variety of glands in various parts of the body. Broadly speaking there are exocrine glands which pour their secretions into the alimentary canal and the endocrine glands (ductless glands) whose secretions enter the blood stream. Lymph nodes, sometimes called lymph glands, are not really glands since they do not secrete hormones or enzymes but they produce lymphocytes and help to protect the body from the spread of infection. The ducts or lymphatic channels which connect these structures and ultimately enter the bloodstream convey tissue fluids which surround the various tissue cells and act as 'middle man' conveying nourishment to and removing waste products from them.

CHAPTER 5

The Skeleton

The internal framework of the human body is its bony skeleton, which gives support and protection and provides levers for locomotion and other movements, such as those concerned with obtaining and eating food. There are animals which possess no backbone and even no rigid skeleton, either internal or external, but they are adapted to their own environment and humans to theirs.

The human being is the only fully upright vertebrate, the term applied to an animal with a backbone. Being upright, and needing to move from place to place or from one position to another, humans have special problems in relation to gravity if their antigravity mechanisms fail, as may happen in old age, for example.

The maintenance of posture and the performance of movements, simple or complicated, necessitates the activity of muscles and of the nervous system, which initiates, controls and coordinates movement. Often the movement has to be coordinated with the organs of special sense, especially the eyes.

Mobility is provided by joints between bones which, especially in the limbs, act as levers. The power to move the bones resides in the muscles which are under the direction and control of the central nervous system. The brain wills the movement (volition), and the message is carried to the appropriate muscles by motor nerve fibers, initially by upper motor neurones in the pyramidal tracts and then, via relay stations in the brain stem and spinal cord, by lower motor neurons in the cranial and spinal nerves. The active muscle (agonist) contracts whilst the antagonist relaxes. For example, in order to flex the arm and convey food to the mouth, the biceps contracts and the triceps relaxes and elongates just the right amount to permit the desired action. Movement is modulated by the extrapyramidal nuclei of the brain and coordinated by the cerebellum.

A distinction is made between bone and bones. Bones are organs, each of which is adapted for its own particular function. Bone is the tissue from which they are made. Bones and muscles are derived from the mesoderm, the middle layer of the embryo. Most bones pass through two stages, a first blastemal stage of condensation of tissue (mesenchyme) and a second, cartilaginous stage. Some bones such as those in the roof and sides of the skull, never go through a cartilaginous stage, calcification occurring directly in the fibrocellular membrane which precedes the bone. Most bones, however, are modelled in cartilage before being mineralized; thus ossification is either intramembranous or, more commonly, intracartilaginous.

Bone is an active living tissue (a specialized type of connective tissue) with several major roles in the body. It is the substance from which bones (the organs) are made and is the body's reservoir of calcium. Apart from forming salts which strengthen bone, calcium is essential for normal cardiac and skeletal muscle contraction, nerve function and blood coagulation. Bone, the tissue, consists of a matrix of collagen fibers impregnated with mineral salts, mainly phosphates of calcium in the form of crystals of hydroxyapatites. Because bone has an extensive network of blood vessels, calcium salts are as easily removed from bone as they are deposited in it.

Bone is constantly being resorbed and reformed and there is a corresponding turnover of calcium which is greatest in infancy. The cells in bone which affect its formation and resumption are the osteoblasts, the osteocytes and the osteoclasts. Osteoblasts secrete the collagen which forms the matrix and are thus bone-forming cells. When they have surrounded themselves with bone (calcified matrix) they become osteocytes. These cells connect with each other and with osteoblasts deep in the bone by means of long protoplasmic processes which extend along the channels (canaliculi) which ramify through the bone. Osteoclasts erode bone, apparently by a phagocytic action (literally eating and digesting bone), and so bring about its resorption.

All of these cells are affected by the hormones which regulate bone structure and calcium metabolism. These hormones are 1,25-dihydroxycholecalciferol formed from vitamin D, parathyroid hormone, calcitonin (secreted by the thyroid gland), glucocorticoids and growth hormone. 1,25-dihydroxycholecalciferol, also called l,25-dihydroxy-D3, and parathyroid hormone both mobilize calcium from bone and increase its concentration in the serum. Calcitonin inhibits bone resorption and thereby tends to reduce serum calcium levels.

1,25-dihydroxycholecalciferol acts not only on bone but also on the small intestine, where it increases the absorption of calcium.

Vitamin D deficiency therefore causes a state of calcium deficiency in which new bone fails to calcify and remains soft, resulting in rickets in children or osteomalacia in adults.

In cases of lead poisoning much of the lead is deposited in bones. Strontium-90, a product of atomic fission, is also deposited in bones. This is radioactive, and continues to be so for a long time after it has been absorbed.

A mature bone is composed of two kinds of bone tissue. Compact bone is the hard dense ivory-like bone which forms the shafts of long bones and the surface layers of flat bones. It is built up of units which are called osteons or Haversian systems. These are cylinders of bone, through the middle of which a minute circular canal, the Haversian canal, runs longitudinally, parallel with the surface of the bone. Blood vessels and lymphatics run in the Haversian canals and nourish the bone substance. In the bone tissue surrounding the Haversian canal are a number of small spaces, called lacunae, arranged in concentric rings, which contain the bone cells. The lacunae communicate with one another and with the central Haversian canal by the minute canals (canaliculi) in which the protoplasmic processes of the bone cells lie.

Trabecular (cancellous or spongy) bone has a microscopic structure similar to that of compact bone but, instead of being dense, it appears spongy, having more and larger spaces and less solid matter. Cancellous bone makes bones lighter without loss of strength. Compact bone is always arranged outside cancellous bone and forms the surfaces of bones. Cancellous bone is trabecular in its internal arrangement, with a criss-crossed pattern of small bars and beams, struts and trusses, determined by mechanical stresses and adding to the strength of the bone. A soft pulpy tissue, bone marrow, is found in the cylindrical cavities of long bones and in the spaces between the trabecular and in the larger Haversian canals of all bones. In early life it is all red marrow (blood-forming) but after about the fifth year it is gradually replaced by yellow marrow (mostly fat cells) until, by the age of 20 to 25 years, red marrow remains only in the vertebrae, sternum, ribs, clavicles, scapulae, cranial bones and proximal ends of the femora and humeri.

Bone surfaces are covered with a tough sheet of fibrous tissue which is known as the periosteum. This clothes a bone all over except where the bone is covered by hyaline cartilage for the formation of a joint.

Bone receives its blood supply from two sources; the surface of the bone from the periosteum; the interior from an artery which enters the shaft, generally about its middle, through a canal known as the nutrient foramen.

In summary, bone has several important functions.
- It is the support tissue for the framework of the body.
- It is a mineral store, containing 97% of the total bodily content of calcium salts.
- It houses the blood-forming bone marrow.

■ DEVELOPMENT OF BONE

In very early fetal life no actual bone is apparent, but the bones of the human skeleton are outlined by other forms of connective tissue, either cartilage or fibrous tissue (membrane). It will be seen later that the majority of bones in the skeleton are described as long bones and these are preceded by cartilage in the embryo; while certain flat bones, such as those of the skull, are developed in membrane.

First of all, therefore, the bones are represented by rods or blocks of cartilage, or sheets of membrane, which resemble in shape the mature bone. The next stage in development is the deposition of calcium salts in the cartilage or membrane (calcification). Later, bone cells or osteoblasts enter the calcified cartilage together with other cells which remove the cartilage. The bone cells proceed to lay down bone in the place of the cartilage which is absorbed. The area in which this process commences is called a center of ossification.

At birth only a proportion of the skeleton is represented by actual bone. The remainder consists of ossifying cartilage, or membrane.

■ GROWTH OF BONES

Most bones go on growing in size for at least twenty years.

Centers of ossification, i.e. areas in which bone cells are replacing cartilage, are necessary for growth in length of a bone. In most long bones there are two such centers, one at each end of the bone. An additional center exists for the shaft of the bone.

The main part or shaft of the bone is called the diaphysis. The portion at each end containing a center of ossification is called the epiphysis (Fig. 5.1). Each epiphysis is joined to the diaphysis by a

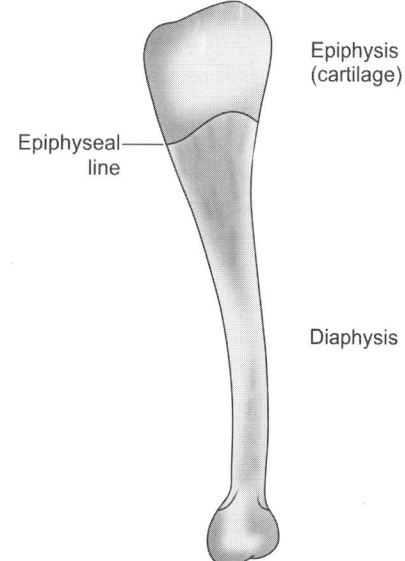

Fig. 5.1: Section of young bone before ossification of the epiphysis has started

layer of cartilage known as the epiphyseal cartilage. This is gradually replaced by bone, and by adult life has disappeared and the epiphysis and diaphysis are completely fused into a single bony structure, but so long as some epiphyseal cartilage remains, growth in the length of the bone is possible.

So far reference has only been made to growth in the length of a bone; increase in circumference takes place by new bone being laid down under the periosteum by osteoblasts situated in this position.

New bone may be formed from time to time in order to repair fractures, without any increase in size of the bone as a whole.

The three main factors which influence the normal growth of bone in children are:
(a) Sex hormones (estrogens and androgens)
(b) Pituitary growth hormone
(c) Thyroid hormone.

Any defect in these hormones may cause stunting of growth.

■ PRACTICAL CONSIDERATIONS

In children, the bones do not contain quite as much calcium salts as in the adult, so that the bones are more elastic and instead of complete fractures resulting from injury, a partial fracture known as the greenstick variety sometimes occurs.

Injuries to the ends of bones in children often result in damage to the epiphysis, which may become displaced rather than the bony substance being broken.

Deficiency in the amount of calcium salts in rickets results in the bones becoming abnormally soft, so that bending with a corresponding deformity of the limbs may take place. Changes in the epiphysis are also apparent.

When a fracture of bone occurs, nature attempts to repair it and the repair is most efficient when the surgeon can place the broken fragments in their natural position. The following process then occurs; the space between the broken ends is filled with blood clot, in which fibrous tissue develops; osteoblasts then migrate from the damaged ends of the bones and from the periosteum and gradually fill up the gap with new bone, known as callus; eventually the continuity of the bone is restored and the callus becomes hard and firm by the deposit of calcium salts in the damaged area. In a healthy individual the repair is usually complete in one to three months.

■ THE SKELETON AS A WHOLE

The skeleton is the framework of the body consisting of bones and, strictly speaking, the cartilages and ligaments which bind them together. It serves to support the soft structures which are grouped around it and to protect the organs of the body. It is so jointed that various parts move on each other and many bones act as levers for the muscles which are attached to them.

The main functions of the skeleton are:
- To act as a framework and to support the soft tissues
- To enable free movement by the action of muscles (i.e. to combine stability with mobility)
- To protect delicate organs and structures
- To form a store of calcium
- To provide for formation of blood cells in the bone marrow.

■ TYPES OF BONE (FIG. 5.2)

The bones of the skeleton are classified according to their shape into long, short, flat and irregular bones.
- *Long bones* are found in the limbs and consist of an elongated shaft with two extremities. The bones of the arm, forearm, thigh and leg are typical examples. The shaft consists of a cylinder of compact bone containing yellow bone marrow. The extremities are formed by a thin outer shell of

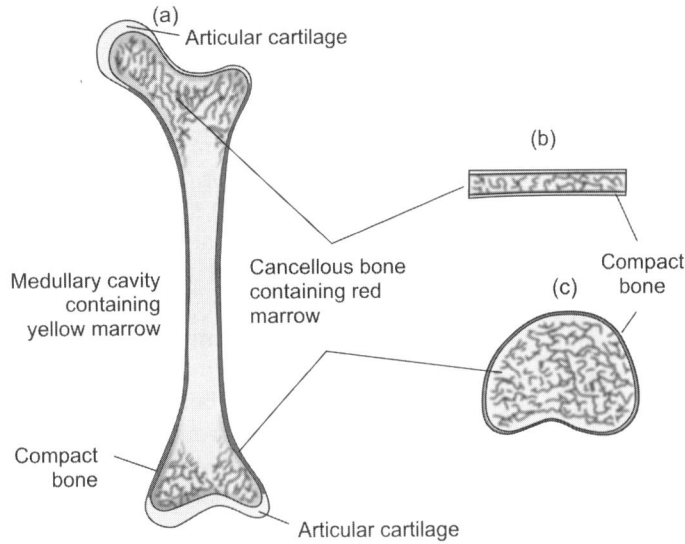

Fig. 5.2: Diagram illustrating the structure of **(a)** a long bone (femur), **(b)** a flat bone (skull) and **(c)** an irregular bone (body of vertebra)

compact tissue with an interior network of spongy or cancellous bone containing red marrow.
- **Short bones** have no shaft but consist of smaller masses of spongy bone surrounded by a shell of compact bone. They are roughly box-like in shape. Examples are found in the small bones of the wrist (carpus) and ankle (tarsus).
- A *flat bone* consists of two layers of compact bone between which is a layer of cancellous bone. Examples are the scapula, innominate bone and bones of the skull.
- *Irregular bones* cannot be placed strictly in any of the previous categories and include the vertebrae and most of the bones of the face.

Sesamoid bones are small bones which are developed in the tendons around certain joints. The patella, in the front of the knee joint, is the largest and most important.

Descriptive Terms

The following terms are used in the description of bones:

- *Articulation:* A joint between two bones, e.g. the humerus articulates with the scapula and the femur with the tibia.
- *Border:* The edge separating two surfaces of a bone, e.g. the vertebral and axillary borders of the scapula separating the anterior from the posterior surfaces.
- *Condyle:* A rounded knuckle-shaped articular surface at the end of a bone, usually covered by cartilage, e.g. the condyles of the femur.
- *Epicondyle:* A small projection adjacent to a condyle and usually giving attachment to ligaments.
- *Crest:* An elevated ridge on a bone, e.g. the crest of the ilium and the crest of the tibia.
- *Facet:* A small articulating surface.
- *Foramen:* An opening or whole perforating a bone, e.g. the obturator foramen in the innominate bone and the nutrient foramen present in all bones.
- *Fossa:* A hollowed-out area or depression in the surface of a bone, e.g. the

olecranon fossa and coronoid fossa of the humerus.
- *Process:* A projection from a bone, e.g. the spinous process of a vertebra.
- *Tubercle, tuberosity, and trochanter:* All terms used to describe various types of process. A tubercle is a small rounded prominence, e.g. the tubercle of the tibia. A tuberosity is a larger protuberance of bone, e.g. the tuberosities of the humerus. A trochanter is a large, round eminence, e.g. the trochanter of the femur. The expanded proximal end of a long bone is often referred to as its head, e.g. the head of the femur, which articulates with the bony pelvis.

■ THE HUMAN SKELETON

The human skeleton, which contains approximately 200 individual bones, is made up of the following parts (Fig. 5.3):
- The skull, viz. the bones of the cranium, face and lower jaw.
- The bones of the trunk, viz. the spinal column, ribs and sternum.
- The bones of the limbs together with the shoulder and pelvic girdles.

The spinal column consists of 33 vertebrae and is divided for purposes of description into cervical (7 vertebrae), thoracic or dorsal (12 vertebrae), lumbar (5 vertebrae), sacral (5 vertebrae) and coccygeal (4 vertebrae) from above downwards. The five sacral vertebrae are fused together to form a single bone, the sacrum; the coccygeal are similarly joined to form the coccyx.

The ribs are twelve in number; they articulate behind with the thoracic vertebrae and, in front, the upper seven articulate with the sternum or breastbone.

The bones of the upper limb, which is attached to the shoulder girdle (clavicle and scapula), are those of the arm (humerus), forearm (radius and ulna), wrist (carpus), hand (metacarpals), and digits or fingers (phalanges).

Included in the lower limb, which is attached to the pelvic girdle, are the thigh bone (femur), the leg bones (tibia and fibula), the ankle bones (tarsus) and those of the foot (metatarsals) and toes (phalanges).

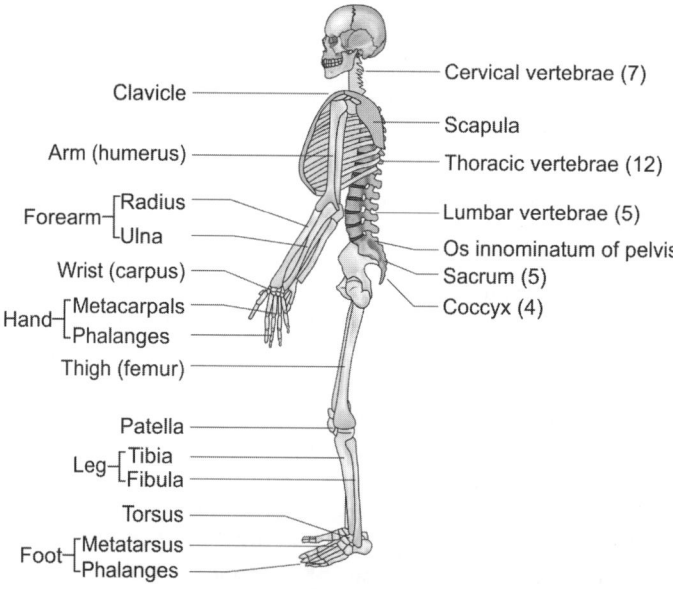

Fig. 5.3: The human skeleton

BONES OF THE SHOULDER GIRDLE AND UPPER LIMB

The Scapula

The scapula or shoulder-blade is a large flat bone which forms a part of the shoulder-girdle and contributes to the wide range of movement of the upper limb, gliding, as it does, across the posterior aspect of the thorax. Parts of its roughly triangular outline can be seen or felt beneath the skin in the living subject.

The processes and thickened parts of the scapula contain cancellous bone and the remainder is a thin layer of compact bone.

The anterior (costal) surface of the scapula is slightly hollowed out in conformity with the nabs which it overlies (Fig. 5.4).

The dorsal surface is slightly convex and is divided into two unequal parts by a large ridge known as the spine of the scapula (Fig. 5.5). The smaller upper part is the supraspinous fossa (supra, L. above) and the larger area below is the infraspinous fossa. These fossae give attachments to the supraspinatus and infraspinatus muscle respectively.

A broad process, known as the acromion, projects forwards almost at right angles from the lateral end of the spine of the scapula (Fig. 5.6). There is a small facet on its medial border for articulation with the collar bone, or clavicle. The upper part of the spine gives attachment to the trapezius muscle of the neck and the lower portion to a part of the deltoid muscle, which abducts the arm.

The large irregular mass of bone which projects forwards from the outer end of the upper (superior) border of the scapula is the coracoid process. Attached to the coracoid process is the coracoclavicular ligament (which binds the clavicle to the process), the short head of biceps and pectoral is minor. These latter two muscles are concerned respectively with flexing the forearm on the upper arm and drawing the scapula forwards around the chest wall.

A smash notch in the superior border of the scapula, the suprascapular notch,

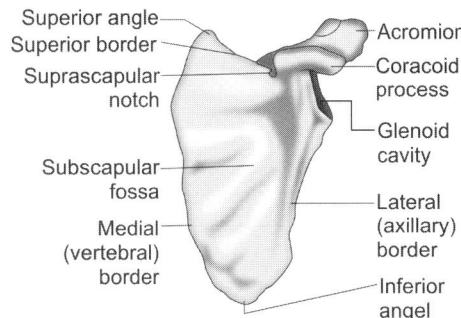

Fig. 5.4: Costal surface of left scapula

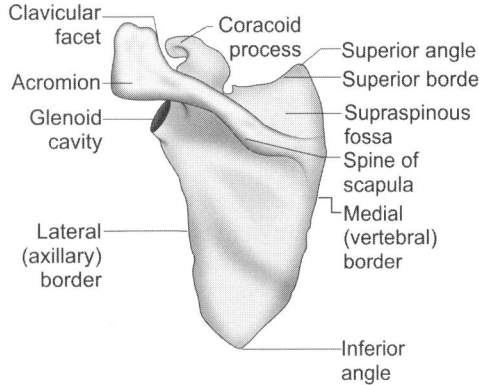

Fig. 5.5: Dorsal surface of left scapula

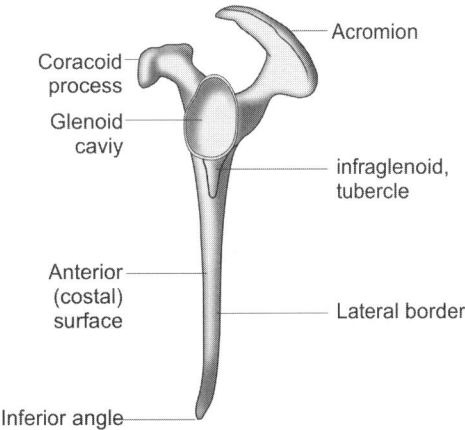

Fig. 5.6: Lateral aspect of the left scapula

transmits the suprascapular nerve to the supraspinous fossa.

The head of the humerus articulates with the scapula at the glenoid cavity to form the shoulder joint. The glenoid cavity is a smooth, shallow pear-shaped cavity at the lateral angle of the scapula. The long head of the biceps muscle is attached just above and triceps just below the glenoid cavity. These two muscles act together in bending and straightening the elbow, the one contracting and, at the same time, the other lengthening an equal amount.

The scapula is so attached by muscles that it can glide across the surface of the thorax. If the shoulders are shrugged backwards and forwards a degree of transverse movement will be felt, and if the arms are raised above the head the inferior angle will be observed to move outwards towards the lower part of the axilla.

The scapula, being covered by muscles and lying flat against the chest wall, is not often exposed to injury and only a direct blow of considerable severity is likely to produce fracture.

The Clavicle

The clavicle (Fig. 5.7) or collar bone is a long bone without a marrow cavity. It consists of cancellous bone within and a layer of compact bone externally. It is situated subcutaneously (just under the skin) at the root of the neck. Its lateral end articulates with the acromion of the scapula and its medial end with the manubrium stern. It acts as a weight-bearing strut or brace for the shoulder and allows the arm to swing clear of the trunk. It also transmits some of the weight of the limb to the axial skeleton. The clavicle has a gently curved shaft, the medial two thirds bowing forwards and the lateral third curving backwards. The bone is weakest at the junction of the two curves and breaks at this point when the collar bone is broken. Such a fracture is common but rarely results from direct trauma despite the exposed superficial position of the clavicle. The fracture is usually the result of indirect injury such as a fall on the outstretched hand or on the shoulder, the force being transmitted to the clavicle and snapping this slender bone. Deformity

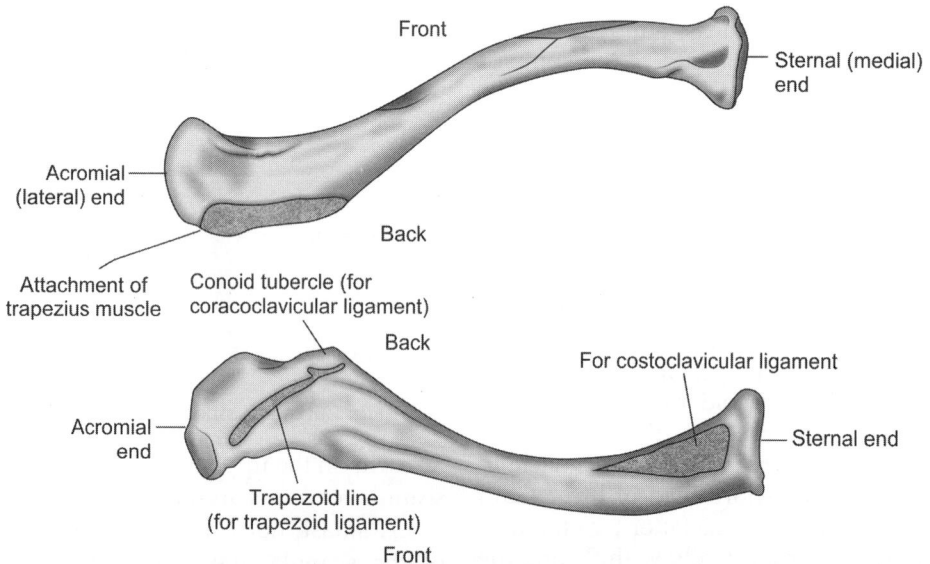

Fig. 5.7: Left clavicle from above (top) and from below

results from the lateral fragment of the clavicle being drawn downwards by the weight of the arm acting on it through the coracoclavicular ligament.

The Humerus

The humerus (Fig. 5.8) is the long bone of the arm. It consists of a shaft and expanded upper and lower extremities. Medially, the upper extremity bears a rounded head, covered with hyaline articular cartilage, which forms a ball and socket joint (the shoulder joint) with the glenoid cavity of the scapula. The slight groove which surrounds the head of the humerus is called the anatomical neck of the humerus. This gives partial attachment to the capsular ligament of the shoulder joint. Laterally the upper extremity of the humerus bears a prominence called the greater tuberosity and in front of this is the lesser tuberosity. A deep groove lying between the tuberosities and extending down. The anterior surface of the upper shaft is known as the intertubercular sulcus. It is about 8 cm long and in it lies the long tendon of the biceps muscle. The tapering region where the upper extremity of the humerus joins the shaft is called the surgical neck of the humerus because it is a common site for fractures to occur. The axillary nerve and posterior humeral circumflex artery are close to it medially.

Nearly halfway down the outer side of the shaft is a roughened elevated area for attachment of the deltoid muscle and known as the deltoid tuberosity. On the posterior surface, passing from above downwards and outwards and having its lower end just below the deltoid tubercle, is a shallow groove, the spiral groove for the radial nerve.

The upper half of the shaft is cylindrical but the lower half is, flattened. Protruberances from the medial and lateral borders of the lower extremity of the bone are known respectively as the medial and lateral epicondyles. The ulnar nerve passes on its way into the forearm in a shallow sulcus behind the medial epicondyle and a blow at this site, jarring the nerve against the epicondyle, gives rise to the expression 'funny bone'.

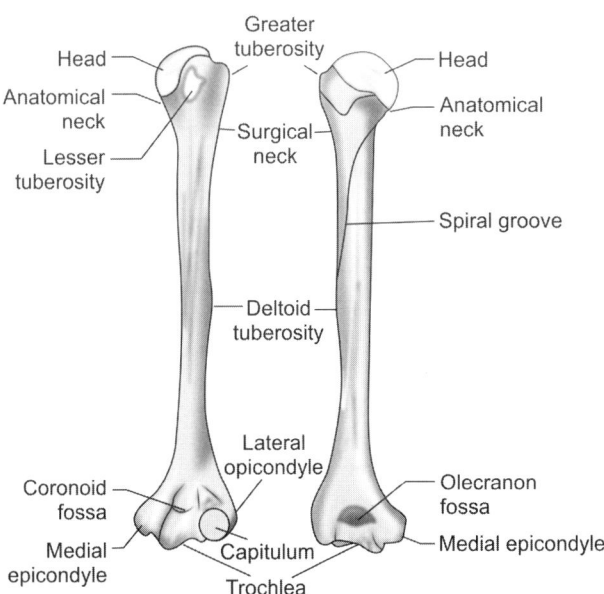

Fig. 5.8: Anterior and posterior aspects of the left humerus

Between the epicondyles is an irregularly shaped area, a modified condyle, which has a smooth articular part shaped for articulation with the radius and ulna at the hinge of the elbow joint. The medial portion, a pulley-shaped surface called the trochlea, articulates with the trochlear notch of the ulna. The lateral portion, a rounded convex projection called the capitalism, articulates with the head of the radius.

Immediately above the articular surface deep depressions are present both on the anterior and posterior surfaces of the bone. On the anterior surface is the coronoid fossa into which the coronoid process of the ulna fits when the elbow is flexed. On the posterior surface is the larger olecranon fossa for the olecranon process of the ulna when the elbow is extended.

When the arm is at rest by the side of the body the head of the humerus is directed backwards and medially towards the glenoid cavity, which faces forwards and laterally. This rotated position of the humerus, with the posterior surface of its shaft facing laterally and backwards, has to be borne in mind when considering movements of the arm and forearm.

The humerus may be fractured at almost any level but is commonly fractured at one of three sites: the surgical neck, sometimes with damage to the axillary nerve; at about mid-shaft just below the attachment of the deltoid muscle, sometimes with damage to the radial nerve in its groove; and at the lower end, when the fracture may extend into the elbow joint or one of the epicondyles may be separated. A fractured medial epicondyle may damage the ulnar nerve. The ossifying medial epicondyle is relatively late in fusing (at about the twentieth year) with the shaft of the humerus and in X-ray films of young people it may therefore look fractured when it is not.

Bones of the Forearm

The forearm contains two long bones, the radius on the lateral (outer) side and the ulna on the medial (inner) side. When the arm is placed in the position for anatomical description, namely with the palm of the hand facing forwards, the radius and ulna (Fig. 5.9) are parallel, and the forearm and hand are said to be in the position of supination. The forearm can, however, be rotated so that the back of the hand is directed forwards. This position is called pronation, and the radius then lies partly across the ulna.

The Radius

The radius is the lateral bone of the forearm. It is a long bone with a shaft and expanded extremities, the lower of which is much the wider of the two.

The smaller upper end of the radius has a circular head which articulates with the capitalism of the humerus and with the radial notch of the ulna, a neck and, medially, a tuberosity for the insertion of the tendon of the biceps muscle. The articular circumference of the head of the radius, is bound to the ulna by an annular ligament, within which it rotates during the movements of pronation and supination of the forearm.

The shaft has a sharp medial border facing the ulna to which it is attached by the interosseous membrane which stretches between the radius and ulna, dividing the forearm into anterior and posterior compartments. The former contains the flexor muscles of the wrists and fingers, the latter the extensor muscles.

The lower extremity of the radius presents an articular surface for the scaphoid and lunate bones of the wrist. At the lateral end of this surface is a downward projection of bone called the styloid process which can be felt through the skin on the lateral aspect of the wrist just above the

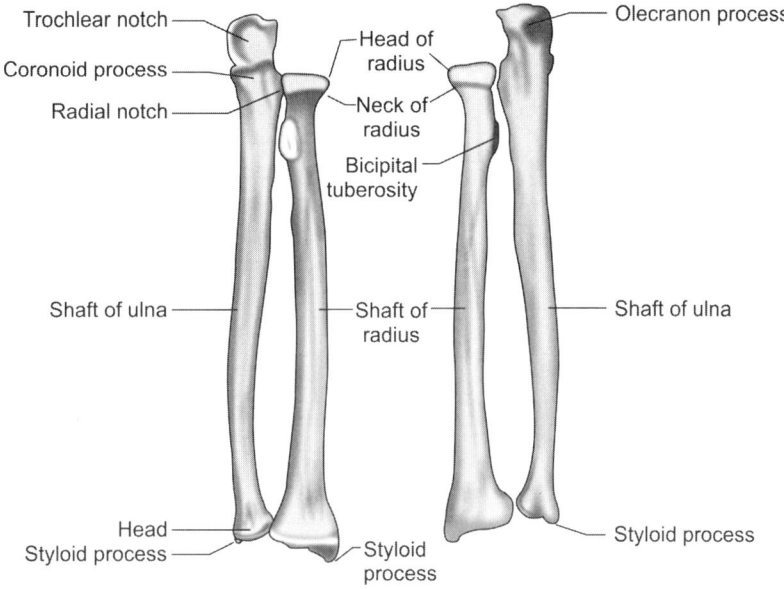

Fig. 5.9: Anterior and posterior aspects of the left radius and ulna

base of the thumb. On the medial aspect of the extremity there is an articular surface for articulation with the ulna.

The Ulna

The ulna is the medial bone of the forearm and is slightly longer than the radius. Like the radius, it is a long bone, with a shaft and upper and lower extremities, but whereas the lower end of the radius is the larger end, it is the upper end of the ulna which is expanded. This extremity is strong and hook-like, with a large C-shaped cavity the trochlear notch, which articulates with the trochlear surface of the humerus. The large mass of bone forming the posterior wall of the trochlear notch and overhanging its upper part rather like a beak is the olecranon process, which fits into the olecranon fossa of the humerus. The posterior surface of the olecranon process can be felt through the skin and its upper limit forms the point of the elbow. The olecranon bursa separates the bone from the skin and may swell with excessive fluid if inflamed (bursitis). The floor of the trochlear notch projects forwards in a process known as the coronoid process, which fits into the coronoid fossa on the front of the humerus when the elbow is flexed. The articular surface of the trochlear notch is continued downwards on the lateral side of the ulna to form the radial notch, which articulates with the circumference of the head of the radius.

The shaft of the ulna narrows as it passes downwards but expands slightly at its lower end to form the head of the ulna, which can be seen projecting on the medial side of the posterior aspect of the wrist. A small downward process at the extreme lower end of the ulna, on its medial side, is called the styloid process; its tip is easily felt through the skin.

With the upper limb hanging straight down by the side, palm facing forwards (i.e. forearm fully extended and hand supinated), the forearm is angulated away laterally from the upper arm. The angle so formed is called the carrying angle and it results from the medial edge of the trochlea of the humerus projecting lower than the lateral edge and from the obliquity of the superior articular surface of the coronoid process. This arrangement adds to the precision with which the hand using, say, a tool or weapon, can be controlled during or after extension of the elbow.

The bones of the forearm are a common site of fracture. Either may be involved in fractures occurring in the region of the elbow joint. Sometimes the olecranon process is separated from the rest of the ulna. Either or both bones may be broken across the shaft. A very common fracture occurs about an inch above the lower end of the radius and is known as Colles' fracture; the styloid process of the ulna is frequently torn off at the same time. This fracture usually results from a fall on the outstretched hand.

The Bones of the Wrist and Hand

The carpus or wrist consists of eight bones arranged in two rows, proximal and distal, with four bones in each.

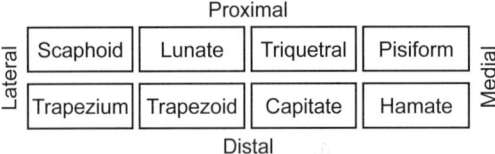

The carpal bones are irregularly shaped bones which articulate with one another and are held in position by ligaments. With the exception of the pisiform, the bones of the proximal row of the carpus articulate with the radius and the articular disk of the inferior radioulnar joint.

The palmar surface of the carpus forms a deep concavity, known as the carpal groove (Fig. 5.10). A strong fibrous band or retinaculum bridges the bony margins of the groove and converts it into a tunnel. The carpal tunnel so formed transmits the flexor tendons and median nerve to the hand. This arrangement increases the strength of the wrist and the efficiency of the flexor muscles. However, if swelling or deformity due to pregnancy, disease or injury compromises the space in the tunnel, the bones and retinaculum being unable to 'give', pressure is exerted on the median nerve which is trapped in the tunnel, thereby damaging it and providing a common example of an entrapment neuropathy. The resulting pain in the hand (particularly at night), sensory loss and weakness and wasting of the short abduction muscle of the thumb (abductor pollicis brevis) is known as the carpal tunnel syndrome.

The metacarpal bones, or bones of the palm of the hand, are long bones, each with a base, a shaft and a head. The bases

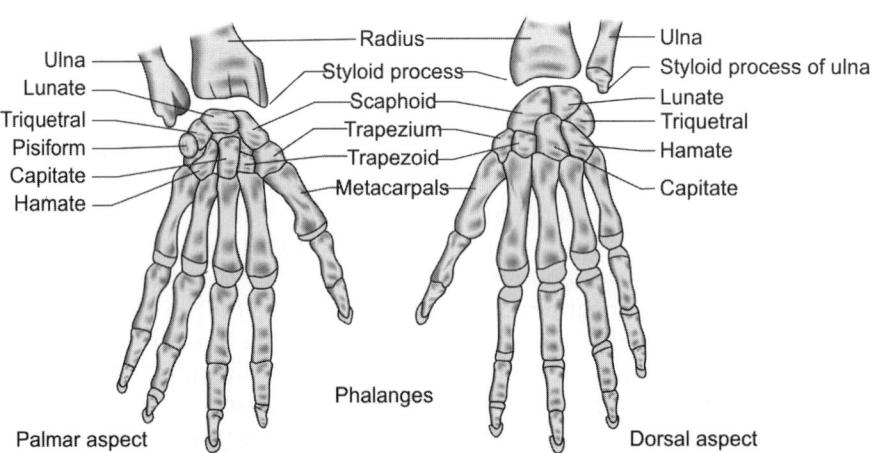

Fig. 5.10: Palmar and dorsal aspects of the left hand

articulate with the distal row of carpal bones, and the heads with the proximal or first row of phalanges. The first metacarpal bone lies anteriorly to the others and is rotated so that its palmar surface faces medially. This makes it possible to oppose the thumb to the fingers and to obtain a good grip with the fingers on one side and the thumb on the other side of an object.

The Phalanges (Singular = Phalanx)

These also are long bones. The thumb has only two phalanges while the fingers have three, proximal, middle and distal, the proximal being the longest. A useful diagnostic clue in the X-rays of patients with acromegaly is that the distal phalanges appear to be 'tufted'.

The joints between the metacarpals and the phalanges are called the metacarpophalangeal joints, those between the phalanges themselves, the interphalangeal joints. The proximal interphalangeal joints are often swollen in patients with rheumatoid arthritis, making the fingers spindle-shaped.

■ BONES OF THE PELVIC GIRDLE

The Innominate Bone (Fig. 5.11)

This is the name given to the hip bone. The two innominate bones join (articulate) together anteriorly at the pubic symphysis and are bridged posteriorly by the sacrum, together with which they form the bony pelvis or pelvic girdle. Each innominate bone is a large irregularly shaped bone which in the child consists of three parts separated by cartilage. In the adult these parts are fused together (i.e. united by bone) but their names are retained for descriptive purposes. The uppermost bone is called the ilium (not to be confused with the ileum, a part of the small intestine). The part situated in front is the pubis, and that posteriorly the ischium. All three bones unite and take part in the formation of the large cup-shaped cavity on the outer surface of the bone, known as the acetabulum, into which fits the head of the femur forming the hip joint.

The Ilium

The ilium, which supports the flank, forms the upper, expanded and flat part of the innominate bone. The external (gluteal) and internal surfaces of the ilium are separated along the upper margin of the bone by the rough iliac crest, which can be felt underlying the flesh at the lower limit of the waist. This is the site from which bone marrow biopsies are frequently taken.

The gluteal surface is marked by three uneven ridges, the posterior, anterior and

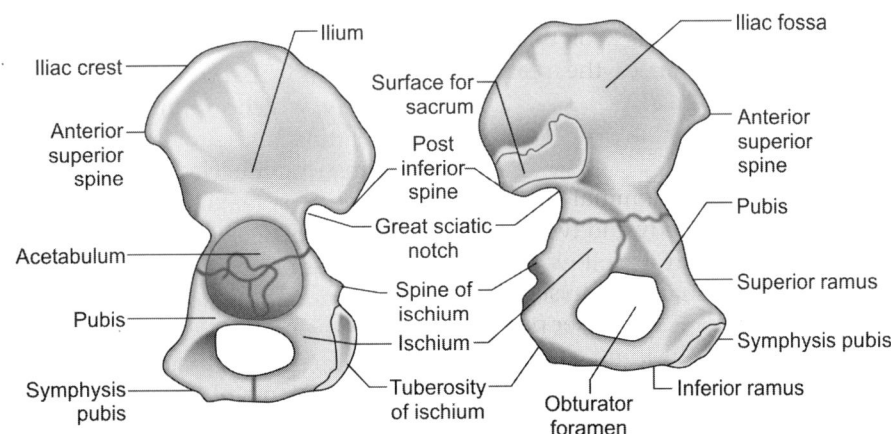

Fig. 5.11: The left innominate bone. External (left) and internal surfaces

inferior gluteal lines. The gluteal muscles arise from this surface of the bone; gluteus maximus behind the posterior gluteal line, gluteus medius between the posterior and anterior lines, and gluteus minimus between the anterior and inferior lines.

The smooth hollow of the internal surface of the ilium is the iliac fossa. Behind and below it is the sacropelvic surface, which is roughened for the attachment of ligaments which bind the ilium to the sacrum and bears an ear-shaped facet where the sacrum articulates.

If the iliac crest is traced forwards, it will be found to end in the anterior superior spine, which gives attachment to the lateral end of the inguinal ligament. The spine can be easily felt in the living subject and is an important landmark in the examination of patients. The posterior end of the iliac crest ends in the posterior superior spine, which cannot be felt in the living subject but which may be marked by a dimple above the medial part of the buttock.

The anterior inferior spine and the posterior inferior spine are situated a little below the corresponding superior spines. Immediately below the posterior inferior spine is a large notch, the greater sciatic notch, which is usually much wider in the female than in the male. Through this notch passes the sciatic nerve, an important nerve which extends down the back of the leg. Damage to this nerve causes the painful condition known as sciatica.

The Pubis

The front portion of the innominate bone is called the pubis. It has a body and two rami. The body articulates with its fellow of the opposite side at the pubic symphysis. The bridge of bone which joins the upper part of the body of the pubis to the ilium, and takes part in the formation of the acetabulum, is called the superior ramus. The bridge which joins the lower part of the body to the ramus of the ischium is the inferior ramus of the pubis.

The free upper border of the body of the pubis is called the pubic crest. At its junction with the superior ramus is a process named the pubic tubercle, to which is attached the medial end of the inguinal ligament.

The urinary bladder lies behind the pubic symphysis and the bodies of the pubic bones and may therefore be injured in fractures of the pelvis involving the pubis. It is more likely to be ruptured if it is full at the time of injury. Rupture of the male urethra must be suspected if blood issues from the external urinary meatus following pelvic injury.

The Ischium

The solid broad portion at the lower, posterior part of the innominate bone is the ischium. It consists of a body and a ramus. The body takes part in the formation of the acetabulum. The ramus of the ischium passes forwards to join with the inferior ramus of the pubis.

Below the acetabulum, the opening bounded by the pubis and the ischium is called the obturator foramen. It is large and oval in the male but is smaller and nearly triangular in the female. In life it is largely occupied by a fibrous sheet called the obturator membrane.

The inferior extremity of the body of the ischium is marked by the rough ischial tuberosity, which supports the body weight when sitting and provides attachment for the hamstring muscles. In life it is obscured by the gluteus maximum muscle when the hip is extended, as in the standing position, but can be easily identified by palpation when the joint is flexed.

The pelvis can be divided into two parts or segments (Fig. 5.12). The upper part, formed mainly by the flanged parts of the two iliac bones, is called the greater pelvis or 'false pelvis.' The cavity of the

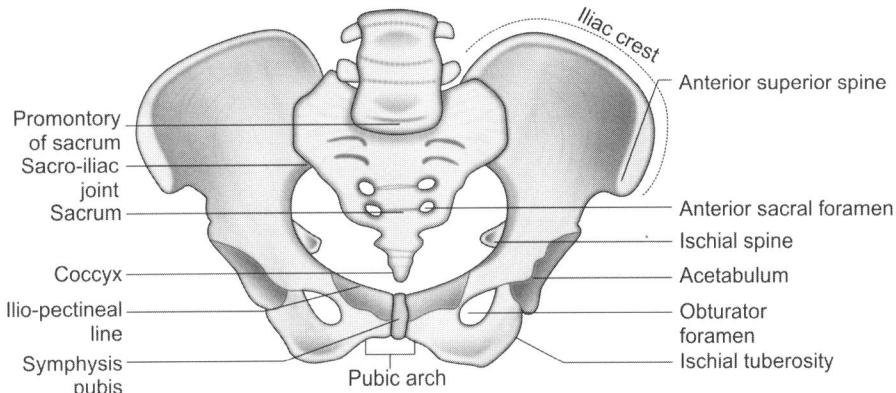

Fig. 5.12: The pelvis

greater pelvis is a part of the abdomen. The smaller segment below, known as the lesser pelvis or 'true pelvis', consists of the rest of the innominate bone (ischium and pubis), on each side and in front, and the sacrum behind. It bounds the pelvic cavity or canal, which is of obstetric importance. The upper or superior opening or aperture of the lesser pelvis is occupied by viscera and the lower or inferior aperture is largely closed in life by the muscular pelvic floor and its sphincters.

The boundary of the superior pelvic aperture, or pelvic inlet, is called the pelvic brim. Its anteroposterior, transverse and oblique diameters are measured for obstetric and anthropological reasons. Each of these three dimensions is greater on average in females than in males, the greatest difference being in the anteroposterior diameter.

The cavity of the lesser pelvis is deeper posteriorly, where it is bounded by the concave surface of the sacrum and coccyx, than it is anteriorly, where it is bounded by the body of the pubis, the pubic rami and the pubic symphysis. On each side, the pelvic cavity is bounded by a smooth quadrangular area formed by the fused ilium and ischium. The pelvic cavity thus enclosed contains the bladder anteriorly, the rectum posteriorly and the uterus in between. Mid-cavity measurements are made, as for the pelvic brim, and again these are greater in the female.

The shape of the inferior pelvic aperture, or pelvic outlet is determined by three wide notches, the pubic arch in front, between the ischiopubic rami, and two large sciatic notches. The three diameters of the pelvic outlets corresponding to those of the pelvic inlet are all greater in the female.

Other pelvic measurements are also used in obstetrics. What matters to the mother and her fetus is the comparison between her pelvic measurements (pelvimetry) and the measurements of the fetal head (cephalometry).

There are differences in shape between the male and female pelvis, the latter having a shape which facilitates the passage of the baby's head during childbirth. The axis of the pelvic cavity follows the curvature of the cavity, which is parallel to the profile of the sacrum and coccyx seen from the side (Fig. 5.13). The backward tilt of the sacrum and the anteroposterior diameter of the pelvic cavity are generally greater in the female. The pelvic axis and the disparity in depth between the anterior and posterior contours of the pelvic cavity are important to the passage of the fetus through the pelvic canal.

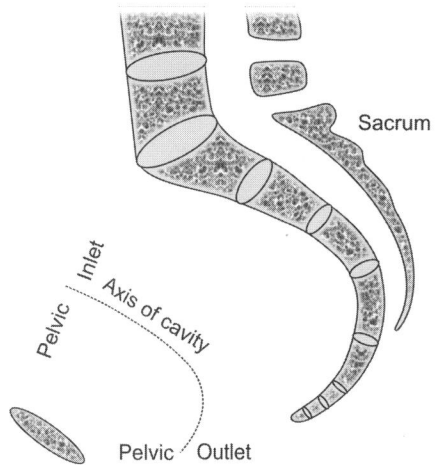

Fig. 5.13: Sagittal section through the female pelvis

In the adult pelvis there are differences between the sexes in linear measurements, angles and shape, of various components of the pelvis. The greater prominence of the hip in the female is probably due to the differences in the ilium between the sexes.

Even in fetal life, the male and female pelves differ from each other, particularly in the suprapubic arch or angle, between the inferior pubic rami, which is greater in the female. Although the female pelvis is adapted for childbirth, the prime function of the pelvis in both sexes is locomotor. The male generally being the more muscular and more heavily built, has a pelvic architecture which is generally stouter than that of the female. The overall dimensions of the male pelvis are greater and its muscular and ligamentous markings are more obvious.

In forensic work involving the identification of human remains, the sex of the deceased can best be determined from examination of the pelvis. Some of its features, especially the iliac crest and the greater sciatic notch, also enable the bone age to be assessed to within a very few years, especially in young adults.

THE BONES OF THE LOWER LIMB

The Femur or Thigh Bone

This is the longest and strongest bone in the skeleton, its length being associated with the striding gait of human beings and its strength being appropriate to the weight and muscular forces to which it is subjected. It has an almost cylindrical shaft, bowed forwards, and two extremities, the upper being a rounded head, a neck and two trochanters and the lower being in the form of a massive double 'knuckle' or condyle (Fig. 5.14).

The head of the femur is hemispherical and its surface is covered with hyaline articular cartilage, except for a small roughened pit for attachment of the ligamentum teres, just below and behind its center. It fits into the acetabulum of the innominate bone to form the hip joint.

The neck extends upwards and medially from the shaft at an angle of about 125° and terminates in the head. The angulation enables the lower limb to swing clear of the pelvis.

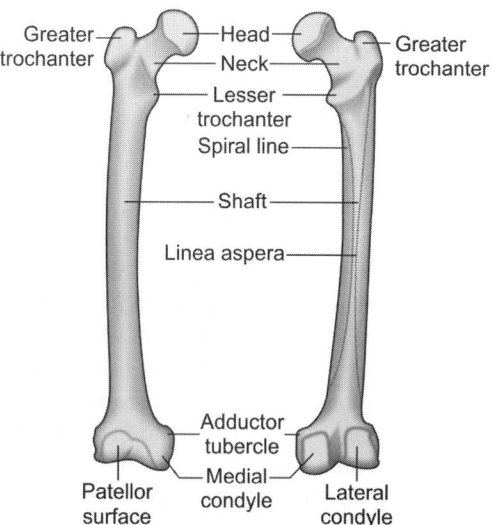

Fig. 5.14: Anterior (left) and posterior views of right femur

The neck of the femur is vulnerable to fracture as a result of tripping, in elderly people, especially women, owing to postmenopausal and senile osteoporotic changes. Twisting (medial rotation) of the thigh due to a similar accident in a person under the age of 16 years may result in a spiral fracture of the shaft of the femur.

The greater trochanter is a large process projecting upwards from the top of the shaft laterally to the neck, which it overhangs, creating a small hollow called the trochanteric fossa, into which is inserted the obturator externus muscle. The outer surface of the greater trochanter and the posterior surface of the upper part of the shaft provide insertion for the gluteal muscles.

The lesser trochanter projects medially from the shaft just below the neck of the femur. It is attached to the psoas muscle. A ridge of bone joining the greater and lesser trochanters on the posterior aspect of the femur is called the intertrochanteric crest.

The shaft of the femur is almost cylindrical except towards its lower end, where it is flattened and expanded. Anteriorly and laterally the shaft is smooth but posteriorly a prominent broad rough ridge, the linea aspera runs vertically, giving attachment to several muscles. In the lower third of the bone, the linea aspera divides into two smaller ridges, one of which passes to each of the condyles. The triangular area enclosed by these two ridges is called the popliteal surface of the femur. The shaft of the femur is surrounded by thick powerful muscles and cannot normally be felt through the skin.

The lower extremity of the femur consists of two (medial and lateral) condyles, separated behind by the intercondylar fossa, which articulate with the corresponding tuberosities of the tibia to form the knee joint. The articular cartilage covering the condyles continues on to the anterior surface of the bone and forms a surface for articulation with the patella or knee-cap. Immediately above the medial condyle is a small tubercle, the adductor tubercle, to which part of the adductor magnus muscle is attached.

The Patella or Knee-cap

The patella is a sesamoid bone developed in the tendon of the quadriceps muscle of the thigh. It is roughly triangular in shape, with its apex directed downwards.

That portion of the quadriceps tendon attaching the apex of the patella to the tuberosity of the tibia is called the patellar ligament. This is tapped by the physician, using a patellar hammer, to elicit the knee jerk, one of the reflexes commonly tested. The rough anterior surface of the patella can be palpated through the skin, from which it is separated by a bursa. Inflammation of this bursa, and of the suprapatellar bursa, gives rise to the condition known as housemaid's knee. The posterior surface of the patella is smooth and covered with articular cartilage; it articulates with the patellar surface of the femur, taking part in the formation of the knee joint.

The patella is quite commonly fractured, being (a) broken transversely into upper and lower portions or (b) shattered into fragments by a direct blow, causing a stellate fracture.

Dislocation of the patella may result from fairly severe violence, frequently involving a twisting injury accompanied by a blow to the inner side of the knee. This is known as acute traumatic dislocation. Alternatively, recurrent dislocation may occur as a result of anatomical abnormalities. Partial dislocation or subluxation is not uncommon, especially in girls.

The Tibia or Shin Bone

The tibia is the second longest bone in the body (the first being the femur) and is the medial and stronger of the two bones of the leg. It has a shaft, shaped like a prism in cross-section, and expanded extremities.

The upper extremity is composed of the medial and lateral condyles, which have weight-bearing surfaces, and a tuberosity. Each condyle has an articular surface for articulation with the corresponding condyle of the femur. Attached to the condyles, in life, are the medial and lateral menisci, which are semi-lunar cartilages.

Between the articular surfaces of the two condyles is the roughened intercondylar area. This gives attachment to the horns of the menisci and to the cruciate ligaments.

On the under surface of the lateral condyle is a small articular facet for the head of the fibula.

The anterior margins of the tibial condyles can be easily felt when the knee is flexed, each forming the lower border of a depression at each side of the patella. The lower part of the tibial tuberosity is subcutaneous and therefore also easily felt.

The shaft of the tibia, being triangular in cross-section, has three borders and three surfaces. The anterior border runs down from the tibial tuberosity to the medial malleolus. It can be felt under the skin and with the exception of the lower quarter, which is rounded and indistinct, it forms a sharp ridge (the 'shin'). It provides attachment for the deep fascia of the leg. The interosseous border gives attachment to the interosseous membrane which stretches between the tibia and the fibula. The medial border is sharp and distinct in the middle and rounded and ill-defined in its upper and lower fourths.

The medial surface of the tibia lies between the anterior and medial borders. It is smooth and situated directly beneath

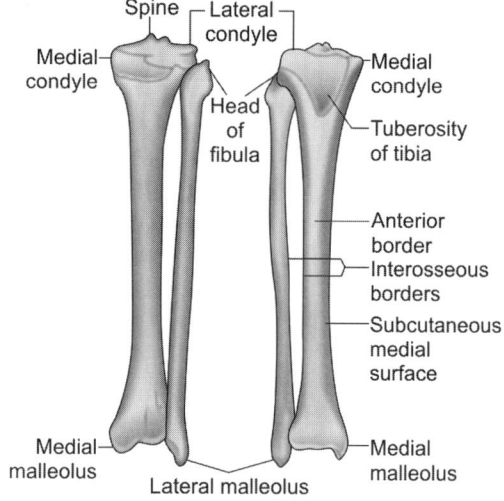

Fig. 5.15: Posterior (left) and anterior views of right tibia and fibula

the skin throughout its length; hence it is sometimes known as the subcutaneous surface. When traced downwards, it is found to end in the medial malleolus. The lower part of the medial surface is crossed obliquely by the great saphenous vein, the profile of which can be seen in some people, especially those with varicose veins.

The posterior surface of the tibia is bounded by the interosseous and medial borders (Fig. 5.15). It gives attachment to the popliteus, soleus and tibia is posterior muscles and to the long flexor muscle of the toes, flexor digitorum longus. The upper part, together with the similar area of the posterior aspect of the lower end of the femur; forms the floor of the popliteal fossa.

The lateral surface of the tibia gives attachment to the tibialis anterior muscle.

The lower extremity of the tibia is slightly expanded. Medially it projects downwards as the medial malleolus. Laterally is found the fibular notch, which is bound by ligaments to the lower end of the fibula. The inferior surface of the lower end of the tibia is smooth and articulates with the talus at the ankle joint.

The Fibula

The fibula is the lateral of the two bones of the leg. Not having to bear weight, it is a slender long bone. It consists of a shaft with upper and lower extremities, named respectively the head and the lateral malleolus.

The head can be felt through the skin as a prominence on the posterolateral aspect of the knee. The common peroneal nerve runs across the neck of the bone just below the head of the fibula and in this superficial position it is vulnerable to injury. This may be direct trauma, such as a blow, or compression of the nerve against the bone by a tight knee bandage or leg plaster or as a result of prolonged sitting with the legs crossed. The result is foot drop with inability to dorsiflex or evert (turn outwards) the foot. Sensation is impaired in the skin over the dorsum of the foot and the front and outer side of the leg.

The head of the fibula has a facet for articulation with the under surface of the lateral condyle of the tibia. (*Note*: This articulation takes no part in the formation of the knee joint.)

The lower end of the fibula is expanded to form the lateral malleolus, which projects downwards to a lower level than the tibia. On the medial surface of the lateral malleolus is a facet for articulation with the lateral surface of the talus in the ankle joint.

The lower ends of the tibia and fibula are firmly held together by ligaments and are also joined throughout their shafts by the interosseous membrane which divides the leg into anterior and posterior compartments.

Fracture of the lower ends of the tibia or fibula, or both, is very common and is sometimes called Potts' fracture. Fracture of the shaft of the tibia also occurs. A fracture of a condyle at the upper end may extend into the knee joint.

Bones of the Foot

The framework of the foot consists of:
- The tarsus
- The metatarsus
- The phalanges

The tarsus consists of a medial and a lateral series of bones (Figs 5.16 and 5.17).
- The medial series comprises the talus, the navicular and the three cuneiform bones.
- The lateral series are composed of the calcaneus and the cuboid.

If the general architecture of the foot is examined it will be seen that there are two arches—a longitudinal one and a transverse one. The longitudinal arch is most marked on the medial aspect of the foot and results from the fact that the talus is placed on top and, therefore, above the level of the calcaneus. The transverse arch is most marked at the level of the base (proximal end) of the metatarsus. These arches are very important in walking and are maintained by strong ligaments aided by muscles. The arches can withstand the very considerable strain caused by an adult jumping from a height of several feet. If the arches become weakened and collapse, the

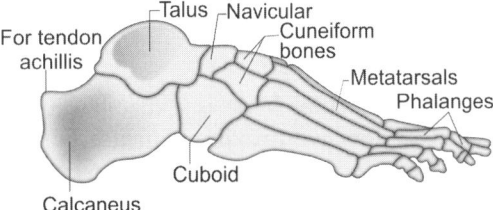

Fig. 5.16: Bones of the right foot—lateral view

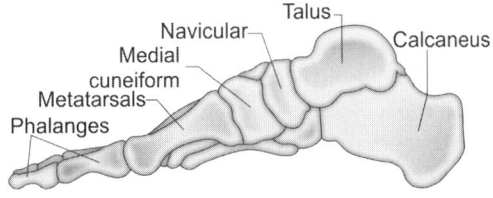

Fig. 5.17: Bones of the right foot—medial view

condition known as 'flat foot' (pes planus) results. An abnormally high-arched foot is called pes cavus.

The talus is a very irregular bone having articular surfaces: (a) above, for the tibia, and on either side for the medial and lateral malleoli forming the ankle joint; (b) below, for the calcaneus; (c) in front for the navicular.

The calcaneus, also an irregular bone, and the largest of the tarsal bones, is situated below the talus. It projects backwards behind the talus, forming the heel, and to its posterior margin is attached the important tendo calcaneus, better known as the Achilles tendon. Projecting backwards, as it does, beyond the bones of the leg, it provides a short lever for the calf muscles acting through the tendo calcaneus. Rupture of the tendon is clearly a serious matter and necessitates surgical repair and immobilization of the ankle in Plaster of Paris.

The calcaneus articulates in front with the cuboid.

The talus and calcaneus are both strong bones and much force is needed to break them. They are fractured usually as a result of falling from a height, depending among other factors upon the weight and muscularity of the victim but usually at least four meters in the case of an athletic man.

The navicular bone is a disc-like bone having a concave proximal surface, where it articulates with the talus, and a convex distal surface where it articulates with the three cuneiform bones. A tuberosity on the medial aspect of the bone provides the principal attachment for the tendon of the tibialis posterior muscle.

The cuboid bone articulates behind with the calcaneus and in front with the fourth and fifth metatarsals. Medially it is in contact with the navicular and lateral cuneiform bones.

The three (medial, intermediate and lateral) cuneiform, or wedge-shaped bones, are placed between the navicular bone behind and the three medial metatarsals in front. The arrangement of the cuneiform bones and the strong ligaments binding them are important factors in maintaining the transverse arch of the foot.

The metatarsus is composed of five metatarsal bones which connect the tarsus to the phalanges of the five toes. They are long bones, each with a proximal base, a shaft and a distal head. The bases of the first three articulate with the cuneiform bones, those of the lateral two with the cuboid. The first metatarsal (of the great toe) is shorter and stouter than the others. The fifth (little toe) has a rough eminence (tuberosity or styloid process) on the lateral side of its base and this can be seen and felt halfway along the lateral border of the foot; sometimes it is fractured when the foot is acutely inverted.

Pain beneath the three middle metatarsal heads is called anterior metatarsalgia and this may be associated with tender calluses under the ball of the foot. An untrained individual undertaking prolonged marching, hiking or running may sustain a stress fracture (march fracture) of a metatarsal.

The phalanges of the foot are also long bones and they correspond in number and general arrangement with the phalanges of the hand. The big toe, like the thumb, has two, a proximal and a distal phalanx. Each of the other toes has three phalanges, the additional one being a middle phalanx.

■ THE SKULL

The most obvious function of the skull is its protective one, the cranium protecting the brain' from externally inflicted injury. The special sense organs are also afforded substantial protection. However, the skull is also involved in a diversity of other functions including the securing and devouring of food and the control of the cerebral circulation. The bony sockets (orbits) housing the eyes ensure a constant distance between these organs and provide a necessary pre-condition for binocular vision. The sockets also provide for rotation of the eyes, utilizing muscles attached to their walls. The fixation of the organs of balance, the labyrinths, within the skull ensures a fixed relationship between the six semicircular canals (three on each side) to each other and to the head, providing the basis for an orderly correlation between these sense organs (receptors) and their central nervous connections.

Strictly speaking the skull consists of the cranium and the mandible, although the term is commonly used for the cranium alone. The upper part of the cranium, forming the brain-box is termed the calvaria and the remainder of the skull forms the facial skeleton.

Bones of the Skull

The bones of the skull are divided into two groups (Fig. 5.18).

1. Those of the calvaria or brain-box, eight in number:
   – 1 frontal (forehead) bone
   – 2 parietal
   – 2 temporal
   – 1 ethmoid
   – 1 sphenoid
   – 1 occipital
2. Those of the face, fourteen in number:
   – 2 maxillae (upper jaw)
   – 2 zygomatic (cheek) bones
   – 2 nasal
   – 2 lacrimal
   – 2 palatine
   – 2 inferior turbinate
   – 1 vomer
   – 1 mandible (lower jaw)

All the bones of the skull, except the lower jaw, are joined together by sutures or immovable joints. The lower jaw or temporomandibular joint is a condyloid joint allowing both hinge-like and side-to-side movements.

Before discussing the individual bones, the skull as a whole must be examined. The top or vault can be removed from an

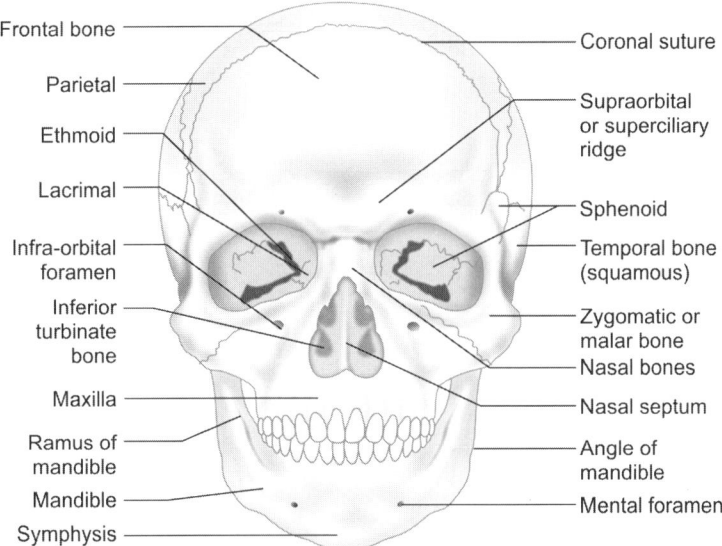

Fig. 5.18: The skull—anterior view

anatomical specimen so that the interior can be examined. The following description is meant to be read with the skull at hand and with the aid of diagrams.

Anterior Aspect (Norma Frontalis)

Looked at from the front, the upper part of the skull is formed by the frontal bone of the forehead. The remainder is formed by the facial bones, including the lower jaw.

The roofs and upper margins of the orbits, or eye-sockets, and the ridges underlying the eyebrows are formed by the frontal bone. The lateral wall of the orbit is formed by the zygomatic bone and the great wing of the sphenoid bone, while several bones, the lacrimal bone and parts of the maxilla, ethmoid and sphenoid bones, form the medial wall. The floor of the orbit is formed mainly by the maxilla. The orbit is cone-shaped, with its wide open base in front (Fig. 5.19) and its narrow apex behind. At its apex is a circular foramen for the passage of the optic nerve. A deep groove, the inferior orbital fissure, extends from the lateral side of this foramen into the floor of the orbit.

The portion of the maxilla which forms the medial margin of the orbit projects upwards to meet the frontal bone. Between these projections of the maxillae are the two nasal bones. Passing vertically downwards from these bones in the midline, the bony nasal septum can be seen dividing the nasal cavity into right and left halves.

On the side walls of the nasal cavity three bony projections are visible, namely the inferior, middle and superior nasal conchae.

Surrounding the opening of the nasal cavity and meeting in the midline below it are the right and left maxillae or upper jaws, which carry the upper set of teeth.

Maxillofacial injuries result from road traffic accidents, acts of violence and accidents in industry, sport and the home. The maxilla, which is less frequently fractured than the mandible, forms with the other bones of the region a mass capable of absorbing considerable violence, thus protecting the brain. Fractures of the middle third of the facial skeleton require prompt and skilled management (reduction and fixation) because of their great physiological and aesthetic importance. The surgeon's work is sometimes facilitated by a tracheostomy but this procedure is generally avoided unless required for associated injuries such as fractures of the larynx or a flail chest.

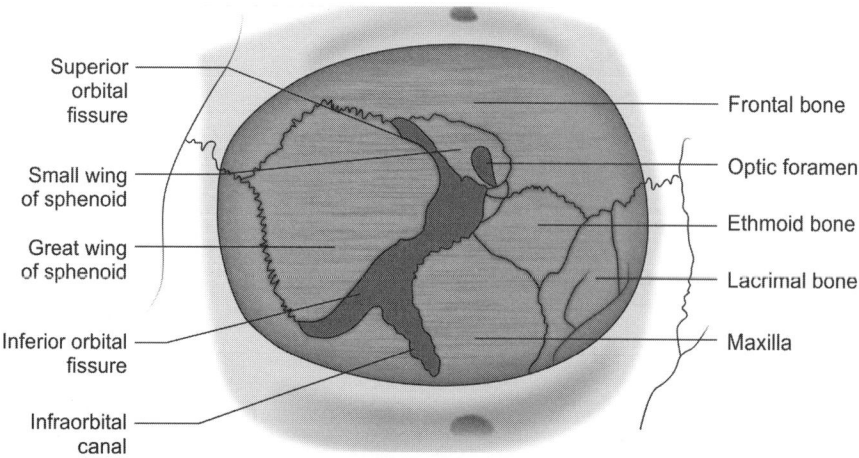

Fig. 5.19: Boundaries of the right orbit viewed from in front

Lateral Aspect (Fig. 5.20)

When viewed from the side the greater mass of the cranial bones can be seen behind the facial bones.

The central part of the lateral aspect is occupied by the temporal bone. A process from this bone passes forward to join the zygomatic (malar) bone, thereby enclosing a fossa (the temporal fossa) in which can be seen a portion of the sphenoid bone. This adjoins the frontal, parietal and temporal bones, so that an irregular H-shaped arrangement of sutures can be seen. A small circle can be drawn enclosing the horizontal limb of the H and portions of all four bones. This area, which overlies the anterior branch of the middle meningeal artery, is called the pterion and its center is an important landmark for the surgeon.

Obvious features of the lateral aspect of the skull are the external acoustic meatus and, behind it, the prominent mastoid process of the temporal bone. Posteriorly, the occipital bone will be seen.

Superior Aspect (Norma Verticalis)

On looking at the skull from above, the frontal bone will be seen to occupy the front of the vault of the cranium and to be separated from the two parietal bones by a suture which runs transversely, the coronal suture. The two parietal bones together form the greater part of the vertex and are separated from each other in the midline by a suture placed at right angles to the coronal suture. This is the sagittal suture. The meeting point of the coronal and sagittal sutures is called the bregma and this marks the site of the anterior fontanelle, a gap filled by membrane in the fetal skull.

The lambdoid suture joins the parietal bones to the occipital bone.

Posterior Aspect (Norma Occipitalis)

The complete lambdoid suture is seen in this view. It is sometimes complicated by a number of small irregular bones appropriately called sutural bones. The most prominent feature of the posterior aspect of the skull is the external occipital protuberance, which can be easily felt in the living subject at the upper end of the median furrow at the back of the neck. Ridges called the superior nuchal lines pass laterally from the protuberance and mark the boundary between the scalp and the neck.

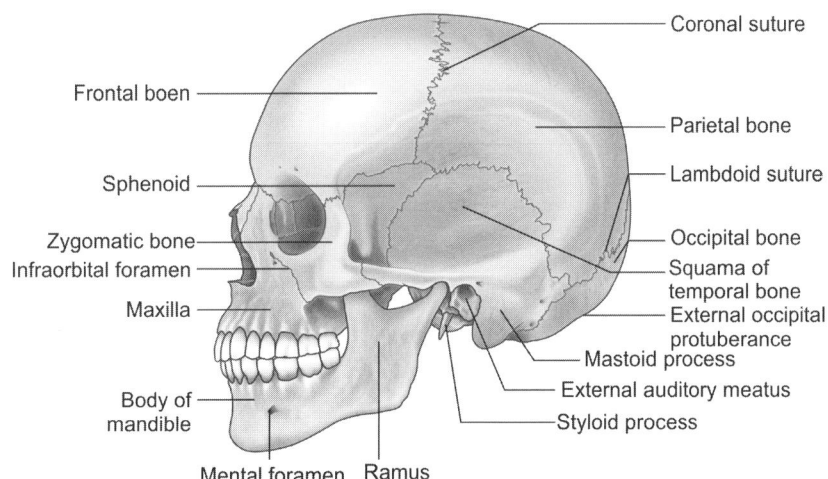

Fig. 5.20: The skull—lateral view

Inferior Aspect (Norma Basalis, Base of the Skull)

The lower jaw should be removed for study of the base of the skull (Fig. 5.21). The anterior part is formed by the hard (bony) palate and the alveolar arches which carry the upper teeth. The hard palate is formed anteriorly by the two maxillae and posteriorly by the two palatine bones, all united together by a cruciform suture. Immediately behind the hard palate, the posterior openings of the nasal cavities (posterior nares) will be seen. Lateral to the maxilla and palate can be seen the fossa or hollow bounded laterally by the zygomatic bone and process of the temporal bone. This is the temporal fossa described in the lateral aspect. A part of the sphenoid bone can be seen here; behind and lateral to it is the mandibular fossa for the articulation of the mandible or lower jaw.

The large oval opening further back in the midline is the foramen magnum, through which passes the spinal cord. This is situated in the occipital bone, a part of which projects forwards to meet the sphenoid bone close to the level of the posterior nares. Two smooth condyles, one on each side of the foramen magnum, articulate with the atlas vertebra. Behind the foramen magnum is the main portion of the occipital bone.

On either side of the occipital bone are portions of the temporal bone including the mastoid process and an irregular portion, the petrous portion, projecting forwards and medially towards the midline. A large round foramen in the petrous portion of the temporal bone leads upwards into the bone and is the opening into the carotid canal, which conveys the internal carotid artery on its course into the cranial cavity. The jugular foramen, a little further back, transmits the internal jugular vein, which returns blood from the brain, and other structures including three cranial nerves (IX, X and XI).

The Interior of the Skull (Fig. 5.22)

The skull cap (calva, cranial vault or vertex) having been removed, it can be appreciated that the walls of the cranial cavity vary in thickness from region to region. Most of the bones have a tough outer table of compact bone separated from a thinner and more brittle inner table by the diploe, which is

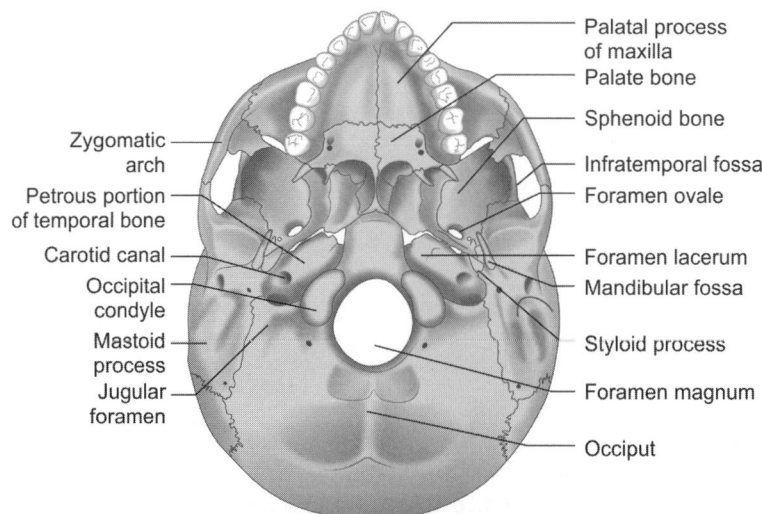

Fig. 5.21: Outline of skull as seen from below

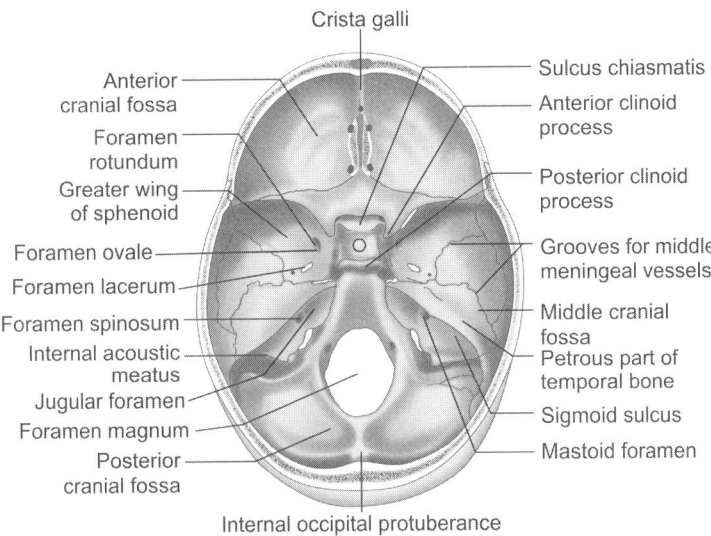

Fig. 5.22: Interior of skull

cancellous bone housing red marrow in its interstices.

The skull cap consists of portions of the frontal, parietal and occipital bones. Its internal surface shows numerous vascular markings. Anteriorly the frontal crest projects backwards in the midline. It gives attachment to the falx cerebri, the thick sheet of dura mater (one of the meninges) which separates the two cerebral hemispheres. It is grooved by the sagittal sulcus which runs backwards in the median plane and accommodates the sagittal sinus. A number of irregular pits on each side of the sagittal sulcus are caused by arachnoid granulations, which are minute projections of the arachnoid mater, one of the membranous coverings (meninges) of the brain. Calcific nodules associated with the arachnoid granulations may sometimes be seen in the skull X-rays of elderly people and are not pathological, i.e. not due to disease.

The internal surface of the base of the skull is clearly divided into three compartments the anterior, middle and posterior; cranial fossae. Impressions for the cerebral gyri are conspicuous in the anterior and middle fossae.

The Anterior Cranial Fossa

In the midline, in front, is a small vertical projection (the crista galli, for attachment of the falx cerebri), on either side of which there is a narrow plate of bone perforated by numerous minute holes and forming part of the roof of the nasal cavity. This is the cribriform plate of the ethmoid and the holes are for the passage of the olfactory nerves. On either side of these plates, a part of the frontal bone forms the roof of the orbits. The posterior margin of the anterior fossa is formed by a sharp edge of bone which is part of the lesser wing of the sphenoid. The medial extremity of this forms the anterior clinoid process, to which is attached the free border of the tentorium cerebelli, the double layer of dura mater which covers the cerebellum.

The Middle Cranial Fossa

In the midline is the sella turcica (like a Turkish saddle) which is hollowed out as the hypophyseal fossa and in life contains the pituitary gland, or hypophysis cerebri.

Enlargement of the fossa, as seen on X-ray pictures, suggests the presence of a pituitary tumor. The sella turcica is part of the body of the sphenoid bone which is traversed anteriorly by a groove, the sulcus chiasmatis, which runs from one optic canal to the other. Posterior to the hypophyseal fossa is the dorsum sellae, a plate of bone which projects upwards and forwards and ends on each side in a posterior clinoid process. Erosion of these processes, as seen on a skull X-ray, is taken as a sign of raised intracranial pressure.

The middle cranial fossa opens out laterally on each side into a deep, wide irregular hollow which supports the temporal lobe of the brain. It is bounded in front by the greater wing of the sphenoid bone and behind by the petrous part of the temporal bone, which contains the internal ear.

The Posterior Cranial Fossa

This is bounded in front by the petrous portions of the temporal bones, with a part of the occipital bone in the midline. Its most conspicuous feature is a large opening, the foramen magnum through which that part of the brain stem known as the medulla oblongata continues down into the spinal cord. Most of the posterior fossa is formed by the occipital bone and it contains the cerebellum, which functions primarily to co-ordinate and adjust movements and make them smooth. In front of the cerebellum lie the pons and medulla which, together with the cerebellum, make up the hindbrain.

Immediately behind and below the petrous portion of the temporal bone, on each side of the posterior fossa, is a deep S-shaped groove called the sigmoid sulcus. This contains the sigmoid sinus which drains venous blood into the internal jugular vein. The junction of these blood vessels lies in the jugular foramen which also transmits the ninth, tenth and eleventh cranial nerves. A number of other holes or foramina will be observed in the cranial fossae and these likewise transmit nerves or blood vessels or both.

Posteriorly in the posterior cranial fossa can be seen the internal occipital protuberance, in front of which lies the confluence of sinuses. On each side is a groove related to the commencement of the transverse sinus.

Having observed the general arrangement of the bones of the skull, some of them require individual study.

The Frontal Bone

This is an irregular flat bone which forms the forehead region, most of the anterior cranial fossa and the roofs of the orbits. In the forehead region, the bone is thick and consists of two compact laminae between which is sandwiched cancellous bone, except in the regions of the frontal sinuses, where the cancellous bone is absent. The frontal sinuses contain instead air which is in continuity with the nasal cavity via the frontonasal canal. The orbital part of the frontal bone consists entirely of compact bone.

On the anterior aspect of the frontal bone are two eminences, one on each side, called the frontal tubers or tuberosities. Below them are two curved superciliary arches joined across the midline by a smooth eminence known as the glabella. The superciliary arches originate as a result of the mechanical stresses imposed upon the frontal bone by the masticatory apparatus (jaws and associated muscles). Below the superciliary arches are the supraorbital margins which form the upper borders of the orbital openings. The supraorbital notch, at the junction of the lateral two-thirds and medial one-third of the supraorbital margin, transmits the supraorbital vessels and nerve. The doctor sometimes applies thumb pressure over this nerve to help in assessing a patient's level of consciousness. The supraorbital margin ends laterally in the zygomatic process which articulates with the zygomatic bone in a suture which can be felt through the skin as a slight depression in the living subject.

A portion of the frontal bone known as the nasal part projects downwards between the supraorbital margins and ends in a sharp nasal spine. Each nasal part articulates with one of the two nasal bones and supports the bridge of the nose.

The Parietal Bone

The right and left parietal bones, joined superiorly in the midline by the sagittal suture, form the greater part of the side walls and roof of the cranium. Each is a four-sided or irregularly quadrilateral bone. The anterior (frontal) border of each parietal bone articulates with the frontal bone at the coronal suture. The posterior margin articulates with the occipital bone at the lambdoid suture and the inferior, margin articulates with the temporal bone. At birth, there are membranous intervals, known as fontanelles, in the skull at the four angles of the parietal bones. The internal surface of the parietal bone is marked by impressions corresponding to the cerebral gyri or convolutions of the brain, and furrows for the middle meningeal blood vessels. A shallow groove for the superior sagittal sinus runs along the superior or sagittal border of the bone.

The Occipital Bone

The occipital bone, situated at the back and base of the skull, forms the greater part of the floor of the posterior cranial fossa. It articulates in front with the two parietal bones, at the lambdoid suture, and on either side with the temporal bone (Fig. 5.23). Its most distinctive feature is the large oval opening known as the foramen magnum, through which passes the lower end of the medulla oblongata.

Behind the foramen magnum is an expanded plate known as the squamous part of the occipital bone. Its internal surface presents four fossae shaped to the two occipital lobes of the cerebrum and the hemispheres of the cerebellum. The internal occipital protuberance is easily identifiable at the junction of the four fossae. The sulcus of the superior sagittal runs upwards from

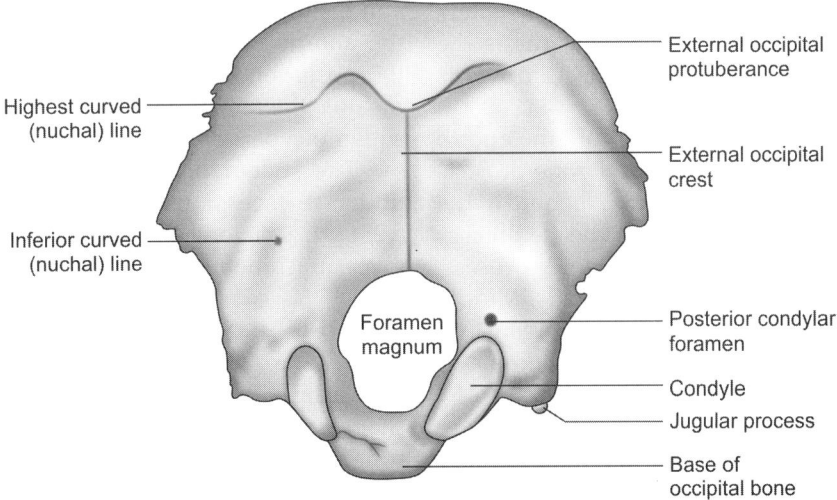

Fig. 5.23: Outer surface of occipital bone

this protuberance and the sulci of the transverse sinuses extend laterally from it. The internal occipital crest runs downwards from the protuberance and gives attachment to the falx cerebelli, a small sickle-shaped process of dura mater containing the occipital sinus. In front of the foramen magnum is the basilar part of the bone which unites with the sphenoid bone. The lateral (condylar) parts of the bone lie on either side of the foramen and on their inferior surfaces are the convex occipital condyles for articulation with the atlas vertebra.

The Temporal Bone

This bone consists of four parts:
1. The squamous part
2. The petromastoid part
3. The tympanic part
4. The styloid process.

The squamous part of the temporal bone forms part of the side wall of the skull. It articulates above mainly with the parietal bone and in front with a part of the sphenoid bone. Behind and below it is continuous with the mastoid portion of the petromastoid part. In its lower part is a circular opening—the external acoustic meatus—which leads by a canal to the cavity of the middle ear. Immediately above the external acoustic meatus is the zygomatic process, which projects forwards to join the zygomatic bone.

The mastoid portion of the petro mastoid part of the temporal bone projects downwards immediately behind the external acoustic meatus in a dense process of bone known as the mastoid process. This contains the mastoid air cells. Middle ear infusion may occasionally spread into these cells, causing mastoiditis and, rarely, further spread may cause a brain abscess. The mastoid process and its air cells are closely related to the groove for the sigmoid sinus in the posterior cranial fossa. The lateral surface of the mastoid process gives attachment to the sternomastoid muscle, amongst others.

The petrous portion projects inwards and forwards at an angle, wedged between the sphenoid and occipital bones, and can be seen on the base of the skull from below and from the interior. As the ends of the petrous portions approach each other they are separated in the midline by the base of the occipital bone. Close to the anterior extremity is the auditory canal (not always easy to make out on the whole skull) or Eustachian tube, which connects the nasopharynx to the middle ear cavity.

The posterior surface of the petrous portion of the temporal bone forms the anterior wall of the posterior cranial fossa and is here grooved by the sigmoid sinus. A well-marked foramen, the opening of the internal acoustic meatus, is seen near the center of the posterior surface. It transmits the eighth cranial nerve which is also known as the vestibulocochlear nerve and subserves hearing and balance. The petrous portion of the temporal bone contains the cochlea, vestibule and semicircular canals.

The tympanic part of the temporal bone is fused internally with the petrous portion and posteriorly with the squamous part and the mastoid process (Fig. 5.24). It forms the anterior wall, floor and lower part of the posterior wall of the external acoustic meatus, the remainder being formed by the squamous part of the temporal bone.

The styloid process projects from the under surface of the temporal bone (Fig. 5.25). It is a long slender process which gives attachment to muscles and ligaments.

The Sphenoid Bone

This bone, which takes part in the formation of the middle cranial fossa, is shaped somewhat like a bat. It has a body, situated in the midline, from which project outwards (a) two greater wings, and (b) two lesser wings.

The Skeleton 65

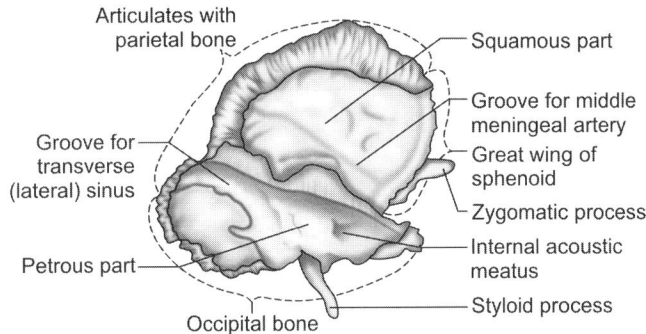

Fig. 5.24: Internal aspect of left temporal bone

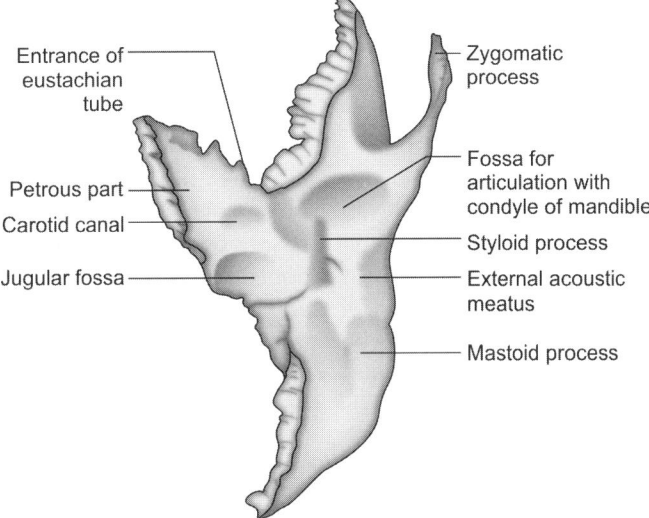

Fig. 5.25: Under surface of left temporal bone

Two pterygoid processes project downwards from the adjoining parts of the body and greater wings (Fig. 5.26).

The body is hollow and contains two large air sinuses. Its upper surface is shaped like a Turkish saddle and is therefore known as the sella turcica. The deepest part of the hollow is the hypophyseal fossa, which houses the hypophysis cerebri or pituitary gland. Behind the sella turcica is the dorsum sellae from the upper angles of which the two posterior clinoid processes project, one on each side and give attachment to the tentorium cerebelli.

From the anterior part of the body the lesser wings spread out on either side to form the posterior margin of the anterior cranial fossa. From the sides of the body the greater wings spread outwards between the frontal and temporal bones, and close to their origin is a well-marked foramen (the foramen ovale) which transmits the mandibular branch of the trigeminal or Vth cranial nerve.

Developmental abnormalities of the sphenoid bone in the fetus can deform the bridge of the nose causing it to be depressed, as in achondroplasia, or abnormally broad

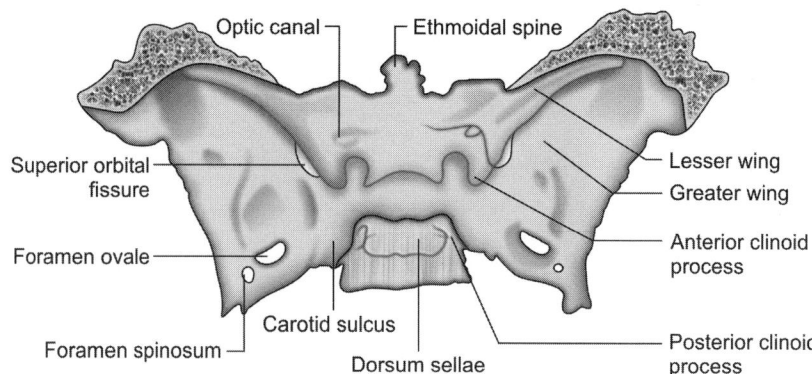

Fig. 5.26: The sphenoid bone viewed from above

with excessive separation of the orbits (hypertelorism), which may be associated with congenital heart disease.

The Ethmoid Bone

This is a box-shaped bone of delicate structure, hollowed out to contain the ethmoidal air cells. Its lateral walls help to form the medial wall of each orbit. Its roof is formed by the cribriform plate which can be seen between the two portions of the frontal bone in the anterior cranial fossa and is perforated by the olfactory nerves. The inferior surface enters into the formation of the roof of the nose.

From the cribriform plate, a perpendicular plate projects downwards to form the upper part of the nasal septum, dividing the cavity of the nose into right and left halves. The septal cartilage is attached to the lower border of the perpendicular plate, so that the nasal septum is bony in its upper part and cartilaginous in its lower anterior part. The nasal septum is usually deflected slightly to one or other side but excessive deflection may cause nasal obstruction and necessitate the surgical operation known as submucous resection (SMR) of the cartilaginous septum, which often appears on an ear, nose and throat (ENT) surgeon's operating list.

Laterally to the perpendicular plate, the superior and middle nasal conchae project from the side walls of the nasal cavities.

The ethmoidal air cells open into fissures (the superior and middle meati of the nose) below these conchae. The inferior nasal conchae have a separate identity as bones and are not a part of the ethmoid or any other bone.

The Maxilla

This is a large irregular bone which unites in the midline with its fellow to form the upper jaw. The upper part of the bone forms the greater part of the floor of the orbit; its lower part, the major portion of the hard palate. Laterally it articulates with the zygomatic bone (Fig. 5.27). Medially it helps to make up the side wall of the nasal cavity and to it is attached the inferior concha (Fig. 5.28).

The body of the maxilla is hollow and contains the important maxillary sinus or antrum, which communicates with the middle meatus of the nose through a small aperture. Each maxilla has an alveolar process containing the sockets for eight teeth. It will be noticed that the roots of the first and second molar teeth are closely related to the floor of the maxillary sinus.

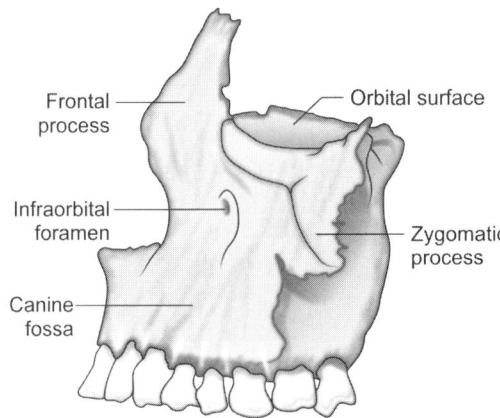

Fig. 5.27: Left maxilla—external or lateral view

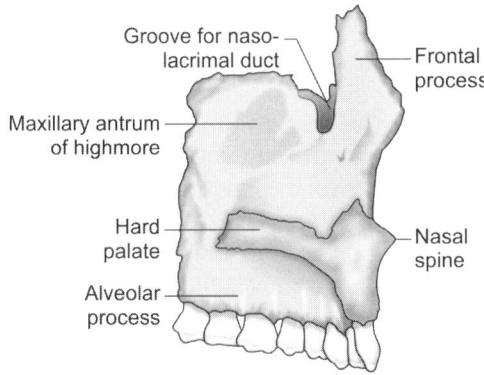

Fig. 5.28: Left maxilla—medial aspect

Inflammation within the nose, resulting from a common cold, may spread to the maxillary sinus so that the cavity becomes filled with mucus. Similar inflammation (sinusitis) may affect the frontal sinus, causing a headache, and much less commonly, the ethmoid and sphenoid air cells.

The Zygomatic Bone

The zygomatic bone (cheek bone) forms the prominence of the cheek, parts of the floor and lateral wall of the orbit and parts of the walls of the temporal and infratemporal fossae. It articulates medially with the maxilla, above with the frontal bone and posteriorly with a process from the temporal bone.

The Lacrimal Bones

These are two small bones which take part in the formation of the medial wall of the orbit (Fig. 5.19).

The Nasal Bones

These are two small bones lying side by side between the frontal processes of the maxilla and forming the bridge of the nose.

The Vomer

This is a thin, flat bone situated in the midline, where it rests on the hard palate and forms the lower and posterior part of the nasal septum. The rest of the septum is formed above by the perpendicular plate of the ethmoid bone and anteriorly by cartilage.

The Palatine Bones

These are irregular in shape and placed between the maxillae and sphenoid bone. Each takes part in the formation of the hard palate, the floor and lateral wall of the nasal cavity and the floor of the orbit.

The Mandible or Lower Jaw

The mandible is the only moving bone in the skull. It consists of a curved horizontal body, which carries the teeth of the lower jaw, and two broad rami which project upwards almost vertically on each side posteriorly. The lower posterior corner of the ramus is called the angle of the jaw (Fig. 5.29). On the inner surface of the ramus is a foramen for the entry of the inferior alveolar nerve and vessels into the mandibular canal, which re-emerges at the mental foramen on the lateral aspect of the bone (Fig. 5.30). The ramus terminates above in two processes: The triangular coronoid process in front, and the convex condylar process of the mandible behind.

The coronoid process provides attachment for the temporalis muscle and the head of the condylar process articulates

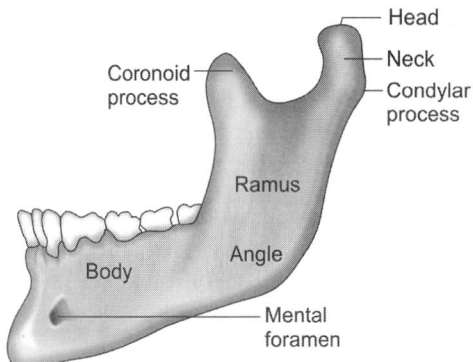

Fig. 5.29: Mandible—outer view of left half

with the temporal bone to form the temporomandibular joint

The mandible becomes smaller and undergoes changes in shape in old age as a is consequence the loss of teeth. Particularly striking is the reduced height (width) of the body of the lower jaw following loss of the teeth and associated absorption of adjacent bone. These edentulous atrophied mandibles are frequently fractured by relatively minor trauma. At the other extreme, mandibular fractures are rare in children with their more resilient lower jaws; loosening or breakage of a tooth is a more common result of trauma in this age group.

Generally, fractures of the mandibular trauma resulting from the blow of a fist, road traffic accidents, and gunshot wounds or falling and hitting the ground (as in the 'parade ground fracture') or another hard stationary object. Such a fracture may cause deformity and loss of function, i.e. difficulty in eating and speaking.

A severe blow to the point of the chin may result not only in mandibular fracture but the condylar heads may be displaced upwards and backwards to enter the middle cranial fossa, resulting in the leakage of cerebrospinal fluid from the ear (CSF otorrhea).

The Fontanelles

It will be recalled that the sagittal suture separating the two parietal bones in the midline meets the frontal and the coronal suture in front and behind meets the lambdoid suture separating them from the occipital bone (Fig. 5.31). At birth, however, the actual bones are not in contact. There is a diamondshaped space covered only by fibrous tissue membrane between the frontal and two parietal bones in the midline—this is called the anterior fontanelle. It lies immediately above the superior longitudinal sinus.

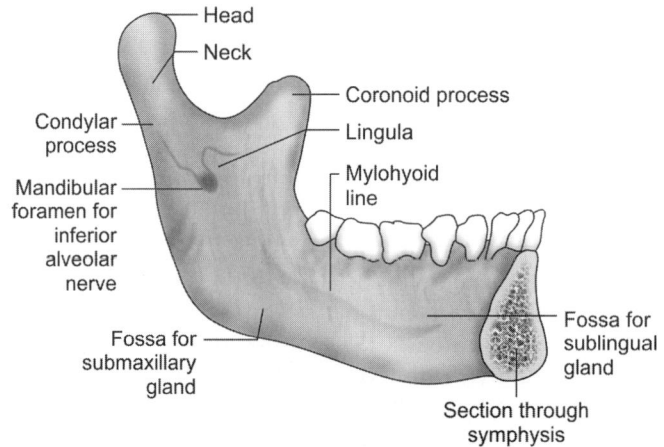

Fig. 5.30: Mandible—inner view of left half

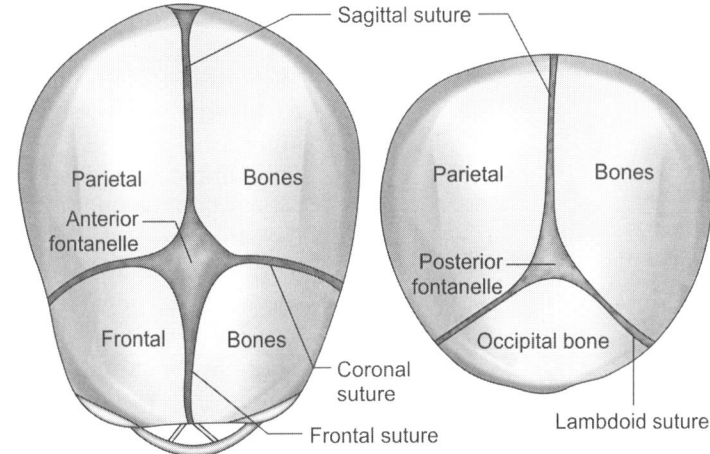

Fig. 5.31: The fetal skull from above (left) and from behind

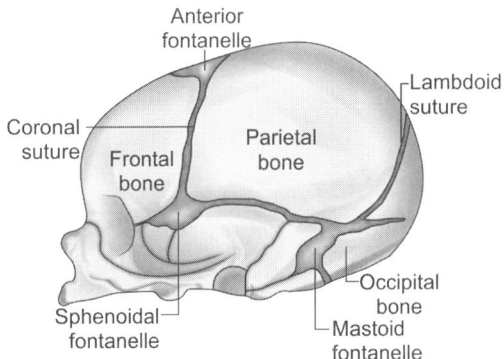

Fig. 5.32: The fetal skull—lateral aspect

The posterior fontanelle is situated at the area of junction between the sagittal and lambdoid sutures. It differs from the anterior fontanelle in being smaller and triangular and in closing a little earlier.

There are four other fontanelles which are small and of irregular shape. They are at the sphenoidal and mastoid angles of the parietal bones and are therefore named the sphenoidal and mastoid fontanelles (one pair of each) (Fig. 5.32).

The presence of the fontanelles and the width of the sutures permit the bones of the cranial vault, or vertex, to overlap slightly, thus facilitating the birth process, during which the skull is slowly compressed into a different shape, or moulded. During this process, the part of the scalp which lies more centrally in the birth canal may temporarily become swollen as a result of impeded venous drainage and edema. The resulting swelling is known as a caput succedaneum.

After birth the size of the fontanelles gradually lessens and the anterior fontanelle is usually closed by the age of eighteen months.

The sutures of the vault of the skull, start to become obliterated in middle age.

■ THE VERTEBRAL COLUMN

The cranium, vertebral column, ribs and sternum constitute the axial skeleton. The bones of the limbs and limb girdles make up the appendicular skeleton.

The vertebral column (spinal column, spine or backbone) is the central part of the skeleton which supports the head and encloses the spinal cord. Its construction combines great strength with a moderate degree of mobility. These features depend on the spine having a number of separate bones united by ligaments and by tough discs of fibrocartilage (the intervertebral discs) which act essentially as hydrostatic 'shock absorbers'. The nucleus of the disc is 85° water and it is bounded by a fibrous

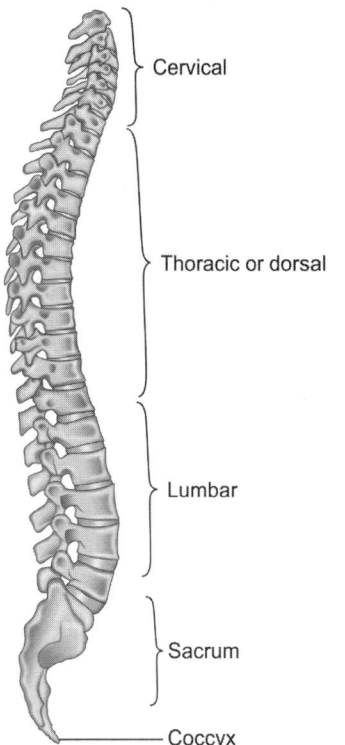

Fig. 5.33: The vertebral column

- It is convex forwards in the cervical or neck region.
- The thoracic region is convex backwards. Excessive curvature is known as kyphosis.
- The lumbar region is markedly convex forwards. When it is excessively convex the term lordosis is used. This term is often also applied to the normal cervical and lumbar curves but this is usually made plain in the text. For example, the normal lumbar lordosis of a pregnant woman acts as a support for the contracting uterus.
- The sacrum and coccyx form a marked forward concavity.

The three main curves in the vertebral column are developed from a single curve in the spine of an infant.

Lateral curvature of the spine is abnormal and is known as scoliosis.

The Vertebrae

The individual vertebrae are all built on the same plan, although there are certain variations in different parts of the spinal column and special vertebrae (atlas and axis), the sacrum and coccyx, which require separate description.

A typical vertebra consists of:
- A body
- The vertebral or neural arch:
  – 2 pedicles
  – 2 laminae
  – 2 transverse processes
  – 1 spine or spinous process
  – 4 articular processes.

The body is the solid box-shaped structure situated anteriorly which has slightly concave upper and lower surfaces. It is separated from the bodies of the vertebrae immediately above and below by the tough intervertebral discs of fibrocartilage.

From either side of the posterior aspect of the body two short, stout bars of bone,

ring, the annulus. The bones give origin to a number of muscles.

The vertebral column is made up of 33 vertebrae which are grouped (from above downwards) as follows (Fig. 5.33):
7 cervical
12 thoracic
5 lumbar
5 sacral forming the sacrum
4 coccygeal forming the coccyx

The Spine as a Whole

It will be noticed that the bones become increasingly larger as the column descends, reaching their maximum width at the upper part of the sacrum, only to become greatly reduced in size as it tapers off into the coccyx.

When looked at from the side the spine will be seen to have several curves.

the pedicles, project backwards. The pedicle has a notch on its upper surface and a similar notch on its lower surface. Each notch forms with its neighbor an intervertebral foramen. The intervertebral foramina transmit the segmental spinal nerves.

From the posterior ends of the pedicles, the two laminae are directed backwards and towards each other and meet in the midline behind. From the junction of the pedicles with the laminae, the transverse processes project outwards on each side of the bone.

Where the laminae unite in the midline behind, the spinous process or spine is formed and projects backwards and, in some parts of the column, downwards.

Two articular processes (zygapophyses) are situated on the upper and lower surface of each vertebra at the junction of the pedicles with the laminae close to the origin of the transverse processes.

The roughly circular opening enclosed by the body in front, the pedicles on either side and the laminae behind, through which passes the spinal cord, is called the vertebral foramen and it forms a part of the vertebral canal. This bony canal helps to protect the spinal cord from injury.

The Cervical Vertebrae

The lower five cervical vertebrae have the same general form, although the seventh has a particularly long spinous process, ending in a single tubercle, and large transverse processes to which cervical ribs are sometimes attached. The upper two vertebrae, the atlas and axis require separate description.

A typical cervical vertebra differs from those of the rest of the spinal column in having (Fig. 5.34)
- A smaller body
- An oblong shape, being broadest from side to side
- A larger and roughly triangular vertebral foramen
- A bifid (double-ended) spurious process, and
- A well-marked foramen in the transverse process for the passage of the vertebral artery.

The Atlas

The first cervical vertebra, or atlas, is specially adapted, together with the axis, to carry the weight of the head and to facilitate its movements. The atlas is easily recognized because it has no body. Instead,

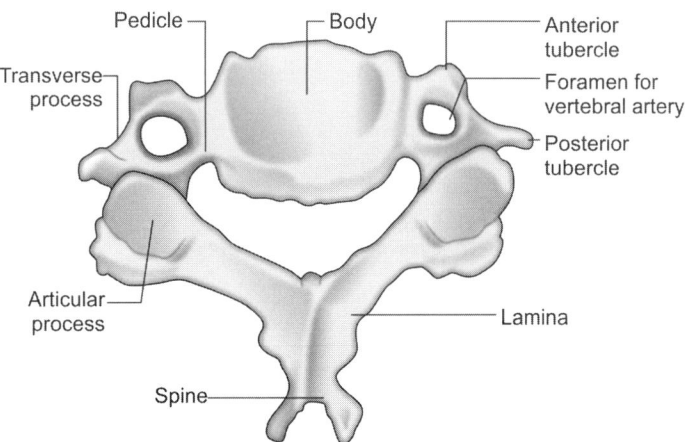

Fig. 5.34: A typical cervical vertebra viewed from above

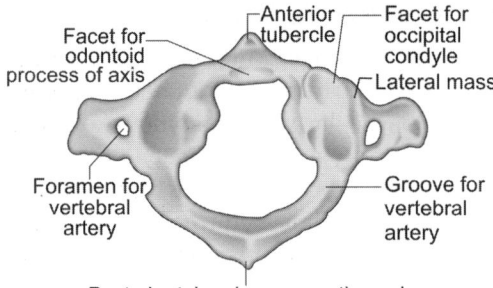

Fig. 5.35: The atlas viewed from above

it consists of a ring of bone enclosing a very large vertebral canal, on the anterior aspect of which is a small facet for articulation with the dens or odontoid process of the axis (Fig. 5.35). The atlas pivots around the dens (at the atlanto-axial joint) when the head is rotated.

The upper surface of the atlas bears on each side a superior articular facet, on a thick lateral mass, for articulation with the occipital condyles of the skull. Nodding movements and lateral flexion are effected at the atlanto-occipital joints so formed. Unlike the other cervical vertebrae, the atlas has no spinous process.

The Axis

The second cervical vertebra, or axis, is characterized by a tooth-like process—the dens or odontoid process—which projects upwards from its body (Fig. 5.36). This process actually represents and occupies the position of the missing body of the atlas. On its anterior surface is a small facet which articulates with the anterior arch of the atlas, an arrangement which permits the rotation of the head. The spinous process of the axis is large and strong; rotate the head.

The Thoracic Vertebrae

Also known as the dorsal vertebrae, these carry the ribs and are twelve in number. Notable features are:

- A gradual increase in size from above downwards, reflecting the progressive increase in load (Fig. 5.37).
- Bodies shaped like those of the cervical region in the case of the upper thoracic vertebrae and like those of the lumbar region in the case of the lower thoracic vertebrae. The fourth thoracic vertebra is heart-shaped. The bodies of the fifth to the eighth thoracic vertebrae are slightly flattened on their left side owing to the pressure of the descending aorta (Fig. 5.38). An aortic aneurysm in this region will erode the bodies of these four vertebrae but leave their intervertebral discs unaffected.
- Costal facets; typically two on each side of the body, for the heads of the ribs

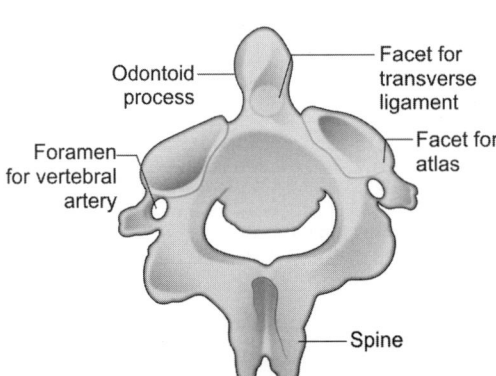

Fig. 5.36: The axis viewed from above and behind

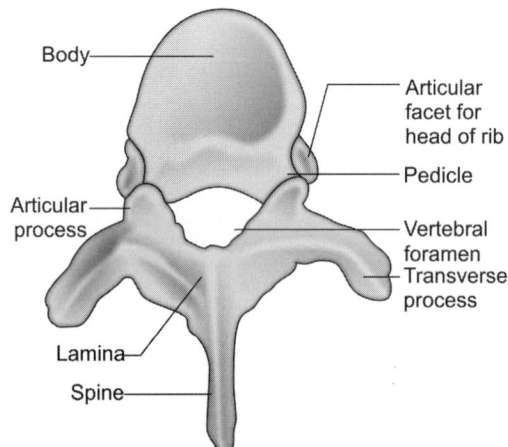

Fig. 5.37: A thoracic or dorsal vertebra seen from above

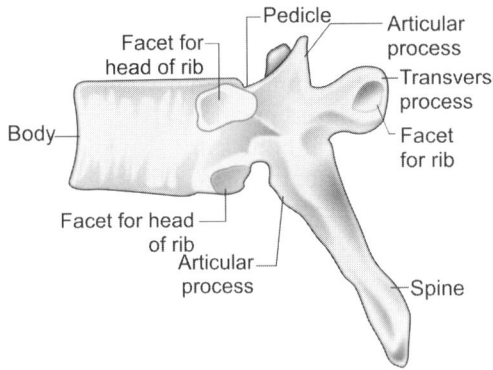

Fig. 5.38: A thoracic or dorsal vertebra seen from the side

and one on the tip of each transverse process, for articulation with the tubercles of the ribs.
- Long, markedly downward-sloping spinous processes.

The Lumbar Vertebrae
- These are the largest vertebrae and are five in number.
- Their bodies are kidney-shaped.
- They have no costal facets.
- Their spinous processes are strong, quadrangular, broad and flat, and almost horizontal.
- The transverse process of the fifth lumbar vertebra is (a) massive and (b) connects with the whole of the lateral aspect of the pedicle and encroaches on the body of the vertebra. The transverse processes of the other lumbar vertebrae are thin and attach only to the junction of pedicle with lamina.

The Sacrum

The sacrum is a large, triangular bone composed of five fused vertebrae, the individual parts of which can be discerned. It articulates above with the fifth lumbar vertebra (forming the lumbosacral angle), below with the coccyx and at the sides with the innominate bones. The dorsal surface of the sacrum is convex and the pelvic surface is concave, thereby increasing the capacity of the true pelvis.

The sacrum has a wide base, articulating with the fifth lumbar vertebra and a narrow blunted apex inferiorly, articulating with the coccyx. The transverse processes project from the central body and those of each side are fused together to form the lateral parts of the sacrum. Between the body and the lateral parts are the four anterior sacral foramina for the passage of nerves.

The upper margin of the body projects forwards and is called the promontory of the sacrum. The upper portion of the lateral part of the sacrum has an ear-shaped surface on its lateral aspect for articulation with the iliac part of the innominate bone, with which it forms the sacro-iliac joint. Behind this surface is a very rough area for the attachment of strong ligaments (Figs 5.12 and 5.13).

On the convex posterior surface is the median sacral crest surmounted by three of four rudimentary spinous tubercles. An each side of the crest are four dorsal sacral foramina for nerves.

The neural canal is continued into the sacrum as the sacral canal and, at its lower end, opens on to the surface of the bone at the sacral hiatus, below the third or fourth spinous tubercle. The sacral canal contains the cauda equina, and the filum terminale and fifth sacral nerves emerge at the sacral hiatus. The inferior part or apex of the sacrum articulates with the coccyx.

Typically, the sacrum is wider in the female than in the male and its ventral concavity is deeper. The pelvic surface of the bone also faces downwards more in the female, thereby further increasing the size of the pelvic cavity and causing the sacrovertebral (lumbosacral) angle to be prior prominent.

The Coccyx (or Tailbone)

This consists of four (sometimes three or five) vertebrae usually fused together so that their individual characteristics are not apparent, although the first coccygeal vertebra may be separate. The coccyx is triangular in shape, articulating at its base with the sacrum and tapering to its apex below. The apex or tip of the coccyx gives origin to the external anal sphincter. The dorsal surface of the coccyx and lower part of the sacrum gives origin to part of the gluteus maximus muscle of the buttock.

Ligaments of the Vertebral Column

The vertebrae are held together by strong ligaments which include:
- Those connecting the bodies. The tough anterior and posterior longitudinal ligaments (Fig. 5.39) run the whole length of the spine, joining the anterior and posterior aspects of the vertebral bodies respectively.
- Those connecting the laminae and the spinous processes.
  - Those connecting the laminae are called the ligamentum flava and consist of elastic tissue.
  - The tough supraspinous ligaments link the spinous processes. They are penetrated by the needle during the performance of lumbar puncture.

These, and to a lesser extent other ligaments, serve to support the vertebral column (spine) when it is in the fully flexed position.
- The vertebral bodies are also joined by the intervertebral discs of fibrocartilage, which are extremely strong and which account for a quarter of the length of the spine. Their atrophy in old age results in shrinkage in height. Each disc consists of a ring-like annulus fibrosus surrounding a gelatinous nucleus pulposus. The annulus fibrosus may rupture posteriorly, as a result of trauma or degeneration, and allow the nucleus pulposus to protrude backwards into the vertebral canal. This is known as a prolapsed intervertebral disc and it occurs most commonly between the fourth and fifth lumbar (L4/5) or fifth lumbar and first sacral (L5/S1) vertebrae. Prolapse at these sites exerts pressure on the roots of the fifth lumbar nerve and first sacral nerve, respectively. Referred pain (sciatica) is felt in the back of the lower limb, along the distribution of the sciatic nerve. Straight leg raising is painful and limited due to the traction exerted on the irritated and already

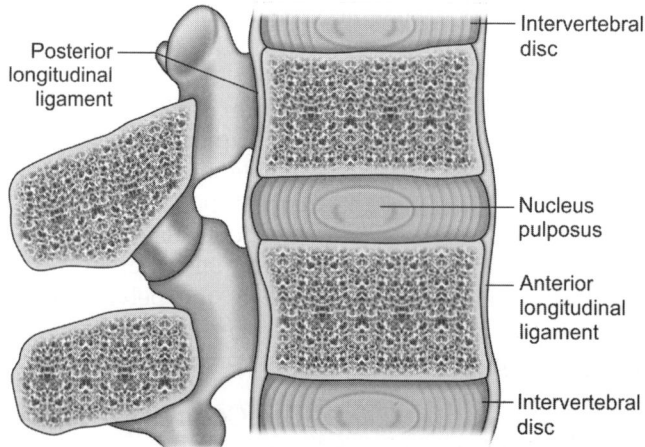

Fig. 5.39: Section of vertebral column showing ligaments and intervertebral discs

stretched nerve root. The ankle jerk may be absent if the first sacral nerve (S1) is affected.

Movements of the Spinal Column

Apart from the movements of nodding and rotation of the head which, it has been seen, take place at the atlas and axis respectively, the movements of the spine as a whole are considerable although the actual range of movement between the individual vertebrae is small. They are:

- (a) Flexion or bending forwards and (b) Extension or bending backwards, in which the maximum movement takes place in the cervical and lumbar regions
- Lateral movement or bending from side to side, well-marked in the neck and also possible in the dorsal region
- Rotation or twisting the spinal column as a whole around its long axis.

It is the elasticity of the intervertebral discs which makes all of these movements possible. The swing of the pelvis from side to side during walking is due to a rotatory movement at the lumbosacral articulation, together with similar movements of the lumbar intervertebral joints. This enables a patient to walk reasonably well even with fixed hip joints.

Notes: The following structures are on a level with various vertebrae:

Structure	On a level with
Oral pharynx	Axis vertebra
Opening of larynx	4th cervical vertebra
Bifurcation of carotid artery	3rd cervical vertebra
Upper margin of sternum	2nd thoracic vertebra
Bifurcation of trachea heart	4th thoracic vertebra 6th, 7th and 8th thoracic vertebrae
Kidneys	12th thoracic, 1st and 2nd lumbar vertebrae
Pancreas	1st and 2nd lumbar vertebrae
Bifurcation of aorta	4th lumbar vertebra

A line joining the highest points of the iliac crests passes between the spines of the fourth and fifth lumbar vertebrae and is a landmark for lumbar puncture.

Fractures of the spine may be accompanied by damage to the spinal cord. Patients with spinal cord injuries suffer from retention of urine, which may be temporary or permanent. If infection is introduced at catheterization, ascending pyelonephritis may result and may be fatal.

■ BONES OF THE THORAX

The skeletal framework of the thorax is formed (a) behind, by the thoracic or dorsal vertebrae; (b) anteriorly, by the sternum and costal cartilages; and (c) the remainder of the circumference, by the ribs (Fig. 5.40). The thoracic cage thus formed communicates above with the root of the neck through the 'thoracic inlet' and is separated below from the abdominal cavity by the diaphragm.

The Sternum

This is an almost flat, dagger-shaped bone which has a slightly convex anterior and a slightly concave posterior surface. It is composed of highly vascular trabecular bone covered by a layer of compact bone.

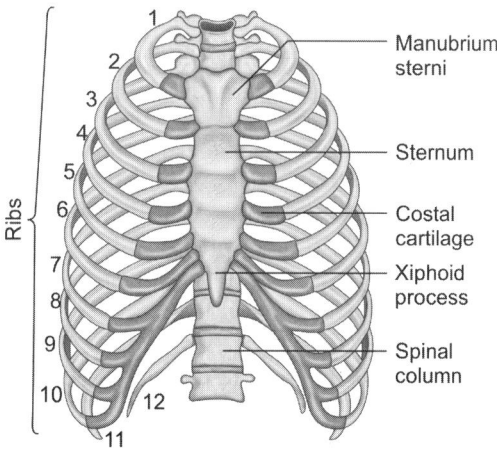

Fig. 5.40: Skeleton of the thorax

The spaces in its spongy interior contain red marrow and a sample of this may be aspirated through a wide-bore needle pushed through the thin cortical bone (sternal puncture). Such a sample may be extremely valuable in the diagnosis of anemias, leukemia's and other diseases affecting the bone marrow.

Along each side of the sternum are seven indent stations where the costal cartilages are attached. The sternum is divided into three parts: (a) the manubrium above; (b) the mesosternum or body in the middle; and (c) the xiphoid process below.

The manubrium is roughly triangular and it articulates on either side with the clavicle, at the sternoclavicular joint, and with the first and second costal cartilages. The adjoining body of the sternum also articulates with the second costal cartilage. The cartilages of the 3rd, 4th, 5th and 6th ribs are attached at intervals, while the seventh is attached at its junction with the xiphoid process.

The xiphoid process forms the lower extremity of the sternum. It sometimes remains cartilaginous but is usually ossified, in its upper part, in adults. It is a small, more or less triangular plate to which are attached the fibers of the linea alba and the rectus abdominis muscle. A part of the diaphragm is attached to its posterior surface.

The sternum is cut vertically down through its midline (median sternotomy) to give access to the heart for cardiac surgery. The sternum is also split in this way in operations on the thymus gland.

The Ribs

The ribs are arches of bone which are directed obliquely forwards and downwards from the spine, with which they articulate, to form the greater part of the thoracic cage. There are usually twelve pairs and they are classified into two groups.

- *True ribs:* The upper seven pairs, which are joined to the sternum by their costal cartilages.
- *False ribs:* The lower five pairs, which have no direct attachment to the sternum. The costal cartilages of the 8th, 9th and 10th fuse with the cartilage immediately above. The 11th and 12th (floating ribs) only partly encircle the thorax and are unattached in front.

The first two ribs and the last three have special features but the intervening seven ribs are similar to each other and are regarded as typical ribs (Fig. 5.41).

Each typical rib is a long bone with (a) a head, (b) a neck posteriorly and (c) a shaft. The head bears two facets for articulation with the numerically corresponding dorsal vertebra and the vertebra above (Fig. 5.42). The neck is stout and lies in front of the transverse process of the corresponding vertebra. There is a well-marked tubercle on the outer surface of the rib where the neck joints the shaft. It has a facet for articulation with the transverse process of the corresponding vertebra.

The shaft of the typical rib is long, thin and flattened. It is not only curved and slightly twisted on itself, but is bent, having an angle about 5 or 6 cm lateral to the tubercle. The shaft has a smooth

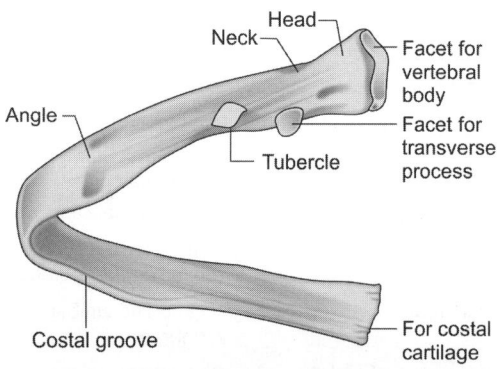

Fig. 5.41: A typical rib

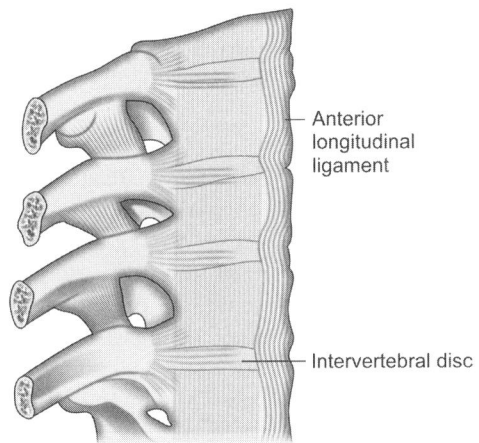

Fig. 5.42: Thoracic vertebrae with ligaments and articulations of ribs

convex external surface, superior and inferior borders, and a smooth internal surface groove inferiorly by the costal groove which is occupied by the intercostal artery and nerve. The borders of the ribs give attachment to the intercostal muscles which pass to the ribs immediately above and below. The internal surface of the rib is lined by parietal pleura, which is firmly adherent to the periosteum of the bone.

The atypical ribs have distinctive features. The first rib is broad and is usually the shortest and flattest of the ribs. It is more curved than all the other ribs but unlike them it is not twisted. Its surfaces face upwards and downwards, i.e. it has upper and lower surfaces. Near the center of the inner border of the upper surface is the scalene tubercle, a small projection to which the scalenus anterior muscle is attached. The subclavian vein crosses the rib in the groove in front of this tubercle and there is a groove for the subclavian artery behind the tubercle. The latter groove is also occupied by the lowest trunk of the brachial plexus; at this site the anesthetist can infiltrate the plexus with a local anesthetic.

The second rib is about twice as long as the first rib and much less curved. It bears a rough tubercle for the serratus anterior muscle. Its costal groove is short and poorly marked.

The eleventh and twelfth ('floating') ribs are short and thin. They have no tubercles and their heads bear only a single facet.

The ribs consist of highly vascular trabecular bone, containing red marrow, enveloped by a thin layer of compact bone.

Rib fractures are common. Sometimes the broken end of the bone is driven into the lung, lacerating it and causing the leakage of air and blood into the pleural cavity, a condition known as hemopneumothorax. A severe crushing injury may fracture several ribs fore and aft so that a portion of the thoracic cage becomes loose ('stove-in chest') and moves paradoxically with breathing, bulging out with expiration and being sucked in with inspiration. The mediastinum swings with the abnormal movement and causes severe shock. Urgent treatment is necessary, a drain being inserted into the chest and connected to an underwater seal, and positive pressure ventilation being given through an endotracheal or tracheostomy tube.

A cervical rib is found in a few people. It articulates with the transverse process of the 7th cervical process. Its anterior end is either free, if the rib is short, or it articulates with the first thoracic rib. It may in part be a fibrous cord. Paraesthesiae ('pins and needles') in the ulnar aspect of the forearm and wasting of the small muscles of the hand may result from the pressure of a cervical rib (even if only a fibrous cord) on the overlying lower trunk of the brachial plexus. Occasionally, pressure on the overlying subclavian artery causes vascular problems (ischemia or even gangrene) in the upper limb.

The Costal Cartilages

These are the flattened bars of hyaline cartilage which connect the upper seven ribs to the sternum and the 8th, 9th and 10th ribs to the cartilages immediately above them. The cartilages of the 11th and 12th ribs are tapered and end in the musculature of the abdominal wall.

The costal cartilages contribute to the mobility, elasticity and resilience of the thoracic cage. Were it not for them, the ribs and sternum would be fractured more frequently.

In old age, the costal cartilages tend to ossify and become less pliable. This makes cardiac massage more difficult (more force being necessary to achieve a useful cardiac output) and more likely to result in fractures of the ribs and sternum.

The Intercostal Spaces

Typically, each intercostal space (Fig. 5.43) contains three muscles and a neurovascular bundle (of intercostal nerve, artery and vein). Irritation of the nerves by diseases of the thoracic spine (e.g. spinal tuberculosis) may cause referred pain in the front of the chest, where the nerves terminate. Pus from a tuberculous vertebra tends to track along the neurovascular bundle and to erupt as a cold abscess at one of the three points of emergence of the cutaneous branches of the intercostal nerves, just lateral to the spine, in the mid-axillary line, or just lateral to the sternum.

The intercostal spaces, being occupied only by soft tissue, provide useful 'windows' for examination of the heart by ultrasound (echocardiography), which cannot be performed through the bone of the ribs.

In a conventional thoracotomy for excision of diseased lung tissue (e.g. lobectomy for bronchial carcinoma or bronchiectasis), access is gained by resecting a portion of the fifth or sixth rib, by a technique which preserves the neurovascular bundle. The elasticity of the thoracic cage permits the surgical intercostal space so created to be widely opened, using rib retractors.

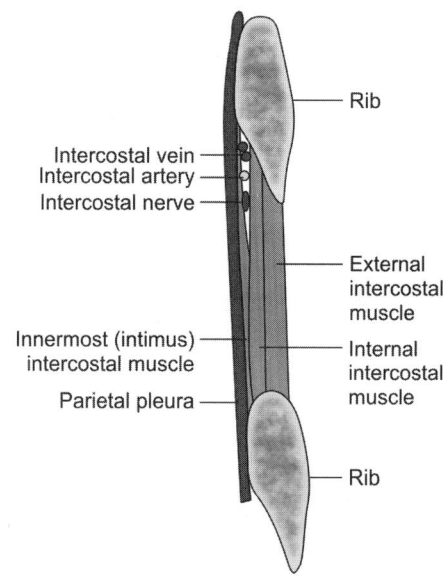

Fig. 5.43: Section through ribs and an intercostal space

CHAPTER 6

Joints or Articulations

Joints are region of the skeleton where two bones meet and articulate. The joints are supported by a variety of soft tissue structures. Joints facilitate growth or transmit forces between bone enabling movement to occur. Simplest classification of joints relate to the range of movements.

Free movement occur in synovial joints and restricted movement occur in synarthroses.

Synarthroses: Subdivided into fibrous joint and cartilaginous joint.

Fibrous joint: Fibrous joints lack intervening cartilage between two bones. The movements are restricted. The three types of articulations are—sutures, gomphoses and syndesmoses.

Suture: Sutures are restricted to skull. In the amount of connective tissue decreases with age and bony ends become opposed.

Schindylesis: It is a specialized suture in which rigid bone fits into a groove.

Gomphoses: Gomphoses is a peg and socket joint between tooth and its socket.

Syndesmoses: Syndesmoses is a fibrous connection between bones. Bones may be connected by interosseus membrane or ligament.

Cartilaginous joint: Cartilaginous joint may be classified as primary (synchondrosis) or secondary (symphysis).

Primary cartilaginous joint: Synchondroses.

In these joints, the centers of ossification are separated by areas of hyaline cartilage. They are present in all post cranial bones.

Secondary cartilaginous joint: In secondary cartilaginous joint, there is an intervening fibrocartilage between the articular ends covered by hyaline cartilage. Collagen fibers blend the fibrocartilage and hyaline cartilage. This blending helps to withstand stress, tension, torsion. All symphysis occur in the midline, e.g. manubriosternal, intervertebral, symphysis menti.

Synovial joint: Bones involved are linked by fibrous capsule, often by accessory ligament. Articulating bony surfaces are covered by hyaline cartilage. Articular cartilage reduce friction and facilitate free movement. Synovial fluid acts as lubricant.

Articular surface: Articular surfaces are formed by hyaline cartilage. Sternoclavicular, acromioclavicular, temperomandibular surfaces are covered by fibrous tissue and so suggest intramembranous ossification. Articular cartilages are resistant to wear and tear and reduce friction. They are compressible and elastic. Young cartilages are white and compressible while older ones are brittle and thinner. Articular cartilages are moulded to bone. It has no penetrating nerves and vessels. Erosion occurs in pathologically dry joints. Changes are extremely slow in healthy joints.

Fibrous capsule: Fibrous capsule encloses joint except at sites of synovial protrusion. It is composed of white collagen fibers and is attached to articular margins. Capsule is perforated by vessels and nerves. It is lined by synovial membrane. Fibrous capsule has local thickening called intrinsic ligaments. Capsule checks excessive movement and abnormal movement.

Synovial membrane: Synovial membrane lines fibrous capsule, intracapsular ligament. They do not line intra-articular discs or menisci. Synovial membrane secretes synovial fluid.

Synovial fluid: Synovial fluid occupy synovial joint, bursa.

Intra-articular menisci: These occur between articular surfaces. It is fibrocartilaginous and is not covered by synovial membrane. Complete disc is seen sternoclavicular and inferior radio-ulnar joint. Function of disc is shock absorption and facilitate combined movement of joint.

Classification of synovial joint: Synovial joint may be classified according to their shape.

Plane joint: Plane joint is an apposition of almost flat surfaces, e.g. intermetacarpal and intermetatarsal.

Hinge joint: These joints resemble hinges because movements are restricted to one plane. They are uniaxial, e.g. humeroulnar, interphalangeal joint. Hinge joints have strong collateral ligaments.

Pivot joint: These are uniaxial joints in which an osseous pivot in an osteocartilaginous ring allows rotation only around the axis of the pivot. Pivot may rotate in ring, e.g. head of radius in annular ligament. Rings may rotate around pivots—atlas rotates around dens of axis vertebra.

Bicondylar joints: They are predominantly uniaxial with main movement happening in one plane. They are called bicondylar because they are formed of 2 convex condyles which articulate with concave or flat surface.

Ellipsoid joint: It is biaxial and consists of an oval convex surface apposed to elliptical concavity, e.g. radiocarpal and metacarpophalangeal joint. Primary movement occur around 2 axis, flexion-extension and abduction-adduction.

Saddle joint: It is biaxial and have concavo-convex surfaces. The convexity is opposed to concavity of opposite surfaces, e.g. carpometacarpal joint of thumb, ankle joint.

Ball and socket joint: These joints are multiaxial joints and formed by the reception of a globoid head into an opposing cup, e.g. hip joint, shoulder joint.

■ JOINTS OF UPPER LIMB

Shoulder Joint (Glenohumeral Joint) (Fig. 6.1)

It is a synovial multiaxial spheroidal joint between roughly hemispherical head of humerus and shallow glenoid fossa of scapula. Its stability depends on surrounding muscular and soft tissue envelop.

It is the most mobile joint in the body and most frequently dislocated.

Articulating surfaces: Articular surfaces are reciprocally curved and are ovoid. Humeral convexity exceeds glenoid concavity. Radius of curvature of glenoid fossa is greater than that of humeral head and is deepened by fibrocartilaginous rim (glenoid labrum). Both articular surfaces are covered by hyaline cartilage, which is thick centrally and thin peripherally on humerus and reverse for glenoid cavity. The curvatures are not fully congruent and so joint is loosely packed. Close packing (full congruence) is reached with the humerus abducted and laterally rotated.

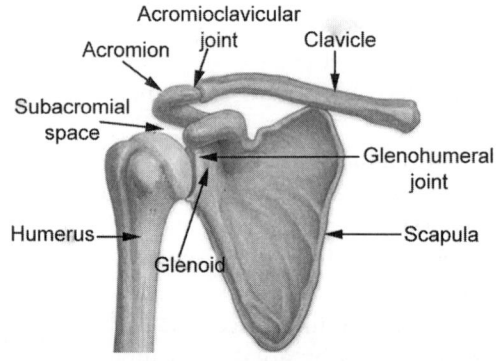

Fig. 6.1: Shoulder joint

Glenoid labrum: It is the fibrocartilaginous rim around glenoid fossa. It is triangular in cross section and varies in thickness. Its base is attached to margins of fossa. Labrum deepens cavity.

Fibrous capsule: It envelops the joint. It is attached medially to glenoid neck. At the glenoid cavity, it includes supraglenoid tubercle inside capsule. Laterally it is attached to anatomical neck. Fibrous capsule is supported by the tendon of supraspinatus (above), infraspinatus and teres minor (behind), subscapularis in front and by the long head of triceps below. Triceps is separated from capsule by axillary nerve. Capsule is least supported inferiorly and subjected to greatest strength in full abduction.

Ligaments of shoulder joint (Fig. 6.2): They are glenohumeral, coracohumeral and transverse humeral.

Synovial membrane: Lines the capsule and covers parts of anatomical neck.

Factors maintaining stability: Tendons of subscapularis, supraspinatus, infraspinatus, teres minor muscles fuse with capsule to form rotator cuff (Fig. 6.3).

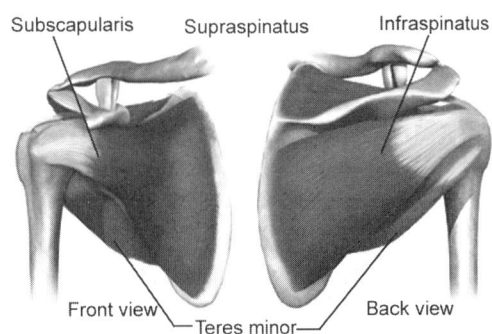

Fig. 6.3: Muscles of the rotator cuff

Movements of shoulder joint: Flexion, extension, abduction, adduction, circumduction, medial rotation and lateral rotation.

Glenohumeral abduction is approximately 90 degree, some 60 degree further abduction occurs at sternoclavicular and acromioclavicular articulation.

Muscles producing movements:
- *Flexion:* Pectoralis major
- *Extension:* Deltoid, teres major
- *Abduction:* Deltoid, supraspinatus
- *Medial rotation:* Pectoralis major, deltoid
- *Lateral rotation:* Infraspinatus, deltoid.

Elbow Joint

It is a synovial joint. Its complexity is increased by continuity with the superior radio-ulnar joint. It includes two articulations, humeroulnar and humeroradial (Fig. 6.4).

Articulating Surfaces

Humeral trochlea and capitulum and ulnar trochlear notch and radial head. The capitulum and radial head are reciprocally curved. Humeroulnar and humeroradial articulations form a largely uniaxial joint and is most congruent and most stable joint.

Fibrous Capsule

It is attached above the coronoid and radial fossa and medial epicondyl anteriorly.

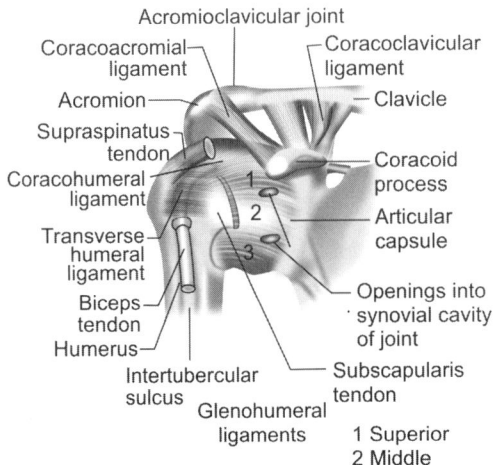

Fig. 6.2: Ligaments of shoulder joint

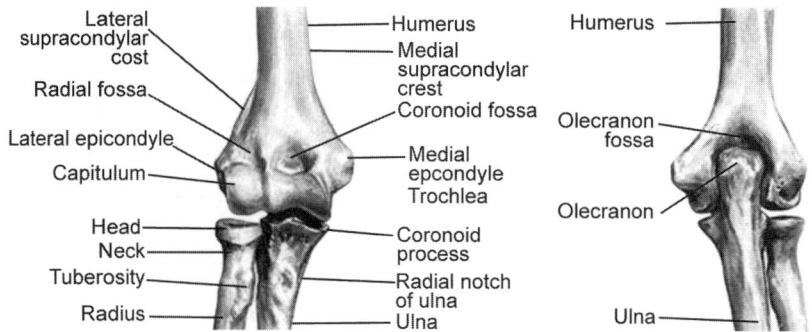

Fig. 6.4: Bones of right elbow joint

Posteriorly is attached to edge of olecranon fossa. Below attached to edge of coronoid process and to the margins of capitulum and trochlea.

Synovial Membrane

Lines humeral articular margins and lines coronoid, radial, olecranon fossa.

Ligaments

These are ulnar collateral ligament and radial collateral ligament.
Movements: Being a uniaxial joint, elbow allows flexion and extension accompanied by slight conjunct rotation.

Carrying Angle

When the forearm is fully extended and supinated, it diverges laterally forming with the upper arm an angle of 163°. This angle is called carrying angle. Its ulnar border cannot touch lateral surface of thigh (Fig. 6.5).

Radioulnar Joints

Superior radioulnar joints (Fig. 6.6): It is a uniaxial pivot joint. Articulating surfaces are between the radial head and annular ligament. Annular ligament is a strong band which encircles radial head holding it against radial notch of ulna.
Synovial membrane: It is continuous with elbow joint.

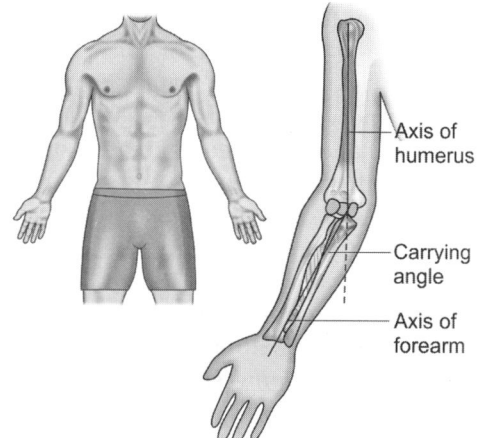

Fig. 6.5: Carrying angle

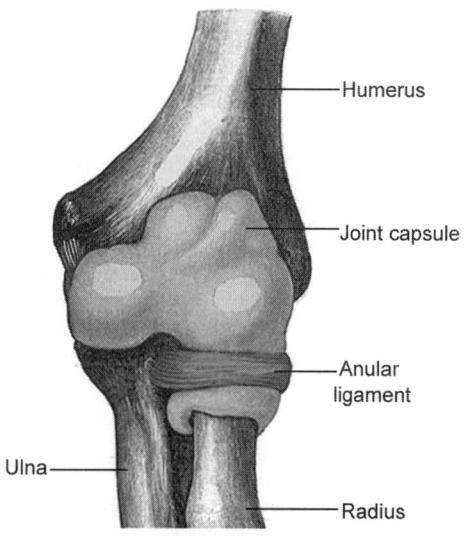

Fig. 6.6: Radioulnar joint

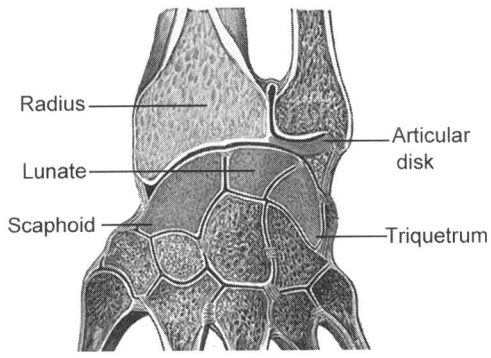

Fig. 6.7: Radiocarpal joint

Factors maintaining stability: It is annular ligament.

Distal Radioulnar joint

Movements taking place are pronation and supination.

Radiocarpal Joint (Wrist joint)

It is a synovial biaxial, and ellipsoid joint formed by articulation of the distal end of radius and the triangular fibrocartilage with scaphoid lunate, triquetrum.

In neutral position of the wrist, only the scaphoid and lunate are in contact with the radius and articular disc (Fig. 6.7).

Fibrous capsule: It is lined by synovial membrane.

Wrist movements: Active movements are flexion, extension, adduction, abduction, circumduction.

■ JOINTS OF PELVIC GIRDLE AND LOWER LIMB

Hip Joint

It is a synovial joint of ball and socket type (multiaxial) (Fig. 6.8).

Articular Surfaces

Femoral head articulates with the cup shaped acetabulum. The articular surfaces are reciprocally curved. The femoral head is covered by articular cartilage except over a rough pit where ligamentum teres is attached. Acetabular articular surface, the lunate surface is an incomplete ring. Acetabular fossa is the central non-articular area in the floor of acetabulum. It is devoid of cartilage and contains fibroelastic fat covered by synovial membrane. Acetabular labrum is a fibrocartilaginous rim attached to acetabular margin.

Fibrous Capsule

Capsule is strong and dense and attached to acetabular margin. It surrounds femoral head and neck and is anteriorly attached to intertrochanteric line, superiorly to

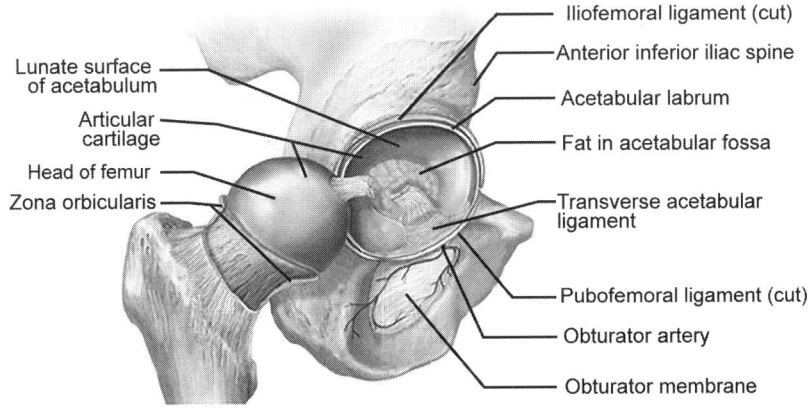

Fig. 6.8: Hip joint

base of femoral neck, posteriorly 1 cm superomedially to intertrochanteric crest.

Ligaments of Hip Joint

Ischiofemoral, Iliofemoral, pubofemoral, transverse acetabular ligament are the ligaments of hip joint.
Iliofemoral ligament: It is a very strong ligament and is inverted Y-shaped in appearance. The stem of the Y is attached to anterior inferior iliac spine and the limbs of the Y are attached to intertrochanteric line.
Pubofemoral ligament: Pubofemoral ligament is triangular in shape, its base attaching to iliopubic eminence and superior pubic ramus. It blends with capsule of hip joint.
Ischiopubic ligament: This ligament thickens the back of the capsule. It attaches deep to iliofemoral ligament.

Ligament of Head of Femur

Apex of the ligament is attached to head of femur and base is attached to acetabular notch (Fig. 6.9).

Relations

Joint capsule is surrounded by muscles.
Anteriorly: Pectineus, psoas major, femoral artery.
Superiorly: Rectus femoris
Inferiorly: Pectineus
Laterally: Gluteus maximus
Posteriorly: Obturator internus

VESSELS AND NERVES

Branches of obturator artery, medial circumflex femoral artery, superior gluteal artery, inferior gluteal artery supply the hip joint.

Nerves are branches of femoral nerve, obturator nerve, accessory obturator nerve, superior gluteal nerve.
Movements produced at hip joint: Movements are categorized as flexion-extension, abduction-adduction, circumduction, medial rotation and lateral rotation.

Muscles Producing Movement (Fig. 6.10)

Flexion: Psoas major and iliacus.
Extension: Gluteus maximus and hamstring muscle
Abduction: Gluteus medius and gluteus minimus. These muscles are involved in walking and running.
Adduction: Adductor longus, adductor brevis, adductor magnus.

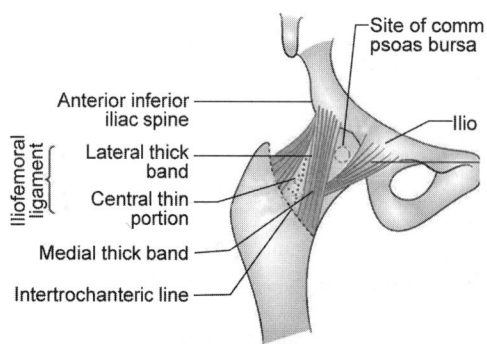

Fig. 6.9: Ligaments of head of femur

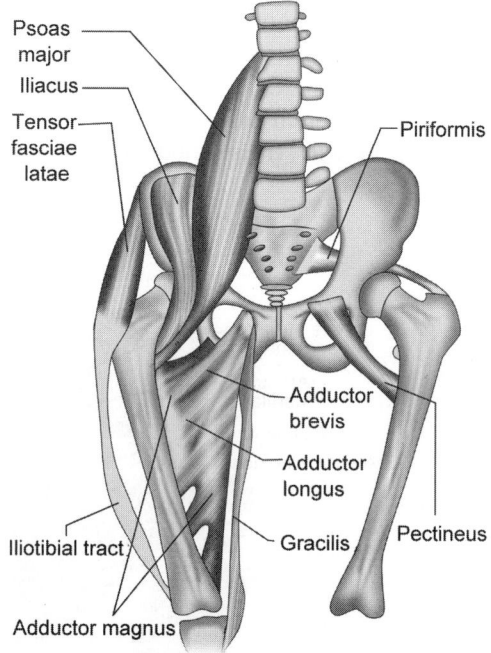

Fig. 6.10: Muscles related to hip joint

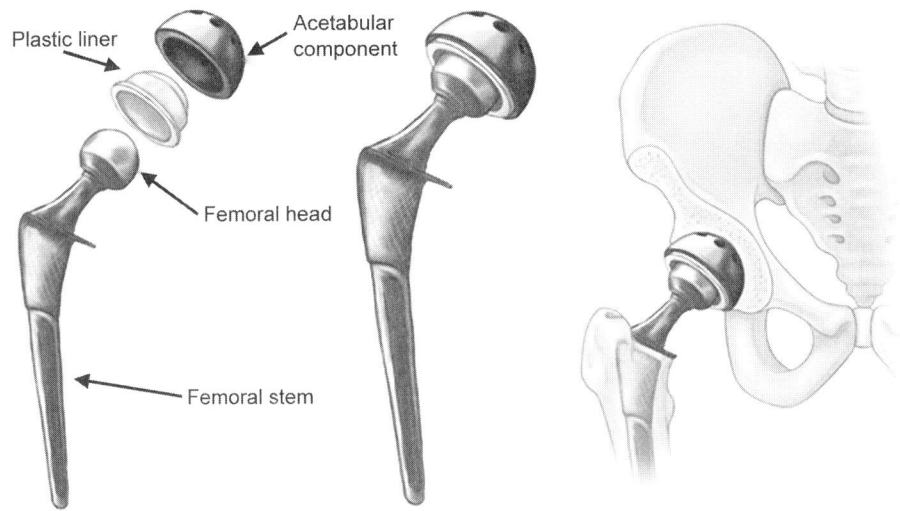

Fig. 6.11: Hip replacement

Medial rotation: Tensor fascia lata, gluteus medius and gluteus minimus.
Lateral rotation: Obturator muscles, gamelli, quadrates femoris.
Clinical anatomy: Iliofemoral ligament is rarely torn during dislocation. Congenital dislocation is more common at hip joint.
Total hip replacement (Fig. 6.11): Conditions requiring total hip replacement are osteoarthritis and rheumatoid arthritis.

Knee Joint

Largest of human joints is knee joint. It is a compound joint. It forms condylar joint with the femur and tibia and forms sellar joint between patella and femur. Strictly the joint is classified as complex (Fig. 6.12).

Articular Surfaces

Femoral condyles are convex and bear articular cartilage. The tibial condyles are also cartilage covered areas. These condyles are separated by intercondylar area. Lateral tibial articular surface is almost circular and smaller. The medial articular surface is oval with long anteroposterior axis. Movements at femerotibial ends are smoothened by menisci and it increases the concavity of tibial surfaces. Patellar articular surface is adapted to femoral surface. An oblique groove divides femoral-patellar surface into large lateral and small medial part into which patella fits in.

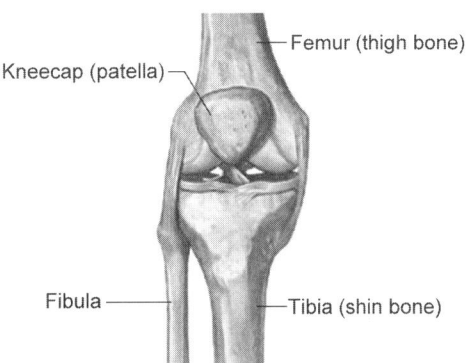

Fig. 6.12: Knee joint

Ligaments of the Joint

Patellar ligament, tibial collateral ligament, fibular collateral ligament, oblique popliteal ligament, arcuate popliteal ligament, anterior and posterior cruciate ligament, transverse ligament.

Fibrous Capsule of Knee Joint

Fibrous capsule is complex, partly deficient partly strengthened by tendons of muscles. Medial capsular fibers blends with tibial collateral ligament. Fibular collateral ligament lies lateral to lateral part of capsule. Anteriorly capsule blends with expansions of vastus muscles and also attached to patellar ligament. Capsule is deficient above and is related to suprapatellar bursa.

Patellar ligament (Ligamentum patella) (Fig. 6.13): It is formed by tendon of quadriceps femoris muscle extending from patella to tibial tuberosity. It is strong, flat, and about 8 cm in length attached proximally to apex of patella medially and laterally it is attached to fibrous capsule.

Tibial collateral ligament: It is a broad flat band and extends from medial femoral epicondyl to medial meniscus and to medial side of upper part of tibia. It is crossed by sartorius, gracilis and semitendinosus muscles.

Ligaments of Knee (Fig. 6.14)

Cruciate ligaments: The ligaments are named so as they cross each other. They are very strong intracapsular structures.

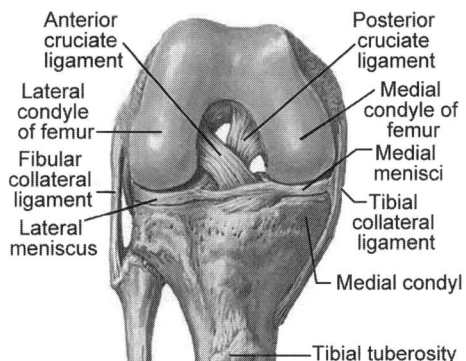

Fig. 6.14: Ligaments of knee

They are named anterior and posterior with reference to their attachments to tibia. Synovial membranes surround the ligaments.

Anterior cruciate ligament: Attached to anterior intercondylar area of tibia and is attached posteriorly to medial surface of lateral femoral condyle.

Posterior cruciate ligaments: It is thicker and stronger than anterior cruciate ligament. It extends from the medial femoral condyle to the posterior part of intercondylar area of tibia.

Menisci

Menisci are intracapsular, fibrocartilaginous structures which deepen the articular surfaces of tibia receiving femoral condyles. The peripheral border of meniscus are thick and convex and the inner border is thin and concave. There peripheral zone is vascularized by capillary loop. Their inner rim is avascular. Tears of menisci are common. Menisci assist lubrication and, facilitate combined sliding, rolling, and cushion extremes of flexion and extension.

Medial menisci: They are broader posteriorly, semicircular in shape. It has anterior horn and posterior horn. Peripheral margin of the menisci is attached to capsule of knee joint and medial collateral ligament.

Lateral meniscus: Forms almost 4/5th of a

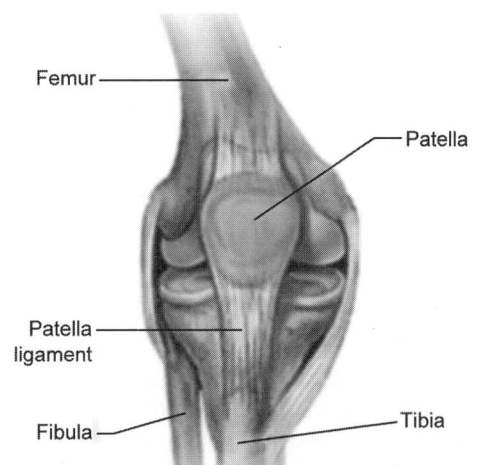

Fig. 6.13: Patellar ligament

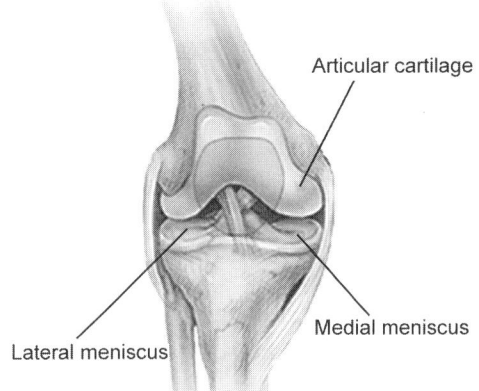

Fig. 6.15: Menisci

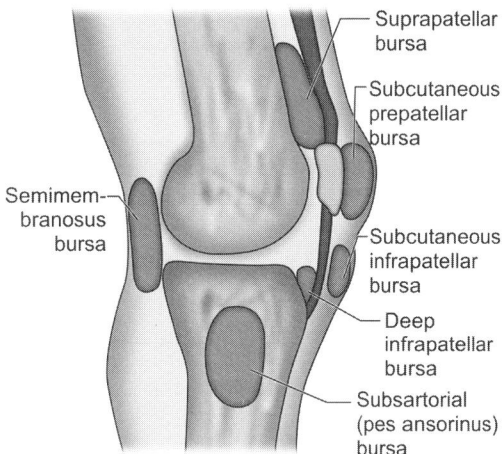

Fig. 6.16: Bursa around knee joint

circle. It is grooved laterally by popliteus muscle which intervenes between the lateral collateral ligament and meniscus (Fig. 6.15).

Bursa Around Knee Joint

Anteriorly subcutaneous prepatellar bursa between patella and skin, deep infrapatellar bursa between patellar tendon and tibia, subcutaneous infrapatellar bursa between tibial tuberosity and skin and a large suprapatellar bursa.

Movements: Movements are flexion, extension, medial and lateral rotation. Rotations can be conjunct (integral with flexion and extension) or adjunct (independent). Conjunct medial rotation of the femur on the tibia in later stages of extension is part of locking of knee. At the beginning of flexion from full extension, lateral femoral rotation occurs which unlocks the joint (Fig. 6.16).

Muscles Producing the Movements

Flexion: Biceps femoris, semitendinosus, semimembranosus.
Extension: Quadriceps femoris
Medial rotation: Popliteus, semitendinosus, semimembranosus
Lateral rotation: Biceps femoris
Blood supply to joint: Genicular branches of femoral artery and popliteal artery (Fig. 6.17).

Arthroscopy of knee: Done using fiber optic video system. Normal findings include suprapatellar pouch, patella-femoral joint, lateral femoral condyle, lateral side of joint, medial femoral condyle, medial compartment with menisci, lateral compartment with lateral menisci (Fig. 6.18).

Clinical anatomy: Knee is an insecure joint. Articular surfaces are poorly congruent. Injuries to menisci are common resulting from twisting strains applied to flexed knee. Injuries to cruciate ligament are also common ranging from sprain to rupture.

Total knee replacement: Surgical replacement required in severe destructive arthritis of joint (Fig. 6.19).

Ankle Joint (Talocrural Joint) (Fig. 6.20)

It is a hinge joint and uniaxial. The lower end of tibia and medial malleolus, lateral malleolus and inferior transverse tibiofibular ligament and body of talus form the articular surfaces.

Articular surfaces: These surfaces are covered by hyaline cartilage. The talar surface is convex and the distal tibial surface is reciprocally curved. The medial malleolar surface is comma-shaped and latreral malleolar surface is triangular. The bones

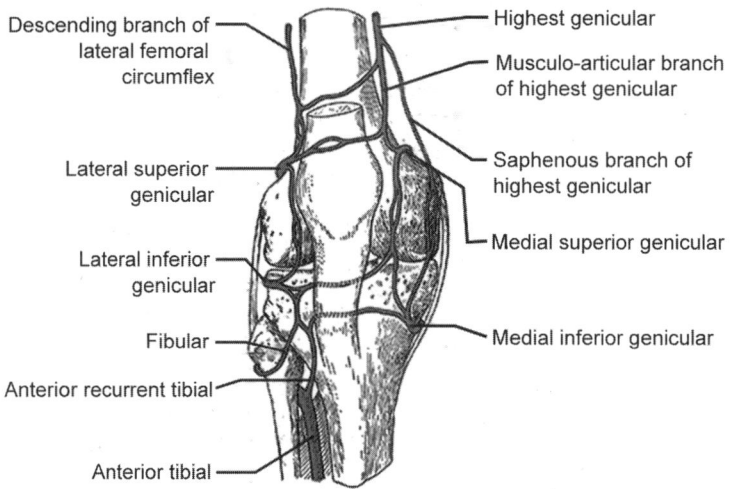

Fig. 6.17: Blood supply of knee joint

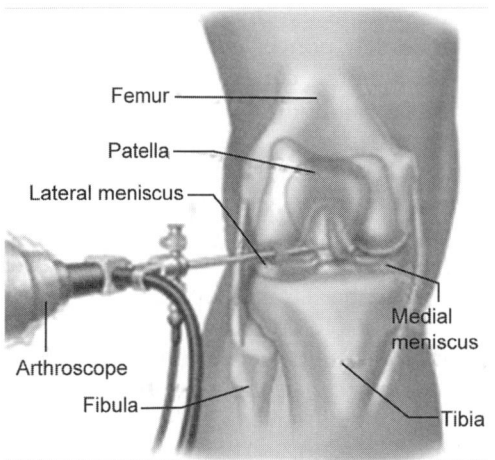

Fig. 6.18: Arthroscopy of knee joint

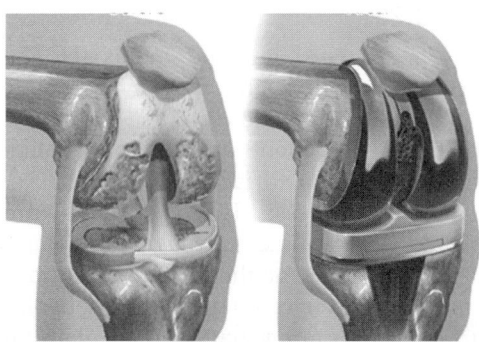

Fig. 6.19: Total knee replacement

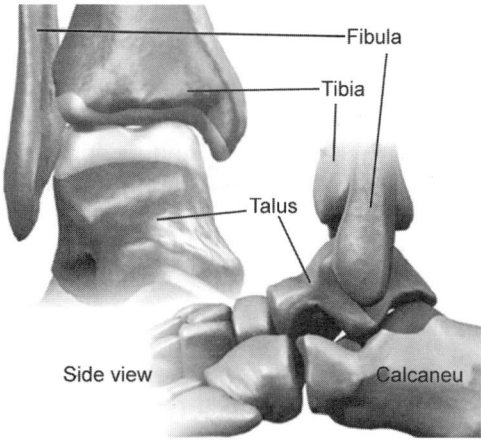

Fig. 6.20: Ankle joint

are held together by fibrous capsule, deltoid ligament (medial ligament), talofibular ligaments, calcaneofibular ligaments.

Movements taking place at the joint: Dorsiflexion and plantar flexion.

Muscles Producing Movements

Dorsiflexion: Tibialis anterior, extensor digitorum longus, extensor hallucis longus.

Plantar flexion: Gastrocnemius, soleus, tibialis posterior.

Applied aspects: Ankle fractures are common and often associated with ligament.

CHAPTER 7

Physiology of Muscle Contraction

Muscle is generally divided into three types skeletal, cardiac and smooth.

The main functions of skeletal muscle tissue are development of tension and shortening. The effect of muscle activity is transferred to the skeleton by means of tendons.

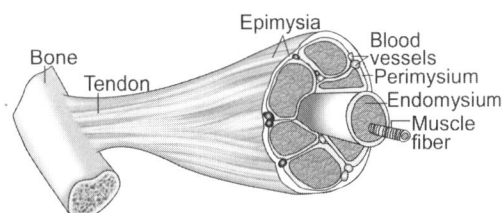

Fig. 7.1: Organization of skeletal muscle

■ SKELETAL MUSCLE

Composed of numerous parallel elongated cells referred to as muscle fibers or myofibers (Fig. 7.1). There are about 10–100 μm in diameter and vary with the length of the muscle often extending its entire length. The muscle fiber is composed of smaller fibrous structures 1 μm in diameter myofibrils. Each myofibril is further subdivided into thick and thin myofilaments.

Thin filaments are about 7 μm wide and 1.0 μm long and thick filaments are about 10–14 mm wide and 1.6 μm long. The arrangement of thick and thin filaments produces the cross striated appearance of the muscle, which results from a regular repetition of dense cross bands (1.6 μm in length) separated by less dense bands (Fig. 7.2). The dense cross bands are referred as A bands (anisotropic) contain the thick filaments, arranged neatly in parallel. The less dense segments the I bands contain this filaments which extend symmetrically in opposite directions from a dense thin line, the Z line.

The width of the I band varies with the degree of stretch or shortening of the

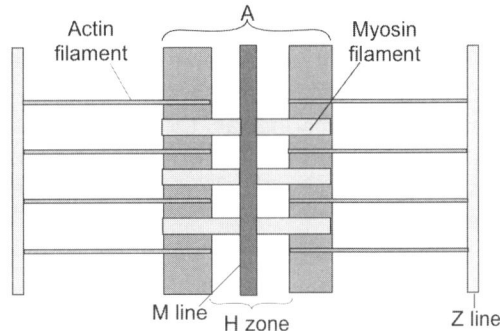

Fig. 7.2: Arrangement of thick and thin filaments in skeletal muscle

muscle fiber. Total width of thin filament Z line complex is 2.05 μm. The gap between the terminations of the thin filaments is called the H zone and the darker area in the center of H zone is the M line.

■ SARCOMERE

Sarcomere is the fundamental contractile unit of muscle. Sarcomere consists of the region between two consecutive Z lines, thus this hrs unit consists of one A band and one half I band at each end of the A band. In cross section at the site of overlap between thick and thin filaments, each thick filament

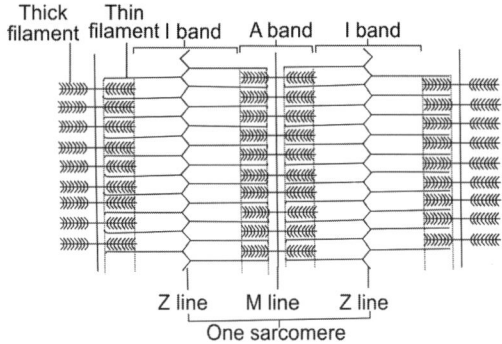

Fig. 7.3: Sarcomere

is surrounded by 6 thin filaments and each thin filament by 3 thick filament (Fig. 7.3).

■ SARCOLEMMA

The sarcolemma is the outer membrane surrounding each muscle fiber. It consists of the membrane proper the plasmalemma and a basement membrane. The plasma membrane conduct the wave of depolarization originating at the motor end plate over the entire cell surface to initiate contraction. It acts as a shield of muscle fiber.

Tubular extensions of sarcolemma called T (transverse) tubules or sarcotubules, extend deep into the fiber at the level of Z line. The spread of excitation to deep lying myofibris rapidly is helped by these membranes.

Sarcoplasm of muscle fiber consists of the contents of the sarcolemma, including mitochondria sarcoplasmic reticulum and Golgi apparatus (Fig. 7.4).

Sarcoplasmic Reticulum—Functions

- Release of Ca^{++} during muscle contraction
- Sequestration and storage of Ca^{++} during muscle relaxation.

Proteins of the Contractile Elements

This filaments are composed primarily of three types of protein, actin, tropomyosin

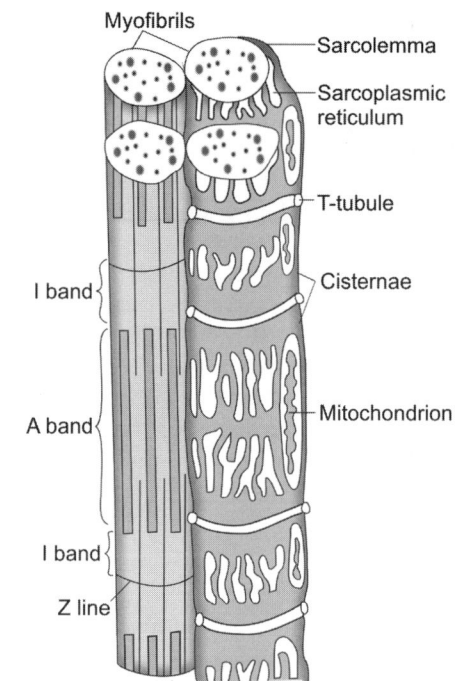

Fig. 7.4: Sarcolemma cut away from muscle fiber to show individual myofibrils

and troponin in a ratio of 7:1:1. The 'functional unit' necessary for relaxation consists of 7 actin monomers.

Tropomyosin

I Troponin Complex

Actin: In vitro actin molecules exist in two states. *G-actin* and *F-actin*.

G-actin: is a monomeric globular protein with a molecular weight of 42,000 and a diameter of 4–5 nm. Actin monomer contains binding sites for other actin monomers, myosin, tropomyosin, troponin I, ATP and cations.

F-actin: It is a fibrous polymer consisting of approximately 300 or more monomers of Gactin is formed in vitro when salts at physiological ionic strengths are added to gactin monomers. Thin filament consists of two strands of factin polymers intertwined as a double stranded helix.

Tropomyosin: Elongated protein which consists of two double helical chains each with a molecular weight of 35,000 wound around each other to form a coil. It lies in each of the two grooves 180° apart formed by the double stranded helix, consisting at factin. Each molecule of tropomyosin extends over seven actin monomers.

Troponin: Troponin consists of a complex of three separate proteins, troponin T, troponin C, and troponin I. Each troponin complex is bound to a tropomyosin molecular. Only actin and myosin are directly involved in tension generation. The tropomyosin troponin complex regulate the actin interaction, hence are called regulatory protein, troponin T binds the other two troponin submits to tropomysin. Troponin C is the Ca^{++} acceptor protein of troponin complex. It binds to troponin T and I which induce inhibitory confirmation of the actin tropomyosin filament.

Other Proteins

- *L-actinin:* Localized at Z line. It has a role in factin getting attached to Z line. Desmin and vimentin are proteins with same function present in Z line.
- *Titin:* Connects Z lines to M line. This provide elasticity to muscle.
- *Dystrophin:* Connects thin filament to glycoprotein to the sarcolemma. It provides structural support and strength to muscle fibril. Congenital defect in it cause muscular dystrophy.

Thick Filament (Fig. 7.5)

Thick filaments consists primarily of myosin and to a lesser extend other proteins.
1. Myosin molecule with 2 heavy chain intertwined and 4 light chains
2. Organization of thick filament
3. Arrangement of tropomyosin actin and troponin in thin filament.

Myosin: It is a dinner of molecular weight 4,80,000. It consists of two globular heads which hydrolyze ATP and interact with actin. It has a rod like regeon which confers stability to the molecule.

Light meromyosin (LMM): Tail portion.
Heavy meromyosin (HMM): Globular end.

Treatment of myosin with trypsin split the protein to above two components.

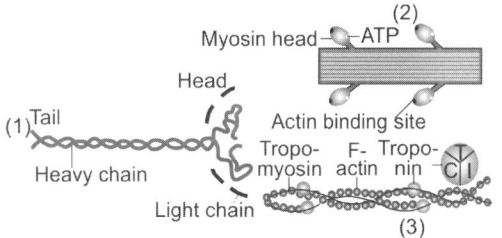

Fig. 7.5: Thick filament and thin filament

Other Proteins of Thick Filament

C-Protein: Associated with A band on either side of M-line.

■ PROPERTIES OF SKELETAL MUSCLE (FIG. 7.6)

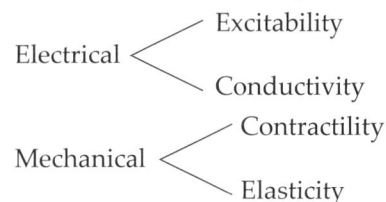

Electrical characteristics: Resting membrane potential (RMP) of skeletal muscle is 90 mv, absolute refractory period 1–3 ms.

Depolarization is a manifestation of Na^+ influx and repolarization a manifestation of K^+ efflux.

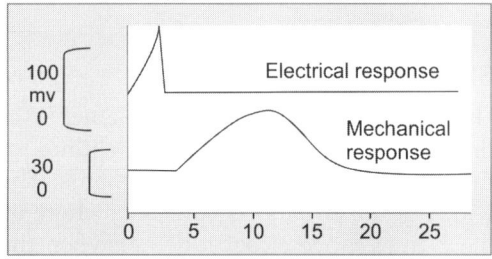

Fig. 7.6: Potential change and tension plotted on the same abscissa

Mechancial characteristics: A single action potential (AP) causes a brief contraction followed by relaxation. This response is called a muscle twitch.

The AP, and the twitch are plotted on the same time scale. Twitch starts about 2 ms after the start of depolarization, before repolarization is complete.

■ MECHANISM OF MUSCLE CONTRACTION

- An AP travel along a motor nerve to its endings on the muscle fibers.
- The nerve seneates the neurotransmitter called acetylcholine at their endings.
- ACh acts on a local area of the muscle fiber membrane to open multiple. ACh gated channels through protein molecules in muscle fiber membrane
- Opening of ACh channels causes influx of Na^+ to muscle fiber which initiates the AP of muscle fiber.
- AP travels along muscle fiber membrane, depolarizes the membrane, travels deeply and causes SR to release large quantities of Ca^{++} ions into myofibrils.
- Ca^{++} ions initiates attractive forces between the actin and myosin filaments, causing them to slide together called contractile process.
- After a fraction of a second, the Ca^{++} ions are pumped back into the SR, where they are stored until new muscle AP come along. This removal of Ca^{++} from myofibrils causes muscle contraction to cease.

Sliding Filament Theory

Shortening of the contractile elements in the muscle brought about by sliding of the thin filament over thick filaments. The width of the A band is constant, where as the Z lines move closer together when the muscle contracts and farther apart when it is stretched.

Power stroke: The sliding during muscle contraction occurs when the myosin heads binds firmly to actin band at the junction of the head with the neck and then detach. Cycling of many myosin heads produce gross muscle contraction. Each power stroke shorten the sarcomere 10 nm.

Excitation Contraction Coupling

The process by which depolarization of the muscle fiber initiates contraction is called excitation contraction coupling. In resting muscle troponin I is tightly bound to actin and tropomyosin corers the sites where myosin heads binds to actin. This troponin–tropomyosin complex constitutes a 'relaxing protein' that inhibit the interaction between actin and myosin. When the Ca^{++} released by the AP binds to troponin C, the binding of troponin I to actin is weakened and it permits the tropomyosin to move laterally. This uncovers binding sites for myosis heads and ATP is then split and contractions occurs. 7 mysosin binding sites are uncovered for each molecule of troponin that binds a Ca^{++} ion. Using Ca^{++} Mg^{++} ATP ase sacroplasmic reticulum reaccumulates Ca^{++} by actively transporting it into the longitudinal portion of reticulum. ATP provides energy for both contraction and relaxation. The ATP of previous contraction used for next relaxation. If transport of Ca^{++} into reticulum is inhibited relaxation does not occur even though there are no more AP. The resulting sustained contraction is called contracture.

Depolarization of the T tubule membrane activates the SR via Dihydropyridine receptors which are voltage gated Ca^{++} channels in the T tubule membrane. DHP receptor serves as a voltage sensor and triggers that unlocks release of Ca^{++} from near by SR. Ca^{++} Channel in the SR that opens to permit the outpouring of Ca^{++} is not voltage gated and is called Ryanodine receptor.

Another name for the sliding filament theory of AF Huxely is cross bridge theory — the thin filaments moving towards the center form cross bridges with the globular heads of myosin also called Ratchet theory.

Mechanics of Skeletal Muscle Contraction

Motor unit: All the muscle fibers innervated by a single motor nerve fiber leaving spinal cord are called a motor unit. Small muscle that react rapidly have a few muscle fibers in each motor unit. Large muscles that do not require very fine control have several hundred muscle fibers in each motor unit.

Simple Muscle Twitch

The contraction followed by relaxation of a skeletal muscle in response to a single stimulus is called a SMT. Duration 0.1 second. LP – 0.01 second, CP – 0.04 second, RP – 0.05 second.

Summation: Means adding together of individual twitch contraction to increase the intensity of overall muscle contraction (Fig. 7.7).
- *Temporal summation:* By increasing the frequency of stimuli also called wave or frequency summation.
- *Multifiber summation:* By increasing the number of motor units contracting simultaneously.

Tetanus (Fig. 7.8)

When the frequency of stimuli increases and reaches a critical level, the successive contractions are so rapid that they fuse together and the contraction appears to be

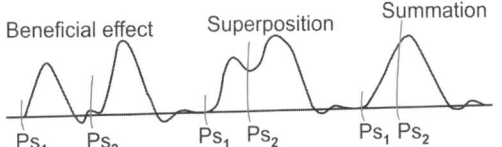

Fig. 7.7: Effect of successive stimuli

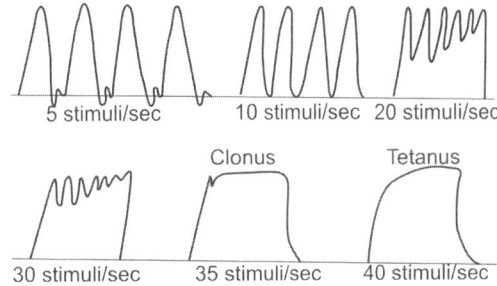

Fig. 7.8: Genesis of tetanus

smooth and continuous called tetanization. CFF (Critical fusion frequency) $\propto \dfrac{1}{CP}$.

Treppe: When a series of maximal stimuli is delivered to skeletal muscle at a frequency just below the tetanizing frequency there is an increase in tension developed during each twitch until after several contractions a uniform tension per contraction is reached. This phenomenon is known as treppe or staircase phenomenon. Increase availability of Ca^{++} for binding to Troponin C is believed to be the cause of treppe. The increase of Ca^{++} ions in the cytosol because of release of more and more ions from the sarcoplasmic reticulum with each muscle action potential and failure to recapture the ions immediately is the physiological basis for this.

Skeletal Muscle Tone

Even when muscles are at rest, a certain amount of tautness remains which is called muscle tone. It result from a low rate of nerve impulse coming from the spinal cord. It is controlled partly by impulses transmitted from brain to exterior motor neurons and partly by impulses originate in muscle spindle of muscle itself.

Muscle Fatigue

Fatigue is defined as the inability of muscle to respond to a stimulus following repeated and strong stimulation for a prolonged period (Fig. 7.9).

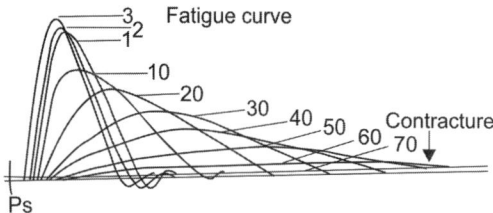

Fig. 7.9: Phenomenon of fatigue in skeletal muscle

Causes of Fatigue

- Depletion of energy producing substances like glycogen, creatine phosphate PO_4, etc.
- Depletion of neurotransmitter ACh
- Anoxia
- Interruption of blood flow through contracting muscle
- Accumulation of metabolic wastes like lactic acid in high concentrations.

Muscular Dystrophy

Mutations in the genes coding for the various components of dystrophies—glycoprotein complex cause muscular dystrophy, charactorized by progressive muscle weakness.

Types

Duchene's muscular dystrophy: X linked fatal usually by 30 years.
Milder form: Becker's muscular dystrophy. Dystrophin is present but altered or of decreased in amount.
Limb: Girdle muscular dystrophy—mutations of genes coding for sarcoglycans.

■ CARDIAC MUSCLE

- Cardiac muscle cells have single nucleus
- Due to presence of gap junctions and intercalated disks the cardiac muscle is behave functionally like a syncitium.
- Each cardiac muscle is 100 μm long, 15–20 μm wide and about 5 μm thick.
- The T tubules have diameter more than twice that of skeletal muscle and lie at Z line. In skeletal muscle T tubule lie at A-I junction.
- Terminal cistern is narrow and form a diad with T. Tubule. In skeletal muscle T tubule and two terminal cisterns form a triad.
- The release of calcium ions from terminal cisterns is Ca^{++} dependent in cardiac muscle (In contrast in skeletal muscle—DHP receptor in the T tubule is a voltage sensor. On the other hand, the terminal cistern of SR contains a ryanodine receptor which is a Ca^{++} channel connected by a foot protein to DHP receptor.

  In cardiac muscle the DHP receptor in T tubules has a calcium channel within it. As the action potential reaches the T tubule DHP receptor Ca^{++} ions are released through the calcium-channel.

  When AP reaches DHP receptor, Ca^{++} released from SR through SERCA to cytosol. In skeletal muscle a conformational change take place leading to displacement of foot protein of ryanodine receptor and opening of Ca^{++} channel in the ryanodine receptor, and this calcium come from the ECF through T tubule.
- The intracellular Ca^{++} concentration can be increased by sympathomimetic agents and digitalis in cardiac muscle.

  But in skeletal muscle contraction all the calcium binding sites on troponin C are saturated by Ca^{++} ions released from terminal cistern. Conversely Ca^{++} Binding sites on troponin C are not saturated by Ca^{++} released into cytosol during normal cardiac muscle contraction (Fig. 7.10).
- Cardiac muscle can not be tetanized. Summation too is not possible because of prolonged refractory period of cardiac muscle.
- Cardiac muscle shows rhythmicity. They show autorhythmicity and pacemaker potential.

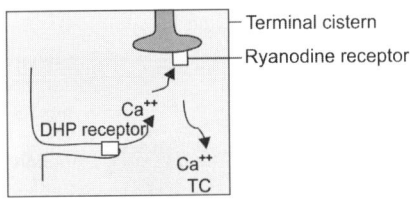

Fig. 7.10: Contraction in cardiac muscle

- Cardiac muscle do not show fatigue. Ca^{++}-dependent Ca^{++}: Release in cardiac muscle cell.

■ SMOOTH MUSCLE

- Smooth muscles are innervated by autonomic nerves—sympathetic or parasympathetic. Postganglionic neurons show swollen ends or varicosities where they end wear the smooth muscle (Figs 7.11A and B). There varicosities contain neurotransmitter contained in vesicles.
- Unlike N-M junction no motor end plate. NT are secreated into interstitial fluid which reach the smooth muscle cell by diffusion.
- SM muscle receptors are muscarinic in contrast to nicotinic skeletal muscle.
- Smooth muscles contain single nucleus. They have a length of 10–500 μm and width of 5–10 μm

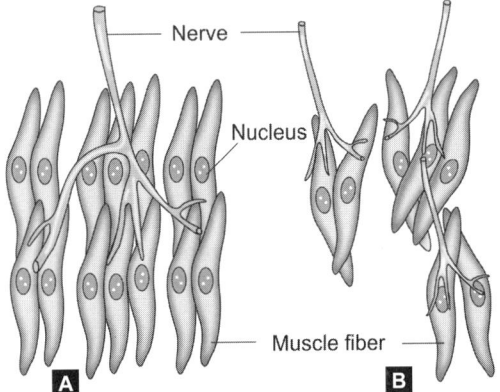

Figs 7.11A and B: Smooth muscle fibers with innervation

- There is no sarcomere. Thick and thin filaments are scattered in cytoplasm.
- Thin filaments are connected to dense bodies and dense bodies are substitutes to Z line.
- The thin filaments lack troponin. Instead a calcium binding protein calmodulin is present.
- T-Tubules are absent. Instead small depressions called caveola present on surface membrane.
- Ca^{++} can enter smooth muscle cell and activates it in 3 ways.
  - NT like ACh on ligand-gated Ca^{++} channel canting entry to Ca++ in to the cell.
  - Voltage gated Ca^{++} channels open in response to AP permitting Ca^{++} entry in to cell
  - Ca^{++} released from SR following activation of IP_3 receptor in skeletal or cardiac muscle
- Interaction between thick and thin filaments of smooth muscle are radically different.
  - One of the 4 light chains around myosin head is phosporelated by MLCK catalyzed by calmodulin which itself is activated by ionic Ca^{++}
  - This reaction leads to cross bridge cycling at a rapid rate using energy from ATP. The enzyme actin–Myosin-ATP ase catalyzes the break down of ATP and releases the energy.
- MLCP (myosin light chain phosphates) causes dephosphorylation. But this does not always lead to relaxation, but slower cycling of cross bridges. The myosin heads stay attached to actin filaments for a longer period. This is known as latch-bridge formation.
- Latch-bridge increases the number of myosin heads attached to actin at a given moment and increase in the

force of contraction. But it requires low expenditure of ATP, and this helps to maintain tone of smooth muscle with almost no requirement of energy.
- The latch-bridges get detached with relaxation of smooth muscle only when cytosolic Ca^{++} concentration is reduced to resting levels or Ca-Calmodulin complex dissociates.
- *Plasticity:* Smooth muscles like those of urinary bladder show plasticity. This is the property by which the tension in smooth muscle return to original level even after prolonged stretching or shortening. Thus, smooth muscles do not show the typical length tension relationship as seen in skeletal or cardiac muscle.

■ NEUROMUSCULAR TRANSMISSION

Skeletal muscle fibers are innervated by large myelinated nerve fibers of motor nervous originating in the anterior horns of spinal cord. The nerve ending makes a junction called neuromuscular junction with the muscle fiber near the midpoint of the muscle fiber. AP in the muscle fiber travels in both directions towards the muscle fiber ends.

N-M Junction (Figs 7.12 and 7.13)

The axons supplying a skeletal muscle fiber losses its myelin sheath and divide into a number of terminal buttons or end feet. End

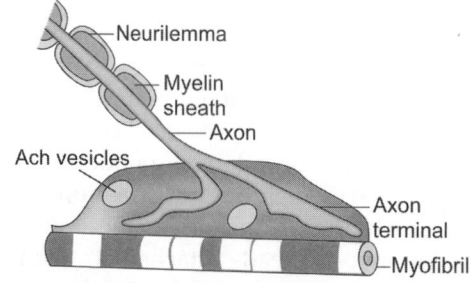

Fig. 7.12: Neuromuscular junction

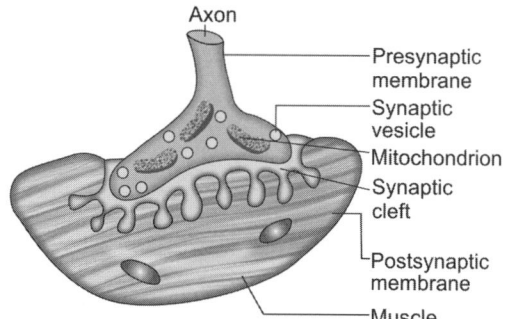

Fig. 7.13: CS neuromuscular junction

feet contain small clear vesicles containing acetylcholine. Motor end plate is the thickened portion of muscle membrane. The end feet fit into depression in the motor end plate. Underneath the nerve ending end plate is thrown into junctional folds. The space between the nerve and end feet is similar to synaptic cleft of synapses and is occupied by spongy reticular fibers. This form the basal lamina along which ECF diffuses. Junctional fold subneural left is formed on the muscle membrane which increases surface area on which neurotransmitter can act. The mitochondria in the axon terminal provide energy for synthesis of NT which is packed into synaptic vesicles. Basal lamina contains large quantities of enzyme anticholinesterase.

This anticholinesterase is capable of destroying ACh. On the inner surface of the neural membrane are linear dense bars. On each side of dense bar voltage gated Ca^{++} channel penetrate the membrane. When the action potential spreads over the terminal these channels open and large quantities of Ca^{++} diffuse into terminal. Ca^{++} ions attract ACh vesicles to neural membrane, some vesicles empty their contents into synaptic space by exocytosis.

Effect of ACh on Postsynaptic Membrane

ACh receptors or ACh gated ion channels located near the mouth of the subneural clefts lying below the dense bar area are present at the end plate. ACh channel remains constricted until 2 ACh molecules attach to the receptor proteins. This attachment produces a conformational charge that opens the channel and Na^+, K^+ and Ca^{++} ions move inside. Negative ions such as Cl^- are repelled by negative charges in the mouth of channel. The negative potential –80 to –90 on the inside of fiber pulls Na^+ inward and prevent K^+ efflux. This produces a local potential charge at the muscle fiber membrane called the end plate potential which initiate AP to cause muscle contraction.

Anticholinestrase Enzyme

ACh released into the synaptic space continue to activate ACh receptors until it get removed. Methods of removal of ACh:
- Destroyed by enzyme anticholinesterase
- Diffuses out of synaptic space

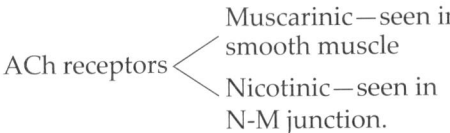

ACh receptors — Muscarinic—seen in smooth muscle
Nicotinic—seen in N-M junction.

Sequence of Events During N-M Transmission

- Spread of AP over nerve terminal opens up Ca^{++} channel opening and diffusion of Ca^{++} from synaptic space into nerve terminal.
- The Ca^{++} attract ACh vesicle to neural membranes adjacent to dense bars.
- Vesicle fuse with neural membrane, exocytosis empty ACh into synaptic space.
- ACh diffuses to ACh receptors; opening of ACh channels cause diffusion of Na^+ to inside muscle fiber.
- Generation of local potential EPP
- Depolarization of muscle membrane to firing level, and AP conducted in both directions along muscle fiber.
- Muscle contraction.

Myasthenia Gravis

It is a serious and fatal disease in which skeletal muscles are weak and tire easily. It is produced due to formation of circulating antibodies to the muscle type of nicotinic acetyl choline receptors. Autoimmunity developing to ACh receptors make the end plate potentials too weak to adequately stimulate the muscle fiber. Usual cause of death in myasthenia gravis is respiratory muscle paralysis.

Treatment: Neostigmine or some other Anticholinesterase drug.

SKELETAL MUSCLES

Bones may be regarded as a series of rigid levers, freely movable about fixed points, the joints, which act as fulcrums. The integration of the muscular and nervous systems, in association with the bones of the skeleton, forms an effective apparatus capable of a wide range of complex activities.

Each muscle is an individual organ, having its own blood supply, lymphatics and nerves. Muscles consist mainly of muscle fibers supported and strengthened by connective tissue. They are attached to each other and to surrounding tissues by the connective tissue components of the fasciae, tendons and aponeurosis.

Fasciae

The whole body is enclosed in an envelope of fibrous connective tissue called fascia. The fascia consists of two layers.

The superficial fascia lies just beneath the surface of the skin and is continuous with the dermis. It is a loose layer composed of fibrous areolar tissue impregnated with adipose tissue. The distribution of the adipose tissue is different in the two sexes, being more abundant in females. It acts as a thermal insulator, protecting the body from loss of heat. The superficial fascia varies in thickness, being thickest over the lower anterior abdominal wall and thinnest over the face, the neck and the dorsal aspects of the hands and feet.

The deep fascia is composed of dense fibrous tissue and lies immediately beneath the superficial layer. It encloses the muscles, blends with ligaments and provides attachment to bony surfaces. Extensions of the deep fascia separate muscles into functioning groups, enclose viscera, blood vessels and nerves, and help to maintain the position of these structures. In some parts of the body the deep fascia is particularly thick and strong, e.g. the pelvic fascia lining the pelvis; the fascia lata surrounding the muscles of the thigh; the palmar fascia in the hand and the plantar fascia in the sole of the foot (see Appendix).

Attachments of Muscle

At the extremities of the muscles the connective tissue of the endomysium, perimysium and epimysium unite to form strong, fibrous, non-elastic cords called tendons. Tendons attach a muscle to the periosteum of a bone, and vary in length from a fraction of an inch to more than a foot (Figs 7.14A and B). Sometimes they form a broad, flat expansion called an aponeurosis.

Most skeletal muscles are attached to bones, although a few, such as the muscles of facial expression, are attached to the soft tissues of the face, and others are attached to cartilage or ligaments.

Some tendons, for example those of the wrist and ankle, which pass under ligamentous bands or through bony tunnels, are enclosed in sheaths of synovial membrane called tendon sheaths. These facilitate smooth, frictionless movement of the tendons.

In situations where a muscle or tendon comes in contact with or moves over a bony prominence, or where the skin moves directly over bone, the pressure is relieved by a small synovial sac called a bursa. Bursae are usually located near joints, for example the olecranon bursa over the olecranon process of the ulna; the prepatellar bursa where the skin moves over the front of the patella.

Bursae may become inflamed, usually as a result of repeated minor injury (e.g. prepatellar bursitis or 'housemaid's knee').

Actions of Muscles

The main mass of a muscle is termed the belly, and lies along the shaft of a bone, never over a joint. Muscles are firmly attached at each end to different bones and it is the tendons which cross a joint. When a muscle contracts, a pull is exerted on both bones but one is stabilized by isometric contractions of other muscles and the contraction pulls the other bone toward it. For example, the belly

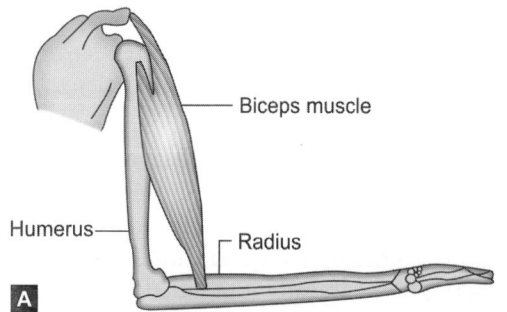
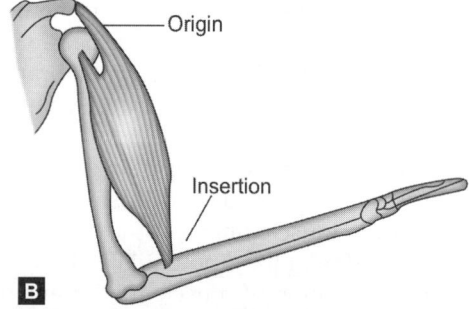

Figs 7.14A and B: Muscles are attached to two bones across a joint. Contraction of the muscle pulls on the bone into which the muscle is inserted, producing movement

of the biceps muscle lies parallel to the shaft of the humerus in the upper arm. The two tendons at the upper end of the biceps are attached to the scapula, while the tendon at the lower end crosses the elbow joint and is attached to the radius. Contraction of the biceps muscle draws the lower arm toward the upper (Fig. 7.5).

The fixed point of muscle attachment is called the origin, while the movable point of attachment is called the insertion. In the example above the muscle attachments into the scapula form the origin of the biceps muscle and the attachment into the radius forms the insertion. Muscles which stabilize the bone giving origin to the muscle are known as fixation muscles.

Muscles which bend a limb at a joint are called flexors. Muscles which straighten a limb at a joint are called extensors. Muscles which move a limb away from the midline of the body are known as abductors, while those that move the limb toward the midline are called adductors. Some muscles cause rotation of a limb. In movements of the wrist joint, supinators turn the hand palm upward and pronators turn the palm frontward. In movements of the ankle joint dorsiflexors turn the foot upward and plantar flexors extend the foot toward the ground. Muscles which raise a part of the body are called elevators and those which lower a part are known as depressors.

Movements are complex and the performance of any given movement, e.g. flexion of the elbow joint, requires the co-ordination of several muscles. Muscles which initiate and maintain a movement are called prime movers or agonists, while those which oppose a movement or reverse it are known as antagonists. Thus when the biceps muscle contracts to raise the lower arm towards the shoulder it is the prime mover. The triceps muscle, which can oppose this action and straighten the elbow, is the antagonist. However, actions which require a joint to be held rigid will cause simultaneous contraction of both prime movers and antagonists.

Synergists are muscles which assist a prime mover by stabilizing a joint crossed by the tendon of the prime mover, thus allowing it to produce a more effective movement.

Muscles may be named according to one or more of the following:
- Function, e.g. flexors, extensors, abductors, etc.
- Attachments, e.g. sternomastoid.
- Shape, e.g. deltoid (like Greek letter D or δ).
- Position or direction, e.g. pectoralis major (large breast muscle), rectus abdominus (straight abdominal muscle), the oblique and straight muscles of the eye.
- Formation e.g. biceps = two heads; triceps = three heads; quadriceps = four heads.

■ PRINCIPAL GROUPS OF MUSCLES
Muscles of the Head and Neck

The muscles of the head, face and neck are too numerous to describe in detail (Fig. 7.15). They can, however, be divided into several main groups.
- Muscles of the scalp (occipito-frontalis) and the ear and of the eye.
- The muscles of facial expression which are supplied by the VIIth cranial nerve.

The orbicularis oculi are circular muscle surrounding each eye which when contracted act as sphincters and close the eyes tightly. The orbicularis oris is situated in the lips between the skin and the mucous membrane of the mouth and has a similar type of action. The buccinator is the principal muscle of the cheek and forms the lateral well of the mouth. It is used in chewing and sucking.

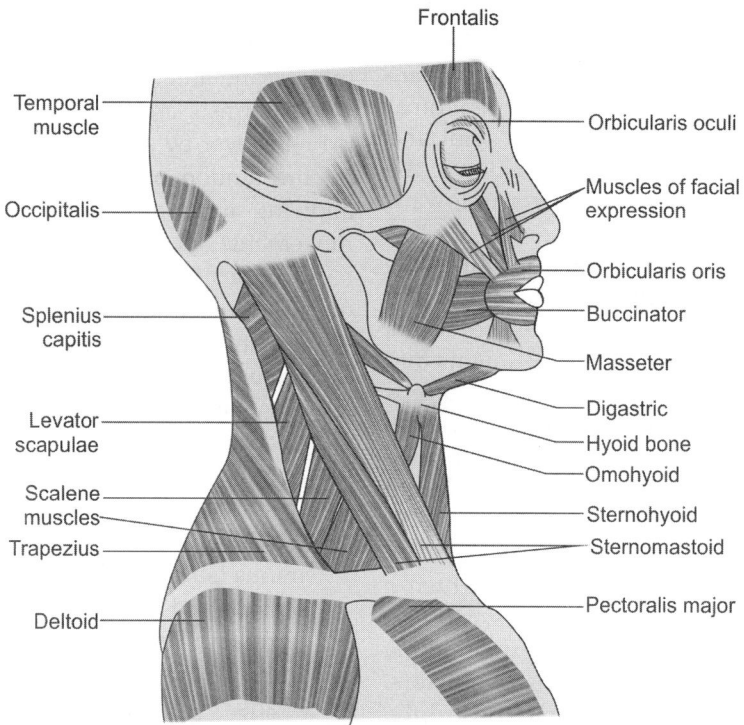

Fig. 7.15: Muscles of the face and neck

- The muscles of mastication which move the lower jaw are supplied by branches of the Vth cranial nerve.

    The temporal muscle arises from the temporal fossa of the skull. Its fibers converge into a strong tendon which is inserted into the coronoid process of the mandible. The masseter muscle is quadrilateral in shape and arises above from the zygomatic arch of the temporal bone. It is inserted into the outer surface of the lower jaw anterior to the angle.
- Muscles of the neck, attaching the head to the trunk.

Superficial Muscles

The platysma extends from the lower jaw in a thin flat sheet to the deep fascia on the front of the chest.

The sternomastoid is an important muscle extending upwards from the manubrium of the sternum and medial end of the clavicle to the mastoid process of the temporal bone. When operating singly each muscle rotates the head towards the opposite side; when acting together they flex the neck.

The trapezius is a large triangular muscle situated at the back of the neck. It arises from the occipital bone of the skull and from the spines of all the cervical and thoracic vertebrae. Its upper fibers are inserted into the lateral third of the clavicle, the middle fibers into the acromion process and the lower fibers into the spine of the scapula. It may also be considered as one of the muscles of the shoulder girdle attaching the scapula to the trunk.

There are also a number of muscles in the front of the neck extending (i) from the lower jaw to the hyoid bone and (ii) from the hyoid bone and thyroid cartilage to the sternum. These are closely related to the trachea and thyroid gland.

Deep Muscles

Examples are the scalene muscles extending from the cervical vertebrae to the first and second ribs.
- *Muscles of:*
  - *The pharynx:* The constrictor muscles which take part in the act of swallowing; also the muscles of the tongue and floor of the mouth
  - *The larynx:* External muscles which move the larynx as a whole and internal muscles which affect the tension of the vocal cords and are used in voice production.

Muscles of the Shoulder Girdle and Upper Limb

- Muscles attaching the scapula to the trunk, e.g. deep rhomboids, superficial—trapezius, serratus anterior.
- Muscles attaching the humerus
  - To the scapula, e.g. supraspinatus, infraspinatus, subscapularis, deltoid.
  - To the chest wall, e.g. pectoralis major and minor, latissimus dorsi.
- Muscles of the arm

  The most important muscles of the arm are:
  - The biceps, which has its origin by two heads, long and short, from the scapula. The long head arises from the top of the glenoid cavity; the short head from the tip of the coracoid process. It is inserted into the bicipital tubercle below the head of the radius. Passing as it does over two joints, it can produce movements at both. Its main actions are to act as a powerful supinator of the forearm and to flex the elbow joint. It also helps in the forward movement of the shoulder joint.

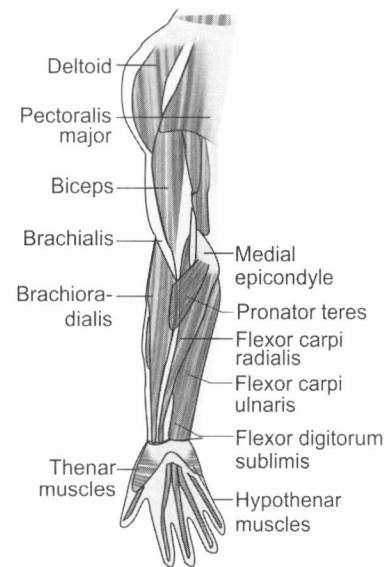

Fig. 7.16: Muscles of the right upper limb—anterior aspect

  - The brachialis, which arises from the front of the shaft of the humerus and is inserted into the ulna (Fig. 7.16).
  - The triceps, situated at the back of the arm, passes from the scapula to the olecranon process of the ulna (Fig. 7.17). It therefore extends the elbow joint, and helps to support the shoulder joint and draw the arm backwards.
- *Muscles of the forearm (Fig. 7.18):* The muscles of the anterior aspect may be divided into three groups:
  1. The main group consists of superficial and deep muscles. The superficial muscles are attached above to the medial epicondyle of the humerus and pass to the fingers; these include the flexor digitorum sublimis, which not only flexes the fingers but also the wrist and elbow joints. The deep muscles include the flexor digitorum profundus arising from the ulna, which does

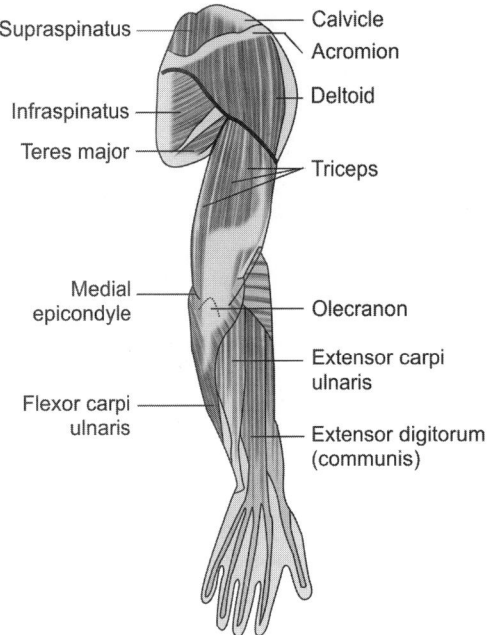

Fig. 7.17: Muscles of the right upper limb—posterior aspect

not move the elbow joint but flexes the wrist and fingers.
2. Muscles which flex the elbow and wrist only, passing from the humerus above to the wrist bones below' (flexor carpi radialis and flexor carpi ulnaris).
3. Muscles whose main action is concerned with pronation and supination (pronator teres, pronator quadratus and brachio-radialis or supinator longus).

The muscles of the posterior aspect may be divided into:
- The extensor muscles of the wrist and fingers (extensor digitorum communis) which, arising from the lateral epicondyle of the humerus, also extend the elbow joint.
- The extensors of the wrist (extensor carpi radialis and extensor carpi ulnaris).

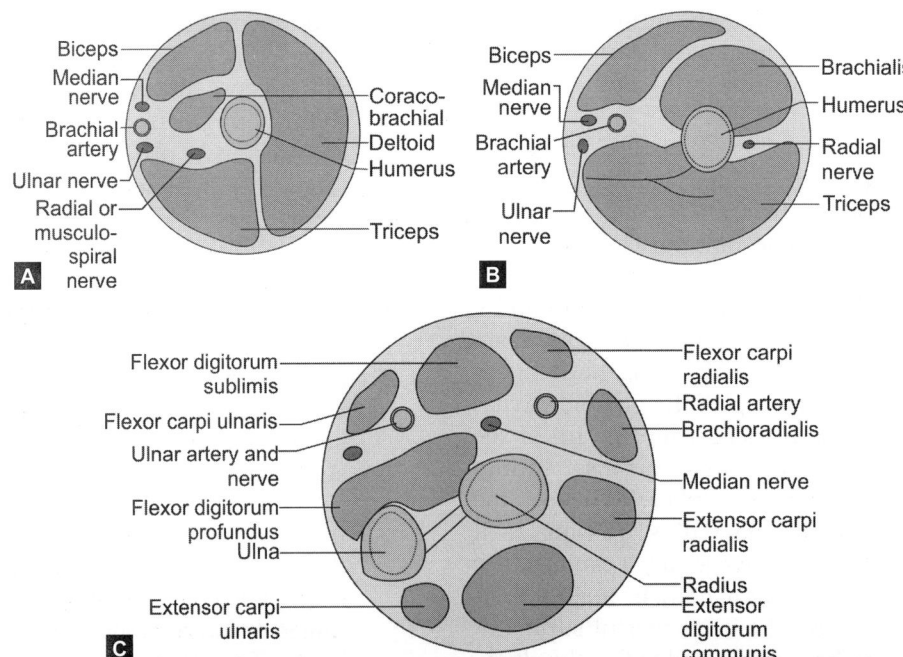

Fig. 7.18: Diagram illustrating the position of the most important structures in the upper limb. **A.** In upper third of arm; **B.** In lower third of arm; **C.** Middle of forearm

- *Muscles of the hand and fingers:* The tendons of the flexor muscles in front and the extensor muscles behind are inserted into the bases of the terminal phalanges of the digits. Slips are also given to the other phalanges.

  The thumb has separate muscles which, however, correspond to the main flexor and extensor groups in the forearm. Special short muscles situated in the palm of the hand move the thumb and form the thenar eminence at the base of the thumb. The prominence on the ulnar side of the hand at the base of the little finger is called the hypothenar eminence. Arising between the metacarpal bones and inserted into the phalanges are the lumbrical and interosseous muscles.

Muscles of the Trunk

The muscles of the trunk may be divided into (i) those of the thorax, and (ii) those of the abdomen.

Muscles of the Thoracic Wall

The superficial muscles include:
- The pectoralis major, a large fan-shaped muscle on the upper anterior part of the chest which also forms the anterior part of the axilla; and the pectoralis minor, a smaller triangular muscle lying deep to the pectoralis major. These muscles arise from the anterior aspect of the sternum, ribs and costal cartilages and are inserted into the upper end of the humerus and coracoid process of the scapula respectively.
- The serratus anterior arising from the ribs passes backwards to the vertebral border of the scapula.
- The intercostal muscles (eleven pairs) which pass from the lower border of one rib to the upper border of the rib below. They are formed by two distinct layers, the fibers of which pass in opposite directions. The internal intercostals are directed downward and backward; the more superficial external intercostals pass downward and forward. They are important muscles of respiration.

The Diaphragm

The diaphragm is the large dome-shaped partition separating the thoracic cavity from the abdominal cavity. It is formed partly by muscle (around the circumference) and partly by a flattened tendon called the central tendon of the diaphragm. It is attached to the circumference of the thoracic cavity:
- In front to the lower end of the sternum (sternal part)
- On either side to the lower six ribs (costal part)
- Posteriorly to the first two lumbar vertebrae by two slips called the crura (legs) of the diaphragm (lumbar part).

The heart and pericardium are related to the central portion of its upper surface. On either side it is covered by pleura and is related to the bases of the lungs. Its lower concave surface, largely covered by peritoneum, is related on the right side and centrally to the upper surface of the liver; on the left side it is in contact with the fundus of the stomach and the spleen.

In the posterior part of the diaphragm, close to its origin from the lumbar vertebrae, are a number of openings (hiatuses) for the passage of the following structures (Fig. 7.19):
- The aorta, in the mid-line
- The esophagus, slightly to the left
- The inferior vena cava, slightly to the right.

The diaphragm is a very important muscle of respiration and is supplied by the phrenic nerve from the cervical plexus. During inspiration the muscle of the diaphragm contracts so that the diaphragm becomes flattened towards the abdomen,

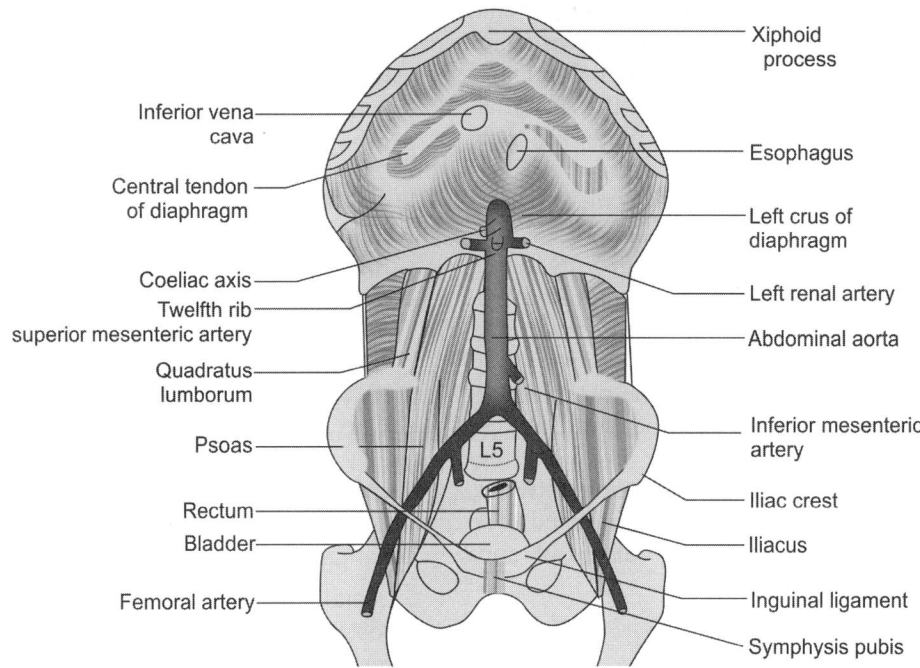

Fig. 7.19: Under surface of diaphragm; muscles of posterior abdominal wall; abdominal aorta dividing into common iliac arteries which give off internal and external iliac arteries

thus helping to enlarge the thoracic cavity. During expiration the diaphragm relaxes and resumes its dome-shaped appearance.

Damage to the phrenic nerve may cause paralysis of the diaphragm. Sometimes abdominal contents herniate through the openings in the diaphragm, the commonest being 'hiatal hernia' in which a portion of the stomach enters the chest through the esophageal opening.

Muscles of the Abdomen

Anterior Abdominal Wall

The muscles of the anterior abdominal wall are arranged in sheets which protect the delicate abdominal organs (Fig. 7.20). Contraction of the abdominal muscles aid in the act of defecation.

- The rectus abdominal is the straight muscle of the anterior abdominal wall. It runs parallel with its fellow of the opposite side and is separated from it by a thin band of fibrous tissue, the linea alba (white line), which extends from the xiphoid process of the sternum to the symphysis pubis. The muscle arises from the pubic bone and is inserted into the xiphoid process and the adjacent costal cartilages. It is enclosed in a dense sheath of fibrous tissue, formed by the aponeuroses of the two oblique muscles, called the rectus sheath. The fibers of the rectus muscle are interrupted by three bands of fibrous tissue which cross it transversely—the tendinous intersections.
- Two oblique muscles help to form the side and anterior walls of the abdominal cavity. The fibers of the external oblique muscle pass downwards and forwards, arising from the lower eight ribs. It is inserted in a fan-shaped manner into the rectus sheath, the iliac crest and the pubic bone. The aponeurosis of

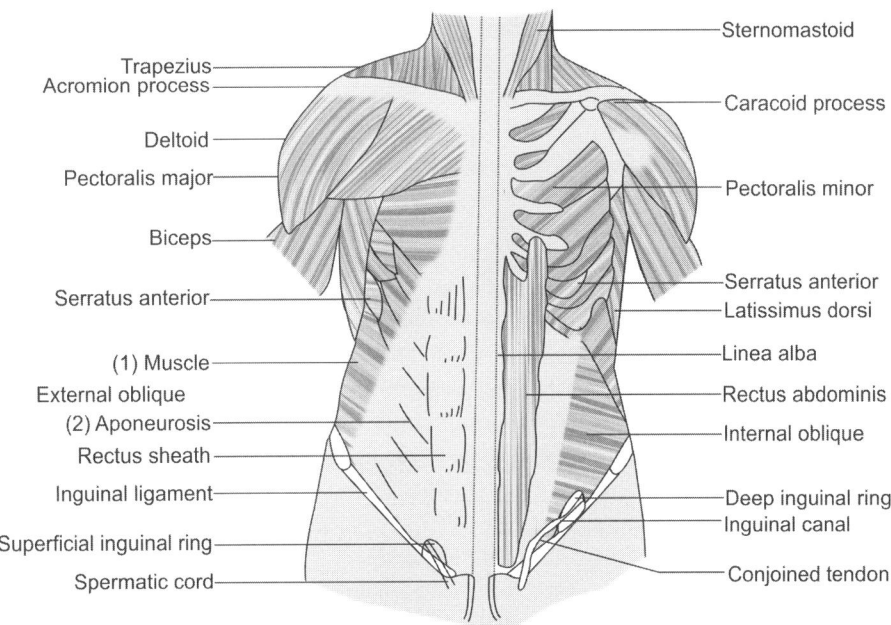

Fig. 7.20: Muscles of the front of the thorax and anterior abdominal wall—left superficial, right deep

the lower border, between the anterior superior iliac spine and the pubic spine, is thickened to form the inguinal ligament (Poupart's ligament).

The internal oblique muscle arises from the iliac crest and the inguinal ligament and is inserted into the rectus sheath and the lower ribs. Its fibers pass upwards and medially and cross those of the external oblique.

The transversus muscle arises from the lower ribs, the iliac crest and the inguinal ligament and is inserted into the linea alba and the pubic bone (Fig. 7.21).

The point at which the aponeuroses of the anterior abdominal wall unite is known as the conjoined tendon. In the inguinal area the aponeuroses of these muscles are pierced by the inguinal canals.

Posterior Abdominal Wall

The psoas muscle arises from the lumbar vertebrae (Fig. 7.22). The iliacus muscle

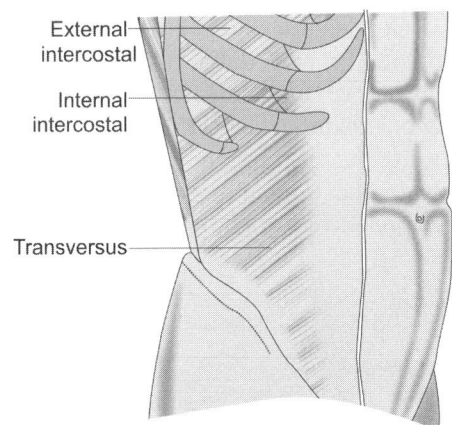

Fig. 7.21: The transversus muscle

arises from the inner surface of the ilium. They are inserted together into the lesser trochanter of the femur.

The quadratus lumborum extends from the iliac crest upwards to the last (12th) rib. The posterior surface of the kidney is closely related to the psoas and quadratus lumborum muscles.

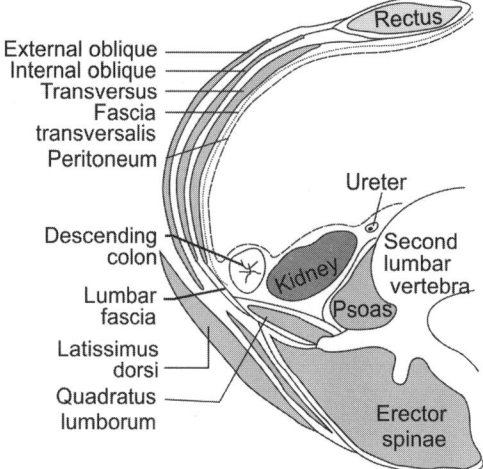

Fig. 7.22: Section of the abdominal wall through the lower part of the second lumbar vertebra

Muscles of the Back

The muscles of the back play an important part in the maintenance of an upright body posture (Fig. 7.23). There are several groups of muscles on either side of the spine which extend for varying distances between the occiput above and the sacrum below. The upper ones extend the neck. The lower ones, including the erector spinae, straighten the spine. In the lumbar region they form a large aponeurosis, the lumbar fascia.

Muscles of the Pelvis

The muscles of the pelvis collectively form the floor of the pelvic cavity. The most important of these muscles is the levator ani, which aids in defecation. It is a muscular sheet extending across the outlet of the pelvis through which passes the rectum, urethra, and in the female, the vagina (Fig. 7.24).

Muscles of the Lower Extremity

The muscles of the lower extremities are among the largest and most powerful in the body.

Muscles of the Buttock

The rounded eminence of the buttock is formed by the gluteal muscles. The gluteus maximus is the most superficial and the largest of this group. It arises from the ilium and is inserted into the gluteal tuberosity of the femur and the iliotibial tract (the fascia which envelops all the muscles of the thigh). The gluteus medius and the gluteus minimus arise from the ilium and are inserted into the greater trochanter of the femur. The main action of these muscles is to extend and abduct the thigh.

Muscles of the Thigh

There are a number of muscles in the thigh which can be described in three groups.

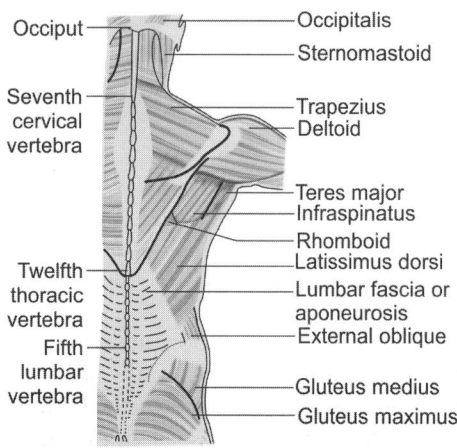

Fig. 7.23: Muscles of the back

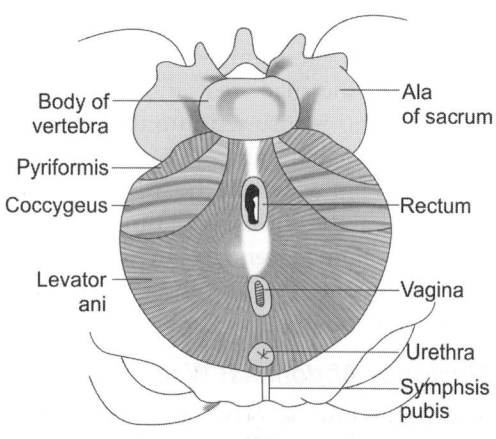

Fig. 7.24: Muscles of the female pelvic floor

Physiology of Muscle Contraction

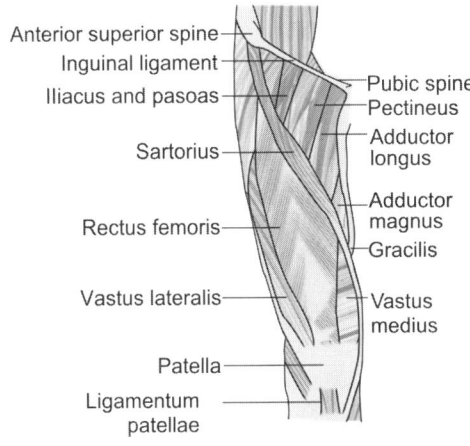

Fig. 7.25: Muscles of the front at the thigh

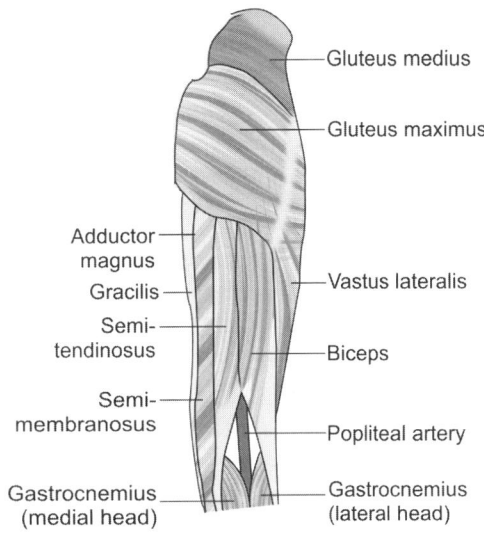

Fig. 7.26: Muscles at the back of the thigh

1. *The anterior group (Fig. 7.25):* The main muscle of this group is the quadriceps extensor, which is made up by the rectus femoris, vastus medialis, vastus lateralis and vastus intermedius, and terminates in a single tendon (the ligamentum patellae), in which the patella is developed as a sesamoid bone. It is inserted into the tuberosity of the tibia and its action is to extend or straighten the knee joint.
   The sartorius muscle arises from the anterior superior spine of the ilium and passes obliquely to be inserted into the medial side of the tibial tuberosity.

2. *The posterior group (Fig. 7.26):* These are also called the hamstring group, which is formed by three muscles, the biceps femoris, semimembranosus and semitendinosus. They arise from the tuberosity of the ischium and are inserted into the upper ends of the tibia and fibula. The biceps femoris passes to the lateral side of the leg and also has a short head arising from the linea aspera of the femur. The other two muscles pass to the medial side of the leg. The biceps, therefore, forms the lateral boundary of the popliteal space, and the semimembranosus and semitendinosus form the medial boundary.
   The hamstring muscles, having their origin above the hip joint and their insertion below the knee joint, are capable of producing movement at both (i.e. they straighten or extend the hip and flex the knee).

3. *The medial group (Fig. 7.27):* This consists of three muscles, the adductors longus, brevis and magnus, which arise from the pubic bone and are inserted mainly into the linea aspera of the femur. Their function is described by their name (i.e. they adduct the thigh towards the midline).

Muscles of the Leg

The muscles of the leg function to provide movement of the foot. They can be described in three groups.

1. *Anterior group:* This is composed of those muscles which lie in front of the interosseous membrane between the tibia and fibula (Fig. 7.28). It includes the tibialis anterior, passing from the tibia to the tarsal bones to dorsiflex the

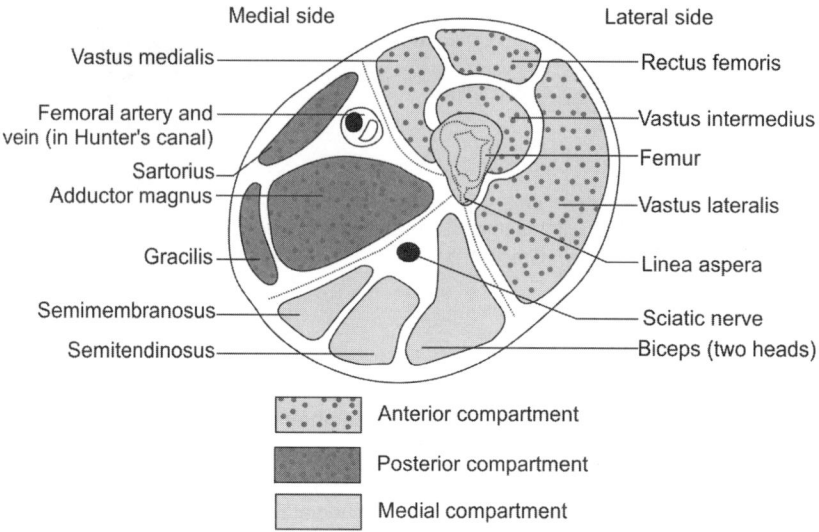

Fig. 7.27: Transverse section of the middle of the thigh

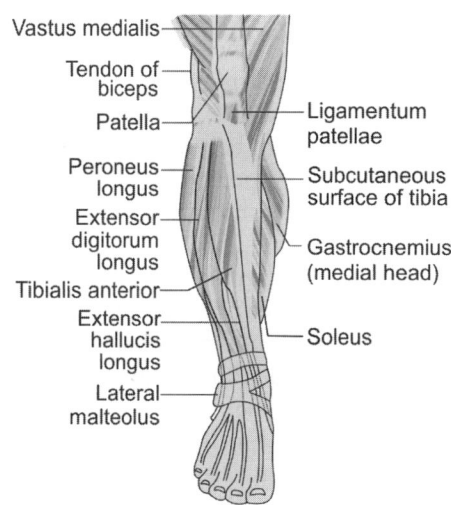

Fig. 7.28: Muscles of the front of the leg

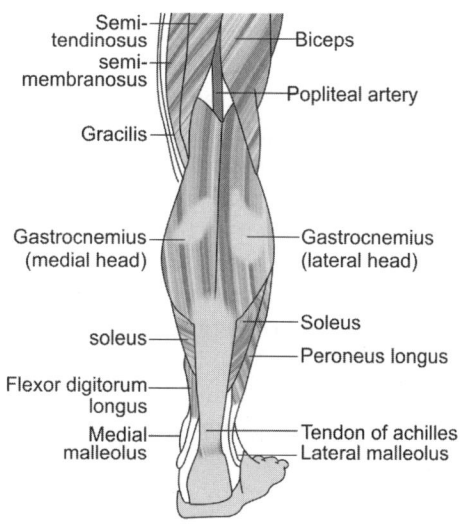

Fig. 7.29: Muscles of the back of the leg

ankle, and the extensor muscles of the toes (extensor digitorum longus).

2. *Posterior group (Fig. 7.29):* This consists of superficial and deep layers. The superficial muscles, i.e. the gastronemius and the soleus, form the back of the calf (Fig. 7.30). The upper end of the gastrocnemius arises from the condyles of the femur, the soleus arises from the posterior aspects of the tibia and fibula. Both are inserted into the calcaneum by the tendo achilles and plantar-flex the ankle joint.

The deep muscles include the tibialis posterior arising from the tibia and fibula, which also plantar-flexes the ankle joint as it passes to its insertion into the tarsal bones, and the flexor muscles of the toes (flexor digitorum longus).

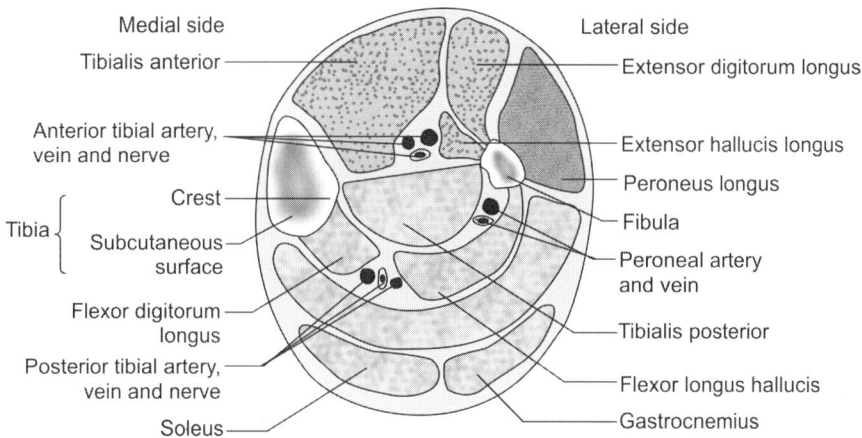

Fig. 7.30: Transverse section of the leg (middle of calf)

In contrast to the muscles of the forearm and hand, the flexor muscles of the toes are situated on the posterior aspect of the leg and the extensors of the toes on the anterior surface. (It must be remembered that the palm of the hand corresponds to the sole of the foot.)

3. *Fibular group:* These are also called the peroneal muscles. They arise from the lateral surface of the fibula and are inserted into the tarsal and metatarsal bones of the foot. Their action is to evert the foot outwards.

There are a number of small muscles in the foot similar to those in the hands, e.g. short muscles in the sole which are attached to the big toe and the interosseous and lumbrical muscles for the toes.

CHAPTER 8

Respiratory System

NASAL CAVITY

Nasal cavity extends from roof of the mouth to cranial base. It is wider below and widest at the central region. The cavity is divided by a median septum vertically. Nasal cavity communicates with frontal, ethmoidal, maxillary and sphenoidal paranasal sinuses. It opens into nasopharynx by a pair of posterior nasal aperture. Each half of nasal cavity has a roof, floor, medial wall (septum), lateral wall, and a vestibule (Figs 8.1 and 8.2).

Roof: Roof is horizontal in central part. Anterior slope is formed by nasal spine (frontal bone) and nasal bone. Central part is formed by cribriform plate of ethmoid bone which separates nasal cavity from anterior cranial fossa. Perforations in cribriform plate transmit olfactory nerves. Posterior slope is formed by sphenoid bone.

Floor: Floor is smooth and concave. Most of the floor is formed by palatine process of maxilla and articulate with horizontal plate of palatine bone posteriorly. Suture formed

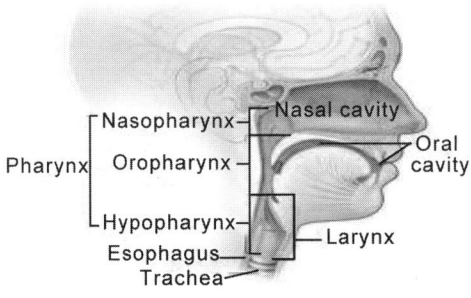

Fig. 8.1: Nasal cavity

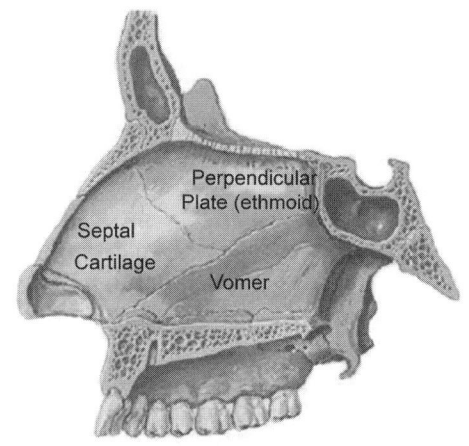

Fig. 8.2: Nasal septum

between these bones is called palatomaxillary suture. Deficiency of bone in the floor of nose is called cleft palate.

Medial wall: Medial wall of each nasal cavity is nasal septum formed by thin sheet of bone (posteriorly) and cartilage (anteriorly). It lies between roof and floor. Major part of bony septum is formed by vomer and perpendicular plate of ethmoid.

Cartilagenous septum: Septal cartilage is quadrilateral located in anterior part and anteroinferior part formed by alar cartilage.

Lateral wall: Lateral wall is formed by maxilla (anteriorly) and by perpendicular plate of palatine bone (posteriorly) and ethmoid bone (superiorly) (Fig. 8.3).

Lateral wall has three projections: The superior, middle, inferior nasal conchae (turbinates). Each concha roofs a groove called meatus. Middle meatus has an

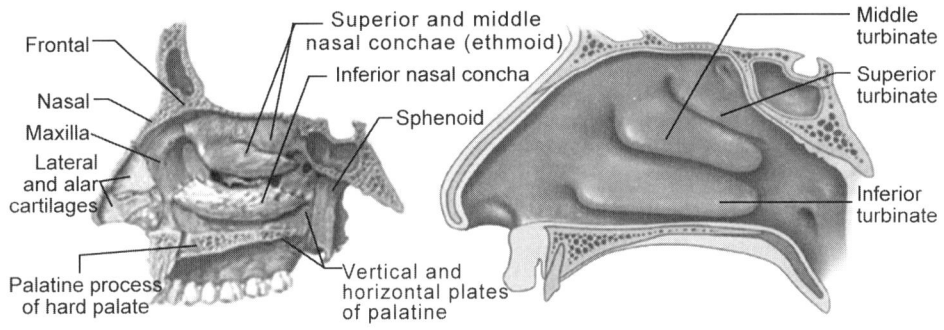

Fig. 8.3: Lateral wall of nasal cavity

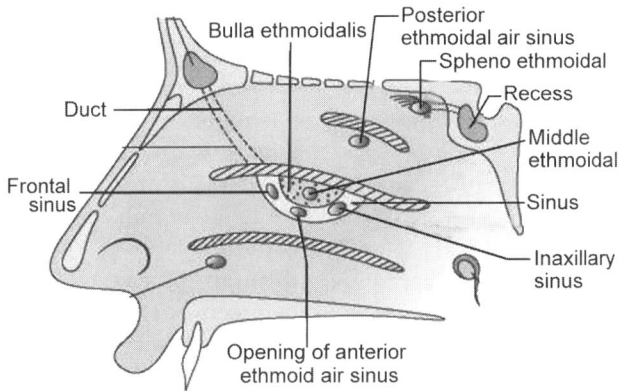

Fig. 8.4: Openings into lateral wall

expanded enclosed air cells called bulla (Fig. 8.4).

Inferior concha and inferior meatus: The inferior concha is thin curved independent bone. Inferior meatus lies below it. It admits the opening of nasolacrimal canal.

Middle concha and middle meatus: Middle concha is the medial process of ethmoid labyrinth and contains air cells. The region beneath it is middle meatus. Anterior part of middle meatus is called atrium. The main feature of middle meatus is the rounded elevation called bulla ethmoidalis and a curved cleft below it called hiatus semilunaris. Middle ethmoidal sinus opens into bulla. Maxillary sinus opens into hiatus semilunaris. Anterior ethmoidal sinus opens at the anterior end of middle meatus.

Superior concha: It is the smallest concha and located in posterior part of nasal cavity. Superior meatus lies between superior and middle concha. Posterior ethmoidal sinus opens into it.

Olfactory mucosa: Olfactory mucosa covers 5 cm sq of posterior upper part of lateral nasal wall. It consists of pigmented pseudostratified epithelium containing olfactory receptor neurons. Axons derived from olfactory receptor neurons course through the mucosa to the cribriform plate. Olfactory receptor neurons are bipolar neurons and their axons converge on the glomerulus in the olfactory bulb and arteries.

Arterial Supply of Nasal Septum

The following arteries supply the septum:
- Anterior and posterior ethmoidal artery
- Superior labial artery (septal branch)
- Sphenopalatine and greater palatine arteries.

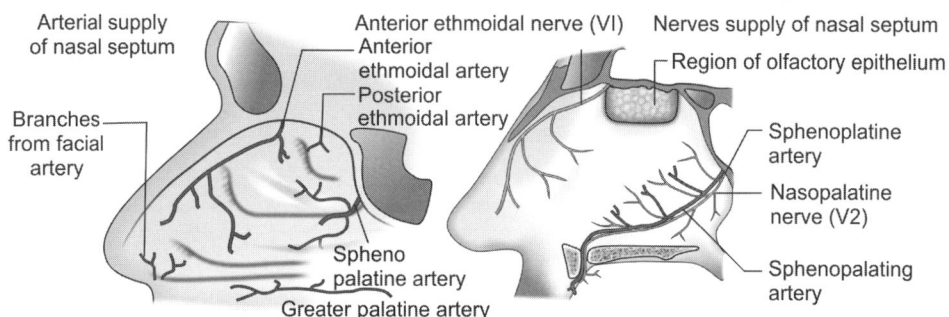

Fig. 8.5: Arterial and nerve supply of nasal septum

Littles area: It is septal area supplied by anterior ethmoidal artery, sphenopalatine artery, greater palatine artery and superior labial artery. Injury to these vessels is common cause of epistaxis (bleeding from nose).

Arterial supply of lateral wall: Anterior ethmoidal artery, sphenopalatine artery, greater palatine artery (Fig. 8.5).

Nerve Supply of Nasal Cavity

Nerves of special sense: Olfactory nerves.
Nerves of general sense: Anterior ethmoidal nerve, branches from sphenopalatine ganglion.
Autonomic nerve supply: Nerve of pterygoid canal.

■ PHARYNX

The pharynx is 12–14 cm long musculomembranous tube. It extends from cranial base to lower border of cricoid cartilage (level of C6) where it becomes continuous with esophagus. The pharynx is limited above by body of sphenoid and base of occipital bone. Posteriorly it is related to cervical part of vertebral column.

Muscles of pharynx are three circular constrictors and three longitudinal elevators. Arterial supply is derived from branches of external carotid artery. Motor and sensory innervations are from branches of pharyngeal plexus.

Interior of pharynx is divided to nasopharynx, oropharynx, laryngopharynx.
Nasopharynx: Nasopharynx lies behind posterior nares and above soft palate. The nasopharynx has a roof, posterior wall, two lateral walls, and floor. Except floor, all other walls are rigid and never obliterated by action of muscle. The nasal and oral parts communicate of pharynx communicate through pharyngeal isthmus which lies between posterior wall of soft palate and posterior pharyngeal wall.

A lymphoid mass, the adenoid lies in the mucosa of the upper part of the roof and the posterior wall.

Lateral walls of nasopharynx receives opening of pharyngotympanic tube (auditory tube, Eustachian tube). Tubal opening is bounded above and behind by tubal elevation. A vertical mucosal fold, the salpingopharyngeal fold descends from tubal elevation behind the auditory tube. Behind the tubal elevation is recess in the lateral wall called pharyngeal recess or fossa of Rosenmuller.

Adenoid or pharyngeal tonsil: Adenoid is a mass of lymphoid tissue situated in roof and posterior wall of nasopharynx. After birth it grows rapidly and undergoes a degree of involution and atrophy by the age of 8–10 years.

Adenoidectomy: It is the surgical resection of enlarged adenoid.

Oropharynx

Boundaries: Oropharynx extends from below the soft palate to upper border of epiglottis. Pharynx opens into mouth through oropharyngeal isthmus demarcated by palatoglossal arch. Its lateral wall consists of the palatopharyngeal arch and palatine tonsil. Posteriorly it is in level with the bodies of 2nd and 3rd cervical vertebra.

Palatoglossal and palatopharyngeal arches: The lateral wall of oropharynx presents two prominent folds, the palatoglossal and palatopharyngeal folds (anterior and posterior pillars respectively). The palatoglossal arch runs from soft palate to sides of tongue and contains the palatoglossus muscle. The palatopharyngeal arch, the posterior fold runs from soft palate to merge with the lateral wall of pharynx and contains palatopharyngeus muscle. A triangular tonsillar fossa lies on each side of oropharynx between the diverging palatopharyngeal and palatoglossal arches and contain palatine tonsil.

Palatine tonsil: Each tonsil is an ovoid mass of lymphoid tissue situated in the lateral wall of oropharynx. Size of tonsil varies with age and pathological conditions. Maximum size is attained at puberty. After puberty it begins to atrophy. Medial surface of tonsil is free surface and has pitted appearance. The lateral aspect of tonsil is covered by fibrous tissue, the tonsillar hemicapsule. The lateral side is related to tonsillar artery and veins accompanying it. A large tonsillar vein called paratonsillar vein is seen lateral to hemicapsule and is susceptible to torrential bleeding during removal of tonsil (tonsillectomy).

Waldeyer's ring: Waldeyer's ring is a circumoropharyngeal ring of mucosa-associated lymphoid tissue (MALT), seen around opening of digestive and respiratory tract. The ring comprises of palatine tonsil, tubal tonsil, nasopharyngeal tonsil.

Laryngopharynx

Laryngopharynx is situated behind the entire length of the larynx extending from superior border of epiglottis to the inferior border of cricoid cartilage.

Piriform fossa: A small piriform fossa lies on each side of the laryngeal inlet bounded medially by aryepiglottic fold and laterally by thyroid cartilage. Branches of internal laryngeal nerve lie in the mucous membrane. Laryngopharynx extend from C3 to C6 vertebra.

Muscles of pharynx: These pharyngeal muscles consist of two groups, circularly disposed muscles called constrictor muscles and longitudinal muscle. Constrictor muscles lie outer to longitudinal muscles.

Constrictor muscles: Superior constrictor, middle constrictor and inferior constrictor are situated in the posterior wall and sides of pharynx. They overlap from below upwards.

Longitudinal muscles: The longitudinal muscles are salpingopharyngeus, palatopharyngeus, stylopharyngeus. These muscles pull the pharynx upwards.

■ LARYNX

It is an air passage, a sphincter and an organ of voice production. It extends from tongue to trachea. Above it opens into laryngopharynx and below it continues as trachea. It lies between C3 and C6 vertebra in adults.

Skeleton of larynx: It is formed by a series of cartilages connected by ligaments and membranes and moved by a number of muscles. The laryngeal cartilages are the epiglottis thyroid cartilage, cricoid cartilage, arytenoid cartilage, corniculate cartilage, cuneiform cartilage.

Epiglottis: Thin leaf like plate of elastic cartilage which projects upward behind the tongue. Its free end is broad and round. Its attached part is attached to the back of laryngeal prominence of thyroid cartilage.

Thyroid cartilage: Largest of laryngeal cartilage. It has two quadrilateral lamina with fused anterior border and free posterior border. Fused anterior border is prominent in males and is called Adam's apple. Shallow oblique line seen on external of lamina. Muscles are inserted to this oblique line. Lamina is related to thyroid gland.

Cricoid cartilage: It is attached below to trachea and articulate with thyroid cartilage and arytenoid cartilage above. It forms a complete ring with narrow anterior arch and broad posterior arch.

Arytenoid cartilage: Articulate with lateral part of superior border of posterior arch of cricoid cartilage. Each is pyramidal in shape and has three surfaces, two processes, a base and an apex. Posterior surface is triangular, smooth and concave. It has two processes— vocal process and muscular process. Vocal ligament is attached to vocal process. Muscles related to movements of arytenoid cartilage attached to muscular process.

Laryngeal cavity (Interior of larynx): Cavity extends from laryngeal inlet (from the pharynx) to the lower border of cricoid cartilage where it continues as trachea. Walls of cavity are formed by fibroelastic membrane and lined by mucous membrane. The continuity of the fibroelastic membrane is interrupted by upper and lower folds. These folds project to lumen of cavity and divide it into upper and lower parts separated by middle portion between the folds which form the ventricle or sinus of larynx. The upper folds are called vestibular folds (false vocal cords) and the lower folds are called true vocal folds. The median aperture between vestibular fold is rima vestibuli and that aperture between vocal folds is rima glottidis. True vocal cords are source of voice production or phonation.

The part above vestibular fold is called vestibule or supraglottic part and comprises of laryngeal inlet formed by laryngeal surface of epiglottis, arytenoid cartilages and aryepiglottic folds.

Laryngeal vestibule: It is the space between laryngeal inlet and vestibular folds. It is wider above and narrow below.

Anterior wall: It is formed by posterior surface of epiglottis.

Lateral walls: Formed by aryepiglottic fold.

Posterior wall: Formed by interarytenoid membrane.

Middle part of laryngeal cavity: It is the smallest part and extends between rima vestibuli and rima glottidis. This part forms ventricle or sinus of larynx and also contains saccule of larynx.

Ventricle (sinus) of the larynx: It is a fusiform recess between vestibular and vocal fold.

Vocal Folds (Vocal Cords) and Ligament

The vocal ligament extends from thyroid angle to vocal process. Vocal ligament is covered by mucosa and then called vocal cord. Mucosa is thin. There is no submucosa and so mucosa appear pearly white.

Reinke's edema: Mucous membrane of larynx is loosely attached throughout larynx and can accommodate considerable amount of swelling. This space is called Reinke's space and fluid accumulation is called Reinke's edema.

Lower part is called subglottic or infraglottic part. It extends from vocal fold to cricoid cartilage. This area accelerates air flow.

Intrinsic muscles of larynx are aryepiglotticus, transverse arytenoids, posterior cricoarytenoid, lateral cricoarytenoid, cricothyroid and vocalis.

Blood supply: Superior laryngeal and inferior laryngeal artery.

Nerve supply: Internal laryngeal, recurrent laryngeal, external laryngeal nerve.

Respiratory System

■ PLEURA AND LUNGS

The lungs are essential organs of respiration. They take oxygen into blood and remove carbon dioxide. The muscles of respiration and the diaphragm increase the volume inside thorax and create negative pressure in the pleural space which surround lung and cause expansion of lungs.

Pleura: Each lung is covered by pleura, a serous membrane arranged as a closed invaginated sac. The visceral or pulmonary pleura adheres closely to the pulmonary surface and its interlobar fissures. The parietal pleura on the outer layer lines, the thoracic wall, diaphragm and structures occupying middle region of thoracic wall.

Visceral and parietal pleura are continuous with each other around hilar structures. They remain in close contact and slide on each other during respiration. The space between them is called pleural cavity in which exists negative pressure. The right and left pleural sacs form separate compartments and touch only behind upper part of sternum. The region between the two pleural sacs is called mediastinum (interpleural space).

The left pleural cavity is smaller than the right because the heart extends to the left side.

Thoracoscopy allows direct inspection of the parietal and visceral pleura. The parietal pleura is transparent and the underlying muscles and blood vessels can be visualized. The visceral pleura is also transparent and appears grey due to underlying lung tissue.

Parietal pleura: At different regions, parietal pleura is distinguished by the name as:
- Costovertebral pleura
- Lining thoracic wall
- Diaphragmatic pleura
- Lining thoracic surface of diaphragm
- Cervical pleura
- Lining upper cervical region of lung
- Mediastinal pleura
- Applied to structures between lungs.

Visceral pleura: This pleura is inseparably adherent to the lung all over its surfaces including lung fissures except at the hilum of lung.

Pulmonary ligaments: Mediastinal pleura is double layered and extends from lateral surface of esophagus to mediastinal surface of the lung.

Pleural recess: Pleura extends beyond the inferior border of lung. The lung is about 5 cm above the lower pleural limit. This space is termed pleural recess.

Vascular supply of pleura: It is by intercostal artery and internal thoracic artery.

Nerve supply: Intercostal nerves and phrenic nerve.

■ LUNGS

The lungs are essential organs of respiration. They are situated on either side of heart and mediastinum. Each lung is free in its pleural cavity except for its attachment to heart and trachea at the hilum. Fresh lung is spongy and can float in water because of air within alveoli. It is also elastic. Its surface is smooth and shiny and separated by fine dark lines. Lungs are heavier in men than women.

Pulmonary surface features: Each lung has an apex, base, three borders, two surfaces. Each lung resembles a half cone.

Apex: It is the upper rounded extremity. It projects above thoracic inlet to the neck. Apex is about 3–4 cm above first rib. The subclavian artery grooves the apex.

Base: It is semilunar in shape and rests on superior surface of diaphragm. The diaphragm separates right lung from right lobe of liver and left lung from liver, stomach, spleen.

Costal surface: Related to ribs.

Medial surface: It is related posteriorly to vertebral column and anteriorly to cardiac surfaces.

Pulmonary Fissures and Lobes

Right lung: It is divided into superior, middle and inferior lobes by oblique and horizontal fissures. The oblique fissure separates the inferior lobe from superior and middle lobes. Short horizontal fissure separates superior from middle lobes.

Left lung: It is divided into a superior and inferior lobe by an oblique fissure. There is a cardiac notch and lingual for superior lobe.

Bronchopulmonary segments: Each principal bronchi divides into lobar bronchi. Primary branches of the right and left are lobar bronchi are termed segmental bronchi. The segmental bronchi are structurally separate and function independently. Such independent units of lung tissue are called bronchopulmonary segments.

Bronchopulmonary Segments (Table 8.1)

Table 8.1: Bronchopulmonary segments of left and right lung

Right lung (3 lobes)	Left lung (2 lobes)
Superior lobe: Apical, anterior, posterior	**Superior lobe:** Apical, anterior, posterior
Middle lobe: Lateral, medial	
Inferior lobe: Apical, medial, basal and lateral basal, anterobasal, posterobasal	**Inferior lobe:** Apical, anterobasal, posterobasal, medial basal, lateral basal

■ RESPIRATORY MOVEMENTS

The renewal of the air in the lungs is secured by the respiratory movements of inspiration (breathing in) and expiration (breathing out). The thorax may be regarded as a completely closed box which alters its size and shape with each ventilation. With inspiration, the cavity of the thorax is enlarged and the lungs, being elastic, expand to fill up the increased space. This expansion of the lungs causes air to be sucked in through the upper air passages and trachea. Inspiration is an active muscular process.

With expiration, the capacity of the thorax returns to its former size and air is expelled from the lungs. Expiration is largely passive in a person at rest.

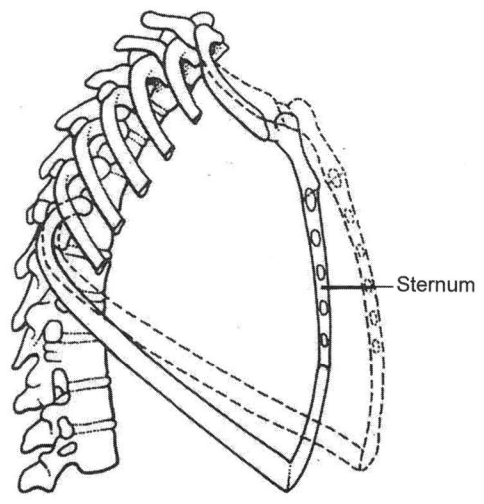

Fig. 8.6: Movements of the ribs and sternum during respiration

The increase in the size of the thoracic cavity during inspiration is brought about by two factors (Fig. 8.6):
1. Upward movement of the ribs.
2. Downward movement of the diaphragm.

Upward movement of the ribs results mainly from contraction of the external intercostal muscles. In forced, deep inspirations the muscles of the neck and shoulder girdle may be brought into operation, *viz.* trapezius, sternomastoid and pectoralis major muscles.

When at rest the diaphragm is dome-shaped, having its concavity towards the abdomen. When the muscle of the diaphragm contracts during inspiration it becomes flattened and, therefore, depressed towards the abdominal cavity (Fig. 8.7).

During quiet expiration the chest returns to its resting size mainly on account of the elasticity of the lungs and the chest wall and by the upward pressure of the abdominal contents on the diaphragm as it relaxes. The internal intercostal muscles provide the small active element of quiet expiration. In forced expiration, such as

Respiratory System

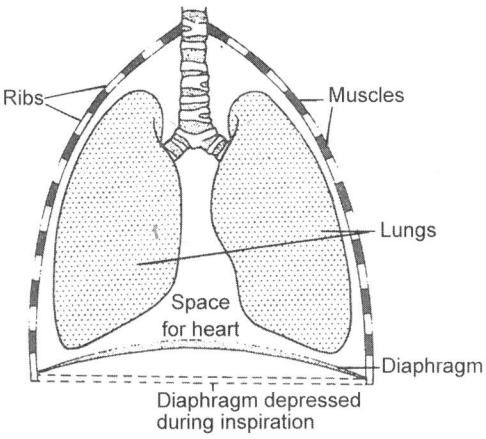

Fig. 8.7: The chest in section

occurs in coughing and during exercise, the abdominal and other accessory muscles are employed.

Normal ventilation, therefore, is a combination of two sets of movements, thoracic and diaphragmatic, sometimes known as thoracic and diaphragmatic or abdominal breathing. In men quiet ventilation is mainly carried out by movements of the diaphragm, while in women the thoracic type of ventilation usually predominates.

Another important function of the respiratory movements is to aid in the return of venous blood to the heart.

Special Respiratory Movements

- Sighs and yawns are types of prolonged inspiration.
- Cough is a forcible expiration usually preceded by a prolonged inspiration. The sound of a cough is produced by forcing air through the narrow opening between the vocal cords.
- Hiccough is a noisy inspiration caused by muscular spasm of the diaphragm at irregular intervals. The noise is produced by the sudden sucking of air through the vocal cords.
- Changes in the breathing pattern can signify emotions.

Movement of Air in the Respiratory Tract

It has been seen that the expansion of the chest by the movements of the thorax and diaphragm causes air to enter the lungs with each inspiration. Further, by an added effort, a forced inspiration will result in still greater expansion and an additional amount of air will enter the lungs.

In the same way, a normal expiration can be supplemented by a forced expiration. Even after a forced expiration, however, some air still remains in the alveoli of the lungs.

The amount of air passing in and out of the lungs with ordinary quiet breathing is called tidal air and measures about 500 mL. The additional volume taken in by forced inspiration is called the inspiratory reserve. That expelled by forced expiration after an ordinary breath is referred to as the expiratory reserve, while that remaining in the alveoli is the residual air.

The term vital capacity may be defined as the volume of air that can be expelled by the deepest possible expiration after the deepest possible inspiration.

It will be seen from Table 8.2 that the vital capacity (VC) is the sum of the tidal volume, the inspiratory reserve and the expiratory reserve also that the total lung capacity (TLC) is the sum of the vital capacity and the residual volume (RV), i.e.

TLC = VC + RV

Table 8.2: An example of respiratory volumes

	Volume in mL	Comment
Tidal volume (TV)	500	Quiet breathing
Inspiratory reserve (IR)	2500	Forced inspiration
Expiratory reserve (ER)	1000	Forced expiration
Vital capacity (VC)	4000	
Residual volume (RV)	1000	Always left in lung
Total lung capacity (TLC)	5000	

The term hyperpnea is sometimes used to express an increased depth of respiratory movement. Apnea means a temporary cessation of breathing. Difficult or labored breathing is called dyspnea.

The stages of respiration are:
- Ventilation of the lungs so that air moves freely in and out.
- Interchange of gases between the blood and the air in the alveoli. The term 'diffusing capacity' or 'gas transfer factor' refers to the ability of each square millimeter of the alveolar-capillary membrane to transfer gas by the process of diffusion. It is measured in mL/min/mm Hg.

In addition there is:
- Loss of water vapor
- Supply of air to the larynx for the purpose of voice production.

Atmospheric air is a mixture of gases and, as a result of oxygen being absorbed and carbon dioxide being excreted by the lungs, it follows that the amount of oxygen in expired air is diminished, while the amount of carbon dioxide is increased. With quiet breathing, the oxygen uptake and carbon dioxide excretion is about 250–300 mL per minute. The percentage of nitrogen remains constant. The amount of carbon dioxide in expired air is 100 times greater than in atmospheric air (Table 8.3).

The following is a summary of the differences between expired air and inspired air:
- Expired air contains less oxygen and more carbon dioxide
- Expired air is nearer to body temperature
- Expired air is saturated with water vapor. The minute droplets of water may pick up bacteria during their passage through the respiratory tract and become a source of infection (droplet infection) to others.

■ VOICE PRODUCTION (FIG. 8.8)

It is convenient to consider this subject in connection with the respiratory system. The voice sounds are produced in the larynx. They are modified in character by the resonance afforded by the nasal cavities and the accessory air sinuses and finally, by means of the tongue, lips and jaw movements, the actual sounds of speech are produced.

The human voice has the following characteristics:
- Loudness
- Pitch
- Quality
- *Loudness:* The variable loudness of the voice is dependent upon the force of the air currents expelled from the lungs through the vocal cords and their consequent vibration. The vibration of the vocal cords is called phonation.
- *Pitch:* By pitch is meant the variation in note, i.e. a high note or a low note. This is dependent on two factors, the length and tension of the vocal cords. In children the vocal cords are relatively short and, therefore, the pitch of the voice is high. Alterations in pitch can be produced by voluntary action by using certain of the muscles of the larynx

Table 8.3: Gas content of inspired and expired air

	Inspired or atmospheric air (%)	Expired air (%)
Oxygen	20	16
Carbon dioxide	0.04	4
Nitrogen	79	79

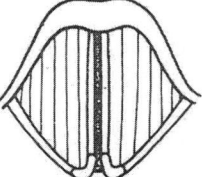 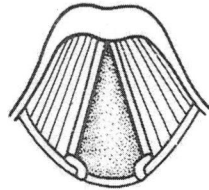

Fig. 8.8: The glottis, showing the vocal cords closed (left) on phonation and open (right) during inspiration

which increase or decrease the tension of the vocal cords. Variation in pitch by the alteration of tension can easily be demonstrated by twanging a stretched string, wire or elastic, *viz.* the greater the tension of the cord or string, the higher the note produced.
- *Quality:* The quality of a note is due to the resonance produced in the mouth, nose and accessory nasal sinuses in the skull. The difference in quality of sound is easily demonstrated by speaking through the mouth and 'speaking through the nose'. The soft palate plays an important part in this act, and if imperfectly formed (cleft palate) or paralyzed (e.g. in diphtheria) a typical nasal voice develops. Full use of the possible variations in quality is made in singing.

Speech

The sounds of the spoken word or articulation are modifications of the primary laryngeal sound which are brought about by movements of the lips, tongue and jaw working either independently or together.

There are two types of broken sound:
1. *Vowels:* Sounds produced with the mouth open and with the vocal cords vibrating continuously without interruption.
2. *Consonants:* There is a sharp interruption or curtailment of the vocal cord vibration. Some consonant sounds are produced mainly by the movement of the tongue against the teeth, for example t and d, are called dentals. The sounds p and b are dependent upon closure of the lips and are called labials. Throaty sounds, g and k, are gutturals.

Whispering: In the act of whispering the sound is produced entirely by movement of the air in the mouth. The vocal cords are relaxed (or open) and do not vibrate, i.e. there is no phonation. The formation of word sounds in whispering is carried out by the movements of the mouth and tongue. Inflammation of the vocal cords interferes with their contraction and vibration and consequently the voice becomes hoarse or is entirely lost, so that whispering only is possible. If it is necessary to rest the vocal cords, the patient must be instructed to speak only in whispers.

■ PHYSIOLOGY OF RESPIRATION

Respiratory system is made up of:
- Gas-exchanging organ the lungs
- A pump that ventilates the lung (Chest wall and respiratory muscles)
- The areas in brain, respiratory centers that control the muscles
- The nerves innervating the muscles of respiration

The amount of air inspired and expired per breath is 6–8 L/min. 250 mL of O_2 enters the body per minute by simple diffusion. 200 mL of CO_2 is excreted. The respiratory rate is 12–15/minutes.

Respiratory Treat Includes

Respiratory tree divides 23 times (generations). Trachea is the 'zero' generation to start with and the 23rd generation is the alveolar sac.

Nose, Mouth
↓
Glottis
↓
Trachea
↓
Two bronchi
↓
Alveoli

There are two zones in the respiratory tree.
1. *Conducting zone:* Up to 16th division, the terminal bronchiole
2. *Respiratory zone:* From the 17th division onwards up to respiratory bronchiole.

HISTOLOGY OF TERMINAL BRONCHIOLE

Cartilage is present in the respiratory tree up to the terminal bronchioles. The cartilage helps to make the respiratory tree patent. Glands are present in the muscles up to terminal bronchiole. Smooth muscles are maximum in terminal bronchiole.

Alveoli

There are about 300 million alveoli. The surface are of these alveoli is 70 sq meters. The peculiarity of alveoli is that it has no glands, cartilage or smooth muscle in the walls. It is lined by simple squamous epithelium.
Two types of cells:
1. *Type I:* Primary lining cells
2. *Type II:* Granular preumocytes.

Surfactant

The type II granular preumocyte secrete surfactant. Surfactant is the surface tension lowering agent. Chemically it is known as dipalmitoylphosphatidylcholine (DPPC). The most important function of surfactant is to prevent collapse of the alveoli when the radius of alveoli is small. The surfactant keeps the alveoli dry and thus promote gas exchange (Fig. 8.9).

According to law of Laplace

$$P = \frac{2T}{r}$$

P = Distending pressure of alveoli
T = Wall tension
r = Radius of the alveoli

Another function of surfactant is to prevent pulmonary edema and keep the alveoli dry.

Approximate Composition of Surfactant

- Dipalmitoylphosphatidylcholine - 62%
- Phosphatidylglycerol - 5%
- Other phospholipids - 10%
- Neutral lipids - 13%
- Proteins - 8%
- Carbohydrate - 2%

The Factors that Prevent Collapse of Alveoli

- Alveolar stability
- Interdependence of alveoli
- Presence of surfactant lining the alveoli.

Alveolar Stability

According to law of Laplace

$$P = \frac{2T}{r}$$

The surface tension (T) is a inward pressure that will help the collapse of the alveoli. The presence of surfactant produces an interface between the fluid in lining the alveoli and the air in the alveolar sac. Thus it reduces the surface tension acting and tendency of alveoli to collapse. When the radius of the alveoli increases it decreases the concentration of surfactant that lines the alveoli. Thus the surface tension acting increases and prevents further distension of alveoli.

In contrast, when the radius of the alveoli decreases, the concentration of surfactant lining the alveoli increases which further decrease the surface tension. Thus collapse of the alveoli is prevented.

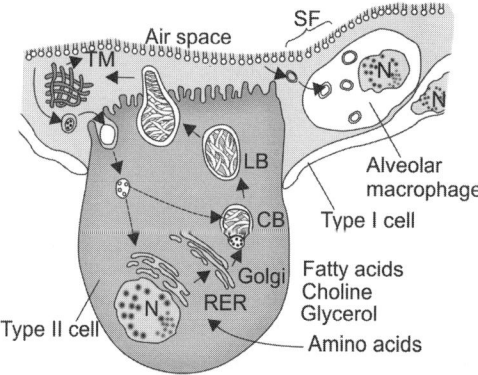

Fig. 8.9: Formation and metabolism of surfactant

Hyaline Membrane Disease

In newborns, especially preterm babies, the maturation of surfactant is not present even at the time of birth. So due to the lack of surface tension lowering agent the expansion of alveoli does not occur at the time of birth. This results in acute respiratory distress syndrome in the newborn. This may lead to death of the newborn. The treatment for this is administration of cortisol to help maturation of surfactant.

Alveoli also contains pulmonary alveolar macrophages. They originate in bone marrow and act as phagocytic cells. These cells process the inhaled antigens to mount immunological effect on them. It releases lysosomal products in the ECF. The manophages stimulate secretion of substances to attract WBCs to lung. Other cells in the alveoli include lymphocytes, plasma cells, mast cells, etc. Mast cells contain heparin and 5 hydroxy tryptamine. Amine precursor uptake and decarboxylation (APUD) cells present in the alveoli store and secrete many substances like vasoactive intestinal peptide (VIP) and substance P.

Nerve Supply

Parasympathetic → Cholinergic → Bronchoconstriction sympathetic → Adrenergic → Bronchodilation
Non-cholinergic, Non-adrenergic nerves that release VIP produce bronchodilation.

The Factors Producing Bronchodilation

- 6 pm
- Inspiration
- Sympathetic stimulation
- VIP.

Factors Producing Bronchoconstriction

- 6 am
- Expiration
- Parasympathetic stimulation
- SO_2
- Cool air
- Exercise
- Adenosine
- Cytokins.

The Structure of Respiratory Membrane

The layers are:
- Alveolar fluid
- Alveolar epithelium
- Basement membrane of alveolar epithelium
- Interstitial space
- Basement membrane of the capillary endothelium
- Capillary endothelium.

It is very thin and 0.5 microns thickness help in instant diffusion of O_2 and CO_2 across the membrane. Increase in thickness or accumulation of fluid results in decreased gaseous exchange.

The Coverings of the Lungs

- Pleura
  - Parietal
  - Visceral.

Parietal pleura: It adheres to chest wall and moves with chest wall.
Visceral pleura: It adheres to lungs and moves along with lungs (Fig. 8.10).

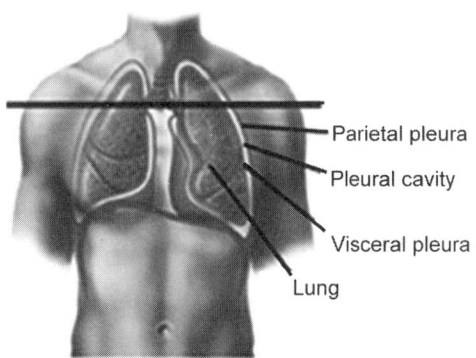

Fig. 8.10: Pleura

FUNCTIONS OF LUNGS

- Respiratory function
- Synthesis of prostaglandins E2 and F2 α, histamine, kallikrein and surfactant
- Removal of prostaglandins E1, E2, F2 α bradykinin, serotonin, noradrenaline, acetylcholine
- Endocrine function
- Angiotensin
  - *Angiotensin I:* Converting enzyme
  - *Angiotensin II:* Lungs
- Fibrinolytic system
- Olfaction
- Vocalization
- Water balance
- Temperature regulation
- Mast cells secrete heparin which act as an anticoagulant.

Pulmonary Ventilation

It is the amount of air which is taken and expelled by the lungs per minute. This process requires the inspiration, and expiration the mechanical process involved in respiration.

Inspiration

It is an active process, in which thoracic cavity expands and parietal pleura and visceral pleura follows it. External intercostals contracts. There is fall in intrapulmonary pressure so air enters the lungs from the atmosphere.

Rib Movements in Inspiration (Fig. 8.11)

1st Rib – Immobile
2nd – 6th – Pump handle movement and bucket handle movement
Assisted by external intercostals muscles innervated by T12. This results the increase in the anteroposterior diameter.

Diaphragmatic Movements

Contraction of the dome of diaphragm 1.5–7 cm descent of dome 75% of tidal volume is inspired due to diaphragmatic movement.
Expiration: It is a passive process in which muscles relax, and the elastic recoil of lung expels the air from the lungs.

Muscles of Expiration

- Anterior abdominal wall muscles
- Internal intercostals

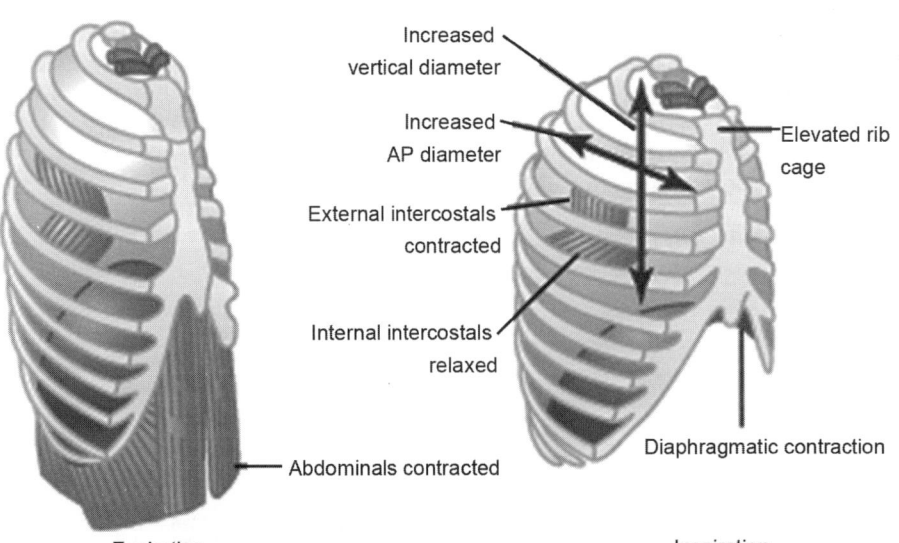

Fig. 8.11: Rib movements during ventilation

- Accessory muscles
- Adductors of vocal cords.

Types of Breathing

It is thoracoabdominal in females and abdominothoracic in males.

Pressure Changes During Respiratory Cycle

Atmospheric pressure = 760 mm Hg

Intrapulmonary Pressure

Beginning of inspiration and end of expiration the intrapulmonary pressure is 760 mm Hg. During inspiration, the volume of the lungs increases and intrapulmonary pressure becomes 3 mm Hg less. During beginning of expiration volume of lung decreases and intrapulmonary pressure becomes 3 mm Hg more (Fig. 8.12).

Intrapleural Pressure Changes

Lungs and chest wall are elastic structures. Lung tends to recoil from chest wall towards the end of expiration. This produces a negative intrapleural pressure of –2 mm Hg. Lung tends to recoil more from the chest wall during peak inspiration. This produces more negative intrapleural pressure of about –6 mm Hg. The intrapleural pressure is more negative at apex of lungs than base of lungs. The negativity increases during standing.

■ MEASUREMENT OF PULMONARY VENTILATION

Lung Volumes and Capacities

There are four pulmonary volumes which when added together, equal the maximum volume to which the lung can be expanded. Combinations of two or more of the lung volumes are called pulmonary capacities.
- Spirometer (Fig. 8.13)
- Spirogram

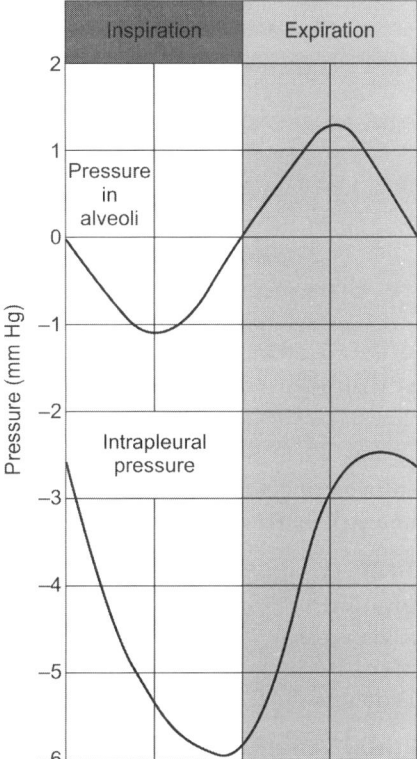
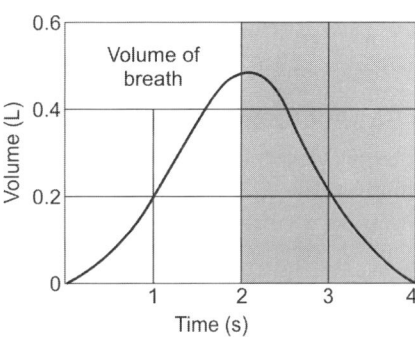

Fig. 8.12: Intrapulmonary pressure

- The pulmonary volumes can be static or dynamic

Static: In a stand still lung.
Dynamic: In a moving lung.

The lung volumes and capacities are about 20–25% less in women than in men. It is greater in large and athletic people than in small and asthamic people.

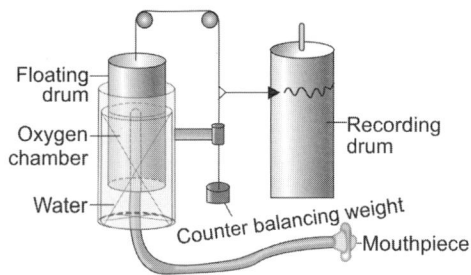

Fig. 8.13: Spirometer with recording drum

■ SPIROGRAM (FIG. 8.14)

Tidal Volume

It is the amount of air that moves into the lungs with each inspiration or the amount that moves out with each expiration. The volume is 500 mL.

Inspiratory Reserve Volume

The air inspired with a maximal inspiratory effort in excess of the tidal volume.
- Men - 3.3 L
- Women - 0.7 L

Residual Volume

Air left in the lungs after a maximal expiratory effort
- Men - 1.2 L
- Women - 1.1 L

The Significance of Residual Volume

- Helps blood to remain aerated after inspiration.
- Maintains contour of lungs.

Lung Capacities

- Inspiratory capacity
- Expiratory capacity
- Functional residual capacity
- Total lung capacity

Vital capacity: It is the largest amount of air that can be expired after a maximal inspiratory effort.

IRV + TV + ERV or IC + ERV
3300 + 500 + 1000 = 4800 mL
Men – 4.8 L
Women – 3.1 L

Variations in Vital Capacity

- More in males
- Standing
- Athletes
- Wind instrumentalists.

Pathological Variations

Decreased in:
- Asthma
- Emphysema
- Pneumonia
- Pneumothorax
- Pulmonary edema

Vital capacity is an index of pulmonary function. It gives useful information about the strength of the respiratory muscles and other aspects of pulmonary function.

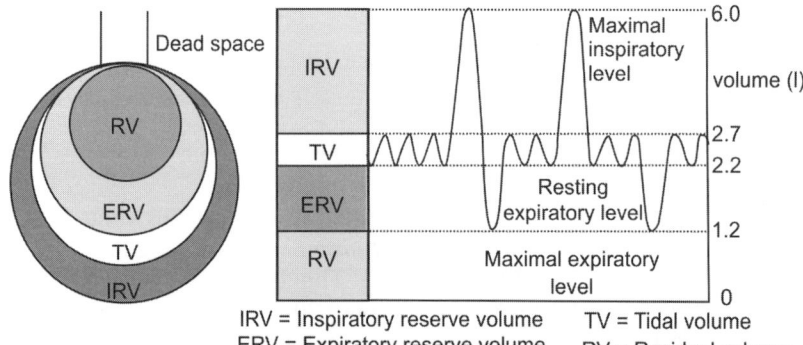

Fig. 8.14: Spirogram showing different lung volumes

Timed Vital Capacity (Fig. 8.15)

Forced expiratory volume 1 (FEV1).
It is the fraction of the vital capacity expired during the first second of a forced expiration.
FEV1 = 83%
FEV2 = 94%
FEV3 = 97%

Importance of FEV1

Vital capacity may be normal, but the FEV1 reduced in asthma and emphysema.

$\frac{FEV1}{FVC}$ = Reduced in obstructive diseases

Both vital capacity and FEV1 reduced in restrictive diseases

So $\frac{FEV1}{FVC}$ may be normal.

Inspiratory Capacity

Tidal volume plus the inspiratory reserve volume,
TV + IRV = IC
This is the amount of air (about 3500 mL) a person can breathe in, beginning at the normal expiratory level and distending the lungs to the maximum amount.

Functional Residual Capacity (FRC)

ERV + RV = FRC
This is the amount of air that remains in the lungs at the end of normal expiration = 2300 mL.

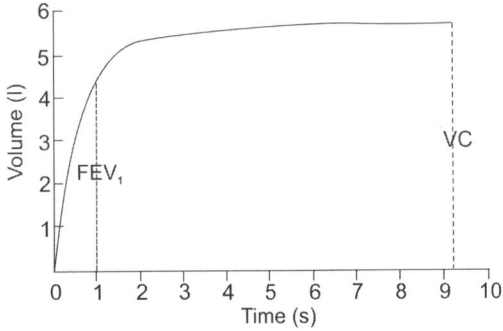

Fig. 8.15: Timed vital capacity

Ventilation perfusion ratio =

$$VP = \frac{\text{Alveolar ventilation}}{\text{Pulmonary blood flow}}$$

$$= \frac{4200}{5000} = 0.84$$

(Alveolar ventilation = Tidal volume × respiratory rate)

Pulmonary Gas Exchange (Tables 8.4 and 8.5)

Oxygen from atmosphere to alveoli and then to blood and tissues.
Carbon dioxide from tissues to alveoli and to atmosphere.
Mechanism - simple diffusion.
Ninety-nine per cent of the O_2 that dissolves in the blood combines with the O_2—carrying protein hemoglobin. Hemoglobin increases O_2 carrying capacity of the blood 70 fold.

Table 8.4: Partial pressure

Gas	Inspired air	Alveolar air	Expired air
O_2	159	104	116
CO_2	0.3	40	27

Table 8.5: Gas composition and partial pressure

Gas	Arterial blood	Venous blood
O_2	100	40
CO_2	40	46

Blood takes 0.75 sec to traverse the pulmonary capillaries at rest.

O_2 Diffusion from Alveolus

PO_2 is 104 mm Hg in alveolus. The PO_2 is 40 mm Hg at the pulmonary arterial end. The PO_2 of blood at the venous end is 104 mm Hg.

CO_2 Diffusion to Alveolus

- PCO_2 is 40 mm Hg at alveolus.
- PCO_2 at the pulmonary arterial end is 45 mm Hg.
- PO_2 of venous blood leaving the lungs is 40 mm Hg.

Oxygen Diffusion from Capillaries to Tissues

- PO_2 at the arterial end is 95 mm Hg and PO_2 of tissues is 40 mm Hg.
- The PO_2 of venous end becomes 40 mm Hg at the tissue level.

Carbon Dioxide Diffusion from Tissues

- PCO_2 at the tissues is 46 mm Hg.
- At the arterial end PCO_2 is 40 mm Hg.
- At the venous end PCO_2 becomes 46 mm Hg when it leaves the organ.

Carbon Dioxide Diffusion to Alveolus

PCO_2 is 40 mm Hg at the alveolus. The pulmonary venous end has PCO_2 45 mm Hg. The PCO_2 decreases to 40 mm Hg at the pulmonary arterial end.

Fate of CO_2 in Blood

In plasma:
- Dissolved
- Formation of carbamino compounds with plasma protein
- Hydration, H^+ buffered, HCO_3^- in plasma.

In RBC:
- Dissolved
- Formation of carbamino Hb
- Hydration, H^+ buffered, 70% of HCO_3^- enters the plasma
- Chloride shifts into cells. Osmolarity of cells increases.

Oxygen Transport in Blood

- Dissolved form
- In combination with Hb.

Dissolved form—0.3 mL/100 mL of blood. This form is directly proportional to arterial PO_2. This is important during exercise.

Oxigenation of Hb helps in the transport of oxygen. Oxygen is transported as oxyhemoglobin. One gram Hb transports 1.34 mL O_2.

So in a person with Hb—15 gm%
15 × 1.34 = 20.1 mL O_2/100 mL blood
But actual O_2 content is only 19 mL/100 mL because Hb can be only 95% saturated.

Oxygen carrying capacity—19 mL O_2/100 mL blood.

ODC (Oxygen-hemoglobin dissociation curve): Graph plotting partial pressure of O_2 against % saturation of Hb. Sigmoid shape.

↑ PO_2—Hb accept O_2
↓ PO_2—Hb release O_2

Factors shifting ODC to left: Show acceptance of O_2
Increase PO_2
Fetal blood
Myoglobin
Alkalinity
Bohr effect—exercising muscle—shift to right.

Carbon Dioxide Transport in Blood

Volume of CO_2 in arterial blood is 48 mL/100 mL. It becomes 52 mL/100 mL in venous blood. PCO_2 increases from 40 mm Hg to 46 mm Hg.

- Dissolved form—3 mL/100 mL plasma
- Carbonic acid—negligible
- Bicarbonate—99.9% of H_2CO_3 dissociates immediately and diffuses out of RBC to plasma, 70% of CO_2 transported this way and it is the most important mechanism of CO_2 transport. The carbonic anhydrase enzyme is present only inside RBC. It accelerates
$$CO_2 + H_2O \rightarrow H_2CO_3$$
- Twenty three per cent of CO_2 transported as carbamino Hb. Carbamino Hb combines with plasma proteins to form carbamino compounds.

Seventy per cent of the HCO_3^- formed in the red cells enters the plasma.

Diffusion Capacity of the Lung

It is the:
- Amount of gas crossing the alveolar capillary membrane.
- Per minute

- Per mm Hg difference in partial pressure of gas on the two sides of the membrane. Normal value = 20–30 mL/min/mm Hg at rest.

Factors Affecting Diffusion Capacity of the Lung

- Surface area of alveolar capillary membrane (directly)
- Thickness of alveolar capillary membrane (inversely proportional)
- Solubility of gas (directly)
- Molecular weight of gas (square root)
    Diffusing capacity for O_2 — 21 mL/min/mm Hg
    Diffusing capacity for CO_2 — 400 mL/min/mm Hg
    Diffusing capacity for CO (DLCO) Co-uptake is diffusion limited
    Diffusing capacity of CO is measured as an index of diffusing capacity.
- *Diffusing capacity increases up to three fold during exercise because of:*
    - Capillary dilation
    - Increase in the number of active capillaries.

Table 8.6: Oxygen content and partial pressure of oxygen in different air spaces

Distribution of O_2	PO_2 (mm Hg)	O_2 content mL%
Inspired air	158	21
Expired air	116	16
Alveolar air	100–104	13–14
Arterial blood	98–100	19
Venous blood	40	14

For each 100 mL of inspired air, 5 mL of O_2 is extracted by the blood (Table 8.6).
For each 100 mL of arterial blood, 5 mL of O_2 is extracted by the tissues.

Oxygen Hb dissociation curve: pH –7.4, temperature 38 °C.
PO_2 (mm Hg) is plotted in the X-axis and percentage O_2 saturation of hemoglobin plotted in Y-axis.

S (sigmoid) shaped curve.
↑ PO_2 — Hb accepts O_2
↓ PO_2 — Hb releases O_2
P50 - partial pressure of O_2 at which Hb is 50% saturated. 26 mm Hg. Hb affinity is inversely related to P50.

Factors Affecting ODC
Shift to Right
Shows Dissociation of O_2
- ↓ PO_2
- ↑ CO_2
- ↑ Body temperature
- ↑ 2, 3-Diphosphoglycerate (2,3-DPG) (By-product of Embden-Meyerhoff pathway).
- ↑ Temperature — shift to right.

2,3-Diphosphoglycerate (2,3-DPG) (Table 8.7)
- By-product of Embden-Meyerhoff pathway
- Present in RBCs
- ↑ in muscular exercise
- Acidosis
- High altitude.

Table 8.7: 2,3-DPG concentration

Decreased in	Increased in
Acidosis	Anemia
atored blood with citrate as anticoagulant	High altitude chronic hypoxia
	Increased:
	• Thyroid hormone
	• Growth hormone
	• Androgen

Shift to Left
- Shows acceptance of O_2
- PO_2 — Hb accepts O_2
- Fetal blood
- Myoglobin
- Alkalinity

Decrease in temperature — shift to left.

Bohr Effect
In exercising muscle, more CO_2 generated.
- Enters the blood by diffusion by pressure gradient

- More PCO_2 decreases the affinity of Hb to O_2
- O_2 is released
- ODC shifted to right ↑ in pH—shift to left.

Myoglobin
- Causes shift to left
- Seen in muscles which are involved in sustained contraction, e.g. leg and heart muscles
- Contains only one atom of iron per molecule
- Readily takes up O_2 at low PO_2
- ODC for myoglobin is a rectangular hyperbola
- Does not show Bohr effect
- Even at PO_2 of 40 mm Hg it is 95% saturated
- Acts as a temporary store house for O_2 in muscles.

Carbon Dioxide Transport (Table 8.8)
- Carbon dioxide has high diffusion coefficient
- Twenty times more than O_2.

Table 8.8: CO_2 distribution

Arterial blood	Venous blood
Volume of CO_2 = 48 mL/100 mL	Volume of CO_2 = 52 mL/100 mL
Partial pressure PCO_2-40 mm Hg	Partial pressure PCO_2 = 46 mm Hg

Carbon Dioxide Transport in the form of Bicarbonate

The important change in CO_2 transport is chloride shift or hamburger phenomenon.

Chloride Shift
- Seventy per cent of the HCO_2 formed in the red cells enters the plasma.
- Plasma is rich in Na and Cl.
- Cl^- comes into the RBC to maintain ionic equilibrium. This exchange is called the chloride shift, mediated by band 3 a membrane protein. Because of chloride shift the Cl^- content of the red cells in venous blood is greater than in arterial blood. Chloride shift occurs rapidly that is in 1 second.

For each CO_2 molecule added to a red cell, there is an increase of one osmotically active particle in the red cell either an HCO_3^- or as Cl^-. The red cell take up water and increase in size. Hematocrit of venous blood is normally 3% greater than that of the arterial blood.

CHANGES OCCURRING IN LUNGS
- Chloride moves out of the cells
- RBCs shrink.

Haldane Effect
Deoxygenated hemoglobin binds more H^+ than oxyhemoglobin.

Forms carbamino compounds more readily.

Binding of O_2 to hemoglobin reduces its affinity for CO_2.

Haldane Effect: Other Effects
- Combination with O_2—Hb becomes more acidic
- H^+ released in excess—bind with HCO_3^- ions
- $HCO_3^- + H^+ - H_2CO_3 - CO_2 + H_2O$
- CO_2 released from blood to alveoli.
- CO_2 uptake is facilitated in the tissues.

CO_2 Dissociation Curve
Graph showing the relationship of:
- Partial pressure of CO_2
- Concentration of CO_2 in blood

More $O_2 \rightarrow CO_2$ Displaces more
More $O_2 \rightarrow$ shifts CO_2 dissociation curve to right.

REGULATION OF RESPIRATION

The normal rate of ventilation in adults is 14 to 18 breaths per minute. In children the rate is more rapid and in infants approaches 40 per minute. The rate is increased in certain diseases, for example pneumonia, and may also be abnormally slowed, especially in some cases of poisoning, for example with morphine.

Respiration is controlled by nervous impulses and by the chemical composition of the blood.

Nervous Control

Although for a short time the rate and depth of respiration can be controlled by the will, ordinarily it is an automatic act under the unconscious control of the nervous system. Situated in the medulla oblongata of the brain is a collection of nerve cells called the respiratory rhythm generator or, in older terminology, the respiratory center. Afferent inputs to the rhythm generator arise from various sources. Those which arise from the stretch receptors in the lungs and which inhibit inspiration travel in vagal nerve fibers. Glossopharyngeal nerve fibers carry impulses from the peripheral chemoreceptors to stimulate breathing. From the medulla efferent nerve fibers pass down the spinal cord to the diaphragm and the respiratory muscles.

A pneumotaxic center in the upper pons inhibits the inspiratory cells of the rhythm generator and provides a rate-controlling mechanism.

Chemical Control

It has been seen that carbon dioxide passes from the tissues into the blood and thence to the lungs, where it is excreted. The central chemoreceptors are particularly sensitive to the amount of carbon dioxide (carbonic acid) in the blood. If the amount rises as a result of more being formed in the tissues, such as during muscular exercise, they are stimulated and send impulses to the rhythm generator. This in turn sends impulses to the respiratory muscles to produce deeper and quicker breathing so that carbon dioxide can be excreted more rapidly by the lungs and the amount in the blood reduced to its normal level. In other words, the function of the rhythm generator is to send out impulses to the respiratory muscles which maintain the rate and depth of breathing so that the level or concentration of carbon dioxide in the blood remains constant.

Chemoreceptors are sensory areas which detect changes in carbon dioxide, hydrogen ion or oxygen in the blood. There are both central and peripheral chemoreceptors.

The central chemoreceptors are on the surface of the medulla, where they are bathed by the cerebrospinal fluid (CSF) in the course of its circulation. Carbon dioxide diffuses through the walls of capillaries from the blood into the CSF and stimulates the receptors, which 'notify' the respiratory rhythm generator. Changes in the blood hydrogen ion (H^+) concentration or partial pressure of oxygen (PO_2) do not influence the medullary chemoreceptors.

The main peripheral chemoreceptors are the carotid bodies and the aortic bodies, situated close to arteries. When stimulated by a decrease in the partial pressure of oxygen in arterial blood (PaO_2), they provoke a reflex increase in breathing. The peripheral chemoreceptors are also stimulated by increases in blood H^+ concentration and increases in the partial pressure of carbon dioxide in arterial blood ($PaCO_2$).

Under normal conditions, the principal chemical factor in the regulation of respiration is the partial pressure of carbon dioxide in the arterial blood ($PaCO_2$), acting mainly through the central chemoreceptors.

Two important practical applications of this fact deserve particular mention.
1. Carbon dioxide may be administered mixed with oxygen during and after a general anesthetic. It will be clear from the facts just mentioned that the effect of inhaling carbon dioxide will be to increase the amount in the alveolar air and, thus, in the blood. The raised level of carbon dioxide in the blood acts as a stimulus to the respiratory center which sends out impulses causing increased ventilation of the lungs, hence a more rapid excretion of the anesthetic and at the same time a greater intake of oxygen. Carbon dioxide is sometimes used to produce increased ventilation of the lungs for other purposes.
2. When administering oxygen, care must be taken to ascertain the percentage of oxygen required and the appropriate type of apparatus for administering it. In some respiratory disorders (e.g. chronic bronchitis) the amount of carbon dioxide in the blood may be persistently raised and the respiratory center no longer sensitive to it. Deficiency oxygen (hypoxia) may then be supplying the main stimulus to the respiratory center. If too high a concentration of oxygen is given, this hypoxic stimulus is removed. Consequently breathing becomes shallower and there is further retention of carbon dioxide, which can result in coma and ultimately death.

- Neural
  - Automatic
  - Voluntary
- A. Chemical
  - Central
  - Peripheral
- B. Neural centers
  - Medullary centers
    - Inspiratory center
    - Expiratory center
  - Pontine centers
    - Pneumotaxic center
    - Apneustic center.

Inspiratory Center

Located in upper medulla formed by Nucleus tractus solitarius. It is called Dorsal Respiratory Group (DRG) which produces the ramp signal.

Ramp signal: Action potentials of increasing amplitude for 2 seconds, then stop.

Gets sensory inputs from:
- Baroreceptors
- Chemoreceptors
- Pulmonary receptors

(via Vagus and Glossopharyngeal Nerves).

Expiratory Center

- Located in lateral medulla
- Formed by nucleus ambiguous and retroambiguous.
- Ventral respiratory group
- Inactive during quite respiration
- Stimulation causes contraction of respiratory muscles
- Gets sensory inputs from:
  - Baroreceptors
  - Chemoreceptors
  - Pulmonary receptor.

Pneumotaxic Center Stimulates Expiratory Center

Automatic Control of Respiration

Medullary respiratory center. The dorsal inspiratory neurons and ventral expiratory neurons are reciprocally inhibited. The medullary respirating center is capable of spontaneous, rhythmic discharge. Irregular discharge which is under the influence of other parts.

Pontine Centers (Fig. 8.16)

- Apneustic center
- Pneumotaxic center

Respiratory System

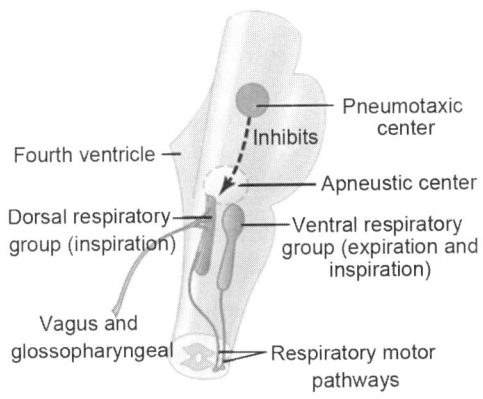

Fig. 8.16: Medullary and pontine centers

Apneustic center: Contain I neurons. So produce apneusis that is prolonged inspiration. Apneustic center is under vagal control. Vagotomy produces apneusis leading to respiratory arrest.

Pneumotaxic center: Situated in upper prons. Contain both E and I neurons. Exact function is unknown. May play a role in switching between inspiration and expiration.

Initiation

Inspiratory center stimulated by apneustic center, stimulus to C3, 4, 5 and T12.

Genesis of Expiration: I neurons send impulses to pneumotaxic center. Inhibit apneustic center.

Pulmonary stretch receptors inhibit apneustic center via vagus.

Pneumotaxic center stimulate expiratory center.

■ CHEMICAL REGULATION

There is a chemosensitive areas controlled by chemical factors.

$$CO_2 + H_2O - H_2CO_3 - H^+ + HCO_3^-$$

H^+ stimulate the inspiratory area

A. Peripheral Chemoreceptors

- *Carotid body:* Glomus cell (Type I)
  Glossopharyngeal
- *Aortic body:* Vagus nerve (Fig. 8.17)

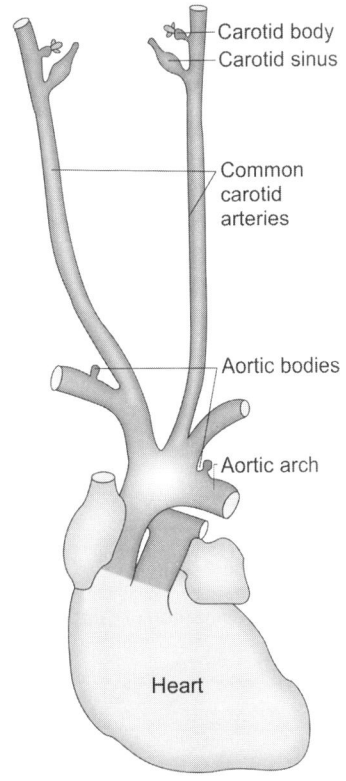

Fig. 8.17: Location of carotid and aortic bodies

Stimulated by
- Hypoxia
- Hypercapnia
- Increased H^+ concentration

Carotid body—Stimulated by (Fig. 8.18)
- Hypoxia
- Vascular stasis
- Asphyxia
- Cyanide poisoning
- Hyperkalemia
  - Highest perfused organ
  - Dissolved O_2 used to meet needs.

B. Central Chemoreceptors

Situated near inspiratory center. Close contact with CSF, Respond to H^+, Blood H^+ cannot cross blood brain barrier (Fig. 8.19). Also respond to CO_2.

Stimulation: Increased H^+ cause hyperventilation and CO_2 washout. Hypoxia does not have effect on central chemoreceptors.

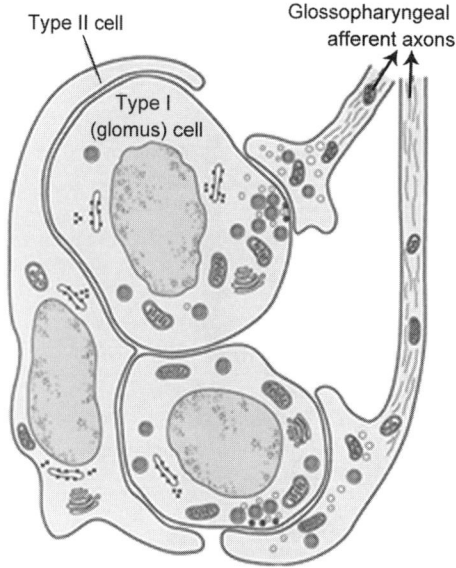

Fig. 8.18: Organization of carotid body

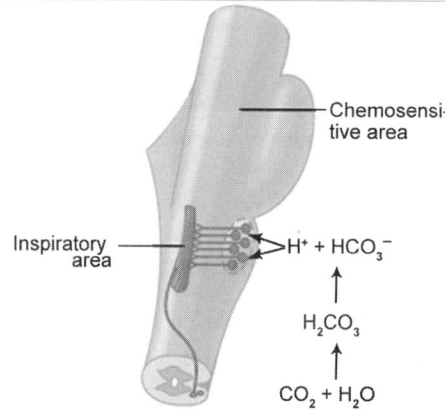

Fig. 8.19: Central chemoreceptor

Aim of Chemical Control

To keep alveolar PO_2 at 40 mm Hg.
Maintains the tension of O_2, CO_2 and H^+ within physiological limits.

Mechanism of Stimulation of Carotid Bodies

Hypoxia:
↓ activity of O_2 sensitive K^+ channel
↓ K^+ efflux
↑ Ca^+ influx

Depolarization
- Release of neurotransmitter
- Stimulate afferent nerve ending
  During hypoxia release catecholamines. Peripheral chemoreceptors respond maximally to reduction in PO_2.

Ventilatory Response to CO_2

- Increase arterial PCO_2
- Chemoreceptor stimulation
- Respiratory center stimulation
- CO_2 washout
- PO_2 becomes normal.

CO_2 Narcosis

CO_2 — Respiratory center stimulation.

Excessive CO_2

- Hypercapnia
- CNS depression
- CO_2 narcosis.

Ventilatory Response to H^+

- ↑ H^+
- Peripheral chemoreceptor stimulation
- Hyperventilation
- CO_2 washout.

Afferents from Higher Centers (Table 8.9)

- Cerebral cortex
  - Corticobulbar tracts
  - Corticospinal tracts
- Hypothalamus and Limbic system
  - Pain
  - Fever
- Hering-Breuer inflation reflex
  - Acts when tidal volume is > 1000 mL
  - Important in exercise

Table 8.9: Factors affecting respiratory centers

Inputs from higher centers	Baroreceptors
Hering-Breuer reflex	Chemoreceptors
J-receptors	Proprioceptors
Irritant receptors	Thermoreceptors
	Pain receptors

- Stretch receptors in smooth muscles of airways act via vagi on apneustic center.
- Hering-Breuer deflation reflex limits deflation.

  J receptors (juxtapulmonary capillary receptors)—impulses travel via unmyelinated vagal fibers.

  This reflex reinforce pneumotaxic center—reflex apnea followed by tachypnea, hypotension and bradycardia.

  —AS Paintal, 1955

Voluntary Control of Respiration

Maximum 45–55 seconds respiration can be voluntarily inhibited—point at which it can no longer be inhibited is called Breaking Point.

Reasons are:
↑ Arterial PCO_2
↓ Arterial PO_2

Voluntary Hyperventilation

Produces apnea followed by resuming respiration
- Hyperventilation—CO_2 washout
- Apnea—PCO_2 increases
- PO_2 falls
- Chemoreceptor stimulation
- Respiratory center stimulated.

Role of Vagus in Respiration

- Inhibits apneustic center
- Stretching of lungs—Vagal stimulation—inhibit inspiration
- Hering-Brauer inflation and deflation reflexes
- Vagotomy results in deep and slow respiration.

Deglutition Apnea

Respiration gets inhibited at any stage if swallowing gets initiated. Afferent impulses travel via glossopharyngeal nerve.

■ HYPOXIA

Hypoxia is the lack of O_2 at tissue level.

Types of Hypoxia
- Hypoxic
- Anemic
- Stagnant
- Histotoxic

Hypoxic hypoxia

Decreased O_2 content in blood.

Causes
- Low O_2 availability, e.g. high altitude
- Decreased pulmonary ventilation. Bronchial asthma, poliomyelitis, pneumothorax
- Cardiac disorders—congestive cardiac failure.

Anemic Hypoxia

Inability of blood to carry sufficient O_2 due to anemia. It is the reduced oxygen carrying capacity.

Stagnant Hypoxia

Decreased rate or velocity of blood flow. Seen in:
- Thromboembolism
- Congestive cardiac failure
- Circulatory shock.

Histotoxic Hypoxia
- Inability to utilize O_2, e.g. cyanide poisoning
- Sulfide poisoning
- Paralysis of cytochrome oxidase system.

Hypoxia: Clinical Features
- Severe hypoxia leads to brain death in 3 minutes
- *Blood:* Erythropoietin secretion
- *CVS:* Reflex stimulation of vasomotor center
- Later depression of VMC.

Respiration: Initially stimulation of chemoreceptors hyperventilation

Later depression of respiration.

GIT: Nausia, thirst
Kidney:
- Erythropoietin secretion ↑
- Alkaline urine

CNS: Loss of self-control, later disorientation, memory impairment, coma and death.

Oxygen Therapy

- Oxygen mask or oxygen tent
- Best in hypoxic hypoxia
  - Can be at atmospheric pressure
  - Can be under high pressure (2–3 atmosphere)
    [Hyperbaric Oxygen therapy]
- Improves dissolved O_2 levels and thereby tissue Oxygenation.

Oxygen Therapy Useful in
- Carbon monoxide poisoning
- Radiation induced tissue injury
- Gas gangrene
- Severe blood loss
- Anemia
- Diabetic leg ulcers
- Wounds that are slow to heal
- Decompression sickness and air embolism.

Effectiveness of O_2 Therapy

- Best in hypoxic hypoxia
- Least effective in histotoxic hypoxia
- Anemic hypoxia—70% effective
- Stagnant hypoxia—50% effective.

Oxygen Toxicity

- Due to production of superoxide anion (O_2^-) a free radical
- H_2O_2
- Abnormality high O_2 content in tissues cause toxicity.
- Prolonged hyperbaric O_2 therapy—excessive amounts of dissolved O_2.

Results in
- Pulmonary edema
- Tissue and cytochrome destruction due to heat

- Retrolental fibroplasias in babies
- Convulsions, coma, death.

Hypercapnea

- Increased CO_2 content of blood
- Asphyxia means Hypoxia + Hypercapnea.

Effects
- Respiratory stimulation initially
- PH become acidic
- *CVS:* Tachycardia, ↑BP, flushing of skin
- Convulsions, loss of consciousness
- Death.

■ ASPHYXIA

Usually due to obstruction of air passage result in hypoxia and hypercapnea.

Stages:
- Hyperpnea
- Convulsions
- Collapse.

Carbon Monoxide Poisoning

- Automobile exhaust
- Coal mines
- Deep wells
- Gun smoke.

Carbon monoxide has 210 times more affinity towards Hb.
Forms carboxy Hb
Anemic hypoxia result
ODC shift to left
Death occurs when Hb saturation with CO goes above 50%.

Cyanosis

Bluish discoloration of skin and mucous membranes due to increased amounts of reduced hemoglobin > 5 gm%.

Depends on
- Amount of Hb
- Degree of Hb unsaturation
- State of capillary circulation.

Two Types
1. Central cyanosis
2. Peripheral cyanosis

Central Cyanosis
Defective oxygenation, e.g. ASD, VSD, PDA, Polycythemia aggravates cyanosis.

Peripheral Cyanosis
Slowing of blood flow → more O_2 extraction → more reduced Hb.
- Cold environment → vasoconstriction → Decreased flow.

Cyanosis—not seen in
Anemic hypoxia: The total Hb content low. So reduced Hb cannot be more than 5 gm%.
CO poisoning: Color of reduced Hb is obscured by the cherry-red color of carbon monoxide Hb.
Histotoxic hypoxia: Blood gas content is normal.

■ DISORDERS OF RESPIRATION
Sequential apnea and respiration.

Types of Periodic Breathing
- Cheyne-Stokes breathing
- Biot's breathing

Cheyne-Stokes Breathing (Fig. 8.20)
Physiological Conditions
- Voluntary hyperventilation
- High altitude
- Sleep.

Pathological Condition
- Cardiac failure
- Brain damage
- Uremia.

Biot's Breathing
Three to four cycles of normal respiration followed by sudden apnea (Fig. 8.21).

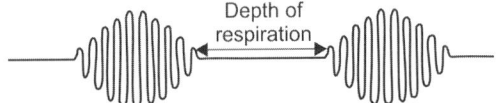

Fig. 8.20: Cheyne-stokes breathing

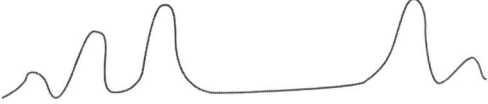

Fig. 8.21: Biot's breathing

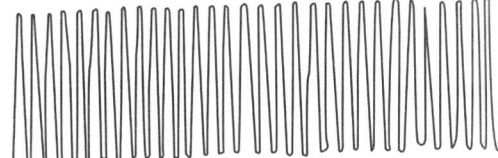

Fig. 8.22: Kussmaul's breathing

Usually Pathological
- Meningitis
- Medullary involvement.

Kussmaul's Breathing
Seen in metabolic acidosis (diabetic keto-acidosis) (Fig. 8.22).

■ ARTIFICIAL RESPIRATION
Tissues of brain, particularly cerebral cortex develop irreversible damage if oxygen supply is stopped for 5 minutes. So the resuscitation must be started quickly without any delay before the development of cardiac failure.

Artificial respiration alone is required as an emergency lifesaving procedure.
- When there is sudden stoppage of breathing as in
  - Drowning
  - Electrocution
  - Anesthetic accidents
  - Carbon monoxide poisoning
  - Strangulation
  - Accidents
- Gradual cessation of breathing as in paralysis of muscles in
  - Poliomyelitis
  - Diphtheria
  - Ascending paralysis.

Methods of Artificial Respiration
Various manual methods of artificial respiration have been described in past and

discarded. The manual method employed is mouth to mouth breathing.

Procedure

- Place the patient in supine position. Provide and maintain a clear airway for the procedure to be effective. Any foreign material present in the mouth cavity must be removed with fingers, e.g. grass, straw, etc. (in case of drowning patients), artificial denture if any, mucus, saliva and blood clots, etc. The tongue must be drawn forward and it must be prevented from falling posteriorly causing airway obstruction. The cloths around the neck and chest region must be loosened. If the mouth is full of blood, mouth to nose respiration should be given.
- Patient's neck is extended by placing one hand under the chin and lifting it and pressing the forehead with the other hand. This prevents the flaccid tongue from falling back into the pharynx.
- Then the patient's nostrils are closed by the thumb and index finger of the hand.
- The resuscitator then takes a deep breath and exhales air into the patient's airway after tightly placing his mouth over patient's mouth and noting the expansion of the chest at the same time. The volume of the air exhaled must be twice the normal tidal volume. This expands the patient's lungs.
- The resuscitator removes his mouth from that of the patient, allowing expiration to occur passively due to the elastic recoil of the lungs and chest.
- Some of the air is likely to enter the stomach through the esophagus. It can be easily expelled by pressure on the epigastrium.
- The above procedure is repeated 12–16 times/minutes till spontaneous breathing returns, or till the patient is shifted to a hospital.
- Mouth to mouth method is most effective manual method because the CO_2 present in the expired air by the resuscitator can also directly stimulate the respiratory centers and facilitate the onset of respiration.

Mechanical Methods of Artificial Respiration

The mechanical respirators are employed when artificial respiration has to be continued for long periods. The mechanical respirators are of two types:
1. Tank respirators
2. Ventilators

Tank respirators: It is also called iron lung chambers as the name indicates consists of an air tight chamber made of iron or steel. The patient is kept inside the tank by placing the head outside the chamber. In drinker method alternate positive and negative pressure breathing machines produce periodic inflation and deflation of the lungs.

Ventilators: They are the artificial respiration machines by which air or oxygen is pumped into the lungs with pressure intermittently through a rubber tube introduced into the patient's trachea. Inflation occurs when air is pumped and expiration occurs by elastic recoil of chest and lungs when it is stopped.

Types of Ventilators

1. Volume ventilator pumps a constant volume of air into the patient's lungs intermittently with minimum pressure.
2. Pressure ventilator pumps the air with a constant high pressure into the patient's lungs.

CHAPTER 9

The Blood (Hemopoietic System)

The blood is a transport system which plays a very important part in the maintenance of life. It flows throughout the body and when in capillaries it is in intimate relationship with the tissues taking oxygen and other nutritive substances to them and at the same time removing their waste products.

■ COMPOSITION AND FUNCTIONS OF BLOOD

It is a complex fluid with different types of cells in suspension. Total blood volume is 8% of body weight. It comes to about 5.6 liter in average young adults. It consists of two parts.

Plasma and Formed Elements

Plasma: It constitute about 55% of blood volume, and 5% of body weight. It is a clear yellowish fluid with 91% of water and 9% of solids. Among solids, about 7.5% are plasma proteins containing S. Albumin, S. Globulin, fibrinogen and prothrombin. Other substances include non-protein nitrogenous substance anions like Cl^-, HCO_3^-, SO_4^-, PO_4^-, I-Cations like Na^+, K^+, Ca^{++}, Mg^{++}, Fe^{++}, P, Cu^{++}, Zn^{++} and also enzymes, hormones, antibodies and bilirubin.

Formed elements: Constitute 45% of blood volume. It includes RBCs (erythrocytes) WBCs (leucocytes) and platelet (thrombocytes).

Functions

- *Respiratory:* Transfer of O_2 from lung to tissues and CO_2 from tissues to lung.
- *Excretory:* The waste products of tissue metabolism such as urea, uric acid, creatinine are transported to kidneys.
- *Nutritional:* Blood carries the products of digestion to tissue cells of various parts.
- *In homeostasis:* The internal environment of our body is almost kept constant. There is extracellular fluid (ECF) bathing the cells the temperature, pH, concentrations of various solutes in it are kept constant. Similarly the solute concentrations of ICF (intracellular fluid) is also kept constant. This phenomenon that the internal environment (milleau interior) is practically kept constant is spoken of as homeostasis. The various physiological arrangements which serve to restore the normal state once it has been disturbed is termed homeostasis. This term was coined by WB Cannon.
- Role of blood in various defence mechanisms.
  WBCs act against invading bacteria and virus. Lymphocytes are connected with the immunity of the body. Plasma carries antibodies which is concerned with humeral immunity.
- Transport of other substances like drugs, hormones, etc. to the various tissues.
- Maintenance of water balance
- Osmotic pressure of tissue fluids are kept constant.

- **Iron balance:** Hemoglobin is the main depot of iron in the body and iron balance is maintained by blood.

Physical Properties

Blood is a red opaque fluid, scarlet red in color when taken from an artery. Venous blood is blue and the normal opacity is due to reflection of light by RBCs.

Specific Gravity

Normal ranges are 1.052–1.062 for whole blood, 1.095–1.101 for cells and 1.022–1.026 for plasma.

Viscosity: Blood is five times more viscous than water.

Osmotic pressure: It is kept constant by the activity of kidneys. Osmotic pressure of plasma is 6.7 atmosphere. 0.9% NaCl solution is isotonic with plasma and it has the same osmotic pressure as plasma. Such a solution is called normal physiological saline.

Plasma can be obtained by centrifuging the anticoagulated blood at a speed of 3000 rev/min for 30 min. Cells are thrown to the bottom of the tube and the upper portion separated is called plasma.

If we keep blood without anticoagulant it clots and serum seperates.

Difference Between Serum and Plasma

Serum = Plasma – (fibrinogen + clotting factors II, V, VIII)

Serum contains large amount of serotonin when compared to plasma. Serotonin is produced by platelets.

Plasma Proteins

About 100 plasma proteins has been recognized. Major component is albumin. Its concentration in plasma is 3.55 gm/dL
    Globulin – 2.2–2.4 gm/dL
    Fibrinogen – 0.3–0.4 gm/dL

Other minor proteins (prothrombin, enzymes) – 50–300 mgm/dL.

Albumin is the major fraction of plasma proteins.

Functions of Albumin

- Eighty percent of osmotic pressure is contributed by albumin. Osmotic pressure is inversely proportional to molecular weight. Osmotic pressure help to retain fluid in the vascular compartment. Osmotic pressure excerted by colloids mainly plasma proteins is called osmotic pressure.
- *Carrier proteins:* It functions as primary carrier for fatty acids, bilirubin and many drugs, and secondary carrier protein for hem part of hemoglobin, thyroxin and cortisol.

Hypoproteinemia—Causes

- Decreased synthesis as in fasting and malnutrition
- Pathological conditions like liver disease, due to decreased synthesis, kidney diseases like nephritis due to increased loss of albumin in urine.

Globulins: Molecular weight of globulin is 1,50,000 – 1,90,000. It includes $\alpha_1, \alpha_2, \beta_1, \beta_2,$ γ globulins. It is mainly produced by the liver. γ globulin is produced by reticuloendothelial system, plasma cells, and lymphoid tissue.

Different Types of Globulins

- *Coagulation proteins:* Prothrombin, thromboplastin
- *Lipoproteins:* α, and β lipoproteins, chylomicrons, HDL, LDL, VLDL, etc.
- *Glycoproteins:* Transferrin, hapatoglobin, hemopexin, ceruloplasmin, etc.
- Aglutinins
- Erythropoietin
- Angeotensinogen
- Anterior pituitary hormones
- Fetuin
- Fibrinogen

Functions of Plasma Proteins

- Osmotic pressure
- Help to maintain peripheral resistance
- Transport function
- Hemostasis
- Defence against infection
- Acid base balance—protein buffer
- Reservoire protein
- Rouleaux formation.

■ FORMED ELEMENTS

RBC (Erythrocytes)

RBCs are the simplest cells in the human body. They exist as biconcave discs in large blood vessels and shape changes to parachute like conformation in the capillaries (Figs 9.1A and B). RBC lose their nuclei before it is released into the circulation. Mature RBCs lack nuclei and cytoplasmic structures like lysosome, ribosome endoplasmic reticulum and mitochondria. It may be considered as a kind living bag containing hemoglobin.

RBC is a living bag that can be deformed to any shape because the cell has grate excess of cells membrane for the quantity of material inside and hence the cell is not ruptured easily. The membrane of the red cell is elastic and can squeeze through capillaries of small size and then return to its original biconcave shape.

Average diameter of RBC 7.5 μm (7.2–7.8 μm). Thickness at the periphery is about 2 μm and at the center 1 μm around. The outer edge appear as a rim around a central depression. The RBC has a high surface area to volume ratio due to its discoid shape. This fascilitate the transport of respiratory gases through it. The RBC in the venous blood are slightly larger because CO_2 content is more in venous blood and so chloride ions enter inside and water moves in along with that.

Advantages of Shape

- Quick exchange of gases because of large surface area
- Changes in volume can be accommodated without changing the membrane integrity
- Can pass through small blood vessels.

Structure of RBC

RBC has an outer cell membrane and an inner stroma. Inside the stroma is the hemoglobin other proteins, lipids and electrolytes (Fig. 9.2).

Major Proteins of RBC Membrane

- Band 3 protein
- Glycophorin
- Spectrin and glycolipids
- Cholesterol and phospholipid
- Enzymes and coenzymes—carbonic anhydrase, glucose 6 phosphate dehydrogenase, glutathione peroxidase, catalase, alkaline phosphatase, urea, amino acids, 2,3-DPG, ATP, reduced glutathione.

Inorganic compounds: Potassium, phosphate, very little sodium.

Metabolism of RBC

Mature RBC has no nuclei, no mitochondria. Hence, ATP can not be produced by citric acid cycle. Ninety percent of glucose entering RBC is metabolized by glycolityc pathway. Ten percent of glucose is utilized by HMP pathway or pentose shunt.

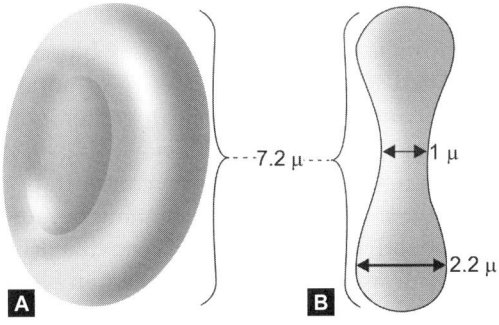

Figs 9.1A and B: Erythrocytes

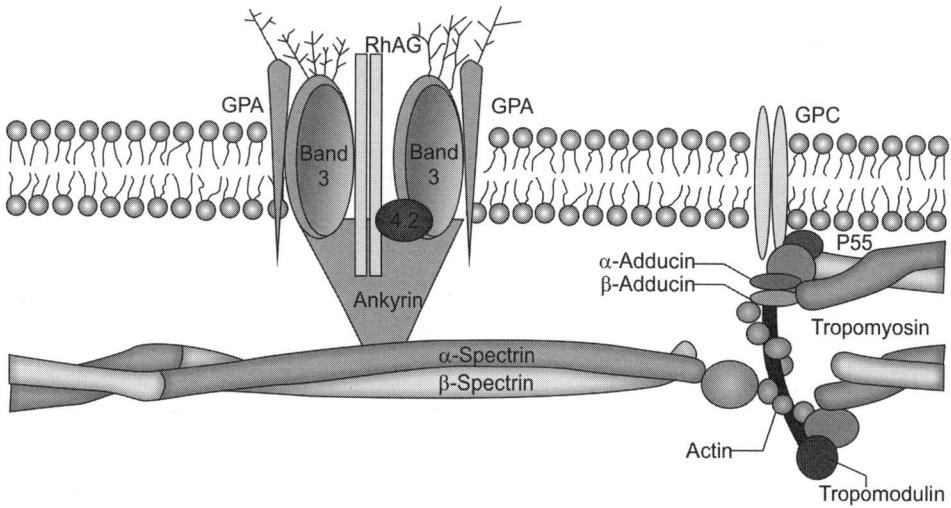

Fig. 9.2: RBC membrane

Functions of Cell Membrane

- Maintenance of cell shape or deformability
- Control intracellular cation concentration i.e. high potassium and low sodium inside.
- Preservation of hem ion in ferrous state.
- Protection of protein against oxidative denaturation.
- Participation in certain metabolic activities.

Functions of RBC

- To transport Hb which in turn carries O_2 from lung to tissues.
- RBC contain large amount of carbonic anhydrase, which catalise the reaction between CO_2 and H_2O. It carries CO_2 as bicarbonate.
  About 1/3rd of CO_2 forms compound with deoxy Hb to form carbamino Hb.
- RBCs are responsible for most of the buffering power of whole blood
- If Hb is free in plasma it will filter through glomeruli and will cause great rise in viscosity and osmotic tension and volume of blood would have been unmanageable.

VARIATIONS IN SIZE, SHAPE, AND STRUCTURE OF RBC

- *Anisocytosis:* Variations in size of RBC
- *Poikilocytosis:* Variations in the shape of RBCs
- *Spherocytosis:* Spherical RBCs—more fragile
- *Anemia:* Reduction in number of RBCs, less than 4 million/mm^3 or their Hb content less than 12 gm% or both
- *Polycythemia:* RBC count increases more than 6 million/cmm.

Properties of RBC

- *Rouleaux formation:* When blood is shed RBC show a tendency to adhere to one another or pile together with their flat surfaces on contact (Fig. 9.3). Increase in fibrinogen concentration increases rouleaux formation because negative charge which keep the RBC widespread in blood is lost when blood is exposed to the atmosphere.

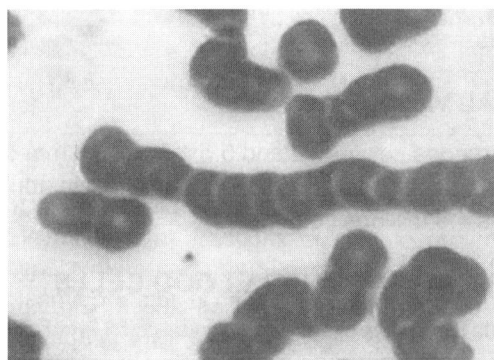

Fig. 9.3: Rouleaux formation

- **PCV:** Anticoagulated blood taken in Wintrobe's tube 2.5 cm bore size, with markings 10–0 and 0–10 centrifuged at 3000 revolutions/mt for 30 minutes. RBCs settle at the bottom, narrow layer of WBC and platelets form buffy coat. Above buffy coat clear straw-colored plasma is formed.

Normal value: Male — 46 ± 5%
Female — 42 ± 5%

Variations
Physiologically
Increase: Male
　　　　　Newborn
　　　　　High altitude
　　　　　After exercise
Decrease: Females
　　　　　Pregnancy

Pathologically
Increase: Polycythemia
　　　　　Dehydration
　　　　　Burns, gastroenteritis
Decrease: Anemia

Erythrocyte Sedimentation Rate (ESR)

The apparatus used to determine ESR is Westergren's pipette, open at both ends, 30 cm in length graduated 0–200. Use 3.8% sodium citrate in the ratio 4:1. Keep the tube mounted in the rack in vertical position undisturbed for 1 hour. Amount of plasma column at top at the end of 1 hour in mm is taken as ESR. Westergren's pipette, length 300 mm, bore size — 2.45 mm.

Lower end of tube closed by removable rubber cap held in position by a spring. 1.6 mL taken in pipette diluted as 4 part blood to 1 part 3.8% solution of sodium citrate.

Value:
Male: 1–3 mm/hr
Female: 3–7 mm/hr
Infants: 0–0.5 mm/hr.
Significance: To assess the prognosis of a disease.
Eserite tube: Also used as an alternate method for ESR.

Factors Affecting ESR
Plasma Factors
Rouleaux formation favors ESR
Fibrinogen: Favors rouleaux formation
Globulin: Increase ESR
Normal biconcave disc shape: Increase ESR
Abnormalities of shape: ESR decreased
Increase in count: ESR decreased
Slanting position of tube: ESR increased.

Variations
Physiological
Increase: In females
　　　　　Lactational
　　　　　Pregnancy from 3rd month
　　　　　Old age
Decrease: Males; newborns.

Pathologically—Inflammation or Tissue Destruction
Increased:
- In a/c infection
- c/c infections like tuberculosis (TB), leukemia, multiple myeloma
- All anemia except sickle cell anemias
- Rheumatic fever
- Rheumatoid arthritis
- Collagen deseases like SLE, polyarthritis nodosa

- Pelvic inflammation, malignancy, trauma
- Nephrosis (low albumin).

Decreased:
In allergy, spherocytosis, sickle cell anemia, afibrinogenemia, polycythemia.

Osmotic Fragility

When suspended in hypotonic saline RBCs undergo rupture and release hemoglobin into surrounding fluid. The ease with which RBCs undergo hemolysis when suspended in hypotonic solution is called osmotic fragility. It is expressed in terms of concentration of hypotonic solution in which the cells are hemolyzed.

Ghost cells: Some hemolytic agents destroy the framework or stroma of the cells partially and the dim colorless outline of the cells can be seen as shadows and is called Ghosts

Blood may be hemolyzed by:
- Fat solvents like ether, chloroform, benzene which dissolve the cell membrane.
- Add distilled water or hypotonic salt solution which increase cell volume and cause hemolysis, by disturbing surface tension (add bile salt and saponin)
- Alternate freezing and thawing
- Temperature of 65 °C
- Treating with acid or alkalis
- Venoms, bacteria, incompatible blood transfusion.

Life Span of RBC

Average: 120 days (Range—90–140 days). In hemolytic diseases reduced to 10–40 days depending on the severity of the disorder.

Destruction and disposal of red cells: By reticulo endothelial system. As RBC grows older due to wear and tear and decreasd metabolic process cell becomes less viable; cell membrane become more fragile and the cell squeezes through a capillary, undergoes deformation and eventually it fragments mainly in spleen. (narrow channels of red pulp). The aging and fragmented cells are ingested by macrophages of the spleen. (liver and bonemarrow) and are lysed. Hb released is degraded.

Protein part: Globin removed and conserved

Iron: Detached from the heme, transported to bone marrow bound to transferring and used for hemoglobin synthesis in the red cell precursors.

Hemoglobin

Normal value:
Male: 14–18 gm/dL
Newborn: 18–23 gm/dL

Variations

Physiological increase: Infants, high altitude, males, excercise

Pathological: Increase—polycythemia Decrease—anemia.

Estimation of Hemoglobin

Direct:
- Depeding on the oxygen carrying capacity.
- Depending on the iron content
- Spectrophotometric method.

Indirect method:
Colorimetric method:
- Sahli's acid hematin method
- Haden Hausser method
- Cyan meth Hb method
- Haldanes carboxy Hb method.

Derivatives of Hemoglobin

- Oxy Hb
- Reduced Hb or deoxy Hb
- Meth Hb
- Carbamino Hb
- Carboxy or carbon monoxy Hb
- Cyan meth Hb
- SulfHb, Acid hematin, Alkali hematin
- Functions of Hb

Functions of Hemoglobin

- *Transport of O_2 efficiently from lung to tissues:* The attachment is loose and reversible.
  - Hb is oxygenated not oxidized.
  - Can carry O_2 to tissues.
  - Liberate O_2 to tissues and become reduced or deoxy Hb.

Heme-Heme Interaction

$Hb_4 + O_2 \rightarrow Hb_4O_2$
$Hb_4O_2 + O_2 \rightarrow Hb_4O_4$
$Hb_4O_4 + O_2 \rightarrow Hb_4O_6$
$Hb_4O_6 + O_2 \rightarrow Hb_4O_8$

This change in oxygen affinity results in a sigmoid shape of the O_2 dissociation curve (Fig. 9.4). In ODC degree of oxygenation or % saturation of Hb with O_2 is plotted against the PO_2.

Oxygen Affinity of Hb

- Changes with Temperature
- pH
- Concentration of 2,3-DPG
- *Concentration of 2,3-DPG:* 2,3 DPG and H ions compete with O_2 for binding with the deoxygenated Hb for O_2 by shifting the position of the 4 peptide chains.
- *Storred blood:* Increased affinity. The cause is decrease in 2,3-DPG
- *High altitude:* Increased O_2 affinity. The cause is decrease in 2,3-DPG
- *Fetal Hb:* Increase in oxygen affinity. The cause is 2.3-DPG binding is less with fetal Hb when compared to adult Hb. Large numbers of receptors for 2,3-DPG is present on beta chain. But the number of receptors are less for gamma chain. This result in movement of O_2 from maternal to fetal circulation.
- *Carbondioxide Transport:* As carbamino hemoglobin
- *Acid-base balance:* Act as a buffer.

Structure, Synthesis and Breakdown of Hb

Hemoglobin is the red carrying pigment in the RBC of vertebrates. It is a protein specially designed for the transport of O_2 with the molecular weight 64,450. Hb is synthesized by erythroblasts present in the bone marrow. Mature RBCs cannot synthesize Hb.

Synthesize Hb

It is a metallo protein with heme as prosthetic group and protein as globins. Hb is a tetramer with 4 submits. Each submit has a prosthetic Heme and globin polypeptide. In addition to Hb, Heme is present as prosthetic group in myoglobin, cytochrome, catalase, etc.

Heme is produced by combination of iron and protoporphyrin 9. Iron is present in it in the form of ferroprotoporphyrin. Prophyrins are cyclic compounds with 4 pyrol rings.

Globin part has 22 polypeptide chains and 2 non α chains (β, γ, δ, etc.)

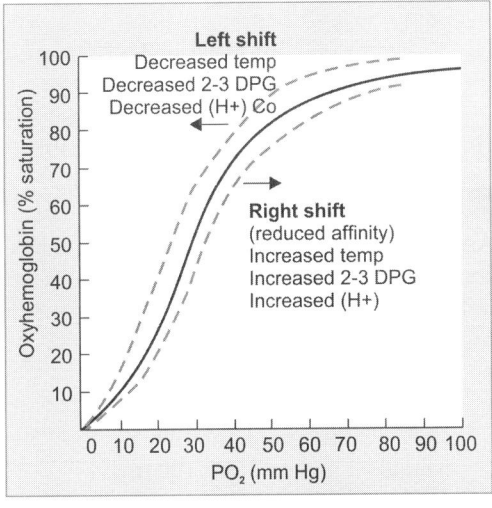

Fig. 9.4: Oxygen hemoglobin dissociation curve

HbA: 97% of adult Hb is HbA having and 2α and 2β chains (Hb $\alpha_2\beta_2$)

HbA₂: 2–5% of adult Hb is HbA₂ having 2α and 2β chains (HbA$_2$–$\gamma_2\delta_2$)

Other Varieties of Hb

HbF: Fetal Hb with $\alpha_2\gamma_2$ special features of HbF is that it has great affinity for O_2 which is beneficial for transport of O_2 from maternal to fetal blood. In the body O_2 content of HbF at a given PO_2 is greater than that of HbA because it bind 2, 3-DPG less avidly.

Iron Metabolism

Iron has to be obtained from food or iron contained in the Hb of dead RBC. Copper and cobalt are also necessary for Hb synthesis.

Essential iron containing compounds in our body are Hb, cytochrome, catalase, peroxidase, Xanthine oxidase.

Storage forms of iron are (a) Ferritin→ apoferritin + iron (b) Hemosiderin transport form Transferrin.

Sources and Requirements of Iron

Liver, heart, kidney, egg yolk are excellent sources, green vegetables are also good sources of iron. Iron in the food may be heme iron or nonheme iron. Heme iron is easily absorbed being soluble. Most of the non-heme iron is ferric and is insoluble. For absorption ferric should be converted to ferrous form by gastric HCL and Vitamin C. So gastrectomy persons and persons with Vitamin C deficiency suffer from iron deficiency. Non-heme iron is ferrous form reach the epithelium of intestinal mucosa and a part of it bind with apoferritin to ferritin. Another part of iron enters plasma, transported as transferrine to various cells which utilize the iron.

Daily requirement:
- Males – 1 mg/day
- Non-pregnant non-lactating woman of reproductive age is 1.5 – 2 mg/day.
- Iron absorption occurs from duodenum and upper part of jejunum.

Abnormalities of Hb

Sickle cell Hb: HbS with α chain is normal. In the β chain there is valin instead of glutamic acid in the 6th position. HbS is insoluble at low O_2 tension. They form tectoids which distort the shape RBCs, and form sickle shaped cells. These are less flexible, more fragile than normal RBC and they harmolyse easily and led to sickle cell anemia. This cause increased viscosity blockage of vessels, and more hemolysis. Manifestations of hemalytic jaundice, tissue infarcts and susceptibility to infection are other features. Sickle cell trait → seen in heterozygous individuals. They are resistant to malaria.

Thalassemia

Defect in globin gene. Polypeptide chains are as such normal. But they are decreased or absent. Individuals with homozygons gene are called Thalassemia major, heterozygous individuals form thalassemia minor.

α-Thalassemia decreased or absent α chain. So synthesis of HbA, HbF, and HbA₂ decreased. But HbH β_4 and Hb art γ_y formed.

β-Thalassemia decreased or absent β chain. So decreased HbA, HbF, and HbA₂.

■ ANEMIA

Anemia is a condition where either the RBC count or the Hb concentration or both are deficient. Females 0 Hb below 11.8 gm/100 mL.

RBC count < 3.8 millions/μL
or
PCV < 37 is called anemia
Males – Hb < 13.2 gm/100 mL
Hematocrit < 40

Androgenic hormones like testosterone is responsible for the higher Hb%, RBC count and hematocrit values in males.

Classification of Anemia (Figs 9.5A to E)

Due to increased destruction → Excessive hemolysis malena, snake bite, G_6PD deficiency spherocytosis, sickle cell anemia.

Polycythemia

Polycythemia is a condition in which Hb concentration, and RBC count or both rise.
- *Primary Polycythemia:* Polycythemia rubravera is a member of the group of diseases known as myeloproliferative syndrome.
- Secondary polycythemia develops in high altitude.
- Emphysema
- Cyanotic heart disease
- COPD.

Break Down of Hb

When the erythrocytes become old they rupture mostly is spleen as well as in liver and bone marrow. The Hb is liberated from the ruptured RBC and phagocytozed by the phagocytes of RE system. Iron and globin is removed, and the remaining tetrapyrrole straight chain compound thus formed is called biliverdin. Biliverdin is oxidized to form bilirubin. All these changes takes place in the phagocyte of RE system.

Bilirubin comes out of phagocyte into plasma.

Bilirubin + Albumin → Bilirubin Albumin complex. This complex is also called free bilirubin complex. It enters liver. In the liver albumin is removed from free bilirubin. Most of bilirubin conjugates with glucuronic acid to form, bilirubin glucuronides, which is water soluble.

Bilirubin + glucuronic acid → Bilirubin glucuronides.

Bilirubin + sulfate radicals → Bilirubin sulfate.

The conjugated water soluble bilirubin sulfate is called conjugated bilirubin. It is discharged into the biliary cenaliculi and get mixed up with bile and gives color to bile. The conjugated bilirubin ultimately enter duodenum. In the intestine, it comes in contact with the intestinal bacteria hydrolyzed to non-conjugated bilirubin, this non-conjugated bilirubin reduced to form urobilinogen and stercobilinogen. Part of urobilinogens and stercobilinogens are absorbed by blood. This urobilinogens and stercobilinogens circulate and get excreted via urine. The rest is excreted via stool.

Conjugation of bilirubin in liver is catalyzed by the enzyme glucuronyl transferase. Unless it is becomes conjugated, it cannot be excreted through bile.

Hemolytic Jaundice

Due to excessive erythrocyte destruction lead to excessive free bilirubin formation and jaundice.

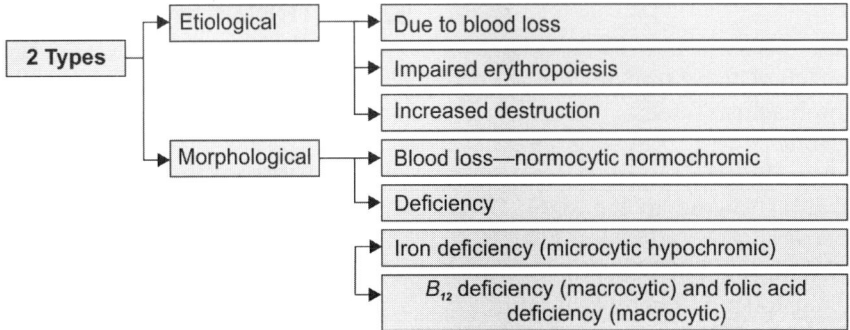

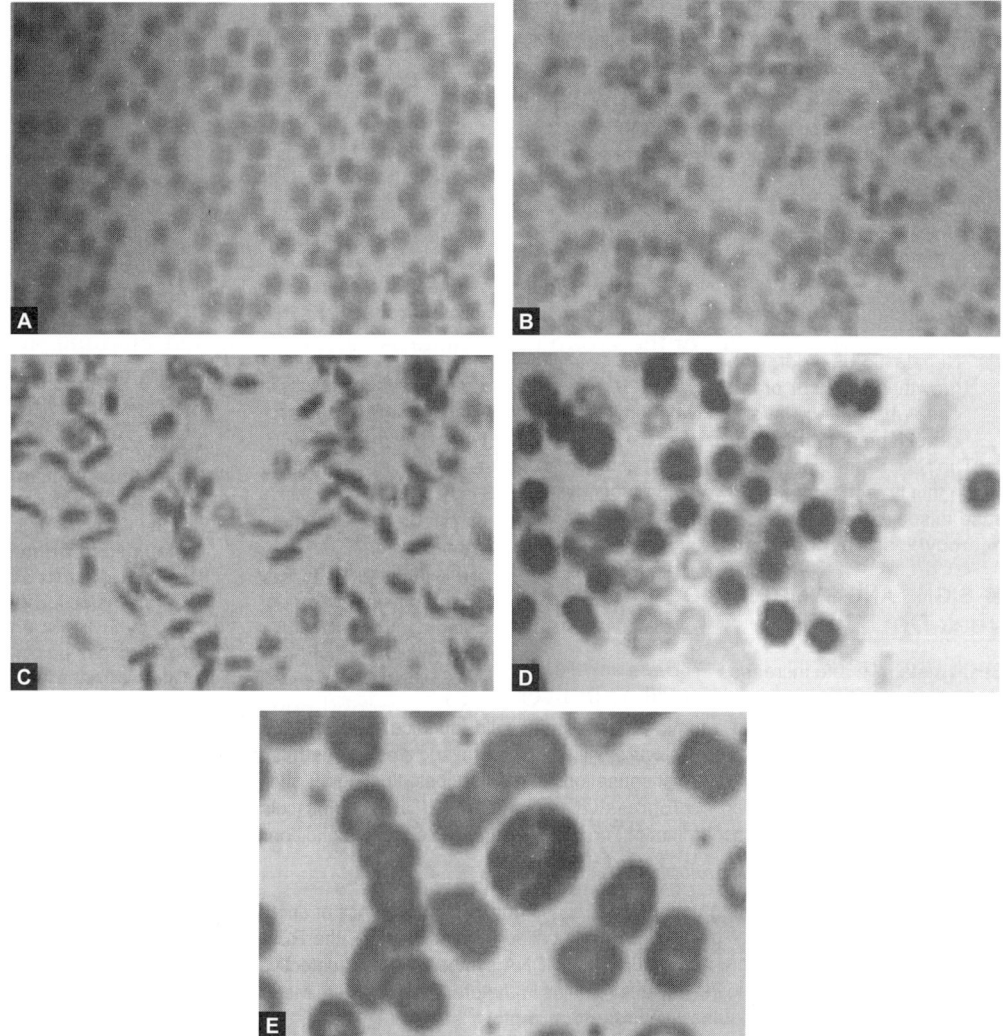

Figs 9.5A to E: A. Normal RBC; **B.** Hypocromic anemia; **C.** Sickle cell anemia; **D.** Thalassemia; **E.** Megaloblastic anemia

Causes
- Malaria
- Mismatched blood transfusion
- Erythroblastosis fetalis
- Snake bite

Bilirubin albumin complex cannot pass the renal filter (owing to big size). Urine contains excessive urobilinogens also.

Normal plasma bilirubin concentration is 0.5–1.0 mg/100 mL in hemolytic jaundice. This level rises greatly.

ERYTHROPOIESIS

The entire process by which RBCs are produced is bone marrow is termed erythropoesis.

Site of Synthesis
- IUL between 0–3 months RBCs are produced in the mesoderm of yolk sac.

Some cells of mesoderm proliferate to form capillary network, a part of which get detached from endothelium

and circulate through the capillaries. This is intravascular erythropoiesis
- After 3rd month of IUL extravascular erythropoeisis occurs mainly is liver also occurs in spleen, thymus, and lymph nodes. This is called hepatic stage.
- From 5th month of IUL onwards RBC formation begins in the red bone marrow. This is myeloid stage.

Extramedullery hemopoiesis → when there is increased used necessity of erythropoiesis yellow marrow is connected to red marrow, and when the necessity is further increased liver and spleen start erythropoiesis, e.g. sclerosis of bone marrow, hereditary spherocytosis leukemia, thalassemia, etc. This is extramedullary enythropoiesis.

Origin of Blood Cells

Two Theories — Monophyletic
                — Polyphyletic

Monophyletic: All types of blood cells are derived from a common premature cell called stem cell.

Polyphyletic: There are separate stem cell for each variety of blood cell.

Stages of Erythropoiesis

All cells in circulating blood is derived from:
- Hemocytoblast or pluripotent uncommitted
- Stem cell diameter—18–23 µ
- Nucleus large, with a rim of basophile cytoplasm.
- Pluripotent stem cell → Give rise to all types of cells (Fig. 9.6).

Myeloid stems cells: Give rise to erythrocyte, granulocyte, monocyte, and platelets

Lymphoid stem cell: Give rise to lymphocytes.

Progenitor cell: As commitment progresses capability of a stem cell for cell renewal decrease and then it is called a progenitor cell. Progenitor cells are more in number than stem cells and also present in bone marrow and blood. Progenitor cells are usually called colony forming units (CFU)
- *CFU (E):* Colony forming unit erythroid series
- *CFU (GM):* Colony forming unit granulocyte monocyte.

There are two types of progenitor for erythroid series.

1st-BFU(E): Burst forming unit Erythrocyte.

2nd-CFU(E): Colony forming unit Erythrocyte. This form is much smaller colonies.

Development of Blood Cells

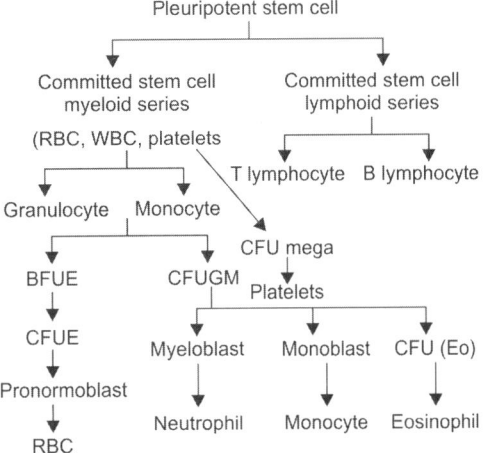

Blast cells: The immediate offspring of the progenitor cells are called blast cells.

Blast Cells Develop to RBC

Pronormoblast (Proerythroblast)
↓
Early normoblast (Early erythroblast)
↓
Intermediate normoblast
(polychromatophilic normoblast)
↓
Late normoblast
↓
Reticulocyte
↓
Mature RBC

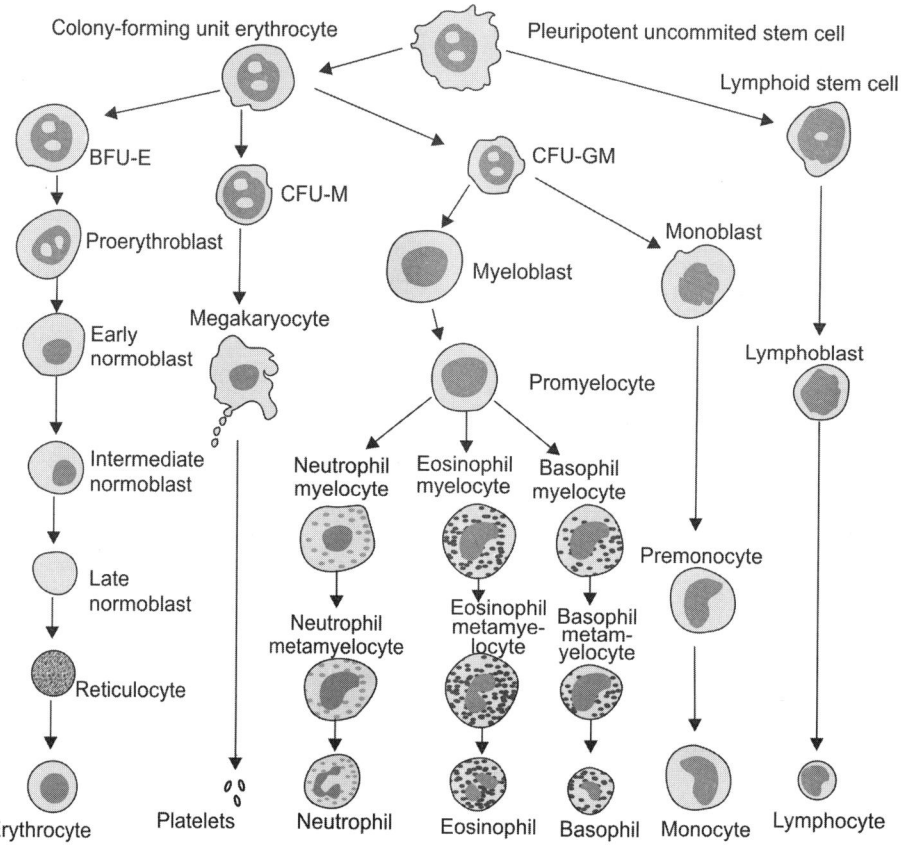

Fig. 9.6: Pluripotent hematopoietic stem cell and cells derived from them

Pronormoblast (Proerythroblast): From the progenitor CFU-E pronormoblast develop size–15–20 m—large round nucleus, Basophilic cytoplasm. Nucleus contain fine punctuate chromatin and several small nucleoli, a rim of scanty cytoplasm.

Early Normoblast (Early erythroblast)

(Basophilic normoblast): Cell is smaller than pronormoblast. 12–16 m nucleus smaller. No nucleoli coarser and more basophilic chromatin strands. Cytoplasm is more basophilic. No Hb active mitosis.

Intermediate normoblast (Polychromatophilic normoblast) still smaller, nuclear chromatin is coarse and form condensation deeply basophilic. Hb begin to appear and its eosinophilic staining give the cytoplasm a polychromatophilic appearance. The basophilic RNA and acidophilic hemoglobin give this polychromatophilic appearance. Proliferative activity stops after this stage.

Late normoblast: [orthochromatic normoblast] size- 7–10 m. Nucleus is smaller, chromatin condensed to firm a cart wheel appearance and stains purplish blue. Nucleus finally disappears. Cytoplasm contain mitochondria and ribosome. Active Hb synthesis no mitosis. Acidophilic cosin stain.

Reticulocyte: Precursor of RBC 7–10 μ Nucleus absent. Large amount of Hb present cytoplasm show a reticulum in supravital staining with brilliant cresyl blue. Remments of RNA appear as clumps of small blue dot or as fine thread connecting the clamp. Reticulocyte mature in 1 or 2 days in bone marrow → enter peripheral blood → reticulocyte lose their mitochondria ribosome with in few days and mature. Mature RBC formed in 1–2 days.

Normal time for maturation of RBC – 5–7 days.

Normal adult reticulocyte count – 0.5–1%.

Newborn – 2–6%.

Factors Influencing and Regulating Erythropoiesis

- Effective O_2 carrying capacity of arterial blood. This is the most important factor in control of erythropoiesis. Any condition causing tissue hypoxia → stimulation of erythropoiesis eggs.
  - Low blood volume as in hemorrhage
  - Poor blood flow as in cardiac failure
  - Decrease in Hb — anemia
  - Decrease in oxygenation of Hb — as in lung disease, heart diseases, high altitude.

  Hypoxia has no direct action on bone marrow. It increase erythropoietin by inducing the production of a hormone erythropoietin.
- *Erythropoietin:* Most important factor to regulate erythropoietin. It is a circulating glycoprotein.

  Site of production — 85% from kidney, 15% from liver.

  Mode of action → erythropoietin increase the number of CFUE → convert it to pronormoblast. Erythropoietin bind to receptor or cell surface → increase calcium uptake → increase RNA → increase glucose, iron uptake → increase Hb synthesis → increase reticulocyte formed → increase red cell production.
- Other factors stimulating erythropoietin
  - Norepinephrin, Alkalosis.
  - Androgens increase erythropoietin by increasing erythropoietin. So increase RBC count in males.
  - Thyroid hormone increase erythropoietin
  - Pituitary GH, prolactin, parathyroid hormone, etc. increase erythropoietin.
  - Estrogen — decrease erythropoietin.
- *Maturation factors:* Vitamin and folic acid are called maturation factors as they are needed for the final maturation of RRC.
- Other vitamins needed for erythropoietin as pyridoxine and Vitamin C.
- *BPA → Burst promoting activity:* Growth of BFU erythrocyte in culture require the presence of one or more growth factors collectively called BPA. both interleukins 3 and granulocyte macrophage CSF stimulate early erythroid progenitor.

  CFU erythrocyte are independent of BPA.
- Protein, amino acid, lipids, etc. are needed for Hb synthesis. Also trace elements, iron, Cu, Co, Zn, etc. are also needed for erythropoietin.
- *Hematopoietic growth factors:* Include (a) erythropoietin, interleukin, stem cell factor granulocyte — macrophage CSF, CSF – I and thrombopoietin.

Applied physiology: Common condition where erythropoietin is deficient.
- Bone marrow hypofunction
- Lack of erythropoietic factors like Vitamin B_{12}, folate, Vitamin C, iron
- Excessive blood transfusion.

Common conditions where erythropoietin become excessive:

- Anemia
- COPD, high attitude where there is excessive erythropoietin generation.

The intensity of erythropoietin can be assessed by noting the reticulocyte count.

A high reticulocyte count (> 3%) indicate excessive erythropoiesis. (< 0.5%) indicate suppression of RBM.

Mechanism: Erythropoietin retards the clearage of DNA that occur in CFUE and cause erythroid cell to survive BFUE are erythropoietin independent for their survival.

In deficiency of erythropoietin: Rapid cleavage proceed to cell death called programed cell death or apoptosis.

WBC (Leukocytes)

Our body has a special system for combating the different infections and toxic agents. This is composed of blood leukocyte and tissue cells originally derived from leukocyte. These cells act in two different ways:

1. By actually destroying invading agent by process of phagocytosis.
2. By forming antibodies and sensitized lymphocytes WBC differ from RBC. WBC possess nucleus, do not contain Hb, and majority of WBC are bigger than RBC. Less in number than RBC.

WBC count—4000–11000/m

Classification (Fig. 9.7)
- Granulocytes granules present in cytoplasm. Nucleus lobulated
- Agranulocytes—no granules are seen under ordinary microscope. Have single lobed nucleus.

Granulocytes

Three types
- Neutrophils
- Eosinophils
- Basophils

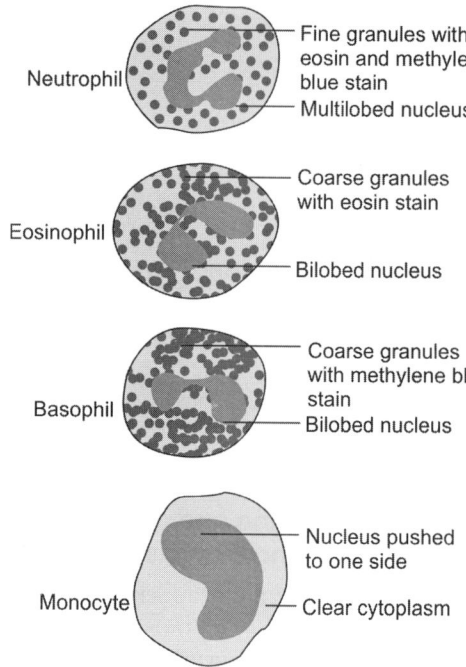

Fig. 9.7: Different classes of leukocytes

Differential Count

This is done by making a smear on a glass slide by using another smooth edged slide to spread the blood drop obtained by finger puncture. It is stained using Leishman stain. Leishman stain is a Romanosky stain which contain acidic dye. Eosin and basic dye methylene blue in acetone free methyl alcohol. The granulocytes can be identified depending on the staining characteristics of granules by Leishman staining. The agranulocytes can be identified by the size and shape of the nucleus and cytoplasm of the entire cell. Differential count is performed by counting 100 cells in the peripheral blood and express the number of each type of cells in percentage.

The acidic dye stain basic part and basic dye stain the acidic part namely nucleus.

Granulocytes

Neutrophil: Contain neutrophilic granules and constitutes 50–70% of leukocytes.

Eosinophil: Contain eosinophilic granules and constitute 1–4% of leukocytes.
Basophil: Contain basophilic granules. They constitute 0–1% of leukocyte.

Agranulocytes

- Lymphocyte: 20–40%
- Monocyte: 2–8%

Neutrophils

Fifty to seventy percent of WBC. Size — 10–14/m in diameter. Nucleus has 2–5 lobes depending on the age of cells. Older cells has more lobes.

Arneth count: Neutrophils in peripheral blood is classified from N_1–N_5 stages depending on the number of lobes present.

Nucleus is purplish blue, cytoplasm pale pink, fine pink granules in cytoplasm. Granules contain enzymes involved in destruction of bacteria.

The Arneth count is expressed in percent of cells with particular number of lobes in peripheral blood from N_1–N_5 stages:

N_1 — 2–10%
N_2 — 20–30%
N_3 — 40–50%
N_4 — 10–15%
N_5 — 2–5%

Shift to left: Younger cells predominate, e.g. A/C infectors, TB, hemorrhage, etc.
Shift to right: Older forms predominate, e.g. megaloblastic anemia, aplastic anemia, septicemia, uremia.

The granules of neutrophil contain enzymes involved in destruction of bacteria, e.g. acid phosphatase myeloperoxidase, lysosomal enzymes and alkaline phosphatase.

The average half-life of a neutrophil in the circulation is 6 hrs; it is therefore necessary to produce over 100 billion neutrophils per day. Many of the neutrophils enter the tissue. They are attracted to the endothelial surface by selecting and roll along the endothelium. This process is margination. They then bind firmly to neutrophil adhesion molecules of integrin family. They next insinuate themselves through the walls of the capillaries between endothelial cells by a process called diapedisis. Many of those that leave circulation enter the gastrointestinal tract and are lost from the body.

Ameboid movement: Neutrophils and macrophage move through the tissue by amoeboid movement.

Invasion of the body by bacteria triggers the inflammatory response.

The bone marrow is stimulated to produce and release large numbers of neutrophils. Bacterial products interact with plasma factors and cells to produce agents that attract neutrophils to the infected area (chemotaxis). The chemotactic agents which are part of a large family of chemokins include component of complement system ($C5_a$), leukotriens, and polypeptides from lymphocytes, mast cells, and basophils. Other plasma factors act on the bacteria to make them tasty to the phagocytes (opsonization). Principal opsonins that coat the bacteria are IgG and complement proteins. The coated bacteria then bind to receptors on the neutrophil cell membrane. This triggers via heterometric G protein mediated responses, increased motor activity of the cell, exocytosis, and respiratory burst. The increased motor activity leads to prompt ingestion of the bacteria by endocytosis (Phagocytosis).

By exocytosis neutrophil granules discharge their contents is to phagocytic vacuoles containing the bacteria and to a degree into the interstitial space (Degranulation).

The granules contains various proteases and antimicrobial proteins called defensins.

Two types of defensines A and B are found in mammals. In addition the cell membrane bound enzyme NADPH oxidase is activated with the production of toxic oxygen metabolites. Toxic oxygen metabolites + proteolytic enzymes from granules—kill the organism.

NADPH oxidase $\xrightarrow{activation}$ sharp increase in O_2 uptake and metabolism in neutrophil (the respiratory burst) and generation of O_2^- by the reaction.

$$NADPH + H^+ + O_2 \to NADP^+ + 2H^+ + O_2^-$$

O_2^- is a free radical formed by the addition of one electron to O_2. Two O_2^- react with $2H^+$ to form H_2O_2 in a reaction catalyzed by the cytoplasmic form of superoxide dismutase (SOD-1).

$$O_2^- + O_2^- + H^+ + H^+ \xrightarrow{SOD-1} H_2O_2 + O_2$$

O_2^- and are H_2O_2 are both oxidants that are effective bactericidal agents, but H_2O_2 is converted to H_2O and O_2 by the enzyme catalase. The cytoplasmic form of SOD contains both Zn and Cu. In amyotrophic lateral sclerosis SOD is defective as a result of genetic mutation. O_2^- accumulates in motor neurons and kills them.

Neutrophils also discharge the enzyme myeloperoxidase which catalyzes conversion of Cl^-, Br^-, I^- and SCN^- to potent oxidants. HOCl is the principal product since Cl^- is abundant in body fluids.

Neutrophil granules contain elastase, and metalloproteinases that attack collagel and other proteases that destroy invading organisms. There enzymes act in a cooperative fashion with the O_2^-, H_2O_2 and HOCl formed by the action of the NADPH oxidase and myeloperoxidase to produce a killing zone around the activated neutrophil. This used to kill invading organisms. But in diseases like rheumatoid arthritis the neutrophils may also cause local destruction of host tissue. The movements of the cell in phagocytosis as well as migration to the site of infection involve microtubules and microfilaments. Proper function of the microfilaments involves the interaction of actin they contain with myosin–I on the inside of the cell membrane.

Neutrophils also release thromboxanes that are vasoconstrictors and platelet aggregating agents, leukotreins that increase vascular permeability and attract other neutrophils to the site and other PG that exert a moderate anti-inflammatory effect.

Genetic Sex and Neutrophil

The female has got 2X chromosome and one inactive sex chromosome. This inactive sex chromosome condenses to form barr body. In neutrophil we can see the barr body as drumstick attached to the nucleus. This is present in 1–15 % of neutrophils in female.

EOSINOPHIL

One to four percent cells present in peripheral circulation diameter—12–16 µ/im. Nucleus bilobed or spectacle shaped with purplish blane color. Cytoplasm contains large coarse crimson red or orange red grannels of uniform size, which are closely packed. Granules does not obscure nuclei. Eosinophilic granules contain:

- *Eosinophilic peroxidase:* Antibacterial property
- *Major basis proteins:* Against parasites
- *Eosinophilic cationic proteins:* Bind and neutralize heparin.

Functions

- Attack parasites by releasing substances that kill parasites
- Inactivate mediators released from mast-cell basophils, and allergic reactions
- Destroy Ag-Ab complex, and involved in detoxification and removal of foreign particles.

Basophil

Size 10–14 µ/im diameter. Nucleus slightly lobulated, purplish bule in color. May be 'S' shaped. Granules are basophilic large coarse bluish black granules fill the cytoplasm and overlies the nucleus obscuring the nucleus. Granules contains large amount of heating and histamine. Basophil resemble large cells in the tissue called mast cells. SRS-A, kallikrein also produced by basophils. Histamine take part in allergic reactions. Heparin is a natural anticoagulant 0–1% of cells and present in peripheral blood.

Agranulocytes

- Lymphocyte
- Monocyte

Lymphocytes: Twenty to forty percent cells are seen is the peripheral blood. Receptors for IgE is present on the surface. Morphologically two types

- Small lymphocytes
- Large lymphocytes–younger forms

Small lymphocyte: 7–10 μm/diameter, nucleus round well-defined, almost completely fill the cell and stains deep purplish blue. Cytoplasm is only a thin rim staining pale blue.

Large Lymphocyte: 10–14 μ/m in diameter. Nucleus is rounded or slightly indented. Stains purplish blue. Cytoplasm is more when compared with small lymphocyte and pale blue in color.

Functionally lymphocytes are classified:

- B Lymphocyte—humoral immunity
- T Lymphocytes—cell mediated immunity.

Monocytes

Largest cell among WBCs 14–18/μm diameter. Nucleus is large intended or kidney-shaped and stain grayish blue. Monocytes gives rise to tissue macrophage.

Functions

Form 2nd line of defense against inflection. Can engulf large particles and more number of particles than neutrophils. They contain lysosomes, with proteolytic enzyme for digesting bacteria and other foreign substances. Also contain bactericidal agents.

Lifespan of WBC

Granulocytes: 4–8 hrs in blood. 4–5 days in tissues.

Monocytes: 12–24 hrs in circulation. In the tissue they become tissue macrophage and remains for months or years.

Variations

- *Leukocytosis:* Physiological, e.g. newborn infants pregnancy, after exercise pathological – A/c bacterial infections like boil, abscess, allergic reaction, asthma, Hay fever, hemorrhage, burns, malignant diseases.
- *Leukopenia:* Typhoid, paratyphoid, ACTH, Cortisone stress, etc.
- *Leukocytosis:* Increase in count above 11,000 cell/mm^3
  Decrease in count below 4000 cell/mm^3
- *Neutrophilia:* Increase in count of neutrophils
- *Basophilia:* Increase in basophils
- *Eosinophilia:* Increase eosinophil count
- *Lymphocytosis:* Increase in lymphocyte count
- *Monocytosis:* Increase in monocytes.

Neutrophilia

- Examples A/C pyogenic infections like streptococci, staphylococci
- Tissue injury due to burns
- Hemorrhage
- Metabolic disorders like diabetic acidosis
- Inflammatory disorders like collagen diseases
- Poisoning with drugs, chemicals, like lead mercury.
- Administration of cortcosteriod.

Eosinophilia

- *Allergic reactions:* Bronchial asthma hay fever

- *Parasitic infestation:* Roundworm, hookworm
- *Skin disease:* Psoriasis, eczema
- *Basophilia:*
  - Smallpox, chikenpox, measles
  - Polycythemia
  - Myxedema
  - After splectomy.
- *Lymphocytosis:* physiological—childhood
- *Pathological:* c/c infections like TB, hepatitis, secondary syphilis, leprosy
- *Monocytosis:* Infectious mononeucleosis
  - TB
  - Protozoal injection—Malaria, Kala-azar
  - Hodgkins disease
  - Monocytic leukemia.

LEUKOPENIA

- *Neutropenia:* Certain infections like typhoid, paratyphoid influenza, measles, malaria, kala-azar aplastic anemia, agranulocytosis
- *Eosinopenia:* Following administration of ACTH, cortisone, stress.
- *Basopenia:* ACTH or cortisone therapy, hyper thyroidism, Cushing's syndrome.
- *Lymphopenia:* Administration of adrenocorticosteroid, aplastic anemia.
- *Agranulocytosis:* Decrease in number or absence of grannulocytes. BM stops producing WBC.
- *Cause:* X-ray irradiation.
- *Drugs:* Chloramphenicol toxicity.
  - Cytotoxic drugs used for malignancy
  - As a part of pancytopenia.
- *Leukemia:* A condition where there is uncontrolled production of WBC by cancerous mutations, characterized by a number of immature cells. Count reach as high as million/mm^3. Leukemia cells are usually nonfunctional.

Disorders of Immunity

- AIDS
- Autoimmunity.

Agranulocytosis

Clinical features: Onset can be sudden or gradual. Patient present with severe sore throat fever, ulceration of throat and mouth. If severe patient dies in a few days.

Rx.

Removal of offending agent.

Supportive treatment with antibiotics. Severe cases – WBC transfusion.

Leukemia

Platelets

Platelets are small colorless granulated bodies which are usually spherical (oval or red shaped). They are non-nucleated 2–4 μm. In a peripheral smear with leishman stain seen as blue dot.

Normal count: 1.5–4 lakhs/mm^3

Average life span: 10 days. (5–12 days) eliminated in reticuloendothelial system mainly spleen.

Electron Microscopic Structure

Cell membrane is made up of two layers. Outer layer—glycoprotein—prevent adherence to normal endothelium and promote adherence to injured area of vessel. Inner layer made of phospholipids layer. Platelet factor plays an important role in clotting mechanism. On the surface of cell membrane specific receptor for certain substances, like collagen, von Willebrand factor, and fibrinogen.

Tubular system: Ring of microtubules seen in periphery, open canalicular system. The contents of the granules are discharged through the canalicular system.

Cytoplasm: Contain action, myosin, glycogen granule called dense and granules. Dense granules contain ATP, ADP, serotonin α granules contain clotting factor → fibrinogen, V, XIII platelets derived growth factor, platelet factor 4, von Willebrand factor. Platelets are derived from giant bone marrow cells called megakaryocytes.

Thrombopoiesis

Pluripotent stem cell
↓
CFU megakaryocyte
↓
Promegakaryoblast
↓
Megakaryoblast → Ist morphologically recognizable unit
↓
Promegakaryocyte
↓
Megakaryocyte (30–60 μ in diameter, light blue cytoplasm and red purple granules)

Platelets

Megakaryocytes extend cytoplasmic pseudopodia into the sinusoids of BM, which detaches into circulation and fragments to form platelets. Single megakaryocyte can give rise to 1000 platelets.

Factors influencing thrombopoiesis: ILN 13, 6 GM CSF, stimulate the production by megakaryocyte. Thrombopoietin is a factor which helps in the maturation of megakaryocyte.

Properties and Functions of Platelets

Normal hemostatic mechanism prevent blood loss from intact vessel. When a blood vessel is injured integrity of vessel wall and presence of adequate number of viable platelets are necessary for hemostasis.
- Plates adhesions
- Platelets activation
- Platelets aggregation
- *Platelet adhesion:* Normally platelets do not adhere to the intact vascular endothelium. When a blood vessel is injured platelets adhere to the exposed collagen underneath endothelium. It requires the participation of von Willebrand factor produced by the endothelial cells and also by megakaryocyte. von Willebrand factor is found in the platelets membrane and in the granules of platelets. It is required for early stages of adhesion.
- *Platelet activation:* The binding of platelet to collagen initiate activation. It is produced by ADP and thrombin accumulating on the platelet membrane. Activated platelets protrude pseudopodia, change shape, discharge granular contents. Phospholipids of platelet membrane converts to arachidonic acid. Arachidonic produce TxA_2 and other prostaglandins.
- *Agregation:* Attachment of activated platelets to one another is facilitated by platelet, activating factor (PAF) produced by platelets, and monocytes. When platelets are activated phospholipids acids of platelet membrane produce arachidonic acid. This arachidonic acid is oxidized by cyclo-oxygenase pathway to yield TxA_2 and PGD_2. These TxA_2 and ADP promotes vasoconstriction and platelet aggregation.

Functions

- Formation of platelet plug and stoppage of bleeding in small vessel wounds.
- Secretion of vasoconstrictors adrenalin and nonadrenalin which is necessary to arrest bleeding in bigger vessels.
- Phospholipids from platelets membrane required for clotting.
- Thrombosthenin is required for clot retraction
- It helps to maintain the intensity of vascular endothelium.
- Phagocytosis of foreign particles.
- It can concentrate, store and transport substances like serotonin, epinephrin and K^+.
- Platelet factor 4, PDGF has role in inflammation and repair.

Disorders

- *Thrombocytosis:* Increase in count after surgery and after child birth. This produce intravascular clotting.
- *Thrombocytopenia:* Decrease in count below 40,000 characterized by hemorrhagic manifestations. It leads to deficient clot retraction and poor contraction of the ruptured vessel. It will lead to spontaneous bleeding into skin, mucus membrane and internal tissue causing multiple subcutaneous hemorrhages.

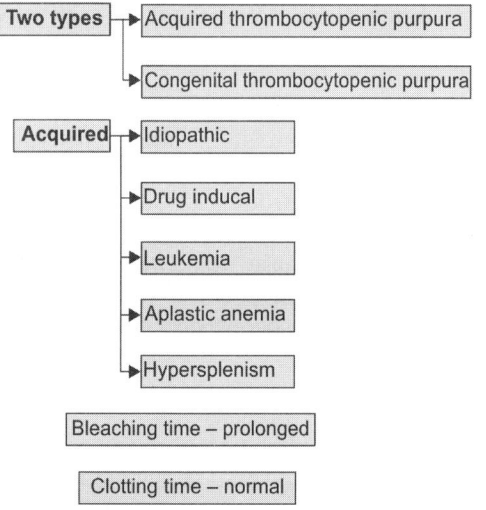

- Thromboasthenic purpura platelet count is normal but platelets are abnormal
- von Wille brand's disease defect of von Wille brand's factor.

Hemostasis

Hemostasis is the process of forming clots in the walls of damaged blood vessel and preventing blood loss while maintaining blood in a fluid state within the vascular system. Hemostasis is attained by different mechanism:
- Vascular spasm (vasoconstriction)
- Formation of a temporary platelet plug
- Blood coagulation
- Growth of fibrous tissue into blood clot and repair of vessel permanently.

Vascular Constriction

Immediately after a blood vessel is cut vessel wall contracts due to:
- Local myogenic contraction of blood vessel initiated by damage to blood vessel
- Nervous reflexes initiated by pain
- Vasoconstriction produced by platelet products TxA_2 and serotonin.

Platelet Plug Formation

Initially platelet plug is a loose plug which is converted to a tight plug by fibrin threads.

Blood Coagulation

Property of blood to lose its fluidity to set into a semisolid jelly when there is injury to endothelial wall, is called coagulation. Clotting is the basic property of plasma aided by platelets. WBCs and RBCs here no direct role, they get entrapped in fibrin meshes of clot. Clotting time 6–8 minute.

After 15–20 minute clot retraction occurs.

Mechanism of coagulation: Involves a cascade of reactions in which inactive enzymes are activated and activated enzymes in turn activate other inactive enzymes. Clotting take place in three essential steps:

1. A complex substance called prothrombin activator is formed in response to the injury either by intrinsic pathway or extrinsic pathway (Table 9.1).
2. *Conversion of prothrombin:* Thrombin by action of prothrombin activator.
3. Conversion of fibrinogen to fibrin by action of thrombin. Fibrin threads are entangled by platelet, RBCs, WBCs.

Intrinsic pathway: Get activated when there is trauma to blood, or exposure of blood or *in vitro* exposure of blood to collagen fibers

Table 9.1: Difference between intrinsic and extrinsic mechanism

Intrinsic	Extrinsic
Initiated by damage to vessel wall or blood itself	Initiated by tissue damage
Occurs both *in vivo* and *in vitro*	Occurs *in vivo* only
Slower usually 1–6 minutes	Rapid in nature within 15 sec
Factors involved XII, XI, IX, X, V, VIII, Ca^{++}, platelet phospholipid	Factors involved VII, X, V, Ca^{++}, tissue, thromboplastin, and phospholipid

under lying endothelium of blood vessels or *in vitro* blood when exposed to negatively charged wettable surfaces like glass.

Extrinsic pathway: Get activated when there is trauma to vessel wall and tissue thromboplastin is released.

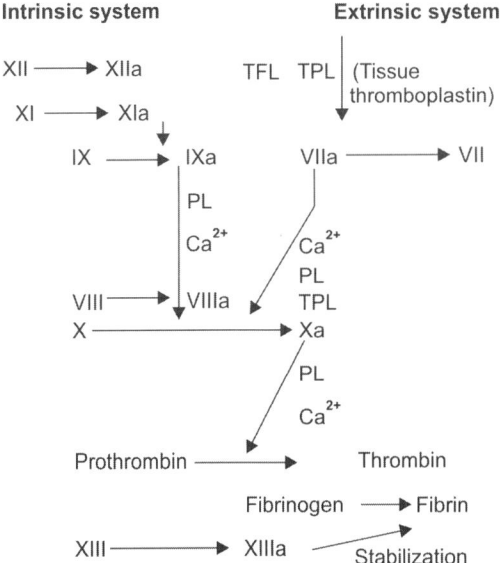

After 15–20 minutes clot retracts extruding a thin clear straw colored fluid called serum. Platelets bind to fibrin thread so as to bind different fibrin thread together. Due to the action of contractile proteins action, myosin, and thrombosthenin present in the platelets there is compression of fibrin mesh work. Contraction of platelets activated by thrombin as well as Ca^{++}.

Clot retractions: After 30–60 minutes the clot contracts and shrinks expressing a thin clear straw colored fluid called serum. This is called clot retraction. This is due to the action of action and myosin present in the platelets.

Actin and myosin pull fibrin threads at the site of adhesion and approximate the edges of the broken vessel.

Normal inhibitors of coagulation produce a mechanism to limit clotting to the vicinity of tissue injury.

Natural substances which prevent intravascular clotting.

(1) endothelial factor. (2) smoothness of endothelium, prostaglandin opposes the action of thromboxane A_2, thrombomodulin a thrombin binding protein this remove thrombin there by slows clotting.

Protein C: A plasma protein—potent in activator of Va and VIIIa proteins promote the activity of protein C—increase the formation of plasmin.

Plasmin lyses fibrin and fibrinogen with the production of fibrinogen degradation products that inhibit thrombin.

Antithrombin III is α globulin can block the effect of thrombin on fibrinogen antithrombin III also inhibit factor IXa, Xa, XIIa.

Heparin: A naturally occurring anticoagulant facilitate the binding of thrombin and antithrombin. Heparin combines with antithrombin III and effectiveness of antithrombin III increase to very high level. Heparin is produced by basophils and mast cells.

Human plasminogen consists of 560 AA heavy chain, and a 241 AA light chain plasminogen receptors are located on the surfaces of many different types of cells and are plentiful on endothelial cells. Plasminogen get activated when it binds its receptor. So intact blood vessel wall is provided with a mechanism that discourages clot formation.

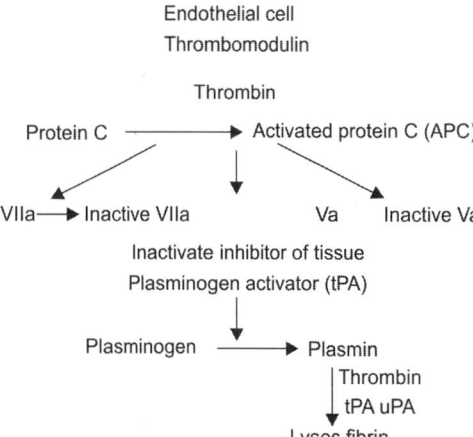

Human +PA is produced by recombinant DNA techniques and is available for lyses of clots in coronary arteries when given to patients, soon after the onset of myocardial infarction.

Anticoagulants

Streptokinase, a bacterial enzyme is also fibrinolytic and is also used in treatment of early myocardial infection. A group of homologous protein now called annexins (annexin II, V) produce fibrinolysis. The physiological role of fibrinolytic enzyme system is to digest intravascular deposits of fibrin in both large and small vessel, which allows reopening of blood vessel.

Anticoagulants: Certain substances can prevent the clotting of blood in *in vitro* and *in vivo.* For example:
- Heparin used as injection, not effective orally. Protamine—used to inactivate heparin.
- Coumarin derivative:
  - Dicumarol
  - Warfarin.

Action: Inhibit the action of vitamin K. Vitamin K is a necessary cofactor for the enzyme that catalyses the conversion of glutamic acid residues to carboxy glutamic acid residues. The six vitamine K dependent proteins involved in clotting are factor II (prothrombin), VII, IX, X, protein C and protein S.

- *Chelating agents:* Which bind Ca^{++} and remove Ca^{++} from blood can be used *in vitro* as anticoagulants, e.g.
  (1) Oxalates of sodium, ammonium and potassium oxalate in 3:2 ratio.
  (2) EDTA—Ethylenediaminetetraacetic acid.

Tests of Hemostasis

Bleeding time: It is the time interval between the onset of bleeding and arrest of bleeding determined by Dukes and Ivy's method.

Dukes method: Ear lobe or finger is pricked and blood is dried every 15 sec with filter paper till no more blood drop stains filter paper.

Normal: 3–6 minutes.

Ivy: BP cuff is tied to upper arm, pressure raised to 40 mm Hg, a wound is made on the forearm (5 mm deep) and the time taken for almost of bleeding determined.

Normal: 3–6 minutes

Arrest of bleeding depends on:
- Platelet plug formation
- Integrity of capillary endothelium
- Degree of capillary constriction
- Size of wound.

1. *Bleeding time is prolonged in:* Thrombocytopenic purpura, defect in platelet function.

   von Willebrand's disease: von Willebrands factor

   Bleeding time is normal in disorders of coagulation time like hemophilia and Christmas disease.

2. *Clotting time:* It is to time taken by blood to clot after it has been shed. It is the time taken for the formation of the clot after withdrawal of blood from the body.

Capillary tube method: Make a finger puncture and using capillary action blood is taken into capillary tube, wait for 2 minuts and then break the tube every 30 seconds. The end point is when the fibrin threads of blood will span a gap of about 5 mm or more between the broken ends. Normal clotting time is 5–8 min prolonged in hemophilia, Christmas disease vitamin K deficiency and hypoprothrombinemia.

3. *Prothrombin time:* Blood is removed and anticoagulants added. Then large excess of Ca^{++} and tissue thromboplastin is added to this oxalated blood. Tissue thromboplastin activate prothrombin to thrombin by means of extrinsic path. The time required for coagulation is the prothrombin time. At the same time prothrombin time of a normal person is tested. Normal value—11–16 sec.

Prolonged prothrombin time is deficiency of factor I, II, V, VII, X.

4. *Clot retraction time:* 30–60 minutes.
5. *Clot lysis time:* 72 hrs.

Abnormalities of Hemostasis

1. Platelet defect — Quantitative / Qualitative
2. Clotting factor deficiency

The use of fresh frozen plasma or concentrates of factor VIII such as cryoprecipitates.

Hemophilia A and Hemophilia B

Hemophilia was the first hereditary bleeding disorder of males transmitted by healthy women. It is caused by deficiency of the blood clotting factor antihemophilic factor or factor VIII, synonyms are true hemophilia, and classical hemophilia.

Inheritance: Inherited as a sex-linked recessive characters as the genes for the disorders are carried by the X chromosome.

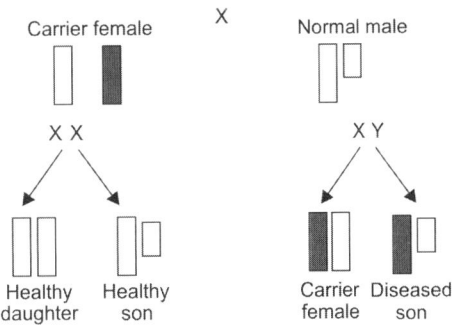

Fig. 9.8: Carrier female married to normal male

Females carrying a gene for hemophilia on one of their two X chromosome transmit the gene to half of their female offspring and to half of their male offspring. The hemophiliacs having only one X chromosome, transmit the gene to all their female offspring, but to none of their male children. Female carrying a gene for hemophilic are called carriers.

Clinical features: Bleeding tendency usually occurs in infancy wound bleeding, tissue bleeding, which may cause formation of hematomas, retroperitoneal and mesenteric bleeding, in addition to pain and swelling they may develop fever, anorexia, and leukocytosis and anemia.

Easy bruising is spontaneous bleeding into skin may occur. Bleeding may occur from mouth and synovial joints intracranial hemorrhage, bleeding into urogenital and gastrointestinal tracts.

The complication of hemorrhage include anemia, constitutional disturbances like fever, anorexia and malaise, etc. Pressure effects of hematoma like hemophilic arthritis and compression of peripheral nerves, respiratory embarrassment.

Diagnosis

Tourniquet test is usually normal
Bleeding time: Normal
Platelet count: Normal
APTT: Prolonged (severe cases exceeds 100 sec then normal)

Clotting time: Prolonged (severe cases exceeds 100 sec than normal) the one stage prothrombin and thrombin time is normal. Thromboplastin generation test used to distinguish between factor VIII and IX deficiency.

Treatment with Blood, Factor VIII Concentrates, Cryoprecipitates

Fresh frozen plasma is an alternative if concentrate or cryoprecipitate is not available disadvantage large doses are required and occurrence of allergies following tooth extraction the fibrinolytic inhibitors with aminocaproic acid or tranexamic acid to reduce factor VIII requirement. Desamino-8-D arginine vasopressin (D DAVP) administration increases the factor VIII activity 3–5 times baseline with 60–120 minutes.

Attenuated androgen danazole used in hemophilia elevated the factor VIII levels significantly.

Hemophilia B

A disorder with deficiency of factors IX is called Christmas disease, plasma thromboplastin component deficiency or hempophilia B inheritance and clinical features same as that of hemophilia.

Diagnosis

Deficiency of factor IX in pa tents plasma but deficiency of factor IX also occurs in newborn infants, liver disease and vitamin K deficiency.

Bleeding time usually normal
- *Platelet count:* Normal
- *APTT:* Prolonged
- *CT:* Prolonged

One stage prothrombine and thrombin time normal thromboplastin generation test distinguishes hemophlia A and B.

Treatment

Infusion of factor IX concentrates:
- PPSB (Factors II, VII, IX, X)
- Prothrombinex (Factor II, IX, X)
- Fresh frozen plasma.

Vitamin K Deficiency

Vitamin K is a fat soluble vitamin essential for synthesis of prothrombin, factor VII, factor IX and factor X. Deficiency of vitamin K is confirmed by showing that the prolonged one stage prothrombin time test is rapidly corrected in 6–24 hrs after the parenteral administration of vitamin K.

Vitamin K deficiency occurs in three disorders. Disorder that impair fat absorption like obstructive jaundice and biliary fistula (due to lack of bile salt) celiac disease, pancreatic diseases, etc.

Sterilization of the bowel by antibiotic drugs of the loss of bastorial flora in the bowel which synthesis vitamin K.

Hemorrhagic disease of the newborn—occurs due to reduced stores of vitamin K, function Imation of the linear, lede of bacterial synthesis of vitamin K or drugs administrated to mother (oral anticoagulants and anticonvulsants).

Treatment

Correction of cause

Administer vitamin K.

Replacement therapy when bleeching is severe.

Liver Disease

The hemostatic defect in liver disease include factors like thrombocytopenia increased fibrinolytic activity and rarely defibrination. Liver is the site of synthesis of clotting factors I, II, V, VII, IX, and X and probably factors XI, XII, and XIII, thrombocytopcnia clinical features are associated with portal hypertension and congestive splenomegaly.

Thromboembolic disorder: Formation of clot inside blood vessel more in side vein.

Congenital: Due to antithrombin III deficiency which is inherited as on autosomed dominant disorder, and protein C deficiency.

Acquired: Following surgery and trauma, pregnancy following use of oral contraceptive.

Mechanism

Thrombin may break away from site of attachment and is carried to blood stream.

Disseminated Intravascular Coagulation

Clotting mechanism is activated in wild spread areas of circulations. It is due to pressure of large amounts of transmatized tissue which releases tissue thromboplastin into tissue, e.g. septicemic should due to bacterial end toxin. Here factors are removed by wild spread clotting. So there will be bleeding tendering.

■ BLOOD GROUP

Membrane of human red cell contain number of blood group antigen. Most important are:
- ABO system
- Rh system

Both systems were discovered by Karl Landsteiner of Germany.

Agglutinogen: The blood group antigens present on human red cell membrane is called as agglutinogen. Aglitinins are antibodies against red cell aglutinogen and is present in plasma.

Antigen: Antibody reaction—consists of clumping or agglutination of the erythrocytes. A single agglutinin binds with several molecules of aglutinogen present on different erythrocytes. IgG type has two binding sites and IgM type has 10 sites.

ABO Systems

The agglutinogens of ABO system belong to a class of iso antigens. There are two such agglutinogen A and B, so that human beings can be divided into four groups.

A group: They have antigen A
B group: They have antigen B
AB group: They have both A and B antigens
O group: A and B antigens are absent.

Group is further divided into A1–80%, A2–20% concentration of antigen rises progressively from birth to puberty and adolescence.

Landsteiner's Law

Landsteiner's Law I: If an agglutinogen is present on the red cell of an individual corresponding aglutinin must be absent in the plasma. This law is applicable to both ABO and Rh system.

Land Steiner's law II: If an agglutinogen is absent in the red cell corresponding agglutinins must be present in the plasma. This law is not applicable to RH systems.

Bl group	Agglutinogen	Agglutinin	Distribution Indian	Western
A	A	Anti B	25%	41%
B	B	Anti A	25%	9%
AB	A & B	Nil	5%	3%
o	A & B Absent	Anti A & Anti B	45%	47%

Blood group substance are also found in other like salivary gland, pancreas, kidney, liver, lungs, etc. in 80% people. They are water soluble and they are called secretors, and the blood group substance appear in gastric juice saliva and other body fluids. In non-secretors the agglutinogen are confined to the cells and will not be present in the secretions.

Chemistry of Blood Group Antigen

A and B antigens are actually oligosaccharides that differ in their terminal sugar on red cell. On red cell they are glycosphingolipids and on other tissues they are glycoproteins.

H antigens are present in individuals of all blood group. H antigen is the precursor of antigen of ABO system, and H gene code for a fucose transferase that put a fucose on the end of the glycosphingolipid.

Blood group A: N acetyl galactosamine on H antigen
Blood group B: Galactose amine on H antigen
Group AB: Both galactosamin and galactose present on H antigen
Group O: Neither on H antigen.

Agglutinins in Plasma

Agglutinin are γ globulins mainly of IgM or IgG. Small amounts of group A and group B antigen enter the body through the food, bacteria etc. This initiate the development of anti A and anti B aglutinin. This anti A and anti B agglutinins are therefore called naturally occurring antibodies and are of IgM class.

The anti Rh antibodies are called acquired antibodies because they are produced by entry of red cell antigen not present on their own red cell either by blood transfusions or pregnancy.

Cold antibody-antigen: Antibody reaction occurs at temperature 5–20 °C. Most of the blood group antibody except ABO and Rh are cold antibodies.

Warm antibody – Ag: AB reaction occur at body temperature, e.g. ABO, Rh antibodies.

Inheritance of Blood Group Substances

A and B antigens are inherited as Mendelian allelomorphs. Allelomorphs means on 2 genes on 2 adjacent chromosome.

A and B genes are dominant, O gene not dominant.

A → AA   B → BB   O → OO   AB → AB AB
 ↳ AO   BO   ↳ AB OO
                                 ↳ AO BO

Information of genotype and inheritance of blood group help in investigations of disputed paternity.

Bombay group: H antigen is absent
Genotype hh

O group with H antigen absent can receive only O group H antigen negative. 99.9%. O blood group are H +ve.

Determination of Blood Group

Make a suspension of blood in citrated saline and put a drop of this suspension in two glass slides. To one slide add anti A and to other anti B agglutinins.

Agglutination in A: A blood group
Agglutination in B: B blood group
Agglutination in both A and B: AB blood group
No agglutination: O blood group

Cross matching
 Major: Donors cells with recipients plasma
 Minor: Donors plasma with recipient's cells

If there is no agglutination donors blood can be transfused to recipient. Major cross matching is more important because donors cells are destroyed in mismatched transfusion. Minor cross matching is less important because donors blood get diluted in recipients large volume of plasma. So less chance of damage to recipient's RBC.

Compatibility in between different blood groups

Donors group	Recipients group			
	A	B	AB	O
O	✓	✓	✓	✓
A	✓	✗	✓	✗
B	✗	✓	✓	✗
AB	✗	✗	✓	✗

✓ No mismatching
✗ Mismatching
O Universal donor (o-ve)
AB Universal recipient

Rh Blood Group

Red cells from a rhesus monkey was injected into a rabbit and antibodies are produced in the serum. It was found that some human red cells are agglutinated by the serum, and some are not. The blood which is agglutinated are Rh +ve, the blood cells that are not agglutinated are Rh –ve blood. More than 40 different antigens have been identified. Rh factor is a system composed of CDE antigens. These antigens are not detected in other tissues. D is the most antigenic component and the individuals having antigen D are termed Rh positive. Individual in which antigen D is absent is Rh –negative.

	Western	Indian
Rh +ve	85%	99%
Rh -ve	15%	1%

Inheritance of Rh System

Inherited by three pairs of gene, C_C, D_D, E_E gene corresponding to antigen D is called D. When D gene is absent in chromosome its place is occupied by alternate gene D. Rh gene is inherited from both father and mother. D is mendelian dominant.

DD Rh +ve

Dd Rh +ve

dd Rh –ve.

Rh typing is done with anti D serum and if there is agglutination Rh +ve.

No agglutination- Rh negative.

Both Rh +ve and Rh –ve individuals do not possess naturally occuring Rh antibodies. They (Rh antibodies) develop in Rh –ve individuals in 2 ways.
1. Transfusion of Rh +ve blood to Rh –ve individual. During Ist transfusion, there will be development of antibodies. No reaction during 2nd exposure agglutination and hemolysis occurs.
2. Transfer of Rh +ve cells from Rh +ve baby to Rh –ve mother at the time of pregnancy, abortion, or delivery through the placenta and development of anti D antibody in the mother after Ist child birth. So during next pregnancy anti D antibody pass transplacentally to 2nd baby (Rh +ve) and induce agglutination and hemolysis.

Importance of Blood Group

- In blood transfusion
- In pregnancy when Rh –ve women conceives a Rh +ve child.
- In cases of disputed paternity.

Erythroblastosis fetalis (hemolytic disease of newborn): When Rh –ve mother conceives a Rh –ve fetus, small amount of blood leak into maternal circulation at the time of delivery or during abortion. If some fetomaternal hemorrhage occur, cells enter the mother. Rh antibodies develop in the mother. No serious effects during Ist pregnancy. During 2nd pregnancy Rh antibody cross the placenta and agglutinate the Rh +ve fetal cells, and cause hemolysis.

Hydrop's fetalis: Death of the fetus due to edema and jaundice.

Icterus gravis neonatorum: Anemia and severe jaundice at birth.

Erythroblastosis fetalis: Erythropoiesis increase. Erythroblasts are seen in circulation.

Kernicterus: Bilirubin level in the blood increases due to excessive RBC destruction and when bilirubin level exceeds 18 mg% bilirubin cross the BBB enter brain get deposited in the basal ganglia. In infants blood brain barrier is not developed. In adults bilirubin can not cross the BBB and so the bilirubin deposited in brain cause neurological symptoms. This condition is called kernicterus.

Treatment

Exchange transfusion in the newborn carried out soon after birth. A polythene catheter is passed along umbilical vein to SVC, small quantities of infant blood withdrawn and replaced by equal volume of compatable Rh –ve blood. Done several times to keep bilirubin level low. Within 6 weeks Rh –ve cells are replaced by baby's own Rh +ve cell. By that time AB that have come from mother's blood would have been destroyed.

Prevention

Injection of anti Rh antibody: Antibody – anti D within 72 hrs after delivery into mother. This destroys the Rh +ve cells that have entered the maternal blood during delivery and prevents AB formation by maternal blood. The immune serum can be given to mother during pregnancy itself, thus preventing sensitization.

- Medicolegal importance as in disputed paternity. If baby's and mother's blood group are known, we can rule out a person being the father but can not say he is the father.

Baby	Genotype	Mother	Father
O	OO	Any gp	Not AB
AB	AB	Any gp	Not O
A	AO/AA	A or O	Not B or O
B	BO/BB	B or O	Nor A or B

- Forensic examination of blood stain, seminal stain or saliva for ABO group substances.
- Increased incidence of spontaneous abortion in blood group incompatible marriages—chances of rejection more if tissue transplantation done in persons with blood group incompatibility.
- Duodenal ulcer common in O group subject.

Ca stomach }
Pernicious anemia } common in group A subjects

Blood Transfusion

Blood transfusion is the administration of whole blood or blood derivatives like plasma or packed cells directly into the vein.

Indication

- To restore blood volume after hemorrhage, surgery
- Severe anemia not responding to usual measures
- Burns
- Hemorrhagic disorder like hemophilia, thrombocytopenic purpura
- Exchange transfusion in hemolytic diseases of newborn due to Rh incompatiblity
- Leukemia.

Substances Used for Transfusion

Whole blood, packed red cell (c/c anemia)
Frozen plasma (burns), (plasma substitutes, clothing factor concentrates, platelets (ITP), leukocytes (Neutropenia.)
Cryoprecipitate: Factor VIII, fibrinogen
Plasma substitutes: Colloids – dextran
Crystalloids: Saline, glucose
Ideal donor: Must be healthy, between 18–60 yrs weight > 45 kg. Not anemic, no history of infections disease like malaria, syphilis, AIDS.

Precautions to be Taken

ABO and Rh typing should be done for donor and recipient cross matching should be done. Tests to rule out infections like hepatitis B, HIV, syphilis, etc. sterile precautions, proper auticoagulant must be added. Venous blood from a healthy donor collected in sterile plastic bag containing anticoagulant.

Anticoagulant Used

- Acid citrate dextrose (ACD)
- Citrate phosphate dextrose (CPD)
- CPD A-1 – CPD

Rate of transfusion depending on requirement usually 15–20 drop/int.

Complications of Blood Transfusion

- Those due to mismatched blood transfusion
- Due to other causes.

Due to mismatched transfusion — A/c, Delayed

Hemolytic transfusion reactions: If one group of blood is transfused into a recipient of another blood group which is not compatible the cells of donor's blood are agglutinated. Recipient cells usually do not agglutinates because the plasma of the donor is diluted very much in recipient. The donor cell agglutinates and lead to hemolysis.

The agglutinated cells may undergo lysis with in the vascular system (hemolysis) and the released Hb due to this rapid hemolysis may block smaller blood vessels in the coronary pulmonary or renal circulation or may appear in renal tubules.

If Hb in renal tubules is sufficiently high it may lead to kidney failure. Renal failure may be caused due to associated shock also.

- Not due to mismatching
  - Excess volume transfusion can cause hypervolemia and cardio respiratory embarassment.
- Donors cells broken down releasing serotonin may cause pulmonary edema
  - Anaphylactic shock like condition may supervene due to release of large amount of histamine from donor's basophiles.
  - Pyrogenic reactions may develop.

Immediate Signs and Symptoms

- Fever
- Chest pain
- Anuria
- Dyspnea or severe fall of BP
  Late → Janndice

Other Hazards

- Development of infections from donor's blood—malaria, syphilis, viral hepatitis, and AIDS.
- Each bottle of blood transfused contain citrate which removes calcium ions of the recipient plasma, rarely especially in cases of liver failure. It may produce tetany or incoagulability of blood.
- Problems due to Rh incompatibility.

CHAPTER 10

Circulatory System

The circulatory system is a transport system, carrying oxygen, nutrients, hormones and other substances to the tissues and conveying carbon dioxide to the lungs and other waste products to the kidneys. The blood is the vehicle or carrier and the blood vessels are the channels along which it travels. The motive power is supplied primarily by the heart, which is a muscular pump. However, the venous return of blood to the heart is assisted by gravity (for those parts which are higher than the heart), skeletal muscle activity squeezing the veins, and the inspiratory phase of breathing, which sucks blood towards the thorax. In addition to the circulation of the blood there is a lymphatic circulation.

Blood is pumped by the heart (left ventricle) into the aorta, from which it is distributed by arteries to all parts of the body. The arteries branch and narrow down to arterioles and these in turn lead to microscopic capillaries which ramify throughout the tissues. The diameter of a capillary is about the same as that of a red blood cell. The walls of the capillaries consist of only one layer of cells, which are joined together but between which there are small spaces through which white blood cells can pass by means of their power of ameboid movement. It is in the capillaries, and in them only, that the blood equilibrates with the interstitial fluid in the tissues; nutrients, water, oxygen, carbon dioxide, and other waste products (arising from the metabolic activities of cells) being exchanged.

The capillaries drain into venules and these unite to form veins, which convey the deoxygenated blood back to the heart (right atrium) to complete the systemic circulation, sometimes referred to as the greater circulation. The lesser circulation (lesser in size but not in importance) is the pulmonary circulation in which venous (deoxygenated) blood is pumped from the right side of the heart (right ventricle) into the pulmonary artery and its branches. Again, after traversing arterioles it reaches capillaries; this time the capillaries of the lungs. Gaseous exchange takes place between the blood in these capillaries and the air in the alveoli, across what is called the alveolar-capillary membrane. The blood thereby loses its excess of carbon dioxide and becomes enriched with oxygen. However, the alveolar-capillary membrane may be thickened by a disease process such as pulmonary edema or fibrosis. Then, oxygen cannot diffuse across it so readily and cannot fully oxygenate the blood so that the patient may show cyanosis, or blueness. Carbon dioxide is a more diffusible gas than oxygen and is not retained in the blood in these cases of what is often called alveolar-capillary block.

Leaving the capillaries of the lungs, the oxygenated blood returns to the, heart via venules which join to form the pulmonary veins. Four large pulmonary veins, two from each lung, enter the receiving chamber (left atrium) of the left side of the heart. In contradistinction to other arteries of the body, the pulmonary artery contains

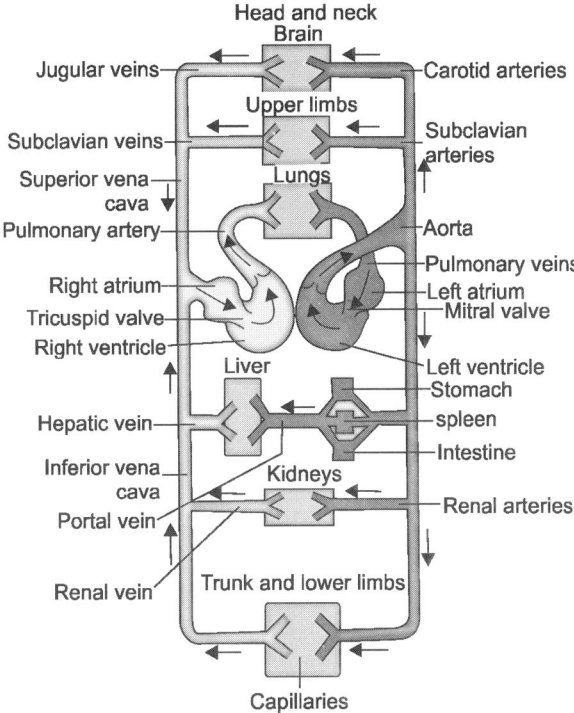

Fig. 10.1: The circulation

deoxygenated or 'venous' blood and the pulmonary veins, unlike any other veins, contain oxygenated or 'arterial' blood (Fig. 10.1).

■ HEART AND GREAT VESSELS

Cardiac differentiation and morphogenesis are intimately related process. The cardiac specific transcription factor is important for cardiac specific gene expression. In man mutation in this factor lead to atrial septal defects, A-V conduction disturbances.

General organization: Heart has a pair of valved muscular pump combined in single organ. It has four cardiac chambers, two atria which receive blood from veins for filling the two ventricles which force blood to arterial trunks. Right heart starts at the right atrium and receives blood via the superior and inferior vena cava along with the main venous inflow from heart itself via coronary sinus. This systemic venous flow passes through the right atrioventricular (AV) orifice which is guarded by tricuspid valve to enter the right ventricle. Contraction of the ventricle closes the tricuspid valve and ejects blood to pulmonary trunk. Blood then flows through pulmonary vascular bed which has low resistance.

Left heart starts as left atrium which receives oxygenated blood via pulmonary veins. It contracts to fill the left ventricle through the left AV orifice which is guarded by mitral valve. Ventricular contraction closes the mitral valve and the pressure developed in left ventricle pumps blood to aorta (left ventricular outflow tract).

From the aorta blood is pumped to the entire systemic arterial tree, including coronary arteries.

The right heart forms the right border and covers most of the anterior aspect of left heart. Thus the right heart forms the largest part of anterior surface. The left heart is mostly posterior in position and is covered by chambers of right heart anteriorly. The inlet of left ventricle (mitral valve) is very close to its outlet (aortic valve). Left ventricular cavity is very narrow and conical and its tip forms cardiac apex. Base of heart is formed by left atrium.

Cardiac shape, size, external features: Heart is a hollow muscular organ with base, apex, series of borders and surfaces. It occupies middle mediastinum between the lungs and their pleura. It lies behind body of sternum and costal cartilages.

Heart is obliquely placed with its base facing posteriorly and to the right and apex facing anteriorly and to the left. Some surfaces of the pyramidal shaped heart are flat, some convex. Therefore heart has a base, apex, sternocostal (anterior) surface, diaphragmatic (inferior) surface, right and left (pulmonary) surfaces.

Its borders are upper, inferior, left and right.

Right atrium: Forms right border and is anterior and inferior to left atrium.

Right ventricle: forms most of the anterior surface.

Left atrium: Forms most of posterior surface and base of heart.

Left ventricle: Its prominent only inferiorly.

Groove on the cardiac surface: Four chambers of the heart produces boundaries that are visible externally as grooves (sulci). The interatrial groove is a shallow groove separating the two atria. The atrioventricular groove (coronary) separates the atria from ventricles. This groove contains the main trunk of coronary arteries.

Right atrium: Its walls form the right border and sternocostal surface. The superior vena cava opens into its dome and inferior vena cava into its lower posterior part. A muscular pouch, the auricle projects anteriorly. A shallow sulcus called sulcus terminalis is present on its surface. The sulcus terminalis extends between the openings of superior vena cava and inferior vena cava. It corresponds internally to crista terminalis which gives origin to pectinate muscles.

Interior of right atrium: It has smooth walled venous component which receives the openings of both superior and inferior vena cava and the coronary sinus. Superior vena cava has no valve whereas inferior vena cava has valve named Eustachian valve. Coronary sinus opens beside opening of inferior vena cava and is guarded by valve.

Openings of small atrial veins are found in the atrial wall. Musculi pectinati are muscular ridges found in atrial wall extending from crista terminalis. Septal wall presents the fossa ovalis which is an oval depression above the opening of inferior vena cava.

Right ventricle: It extends from the right atrioventricular opening to almost cardiac apex. Its upper end forms infundibulum or conus arteriosus.

External features: It forms major part of sternocostal surface. Inferior surface is related to pericardium and central tendon of diaphragm. The wall of right ventricle is significantly thinner than left ventricle, the ratio of thickness being 1:3.

Internal features: The inlet and outlet components are separated by an arched crest called supraventricular crest.

Tricuspid valve: It is the atrioventricular valve between right atria and right ventricle. It consists of the orifice, annulus, cusps, supporting chorda tendinae and papillary muscles.

Left atrium: It is smaller in volume than right atrium and has thicker wall. Left atrium is cuboidal in shape and lies behind right atrium. It forms the base of heart and receives termination of four pulmonary veins.

Left Ventricle

General and external features: Left ventricle is a powerful pump. It pumps blood to high pressured systemic arteries. It is cone-shaped and narrower than right ventricle. Its walls are three times thicker than that of right ventricle. It forms sternocostal, left and inferior surfaces of heart.

Internal features: Inlet of left ventricle is guarded by mitral valve and outlet guarded by aortic valve (Fig. 10.2).

Vascular Supply

Coronary arterial supply: Right and left coronary arteries arise from ascending aorta from the aortic sinuses. The main arteries and major arteries are subepicardial.

Right coronary artery: It arises from anterior aortic sinus. It lies between right auricle and pulmonary trunk. Then it lies in A-V groove and descends in right cardiac border curves posteriorly to crux of heart.

Main branches are marginal artery and posterior interventricular artery.

Left coronary artery: It is larger than right coronary artery. Left coronary artery supplies greater volume of myocardium. Most of the interventricular septum is supplied by left coronary artery. It supplies from left posterior aortic sinus. The artery lies between pulmonary trunk and left auricle and emerge into AV groove. Main branches of left coronary artery are anterior interventricular artery, diagonal artery, circumflex artery.

Coronary distribution: Right coronary supplies all of the right ventricle, a variable part of diaphragmatic surface of left ventricle, posteroinferior 1/3 of interventricular septum, right atrium and part of left atrium. Left coronary artery supplies most of the left ventricle and a narrow strip of right ventricle, anterior 2/3 of interventricular septum and most of left atrium.

Coronary artery disease: Atherosclerosis characterized by deposition of lipid and accumulation of macrophages in tunica intima. Lipid accumulation lead to formation of atherosclerotic plaque. Formation of plaque narrows the arteries and reduces coronary blood flow. Plaque may rupture and also form thrombus. Sudden blockage of coronary artery leads to myocardial infarction.

Cardiac veins: Heart is drained by coronary sinus and its tributaries, the anterior cardiac

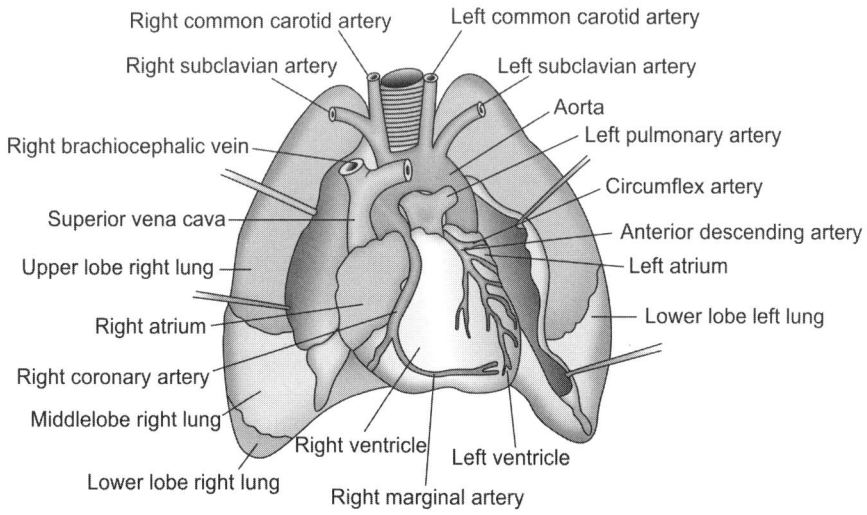

Fig. 10.2: The lungs, heart and great vessels

veins and the small cardiac veins. The coronary sinus and its tributaries return blood to the right atrium from the entire heart including septa.

Coronary sinus: Large majority of cardiac veins drain into the wide coronary sinus. It is 2–3 cm long and lies in the posterior atrio-ventricular groove between the left atrium and ventricle. The coronary sinus opens into right atrium. Its tributaries are great cardiac vein, small cardiac vein and middle cardiac vein.

CARDIOVASCULAR PHYSIOLOGY

Cardiovascular system comprises of heart and blood vessels. The function of cardiovascular system is to supply oxygen, nutrients and other essential substances to the tissues of the body and to remove carbon dioxide and other metabolic end products from the tissues.

HEART

Heart is a muscular organ situated in between the two lungs in the mediastinum. It is made up of two atria and two ventricles. The right atrium has got the pacemaker known as Sinoatrial node that produces cardiac impulses and AV node that conduct these impulses to the ventricles. Two veins drains into that:
1. Superior vena cava that returns the venous blood from the head, neck and upper limbs.
2. Inferior vena cava that returns the venous blood from the lower parts of the body.

Right atrium communicates with the right ventricle through the tricuspid valve. Venous blood from the right atrium enters the right ventricle through this valve (Fig. 10.3). From the right ventricle pulmonary artery arises. This carries the venous blood to the lungs. Blood is oxygenated in the lungs and returned to the left atrium as arterial blood through pulmonary veins.

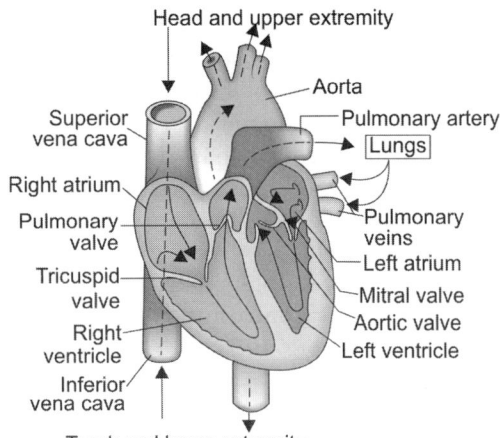

Fig. 10.3: Directions of blood flow in various chambers and vessels of heart

This is the only exception in the body where artery carries venous blood and veins carries arterial blood. The left atrium communicate with the left ventricle through the mitral valve. Left atrium empties the arterial blood into the left ventricle through this valve. Left ventricle pumps the arterial blood to different parts of the body through systemic aorta. That part of circulation which involves the pulmonary artery lungs and pulmonary veins is called the pulmonary circulation also called the lesser circulation. That involving the aorta other viscera and veins which drain into superior and inferior vena cava are called the systemic circulation.

The ventricles are thickly muscular structures and their force of contraction is powerful. Of the two the left ventricular wall is much thicker than the right. In between the two atria lies inter atria septum which forms the common wall between the atria whereas the interventricular septum separate the left from the right ventricle. The cavities of the cardiac chambers are lined by endothelial lining and lining is called endocardium. A bundle called AV bundle begins from AV node courses along the

Circulatory System

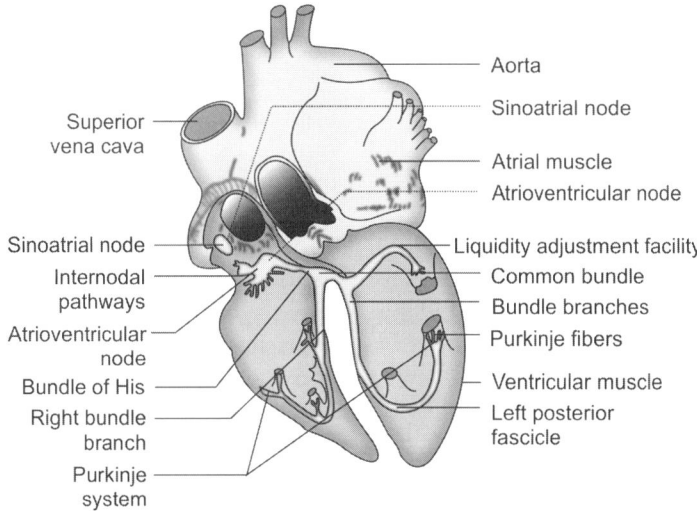

Fig. 10.4: Conducting system of heart

interventricular septum for a short distance then splits into a right and left branch called the right and left bundle branch (Fig. 10.4). The individual branches then turned to enter the myocardium where they branch extensively and are called fibers of Purkinje.

Layers of Wall of the Heart

Heart is made up of three layers of tissues (Fig. 10.5):
1. Outer pericardium
2. Middle myocardium
3. Inner endocardium

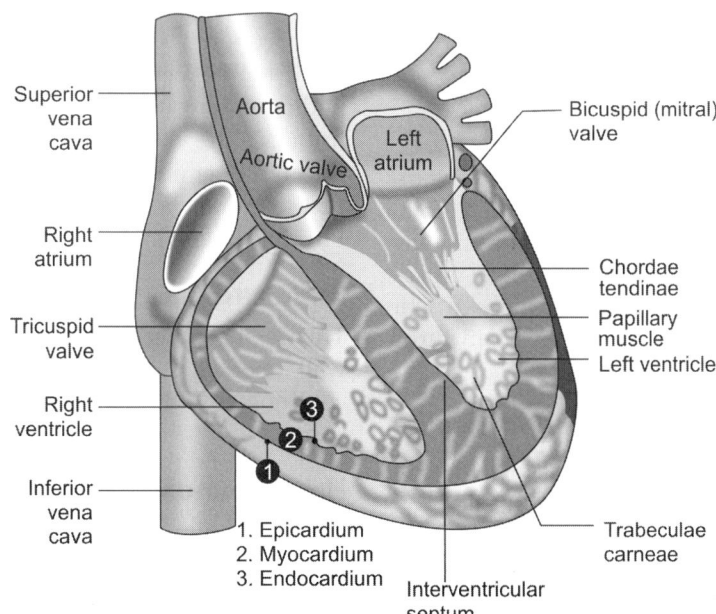

Fig. 10.5: Section of heart and great vessels showing chordae tendinae and papillary muscle

1. *Pericardium:* Pericardium is the outer covering of the heart, it has outer fibrous layers and inner serous layer. The outer fibrous layer continuous as tunica adventitia of the large blood vessels. It is attached with diaphragm below. Because of the fibrous nature it protects the heart from overstretching. Serous layer is a membranous sheath made of outer parietal pericardium and inner visceral pericardium. The visceral pericardium is also called epicardium.

   In between the parietal and visceral pericardium there is a thin space called pericardial space—which contains a film of pericardial fluid.

2. *Myocardium:* This is the middle layer of the wall of the heart. Myocardium is constituted by three types of cardiac muscle fibers:
   a. Muscle fibers forming contractile unit.
   b. Muscle fibers forming pacemakers which initiate the impulses for contraction.
   c. The muscle forming the conductive system.

Muscle Fibers Forming the Contractile Unit of the Heart

They are striated and involuntary. The cardiac muscle fiber is bound by sarcolemma. The sarcomere of the cardiac muscle have structures similar to those in skeletal muscle. It has all the muscle proteins namely actin, myosin, troponin and tropomyosin throughout the musculature.

Pacemaker and Conducting Tissue

Heart has well-developed pacemaker tissue which can generate rhythmic impulses.

Cardiac muscle fiber is branched and at the point of the union of the branches, the membrane of both muscle fiber fuse together and forms a tough structure called intercalated disk. The intercalated discs form tight junctions between the muscle fibers and do not permit any ions to pass through. However, these disks play an important role during the contraction of muscle by pulling the muscle fibers with one another. At the sides membranes of adjacent muscle cells fuse together to form gap junctions. The gap junction is permeable to ions, and help all muscle fibers to act like a syncytium. The syncytium in human heart has two potions, syncytium of atria and the syncytium of ventricle. These two are connected by a thick nonconducting fibrous ring called the atrioventricular ring.

Muscle Fibers Forming Pacemakers

They are less striated and generates the impulses which form heartbeat. Sinoatrial node is the pacemaker in human heart and it is situated in the posterior wall of the right atrium near the opening of superior vena cava.

Muscle Fibers Forming Conductive System

They conduct impulses rapidly from SA node to the ventricle. Impulses from SA node are transmitted to the atria directly. Impulses are transmitted to the ventricles through inter nodal fibers, AV node, bundle of His, branches of bundle of His and Purkinje fibers.

Endocardium

This is the inner most layer of the heart wall, made of endothelial cells which is continuous with the endothelium of blood vessels.

Heart Sounds

Heart sounds are like a chorus sung by two AV valves and two semilunar valves. There are specific areas on the chestwall over which sounds from each of the four valves are best heard.

Tricuspid area is in the fourth intercostals space along the right border of sternum

Mitral area is in the 5th intercostal space about 1 cm medial to midclavicular line, i.e. over the apex beat.

Pulmonary area is in the second intercostal space along the left border of sternum.

Aortic area is in the 2nd intercostal space along the right border of sternum

A total of four heart sounds,1st, 2nd, 3rd, and 4th are produced by certain mechanical activities during each cardiac cycle.

First Heart Sound: It is produced by the vibrations setup by the sudden closure of AV valves at the start of ventricular systole during each cardiac cycle. First heart sound is long and soft when heart rate is low and loud when the heart rate is high.

Duration is about 0.15 s

Frequency is 25–45 Hz. Sounds like LUBB

Second Heart Sound: It is caused by the vibrations associated with closure of the semilunar valves just at the onset of ventricular diastole. Second heart sound is short, loud, high-pitched sound.

Duration is 0.12 s

Frequency is 50 Hz. Sounds like the spoken word DUBB

- First heart sound becomes more intense when the force of the ventricular contraction increases.
- Where the PR internal is very prolonged AV values approximate before the onset of ventricular contraction. The first heart sound becomes faint.
- In bundle branch block the 2nd sound is frankly split.

Third Heart Sound: It is produced by the vibration of ventricular wall produced in the first rapid filling phase of the ventricle.

Fourth Sound: Atrial sound produced by the last rapid filling phase. When the 3rd heart sounds clearly audible it produces a triple rhythm. Fourth heart sound when audible similarly produce a presystolic gallop. All gallop rhythms are triple rhythms.

Arterial Pulse

Genesis and characters of normal pulse: The blood forced into the aorta during systole not only moves the blood in the vessels forward but also sets up a pressure wave that travels along the arteries. The pressure wave expands the arterial walls as it travels and the expansion is palpable as a pulse.

Rate of travel – 4 m/s in the aorta, 8 m/s in the large arteries and 16 m/s in small arteries of young adults. With advancing age the arteries become more rigid and the pulse wave moves faster.

The strength is of pulse is determined by pulse pressures and bears little relation to the mean pressure. The pulse is weak (thready) in shock. When pulse pressure is high the pulse waves may be large enough to be felt or even heard by the individual (palpitation, pounding heart). When aortic valve is incompetent (AI) pulse becomes particularly strong and the force of systolic ejection may be sufficient to make the head nod with each heartbeat collapsing pulse. Corrigan or water-hammer pulse. A water hammer is an evacuated glass tube half-filled with water that was a popular joy in the 19th century. When held in the hand and inverted, it delivers a short hand knock.

The dicrotic notch a small oscillation on the falling phase of the pulse wave caused by vibration set up when aortic valve snaps shut, is visible if the pressure wave is recorded but is not palpable at the wrist. The pulmonary artery pressure curve also has a dicrotic notch produced by the closure of the pulmonary valves.

The arterial pulses are used usually for the evaluation of:

- *Rate:* Right radial pulse
- Rhythm
- *Character:* Right carotid artery

- *Symmetry:* Radial, bracheal, carotid, femoral popliteal and pedal pulses should be confirmed.

Jugular venous pressure (JVP): Atrial pressure rises during atrial systole and continuous to rise during isovolumetric ventricular contraction when the AV valves bulge into the atria. When the AV valves are pulled down by the contracting ventricular muscle, pressure falls rapidly and then rises as blood flows into the atria until the AV valves open early in diastole. The return of the AV valves to their relaxed position also contributes this pressure rise by reducing atrial capacity. Atrial pressure changes are transmitted to the great veins producing a wave, C wave, V wave. Jugular venous pressure is transmitted backward into jugular veins. It is best examining the JVP while patient reclines at 45 degree.

Wave form of Jugular Venous Pulses

- A and V waves separated by X and Y descents.
- A atrial systole precedes tricuspid valve closure.
- *X descend:* Descend of the tricuspid valve ring.
- *C wave:* Tricuspid valve closure.
- *V wave:* Atrial filling during ventricular systole.
- *Y descend:* Decline in atrial pressure as tricuspid valve opened to allow ventricular filling produces the Y descent.

Echocardiography: Work, movement and other aspects of cardiac function can be evaluated by echocardiography a noninvasive technique that does not involve injections or insertion of a catheter.

In a echocardiography, pulses of ultrasonic waves commonly at a frequency of 2.25 MHz are emitted from a transducer that also functions as a receiver to detect waves reflected back from various parts of the heart. Reflection occur whenever acoustic impedance changes and a recording of the echoes displayed against time on an oscilloscope provides a record of the movements of the ventricular wall, septum and valves during the cardiac cycle. When combined with Doppler technique echocardiography can be used to measure velocity and volume of flow through valves. It has considerable clinical usefulness. Particularly in evaluating and planning therapy in patients with valvular lesions.

First Heart Sound

Causes

Other important contributing factors are turbulence of the blood, vibration of the ventricular, aortic and pulmonary walls.

Applied Physiology

Vibration set up by the closure of the mitral and tricuspid valves. It is the closure of the mitral and tricuspid valves. Therefore, ultimately it is the closure of the valves that is mainly responsible for the sound.

- The 1st heart sound becomes more intense when the force of the ventricular contraction increases.
- Where the PR interval is very prolonged the AV valves approximate before the onset of ventricular contraction, the 1st heart sound becomes faint.
- In bundle branch block the sound is frankly split.

Second Heart Sound

- At the end of the protodiastole the semilunar valves close abruptly and column of the blood in the great vessels rebounds abruptly. This causes vibration in the:
  - Semilunar valves.
  - In the blood within the great vessels
  - The tense vessel walls.

Applied Physiology: The intensity of the 2nd heart sound increases with the increase of the hydrostatic pressure within the great vessels. Thus in systemic hypertension, the intensity of the 2nd heart sound in clinical aortic area increases and often acquires a character called metallic. Conversely in pulmonary hypertension the intensity of 2nd heart sound in the pulmonary area is accentuated.

Heart Sounds Causes, Character and Abnormalities

In each cardiac cycle the heart produces four sounds. Extra sound is called an adventitious sound. Except in some special conditions adventitious sounds indicate some abnormalities. Further the characteristics of the heart sound are fairly stereotyped in a normal heart. Therefore any alteration of their characteristics may be due to pathological reasons. Only 1st and 2nd sounds can be heard by the stethoscope. Phonocardiograph however can pick up and record all the four heart sounds in a normal individual.

Mechanism of Production of Heart Sounds

The vibration of wall as well as the water generate sounds—according to Rushmer famous American cardiologist—The acceleration and deceleration produce the vibration of the wall of the heart and vessels. Vibrations of the closing valves strongly contribute to heart sounds.

The acceleration and deceleration are produced by:
- Contraction of ventricle
- Closure of the valves.
- Another important factor for the generation of the sounds is turbulence in the blood.

■ ECG

History

William Einthoven a Dutch physiologist originally developed the techniques of echocardiography. He was awarded Nobel Prize in 1924 for his contribution and is called the father of modern electrocardiography.

Electrocardiography refers to extra cellular recording of the summed-up electrical events of all the cardiac muscle fibers generated with each heartbeat. Electrically heart behaves like a dipole. The record of the potential fluctuations during the cardiac cycle is called ECG. The machine used to record these potential fluctuations is called Electrocardiograph which is essentially a sensitive galvanometer.

Recording of ECG: Recorded using two types of leads (Fig. 10.6):

Bipolar Leads

Both electrodes are active and one of the active electrode is connected to negative terminal of the ECG machine and the other to the positive terminal. Three standard limbs leads used in bipolar recording are based on Einthoven's postulate. According

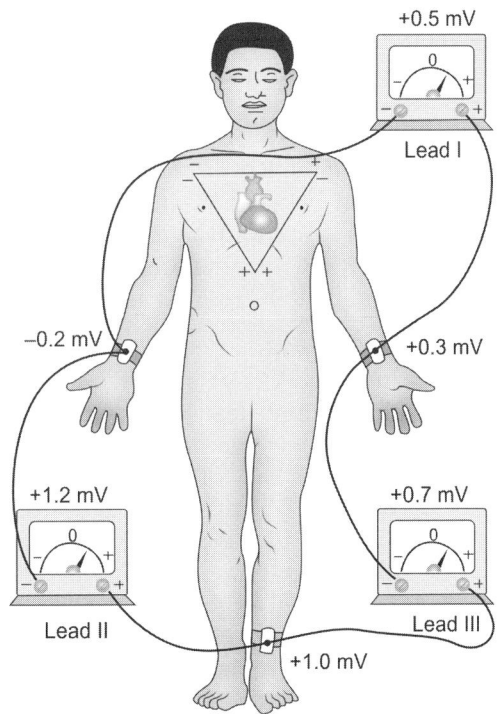

Fig. 10.6: Classical leads of ECG

to this body is like an electrically homogenous plate in which the right and left shoulders and the pubic region form the corners of an equilateral triangle with heart in the center (Einthoven's triangle) and that two active electrodes need to be placed at two corners of this triangle. Electrodes are connected to the:
- Left Arm (LA)
- Right Arm (RA)
- Left Foot (LF)

Instead of the shoulders and pubic region.

Unipolar Leads

In unipolar recording one electrode is active of the exploring electrode and the other is an indifferent electrode at zero potential. So in unipolar recording potential fluctuations occurring at the site of exploring electrode is the record of the potential.

Unipolar Chest Leads

Six unipolar chest leads (precordial leads)
V1-V6: Indifferent electrode—at potential
Active electrode placed on six points on the chest as:
LV1—Right 4th ICS near sternum
LV2—In the left 4th ICS just near sternum
LV3—Half way between V2 and V4
LV4—Left 5th ICS at Midclavicular line
LV5—In left 5th ICS at anterior axillary line
LV6—In the left 5th ICS at mid axillary line.

Unipolar Limb Leads

These include lead VL, VF and VR.
In unipolar limb leads one exploring (active) electrode is placed over a limb. (In lead VL over the left arm. VF over left foot and lead VR over the right arm) and is connected to the positive terminal of electrocardiograph. The indifferent electrode is obtained as above connected to the negative terminal of electrocardiograph. Now these leads are replaced by augmented limb leads.

Augmented Unipolar Limb Leads

aVR, aVL, aVF
The augmentation by 50% obtained by increasing size of potential 50% without any change in the configuration from non-augmented record. Active electrode is from one of the limbs and the indifferent electrode is obtained by connecting the other two limbs through 5000 Ohms resistance as:

Lead aVR
- Active electrode – RA
- Indifferent electrode – LA + LF

Lead aVL
- Active electrode from – LA
- Indifferent electrode – RA + LF

Lead aVF
- Active electrode – LF
- Indifferent electrode – RA + LA

Correlation of the events during cardiac cycle: Right AS occurs before left AS because SA node in the right atrium. Left ventricular systole occurs before right ventricular systole. But RVS completes first.

Electrocardiograph

It is a sophisticated string galvanometer. A modern electrocardiograph amplifies and records the potential fluctuation on a moving strip of paper.

Some machines have a writing ink pen that records directly on the moving sheet of paper.

In some others, instead of ink pen special paper is used which turns black on exposure to heat. The stylus (recording pen) is made hot by electrical current flowing through it.

X Axis – Time
Y Axis – Voltage

Horizontal: One small division = 0.04 sec
One large division – 0.2 sec
Vertical: One small division = 0.1 mv
One large division = 0.5 mv

Calibration of Time and Voltage on ECG Paper

Special ECG paper having 1 and 5 mm squares are used recording is normally made at a standard speed of 25 mm/sec.

On horizontal axis therefore, each millimeter represents 0.04 sec.

The sensitivity of ECG is adjusted in a way that a potential fluctuation of 1 Volt causes a vertical deflection of 1 cm. On vertical axis each mm represents 0.1 Volt magnitude of potential.

Normal ECG (Fig. 10.7)

Electrocardiogram refers to the record of the potential fluctuations during the cardiac cycle. As a result of sequential spread of excitation in the atria, the ventricular walls and finally repolarization of the myocardium, a series of positive and negative waves designated as PQRS and T are recorded during each cardiac cycle. Depolarization moving toward an active electrode in a volume conductor produces a positive deflection, whereas depolarization moving in the opposite direction produces a negative deflection.

The spread of cardiac Impulse: The cardiac impulse which originates in the SA node in the form of AP spreads throughout the heart through the conduction system.

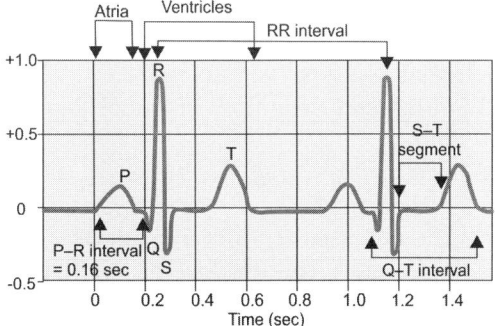

Fig. 10.7: Normal ECG showing different intervals and segments

SA Node and atria: The impulse spreads over the muscle fibers of atria with which the ends of SA nodal fibers are fused and through the interatrial tract to the left atrium. Conduction through these causes simultaneous depolarization of both the atria. Atrial depolarization is completed in about 0–1 sec. Through the inter nodal tracts (anterior middle and posterior) the impulse reaches to AV node from SA node with in 0.03 sec after it is origin.

AV node: Conduction through AV node is slow, there is a delay of about 0.1 sec. The causes of AV nodal delay are:
- Transitional fibers connecting inter nodal tracts and AV node are very small and they, and the AV nodal fibers conduct the impulse at a very slow rate 0.02–0.05 m/s.
- RMP of transitional fibers and AV nodal fibers is much less negative than rest of the cardiac muscle fibers.
- There are very few gap junctions connecting successive fibers in the pathway. AV nodal delay is useful for it provides time for completion of atrial contraction and their emptying, before ventricular contraction.

Ventricular Conduction: The impulse conducted through the AV node are distributed to ventricles through bundle of His, it's branches and Purkinje fibers in 0.08 to 0.15 sec. In humans depolarization of the ventricular muscle proceeds as:
- Starts at the left side of inter ventricular septum
- Moves first to the right across the mid portion of the septum
- The wave of depolarization then spreads down the septum to apex of heart
- It then returns along the ventricular walls to the AV grove, proceeding from the endocardial to epicardial surface.
- The last parts of the heart to be depolarized are the posterobasal portion of

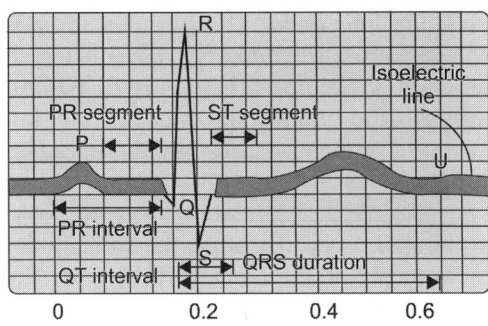

Fig. 10.8: Waves of ECG

the left ventricles, the pulmonary conus and the upper most portion of the septum.

Waves of ECG (Fig. 10.8)

P Wave
Configuration: P Wave is the positive deflection
Cause: It is produced by the depolarization of atrial musculature so also called atrial complex.
Duration: Of P wave is not more than 0.1 sec.
Amplitude: Of P wave is from 0.1 to 0.12 mV
Clinical significance: Magnitude of P wave is a guide to the functional activity of atria.

QRS Complex
Configuration: QRS complex consists of three consecutive waves. Q wave is a small negative wave which may be absent normally quite often. It is continued as a tall positive R wave which is followed by a small negative S wave.
Cause: QRS complex is caused by ventricular depolarization.
Duration: Less than 0.08 sec. It is a measure of intraventricular conduction time.
Amplitude: Of Q wave is 0.1 to 0.2 mV R Wave is 1.0 mV and S wave is 0.4 mV (Total 1.4–1.6 mV)

Clinical Significance
QRS complex from precordial leads are more important than limb leads.

Deep Q wave (more than 0.2 mV) – MI.
Tall R wave (more than 1.3 mV) Ventricular – hypertrophy.
Low voltage QRS complex (sum < 1.5 mV) seen in hypothyroidism and pericardial effusion.
QRS complex is prolonged in bundle branch block.

T Wave
Configuration: Last, positive, dome-shaped deflection. Same direction as QRS complex.
Cause: T wave represents ventricular repolarization.
Duration: 0.27 sec
Amplitude: 0.3 mV

Clinical Significance
Old age: T wave flattered
Inverted T wave: MI
Tall peaked T wave: hyperkalemia.

U Wave
Configuration: Small round positive wave
Duration: 0.08 sec
Amplitude: 0.2 mV
Significance: Rarely seen normally. It becomes prominent in hypocalcemia.

Einthoven's Law
Potential at L II = L I + L III
In closed circuit the total sum will be 0, i.e L I + L II + L III = 0 (Kirchhoff's law) Einthoven reversed the polarity of L II.
so L I – II + L III = 0.
Unipolar recording: We measures the actual potential two types of electrodes:
1. *Indifferent electrode:* Potential kept at zero.
2. *Active (exploring) electrode:* It act as +ve electrode.

The potential of indifferent electrode is kept as follows. The wires from L I, L II, L III is connected to a high resistance wire of 5000 Ω. This electrode is first made by Wilson and so called Wilson's central electrode.

Unipolar limb leads: VR, VL, VF.
Unipolar chest leads: V1, V2, V3, V4, V5, V6.

Altogether there are 9 chest leads but only 6 are commonly used.

Augmented unipolar limb leads: Hence the voltage is increased here, the amplitude of wave is increased 1.5 times. We get aVR, aVL, aVF. In aVR instead of connecting VR, VL, VF to Wilson's central electrode, we disconnects the right arm from Wilson's central electrode:

$$aVR = VR - \frac{VL + VF}{2}$$

$2aVR = 2VR - (VL + VF)$
In closed circuit $VR + VL + VF = 0$
$VR = -(VL + VF)$
$2aVR = 2VR + VR = 3VR$
$aVR = 3/2\ VR$

Unipolar chest leads: Positions of leads in the chest:
- V1 – Electronic placed at the 4th ICS on right of sternum.
- V2 – 4th ICS to the left of sternum.
- V3 – Midway between V2 and V4.
- V4 – 5th ICS to left of sternum at MCL
- V5 – left 5th ICS at anterior axillary line.
- V6 – Left 5th ICS at Mid axillary line.

PR segment or PQ segment: It is in iso electric Line – End of P wave to beginning of Q wave. In certain leads Q wave will be absent. So called PR segment.

Q wave: Followed by large R waves and small S wave.

QRS Complex: Due to ventricular depolarization precedes ventricular systole. Magnitude and configuration of QRS will change accordingly to position of leads.

Transmission of depolarization: SA node to AV node through atrial pathways shifting depolarization from left to right of inter ventricular septum.

Downwards through inter ventricular septum myocardium of left and right ventricular.

ST Segment: After QRS complex an isoelectric segment from end of S wave to beginning of T wave – ventricle is completely depolarized at the end of QRS complex for some time.

T wave: ST segment is followed by another +ve deflection, which represent ventricular repolarization.

Duration > QRS 0.1–0.3 sec (0.27 sec average)
Amplitude > P wave 0.2–0.3 mV

Wave	Duration (sec)	Amplitude (mv)
P	0.1	0.1
QRS	0.1	1.0
T	0.2	0.2

PR Interval: Interval from beginning of P wave to beginning of QRS complex (P wave is included).

Duration: 0.12–02 sec (0.16 sec).

Denotes: P wave atrial depolarization upto QRS complex – beginning of ventricular depolarization so atrial depolarization of conduction through AV node and bundle of His.

Prolongation of PR interval: means > 0.2 sec. Heart block usually blocks occurs in bundle of his.

PR interval shortened: In WPW syndrome (Wolf Parkinson) white syndrome. Here, there is an additional pathway connecting atrium to ventricle called bundle of Kent conduction velocity in this pathway is very high.

QT interval: Beginning of Q wave to end of T wave 0.4 sec include ventricular depolarization and repolarization.

ST interval: End of S wave to end of T wave ventricular repolarization 0.32 sec.

RR interval: Important to calculate no of heartbeat per minute.

$$HR = \frac{60}{PR\ interval\ in\ sec} = \frac{1500}{No.\ of\ small\ segments\ between\ PR}$$

One cardiac cycle = 0.8 sec

Uses of ECG

- Disorders of cardiac rhythm
- Enlargement of heart

- Myocardial infarction
- Heart block + electrolyte imbalance

Disorders of rhythm: Arrhythmias—causes
- Extra systole.
- Paroxysmal tachycardia
- Flutter or fibrillation

Extra systole: Extra contraction of heart other than normal pattern can arise at: (a) Atrial level (b) Nodal (c) Ventricular usually the cause is ectopic focus may be due to:
- Ischemia
- Lack of sleep
- Toxins – caffeine, nicotine.

	P wave	QRST	
Atrial	Abnormal	N	P wave abnormal ventricular waves normal
Nodal	Inverted	N	From AV node impulse pass up and down
Ventricular	Buried in QRS	Abnormal	P waves not seen

Ventricular Extra Systole

QRS: Amplitude ↑
- Duration ↑
- T wave inverted
- Compensatory pause.

Before ventricle is repolarized ventricular depolarization prolonged for some more time.

Compensatory Pause: After ventricular extra systole a long pause. Then P of next impulse. When impulse comes ventricle is in absolute refractory period of extra systole. So no response ventricle waits for next impulse when next normal impulse come normal response. Total duration from P wave preceding extrasystole to next P waves is two cardiac cycle.

PAT: Arise spontaneously, last for some time and disappear. No of impulses arises from the ectopic focus in the atria. HR will be 150–220/mt. But it is conducted to atria.

PVT

- *Cause:* Ectopic focus is ventricle ischemic or irritant focus in ventricle.
- Circus movement.

Ventricular Fibrillation: Ineffective, incoordinate, irregular type of ventricular contraction occurs is a complication of PVT.

Atrial Flutter: 200–350/mt. Heart rate is more than PAT.

Cause

- Ectopic focus
- Circus movement

Atrial Fibrillation: Ineffective contraction. Some muscle contracting some relaxing. Small fibrillary type of P wave in ECG.

Ventricular fibrillation: Common complication of myocardial infarction. Also occurs in electrocution.

Rx: Defibrillators.

Heart Block

In complete heart block.

Complete heart block: Impulses are not conducted to ventricles. Atrium will be contracting ≤ it's own rhythm. Ventricles ≥ it's own rhythm.

First Degree HB: Prolongation of PR interval > 0.2 sec.

Second Degree HB: Prolongation of PR interval 2:1 or 3:1 block. In the case of 2:1 block, out of 2 impulse produced by atrium only one is conducted to ventricles. In the case of 3:1 block, out of 3 impulse produced by atria only one is conducted to ventricle.

Third Degree HB: Heart rate will be 40–45/min. No impulse transmission from atria to ventricle. It is called idioventricular rhythm.

Stokes–Adams Syndrome: Severe heart block. Heart rate – 15/min. Blood supply to brain very much decreased. Patient feels dizziness.

Cardiac Cycle (Figs 10.9 and 10.10)

Duration of one cardiac cycle = $\frac{60}{72}$ = 0.8 sec.

When atrium is contracting ventricle is relaxed. When ventricle contract atrium is relaxed.

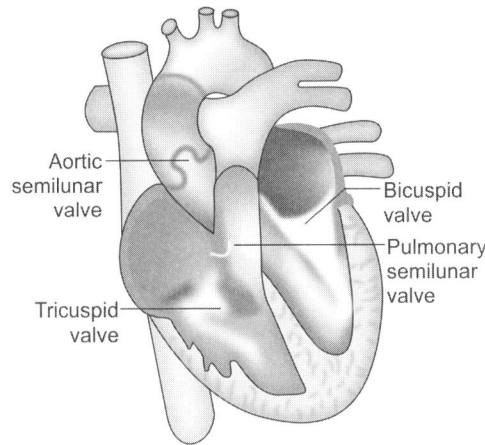

Fig. 10.9: Diagram of heart showing the valves of heart

Atrial systole – 0.1 sec
Atrial diastole – 0.7 sec
Ventricle systole – 0.3 sec
Ventricle diastole – 0.5 sec

Ventricular Systole
- Isovolumetric contraction – 0.05
- Rapid ejection phase – 0.1
- Reduced ejection phase – 0.15.

Ventricular Diastole – 0.5 sec
- Protodiastolic phase – 0.04 sec
- Isometric relaxation phase – 0.06 sec

- Rapid inflow phase – 0.1
- Reduced inflow phase – 0.2 sec
- Last rapid inflow – 0.1.

Atrial systole: Atrium contracts. Atrial pressure is 0–10 mm Hg.

Atrioventricular valves are open now.

Ventricular Systole
- *Isometric Contraction Phase:* 0.05 sec there is closure of AV valves. 1st heart sound is heard in this phase. Semilunar valves (pulmonary and aortic) are in a closed state. Ventricle is contracting on incompressible blood. There is a sharp rise in ventricular pressure from 0–80 mm Hg, on right side pressure rises from 0.10 mm Hg.
- At the end of isometric contraction phase the semilunar valves are open since the pressure rises to 120 mm Hg. Aortic pressure is only 80 mm Hg. Ventricle is still contracting and blood is ejected to aorta and pulmonary artery. This phase is rapid ejection phase.
- *Reduced ejection phase:* Ejection continues but pressure is reducing from 120–80 mm Hg (0.15 sec). There is a tendency of blood flowing back from

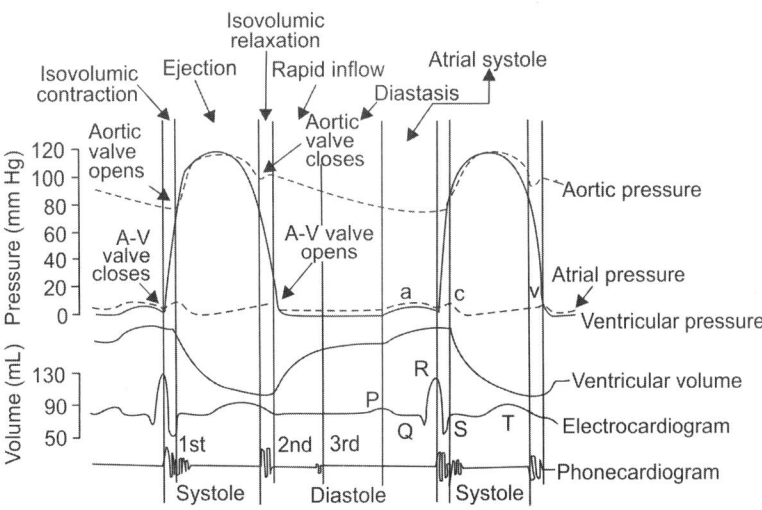

Fig. 10.10: Events of cardiac cycle

aorta to ventricle. Since the ventricular pressure is less than aortic pressure.

Ventricular Diastole

- *Proto diastole:* (0.04 sec) back flow to ventricle from aorta. Semilunar valves close, closure of semilunar valve produce 2nd HS.
- *Isometric relaxation:* 0.06 sec. All the valves are closed. Sharp reduction in pressure. Sharp reduction in pressure from 80–0 mm Hg. Comparatively high pressure in the aorta. AV valve open at the end of isometric relaxation.
- *Rapid inflow phase:* 0.1 sec. There is rapid inflow of blood into ventricle. Only slight increase in pressure in ventricle from 0–10 mm Hg.
- Reduced inflow phase (0.2 sec) Period of diastasis.
- *Last rapid inflow phase:* Additional 20–30% of blood flow into ventricle due to atrial contraction (0.1 sec). Seventy to eighty percent of blood is pumped from atrium to ventricle when atrium is relaxed.

Atrial systole: AV valve remains open. Thirty percent ventricular filling is due to atrial systole. Corresponds to 'a' wave of atrial pressure curve.

Ventricular systole: AV valve closes, atrial pressure increases and 1st heart sound is heard.

Mechanical Changes (Fig. 10.11)

Pressure change: Ventricle
- Aorta – pulmonary artery
- Right atrium, Jugular vein.

Volume changes: ventricle
- Production of heart sound
- Apex beat.

Ventricle: Pressure at the end of ventricular diastole 10 mm Hg. During diastole varies from 0–10 mm Hg.

Atrial systole or ventricular diastole 0–10 mm.

Isometric contraction phase: pressure increase from 10–80 mm Hg.

Rapid ejection: Pressure increase from 80–120 mm Hg.

Reduced ejection: Ejection from left ventricle to aorta. Aortic pressure is lower than left ventricular pressure. At the end of reduced ejection the aortic pressure increase more than left ventricular pressure. But there is some ejection of blood into aortic due to momentum.

Proto Diastole

Back flow of blood from aorta to left ventricle. Due to this semilunar valve closes.

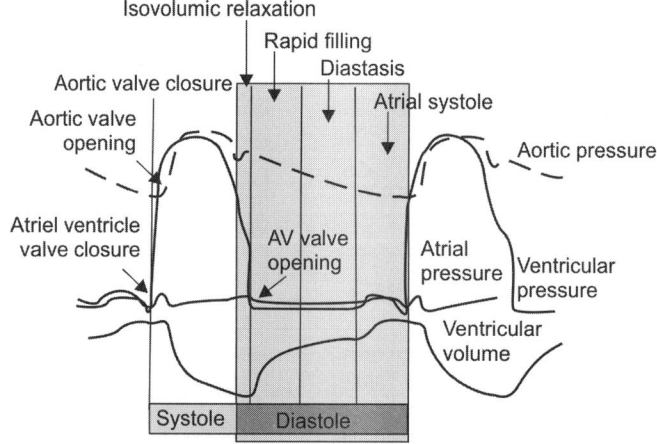

Fig. 10.11: Pressure and volume changes in different phases of cardiac cycle

Isometric Relaxation Phase

From 80 mm Hg pressure it comes back to zero at the end of IRP.

Atrial pressure is 7–8 mm Hg is more than ventricular pressure during the end of IRP and AV valve opens.

Due to increase in volume slight increase in pressure in ventricle 0–10 mm Hg. *Right ventricular pressure:* Maximum pressure is 25. At the end of isometric contraction 10 mm Hg.

Pathologically

Left ventricular pressure increase:
- Aystemic hypertension
- Aortic stenosis.

Aortic Pressure Changes

Minimum pressure in diastole: A total of 80 mm Hg. Aorta contain elastic fibers and has the recoiling tendency. So aortic pressure does not fall to 0 mm Hg during diastole.
Isometric contraction phase: Towards the end of this phase aortic valve open.

Rapid Ejection Phase

During rapid ejection phase (REP) pressure in aorta rises from 80–120 mm Hg. But remain slightly less than left ventricular pressure.
Reduced ejection: Amount of blood ejected into aorta will decrease.

Toward the end of reduced ejection, pressure in the aorta becomes slightly greater than left ventricular pressure.

Towards the end of proto diastole the pressure in aorta is more than left ventricular pressure and blood will be regurgitated back into ventricle. So aortic valve closes. There is a reduction in aortic pressure curve. This is incisura (due to back flow of blood).

Pulmonary Artery

Isometric contraction phase—9 mm Hg.
Maximum ejection phase—25 mm Hg.

Atrial Pressure Changes

Atrial systole: It produces a wave. Up stroke is due to atrial contraction, down stroke only few fibers are contracting.

Isometric Contraction

Pressure in atrium is increased. It is due to the bulging of the AV valve into atrium. This produce C wave (closure of AV valve). Upstroke is produced by the shortening of ventricular muscle pulling the AV valve down.
V wave: Venous filling of atrium.

Jugular Venous Pressure

The pressure changes in the atrium is reflected to the jugular veins and one can record the a, c, v waves in jugular vein.

Pressure changes in right atrium ranges from 0–1 mm Hg during diastole, 0–5 mm Hg during systole.

Left atrium	2	12
Right atrium	0–1	5

Volume Changes in the Ventricle

Twenty-five to thirty percent of blood ejected in atrial systole to ventricle.

End diastole volume – 130 mL.

At the end of systole blood remaining in ventricle is 50–60 mL.

Heart Sounds

The heart sounds and their pathological alterations are of great diagnostic value in clinical medicine.

Production of Heart Sounds

The even flow of blood is interrupted during the beginning of the contraction phase and this is signaled by first heart sound. The vibrations of the valves and more especially of the muscles are also significant factors in the production of the first sound. The turbulence of the flow of blood may also play a role. In most people closure of mitral and tricuspid valves is not at the same time and this produce splitting of 1st heart sound.

Second Sound

The second sound is heard when the intraventricular pressure falls below the aortic and pulmonary pressure and the back pressure forcibly shuts the semilunar valves. The splitting of 2nd heart sound is caused by the difference in the end of left and right ventricular systole.

Third and Fourth Sounds

Subsequent to the opening of the AV valves blood rushed into the ventricle and this sudden movement may produce vibration of the ventricular wall, corresponding to the termination of the rapid filling phase and it cause faint third sound. Simultaneously a faint sound may also result in the very beginning phase of cardiac cycle. When the blood is flowing from atria to ventricles. This is an atrial sound and the turbulence of blood may be a factor. Normally 3rd and 4th heart sounds are not audible. They can be recorded only by phonocardiogram.

The 1st and 2nd heart sounds can be heard by stethoscope. The pulmonary valve sounds can be heard best in the 3rd left intercostal area near the sternum while aortic area is on the 2nd right ICS. Tricuspid valve is loudest in the fourth right ICS while mitral area corresponds to the apex beat. The 1st and 2nd sounds can be heard over all these areas.

Murmurs: When fluid flows slowly through a tube of uniform diameter no sound is produced. But the moment the flow loses it is uniform character and becomes turbulent a murmur is heard.

Cardiac Output

Methods of Measurement

Based on Ficks principle

The amount of substance taken in or given out by an organ is equal to arteriovenous difference in concentration of substance × blood flow.

$Q = (A–V) \times$ blood flow
$Q =$ Substance taken in or given out
$A =$ Arterial concentration of substance
$V =$ Venous concentration of substance.

$$\text{Blood flow} = \frac{Q}{A-V}$$

$Q = O_2$ consumption $= 250$ mL/min (using computerized O_2 detectors)

Arterial O_2 content $= 19$ mL/100 mL.

Venous O_2 content $=$ (different for different organs) we have to collect pulmonary artery blood by cardiac catheterization 14 mL/100 mL.

Atrial = venous difference = 5 mL/100 mL

$$COP = \frac{100}{5} \times 250 = 5000 \text{ mL}$$

Thermo Dilution

Inject chilled saline into right atrium by using a double lumen catheter. One end contain thermistor to detect the temperature change before and after injection of chilled saline at the pulmonary artery level. From this, we can calculate (right) ventricular output.

Cardiac Output

Ref: Volume of blood ejected per ventricle per minute 5 L/min

COP = stroke volume × heart rate
= 70 × 72 = 5 L

Systolic discharge: Blood ejected per ventricle per minute. COP—also called minute volume. Stroke volume—is the output of the ventricle per beat and is about 70–80 mL. The minute volume or COP is the output of each ventricle per minute. This is obtained by multiplying the stroke volume by the heart rate and is 5 L (70 × 72 mL).

Regulation of COP

Sympathetic stimulation increases HR.
Increase temperature – increase HR
Hormones EN, NEN increase HR

Circulatory System

Upto the HR 180 beats/min – COP increasing correspondingly.

Above 180 – COP will not increase.

Two type of regulation:

Homometric Regulation

Independent of fiber length, e.g. +ve inotropic effect of sympathetic stimulation. EN and NEN cause increase myocardial contractility.

Drugs: Digitalis increase force of contraction, phenobarbitone decrease force of contraction. Acidosis, hypercapnia, hypoxia, etc. inversely affect stoke volume and cardiac output.

Heterometric Autoregulation

Increase end diastolic volume: Stretching and increase in length of muscle fiber increase force of contraction increase COP.

End diastolic volume (EDV): Stretching and increase in length of muscle fiber increase force of contraction increase COP.

End diastolic volume act as a free load or preload act on muscle before muscle start contracting. Aortic impedance or arterial resistance act as after load. Venous return directly affect end diastolic volume. Venous return is in turn influenced by several factors.

- Skeletal muscle pump.
- Venous force which depend on sympathetic discharge.
- Negative intrathoracic pressure which acts as a sucking force for venous return.
- *Posture:* Venous return more on lying down position.
- *Blood volume:* When blood volume is less venous return also decrease.
- Cardiac pump
- Exercise increase in HR.

EDV: When increased heart is contracting with greater force and emptying more. Starling law is not applicable in exercise.

Heart rate ⟨ Physiological variations / Pathological variations

Old age: Increase
Meals: Slight increase
Emotion: Anxiety increase
Exercise: Increase
Inspiration: HR increased
Expiration: Decreased
Temp: For 1°F, 10 beat increase in HR
Sleep: Decrease HR
Athletes: HR decrease.

Pathological
Shock, hemorrhage: Increase HR
Hyperthyroidism, fever: Increase HR
Arrhythmia: Increase HR

Regulation of HR ⟨ Nervous and hormonal control / Chemical / Long-term

Variations of Cardiac Output

- *Sleep:* No change
- *Meal:* Increase
- *Temp:* Increase
- *Exercise:* Increase.

Physiological
- Hyperthyroidism
- Anemia
- *Fever:* Increase COP.

Pathological
- Hypothyroidism ⎫
- Hemorrhage ⎬ decrease

Distribution of COP

Liver – 1500 mL/mt
Kidney – 1250 mL/mt
Brain – 750 mL/mt
Heart – 250 mL/mt
Skeletal muscle – 750 mL/mt
Skin – 450 mL/mt
Rest of body – 350 mL/mt

Preganglionic fibers originate from intermediolateral grey column of T1–T5. This is controlled by vasomotor center (VMC).

Vasomotor Center: Situated in the medulla.

In the rostral part, certain neurons in C1 area – presser area is vasoconstrictor.

Caudal and Intermediate Part of Medulla

Sets of neurons:
A1 (depressor)–Nucleus of tractus solitarius
A2 area.
C1 pressor area stimulate heart and vessels.
A1 area – inhibit the pressor area, so inhibit sympathetic system.

Regulation of COP

Role of heart in COP is called permissive role. Normal COP = 5 L/min. But the heart is capable of pumping much more than that even at rest, i.e. 10–13 L depending upon the blood returning to heart.

Factors increasing permissive role: Called hyper effective factors.
Factors decreasing permissive role: Hypo effective factors.

Hyper Effective Factors

- Sympathetic stimulation. Exercise causes this. COP increased to 25 L.
- Heart is hypertrophied in an athlete. The permissive role is increased. It can be increased to 35 L in an athlete.
- Factors inhibiting parasympathetic activity can increase the activity of heart.
- Thyroid hormone can increase COP, e.g, hyperthyroidism.

Hypo Effective Factors

- Parasympathetic stimulation.
- Decrease in thyroid hormone
- Defeats of myocardium. Myocardial infarction, valve defect. Septal defect, etc.

COP = stroke volume × heart rate
∴ Any factor which influences stroke volume and heart rate can influence COP.

Stroke volume depends upon how much of blood returns to atria and then to ventricle. Thus venous return influences stroke volume. Thus the factors influencing venous return influences stroke volume. SV will depend upon end diastolic volume. Also on myocardial contractility (force of contraction). COP also depends on aortic impedance (aortic resistance). This in turn depends on systemic blood pressure. Aortic impedance influences the blood pumping and there by COP. Factors influencing the length of muscle fiber also affect COP this is known as heterometric regulation. All other factors which influence COP without affecting the length of myocardium are homometric regulation. All the factor influencing heart rate also affects COP.

Effect of End Diastolic Volume on COP

Factors influencing EDV are:

- *Intrapericardial pressure:* Increase in Intrapericardial pressure decreases the venous return, EDV, SV, and COP and vice versa. Increase in pericardial fluid, pericarditis, and causes that increase intrapleural pressure will decrease EDV by decreasing venous return.
- *Atrial systole:* Increase in force of atrial contraction increase the filling of left ventricle increase EDV, SV, and COP.
- *Blood volume:* Increase in blood volume increase VR increase EDV, SV, and COP.
- *Body position:* VR decrease in standing posture (gravitational effect pulls the blood down) decreases EDV, SV, and COP, vice versa in lying posture.
- *Pumping action of skeletal muscle of lower limb:* When it is increased as in exercise VR increases SV, EDV and COP increase.
- *Sympathetic stimulation:* Venous tone is increased. Venous constriction results, more blood will be pumped up. This occurs in exercise. Abdominal

muscle contraction also increases in exercise. Veins are compressed increase in VR, EDV, SV, and COP.
- *Peripheral resistance:* Resistance offered to the flow of blood mainly by arterioles. This is decreased in exercises. This increases VR, EDV, SV, and COP.
- Increase in negativity of intrathoracic pressure during inspiration increases VR, EDV, SV, and COP.

Myocardial Contractility

- *Sympathetic stimulation:* Nervous influence (Tonic influence) can be either +ve or –ve with sympathetic stimulation. There is +ve tonic influence. There are four tonic influences.
    1. *+ve ionotropic effect:* Increase in the contractility.
    2. *+ve chronotropic effect:* Increase in the rate of heart.
    3. *+ve chronotropic effect:* Increase in the conduction velocity.
    4. *+ve bathmotropic effect:* Increase in excitability/irritability.

    Parasympathetics cause all 4 –ve tropic effects.
- *Influence of hormones:* Thyroid hormone increase myocardial activity. Glucagon, ACTH, pituitary hormone, etc. effect the contraction.
- Drugs increasing the heart rate caffeine, theophylline, digitalis increase the force of contraction in a failing heart. Drugs like Quinidine decreased the force of contraction.
- Increase in [CO_2]
- In acidity
- In [O_2]

  } decrease myocardial contraction.

- Intrinsic myocardial defects (MI) also decrease myocardial contractility.

Aortic Impedance

This is the after load against which heart has to work. If BP is increased COP is decreased because the heart has to overcome this resistance. But this negativity is overcome by an increase in EDV which will return COP. Thus to a limit increased EDV will overcome the aortic impedance.

Factors Influencing Heart Rate

All the factors influencing the pacemaker activity will increase the heart rate.

Temperature, anxiety, emotion, etc. increase the heart rate, sleep, pain, etc. decrease this heart rate.

- Sympathetic stimulation increase the HR. Spinal center for increasing HR is in upper five thoracic segments. This is the sympathetic center.
- Parasympathetic center is in the medulla (Dorsal nucleus of Vagus – cardio-inhibitory center).

  Spinal center is influenced by the vasomotor center/area in the medulla these two are again influenced by higher centers from cerebral cortex, hypothalamus, limbic system.

  Inhibition of cardio inhibitory center or stimulation of VMC increases HR.

  Marey's reflex: Inverse relationship between BP and HR. When BP increase HR decreases. This is due to reflex mechanism (Baroreceptor mechanism)

  Brain bridge reflex: When there is an increase in VR to heart (increase in right atrial pressure) which can be done by infusion, atrial volume receptors are stretched. Impulses pass by the vagus resulting in an increase in HR when initial HR was low.

- Heart rate is also increased by hormones, thyroid hormones glucagon, nor adrenaline, adrenaline. Decrease in HR can be due to a decrease in baroreceptor activity.
- Toward the end of expiration, HR decrease inspiration increase HR.
- Lack of hormones (thyroid, glucagon) decreases HR.

- Premature beat in extra-systole decreases HR. But the beat after compensatory pause increases HR. Post extra-systolic potentiation.

■ VASCULAR SYSTEM

Systemic circulation: Greater circulation
Pulmonary circulation: Lesser circulation

Parts of Systemic Circulation

Aorta: Large arteries (Windkessel vessels). They have three layers in the vessel wall:
1. Tunica intima
2. Tunica media
3. Tunica adventitia

Windkessel effect: During systole blood is ejected into already filled aorta and great vessels. During diastole blood is pumped from atria to ventricle. But due to inertia and elastic recoil blood flows in the vessels during diastole. This is called the Windkessel effect and the vessels showing this effect are called Windkessel vessels. Cross sectional area of aorta – 4.5 sq cm.

Arterioles: Otherwise so called resistance vessels. The driving force for forward flow occurring in arteries is pumping action of heart and elastic recoil of vessels. Arterioles has thick muscular tube wall with abundant smooth muscle fibers. The pulsatile flow in aorta and larger arteries are converted to steady flow in arterioles. Aorta and arteries systolic pressure 120, diastolic pressure 80 maximum drop of BP at the level of arteriole and both systolic and diastolic pressure become equal in capillaries. Arteriole controls the flow of blood from arteries to capillaries.

Capillaries: Exchange vessels have only a single layer of endothelial cells concerned with exchange of gases and nutrients.

Veins: Called capacitance vessels and have capacity to accommodate more blood.

2% blood	-	Aorta	} 10%
8%	-	other arteries	
1%	-	Arterioles	
5%	-	Capillaries	
54%	-	Venous side	
18%	-	Pulmonary artery	
12%	-	Lung	

Blood flow: Reynolds's No: 2000. Beyond which streamlined flow become turbulent.

■ POISEUILLE'S LAW

$$Re = \frac{\rho(rho) \, DV}{\eta(eta) \text{ viscosity of fluid}}$$

Re – Reynolds's number
ρ(rho) – Density of fluid
D – Diameter of tube
V – Velocity of flow
Velocity of flow = Rate of displacement cm/sec
Blood flow = Volume (cm^3)/sec

Pressure Change in Vessels

Aorta	– 120 mm Hg
Large artery	– 95 mm Hg
Small artery	– 85 mm Hg
Arteriolar end of capillary	– 30 mm Hg
Venous end of capillary	– 10 mm Hg
Vena cava	– 0 mm Hg.

Pressure in right atrium is also called central venous pressure. It is almost 0 mm Hg.

Veins: Veins of the lower limbs are provided with valves that direct the blood flow to the heart. The veins are surrounded by the muscles of the limb. They have a tone, and when they contract blood is pumped up called venous pump or muscle pump. Sometimes the valves may fail to function. Blood will not return properly to heart. This causes distension of veins varicose veins. Junction where arteriole divide into capillaries there is muscle cuff, which control the blood flow this is called pre-capillary sphincter. In some cases arterioles are not dividing directly to capillaries. Arterioles are connected to capillaries by metarteriole. Metarteriole have several capillaries which have precapillary sphincter. When there is activity, more of precapillary sphincters will open. This is called vasomotion.

Innervations of blood vessels: Sympathetic fibers are the adrenergic fibers secreting noradrenalin at nerve ending. There are sympathetic cholinergic fibers which secrete acetyl choline.

$$\text{Adrenergic} \begin{cases} \alpha \text{ adrenergic} \\ \beta \text{ adrenergic} \end{cases}$$

Thoracolumbar division of sympathetic nervous system is controlled by vasomotor center which in turn is controlled by hypothalamus and higher center at cerebral cortex.

Parasympathetic: Cranial division supplies upper part of the body. Sacral division supplies pelvic region. There is no parasympathetic supply to the blood vessel of skeletal muscle.

Sympathetic cholinergic supply skin and skeletal muscle. They are sympathetic vasodilator fibers arising from cerebral cortex. These are arising from areas called motor and premotor areas: Hypothalamus → Mid brain → spinal center.

Factors Affecting Blood Flow

Velocity of flow rate of displacement cm/sec:

Physical Factors

$$\text{Blood flow} = \frac{\text{Pressure gradient}}{\text{Resistance (mL/min)}} = \frac{P}{R}$$

Velocity (cm/sec) Blood flow = volume (cm³)/sec

Pressure also depends on physical factors like (1) velocity. of flow (2) viscosity of blood (3) Diameter of the vessel (4) Resistance (5) elasticity of blood vessels also affect pressure, e.g. atherosclerosis. Normal flow in a vessel is said to be laminar flow or streamline flow. A thin layer of blood in contract with the wall of BV is at rest. The speed of flow increases with increasing distance from the vessel wall so that maximum speed is seen in the layer at the center of the vessel. Streamline flow does not produce any sound. There is turbulence when there is a constriction in the blood vessel.

■ NERVOUS CONTROL OF THE HEARTBEAT

The electrical stimulus for contraction of cardiac muscle is generated spontaneously within the heart and this continues to occur if the heart is stripped of its nerve supply. In other words, the heartbeat is spontaneous and continues in the denervated heart. However, the autonomic nervous system exercises control over the rate of the heartbeat. Impulses passing down the parasympathetic fibers of the vague nerve are inhibitory to the heart and slow it. The heart also has a sympathetic nerve supply, however, from the cervical and upper sympathetic ganglia, and sympathetic nerve impulses quicken the heart. If the effects are balanced, the 'normal' heart rate is maintained. If there is sympathetic over activity, possibly due to acute anxiety, tachycardia occurs. On the other hand, increased parasympathetic tone results in bradycardia. Strong vagal stimulation may even abolish spontaneous nodal discharge temporarily so that fainting (syncope) occurs. The pulse of a person who is recovering from a simple faint is slow.

The autonomic nerve fibers exert their effects upon the cardiac cells via neurotransmitters or chemical messengers. Certain proteins at the cell surface are receptors for these neurotransmitters. The parasympathetic fibers of the vagus nerve act by releasing acetylcholine which is taken up by acetylcholine receptors at the surface of the cardiac cell. These are also called muscarinic receptors because the actions of acetylcholine on them is similar to that of muscarinic, an alkaloid which is present in toadstools in poisonous amounts. The chemical mediators for the action of the sympathetic nervous system on cells are adrenalin and noradrenalin and the receptors are known as adrenergic receptors, of which there are two types, alpha (α) and beta (β), each with two subtypes. The adrenergic receptors of the heart are $β_1$ receptors. Drugs which block these receptors are used to treat several cardiovascular diseases, particularly coronary heart disease in which they reduce the rate and force of cardiac contraction and shield the heart from the effects of stress, which causes the release of catecholamines (adrenalin and noradrenalin) from sympathetic nerve endings and from the suprarenal glands.

Cardiac Investigations

The electrical events of the heart are recorded on the elertrocardiogram which may be altered in a variety of ways by disease. Diagnostic changes occur in some conditions, such as acute myocardial infarction, and the electrocardiogram is invaluable in the detection of disturbances of cardiac rhythm, or arrhythmia. Echocardiography is the examination of the heart by means of ultrasound which is directed through the heart from a transducer placed on the skin and which is echoed back by the structures which it encounters. By this means, pictures are obtained of the four cardiac chambers and of the valves of the heart. The movements of the valves and of the walls of the heart may be studied and measurements may be made of the size of the cardiac chambers and of the thickness of their walls. Atrial and ventricular septal defects and other congenital abnormalities may be diagnosed. Pericardial effusions and tumors or thrombi inside the heart may be detected. A variety of further investigations is available for studying the alterations in anatomy and physiology in diseases of the heart.

■ THE BLOOD PRESSURE

Blood pressure may be defined as the force or pressure which the blood exerts on the walls of the artery in which it is contained.

When an artery is cut across, the blood spurts out from the end nearest the heart with considerable force and is obviously under high pressure within the artery. It will further be observed that, in addition to the continuous stream, there will be regular spurts of increased pressure corresponding with each heartbeat. The continuous pressure is partly dependent on the elasticity of the arteries and is called the diastolic pressure. The increased pressure occurring with each beat of the heart is the systolic blood pressure.

If definite amount of fluid is pumped through a large tube with a certain amount of force it will flow out at the far end at a definite rate and pressure. If the same amount of fluid is pumped through a narrower tube with the same force the pressure with which it leaves the tube will be increased. The narrower the opening of the tube the greater will be the friction of the fluid on the walls of the tube.

An illustration of this can be seen in the use of the ordinary garden hose. If no nozzle is attached and water is turned on at moderate pressure a steady stream will emerge from the end of the hose and project for about a foot. If a narrow nozzle is then attached without altering the supply of water this will leave the nozzle in a fine jet projected for a number of yards with much friction against the walls of the nozzle as it leaves. Compression of any part of the hose without the nozzle will be easy, in other words, the pressure within is relatively low. The application of the nozzle, by narrowing the opening and causing resistance to the outflow, will cause an increase in the pressure within the whole of the rest of the hose which can no longer be so easily compressed.

The same mechanical factors are applicable in regard to the blood pressure within the arteries. The heart may pump with a constant force. The aorta is a relatively wide channel but the arteries gradually become smaller and by their resistance to the flow of blood maintain a high pressure in the whole of the arterial system. If the heart beats more strongly the pressure will be increased, but it will fall if the force of the heartbeat is reduced. Again, if the normal size of the arteries is reduced the resistance will be increased and the blood pressure will rise. Lastly, if the volume of circulating blood is diminished (e.g. after hemorrhage) the blood pressure will fall.

Blood pressure is therefore maintained by the following factors:
- The force of the heartbeat;
- The resistance to blood flow in the arterioles, i.e. the peripheral resistance; and
- The volume of circulating blood.

The Measurement of Blood Pressure

Clinically, the blood pressure is measured by an instrument called the sphygmomanometer. This consists of a rubber bag which is placed around the arm. The interior of the bag is connected by a rubber tube to a mercury pressure-gauge. When the pressure in the bag equals the pressure in the artery, the latter is compressed flat and the flow through it temporarily arrested. The pulse, therefore, disappears. This may be appreciated either by the finger or by listening over the brachial artery at the bend of the elbow with a stethoscope. The height to which the column of mercury has been forced at this moment is therefore the systolic blood pressure. The height is measured in millimeters and the blood pressure is referred to as being so many millimeters of mercury (mm Hg).

As the column of mercury is allowed to fall there comes a point at which the stethoscope sounds suddenly become muffled or disappear. The height of the mercury column at this point is taken as the diastolic blood pressure.

The blood pressure varies with rest and activity, emotion and age. A resting young adult would be expected to have a blood pressure of about 120/80 mm Hg, the numerator being the systolic pressure and the denominator the diastolic pressure. There is, however, a wide range of normality. A WHO guideline asserts that a normotensive individual has a systolic blood pressure of less than 140 and a diastolic-pressure of less than 90 mm Hg at rest. Repeated readings above 160/95 mm Hg may indicate hypertension and intermediate readings are described as 'borderline.'

A high blood pressure, or hypertension, may damage the arteries and eventually lead to stroke or a heart attack (myocardial infarction). A low blood pressure, or hypotension, occurs acutely in cases of shock due to blood loss, septicemia, myocardial infarction or other causes. Renal perfusion may be threatened if the systolic pressure falls below 80 mm Hg and renal failure may ensue. Chronic hypotension may result from Addison's disease of the adrenal gland.

The difference between the diastolic and systolic arterial pressures is called the pulse pressure. This may also be affected by disease.

The Pulse

Each time the left ventricle contracts it forces its contained blood into the aorta. The aorta being elastic expands in order to accommodate this additional amount of blood. At the same time, the blood which was present before the ventricular contraction is now pushed on into the next section which, in turn, also expands, and so on. Thus a wave of expansion is created which starts at the root of the aorta and spreads over the whole of the arterial system, gradually dying away as it reaches the capillaries. This wave of expansion constitutes the pulse and it travels rapidly over the arteries, much more rapidly, in fact, than the velocity of the bloodstream.

The pulse can be felt and often seen in the superficial arteries of the body, but it is customary to study it in the radial artery. The other arteries in which it can be felt with ease are the temporal in front of the ear, the facial as it passes over the lower jaw, the carotid artery in the neck and the dorsal is pedis on the dorsum of the foot.

Nervous Control of the Blood Vessels

Most of the arteries of the body are directly under the control of the autonomic nervous system. Special centres, known as the vasomotor centers, exist in the hypothalamus and medulla oblongata to exercise this control. Two sets of nerves are present.
1. Vasoconstrictor
2. Vasodilator.

These nerves may affect the whole of the circulatory system at a time, or their action may be limited to a localized organ or part.

Vasoconstrictor nerves: As their name suggests, these nerves narrow the lumen of a blood vessel and thereby diminish the amount of blood to the part or organ which it supplies. If all the vasoconstrictor nerves are sending out impulses, a general effect will be produced; the whole of the arterial system will be narrowed and therefore the blood pressure will be raised (see p. 147).

Vasodilator nerves: These act by dilating the blood vessels and allowing a greater blood supply to the organ. Thus, the blood vessels of the alimentary tract are dilated by this action during the process of digestion; also during muscular exercise the blood vessels to the muscles are dilated so that they are able to carry more blood.

In the serious condition known as 'shock' the blood vessels as a whole become dilated and, in consequence, the blood pressure falls. One of the methods of treatment is to give drugs which stimulate the α-adrenergic receptors causing the arteries to narrow, thereby raising the blood pressure.

Most sympathetic impulses stimulate vasoconstriction and parasympathectic impulses result in vasodilatation.

An example of the nervous control of blood vessels which everyone has either felt or observed is the phenomenon of blushing. This is a purely local modification of the circulation and variation in the amount of blood in the skin of the face, and surrounding parts if the blush is extensive. An emotion, pleasure, embarrassment, disgust, or offended modesty perchance, possesses the mind and with inconsiderate haste the skin grows red and a hot flush is felt. This is due to the conscious nervous system affecting the vasomotor center over which the individual has no control. Vasodilator impulses are sent out and the small arteries in the skin of the affected part dilate, bringing an excess of blood to the surface.

Conversely, in extreme terror or rage the face may become very pale and cold ('white with rage'). In this case the vasoconstrictor nerves are limiting the flow of blood through the arteries.

BP—Control, Factors Influencing, Hypertension

Regulation of Blood Pressure

Divided into:
- Short-term – within seconds
- Intermediate-term – within minutes
- Long-term – within days.

Short-term Mechanism

- *Baroreceptors:* Situated in the carotid sinus, aortic arch and chambers of heart. They are most useful in regulation of BP in the pressure range of 70–150 mm Hg.
- *Chemoreceptors:* They are working in pressure range of 40–70 mm Hg.

  The chemoreceptors are aortic bodies and carotid bodies and the factors responsible for stimulation of chemoreceptors are:
  - Hypoxia
  - Hyper apnea
  - Acidosis.

  This will stimulate the vasomotor center (VMC) and will cause increase in blood pressure.

  Primary response: Vagal center nucleus ambiguous and dorsal motor nucleus of vagus get stimulated and produce bradycardia.

  Secondary response: Inhibition of vagal center by respiratory system cause tachycardia.
- *Hormonal mechanism:* Secretion of adrenalin and noradrenalin cause increase in heart rate.

  These changes in heart rate cancel and so the heart rate is not much affected.

  But blood pressure is definitely increased.
- *CNS ischemic response:* BP below 40 mm Hg. Cushing response cause increase in BP when increase ICP compress arteries.

Intermediate-term Mechanism

- Renal mechanism
  - By increasing peripheral resistance (vasopressin or ADH)
  - By increasing blood volume (ADH)
- Catecholamine from adrenal medulla
  - Adrenalin
  - Nonadrenalin
  - Dopamine.
- Intrinsic vascular mechanism
  - Capillary fluid shift
  - Stress relaxation.
- Renin Angiotensin mechanism:

  Capillary fluid shift: Whenever the mean blood pressure increases more fluid is lost at the arterial end of capillaries, circulating blood volume is reduced and blood pressure returns to normal.

  Stress relaxation: When blood volume changes in the range of +30% to –15%, e.g. due to transfusion or hemorrhage blood pressure shows only a transient change.

  This is because blood pressure returns to normal by local vascular tone adjustments even in the absence of other regulating mechanisms.

Long-term Mechanism

Regulation of Blood Volume

Accomplished by humeral mechanisms involving kidneys hormones are:

- *Antidiuretic hormone:* Secreted from posterior pituitary in response to thirst mechanism which conserve water by its action on distal convoluted tubule and collecting duct of kidney.
- *Aldosterone:* Secreted from the adrenal cortex which produce salt and water conservation by acting on the distal convoluted tubule and collecting duct of kidneys.

Renin Angiotensin Mechanism

- Rennin is secreted by the JG cells in response to decrease in renal blood flow. It produce vasoconstriction.

  Renin converts angiotensinogen to angiotension I

  Angiotensin I: ACE angiotensin II

  Angiotensin II: It is a potent vasoconstrictor, and it helps to maintain BP when extracellular fluid volume is reduced.
- Atrial natriuretic peptide.

Factors Maintaining BP
- Cardiac output
- Peripheral resistance
- Elasticity of the arterial walls (continuous flow)
- *Blood volume:* It affect both systolic and diastolic pressure.
- Volume of vascular space. When there is vasodilatation, BP decreases.

Hypertension
Sustained elevation of blood pressure.
- *Primary:* Essential hypertension –90%
- *Secondary:* Due to some other deceases –10%.

Primary or Essential hypertension: Cause is not known. But associated with atherosclerosis.

Secondary Hypertension:
- Endocrine
- Renal hypertension
- Coarctation of aorta
- Toxemia of pregnancy.

Endocrine
- Adrenal medullary tumor. For example, pheochromocytoma which secretes catecholamine. This will increase blood pressure.
- Cushing syndrome increased secretion of glucocorticoids.
- Conn's syndrome → Increase mineralocorticoids, e.g. aldosterone.

Renal Hypertension
Renal artery stenosis increase renin secretion.

Pyelonephritis, nephritic syndrome also increase blood pressure.

Coarctation of Aorta
High blood pressure in upper portion of body.

Treatment of Hypertension
β Blockers
Ca^{++} channel blockers
Angiotensin converting enzyme inhibitors.

■ CARDIAC FAILURE
Causes of Cardiac Failure
- *Increase preload:* According to Starling's law increase end diastolic volume which augments cardiac failure. Too much increase in preload lead to ventricular dilation and heart failure.
- *Increase in after load:* For example, hypertension. There is resistance to outflow of blood which leads to ventricular dilation and heart failure.
- *Decreased myocardial contractility:* Also leads to decreased pumping and failure of heart.

Left Heart Failure
Features: Cardiomegaly, arrhythmia dysphea and orthopnea.

Fatigue, hypertension, poor tolerance to stress and oliguria. Decreased left ventricular output leading to elevation of left ventricular volume and pressure and its transmission to left atrium and pulmonary veins.

Conditions Causing Left Heart Failure
- Left ventricular outflow obstruction due to:
  - Systemic hypertension
  - Aortic valve stenosis
  - Coarctation of aorta
- Left ventricular inflow obstruction due to mitral stenosis.
- Reduced ventricular contractility:
  - Cardiomyopathy
  - Anterior wall myocardial infarction.

Right Heart Failure
Decreased right ventricular output which leads to increased right ventricular pressure which lead to increased right atrial pressure. When right atrial pressure increases, manifest as increased jugular venous pulse, edema, congestion of viscera and hepatomegaly.

Forward failure: Due to inadequate chronic obstructive pulmonary (COP).

Backward failure: Increased end diastolic volume (due to decreased COP) ventricular pressure increased. The elevation of left and right ventricular pressure results in pulmonary and systemic congestion, respectively.

■ SHOCK

Cardiovascular shock is characterized by insufficient cardiac output so that the circulation fails to meet the oxygen and nutritional elements of the tissue. It is due to insufficiency of the cardiac output which is not necessarily due to fault of the heart.

Causes of Shock

- *Hypovolemia:* Hemorrhage or diarrhea.
- *Cardiogenic shock:* Shock in myocardial infarction in which cardiac output is insufficient.
- *Septicemic shock:* Caused by arteriolar and venodilation due to bacterial toxins leading to reduction in cardiac inflow resulting in fall of cardiac output.

Dangers of shock: Reduction of cardiac output fall of → perfusion pressure → fall of tissue perfusion → tissue anoxia → death of the brain → death of individual. There may → be insufficient filtration by the kidneys → accumulation of waste products.

Common factors of shock are cold clammy skin, low BP, tachycardia oliguria. There may be also mental confusion.

Compensatory Mechanism

The aim of compensatory mechanism is to restore the perfusion pressure. Three types of compensatory mechanism:
1. Vasoconstriction – (a) Neural mechanism, endogenous chemicals.
2. Tissue fluid shift
3. Body water conservation.

Vasoconstriction

- Neural mechanism—in hemorrhagic shock there is withdrawal of normal stimulation of baroreceptors withdrawal of inhibition of vascular mural cells (VMC), sympathetic stimulation elevation of BP and tachycardia → perfusion of the tissues is restored.
- Sympathetic stimulation also causes carotid chemoreceptor stimulation by causing vasoconstriction of the artery feeding the carotid chemoreceptor. Chemoreceptor stimulation produce VMC stimulation.
- Fall of BP results in ischemia of the VMC and in turn produces stimulation of VMC. So, there is sympathetic stimulation of VMC. It causes elevation of BP and restoration of perfusion. Also sympathetic stimulation causes redistribution of blood flow, the continuous splanchnic and muscle blood flow are cut and the available blood is directed to the brain and heart.

Sympathetic stimulation produces the signs of shock like pallor and sweating. Endogenous substances like adrenalin are also liberated which reinforces the sympathetic activity.

Tissue Fluid Shift

As BP falls the capillary blood pressure also falls, but there is no fall of the colloidal osmotic tension. This causes stoppage of flow of fluid from the capillary to the tissue. If fall of BP is greater the return of tissue fluid to the capillary is enhanced and this corrects the hypervolemia within the vascular compartment.

Conservation of Body Water

Fall of BP leads to lowering of perfusion pressure of the kidney → production → of renin production of angiotensin → production of addosterone → Sodium retention → body water retention.

In stress the hormone antidiuretic hormone (ADH) is also secreted in greater amount. This reduces the volume of the urinary output. Body water conserved → hypovolemia corrected. ADH in high concentration acts as vasopressin which is a powerful vasoconstrictor. Compensatory mechanism are often called negative feedback mechanism.

Irreversible shock: If the shock continuous and is not treated promptly the stage of irreversible shock develops. The +ve feedback mechanism appear in the screen with the result that there develops a vicious cycle.

- *Cardiac damage:* The subendocardial region of myocardium is susceptible to anoxia. When the BP is falling this danger increases and ultimately subendocardial damages occur.

    → faster fall of cardiac output vicious cycle operates.

    A myocardial depressing factor appear in the circulation during advanced stages of shock, this reduces cardiac contractility.

    In advanced stages of shock acidosis → develops and depresses the myocardial contractility still further → further fall of BP vicious cycle.

- *Acidosis:* Tissue anoxia leads to accumulation of lactic acid → acidosis.

    The fall of pH causes relaxation of the arteriolar and precapillary sphincter → muscles → vasodilatation vicious cycle.

- *Toxemia:* Prolonged spasm of the splanchnic vessels → intestinal ischemic damage due to lack of O_2 → massive entry of the intestinal → bacteria → release of toxin vascular smooth muscle relaxation.

- *VMC ischemic:* Slight ischemia stimulates the VMC but massive ischemia kills it. Which produce sympathetic paralysis and fall of BP.

- Atherosclerotic lesions in the coronary or cerebral arteries.

REGIONAL CIRCULATIONS

Coronary Circulation

Factors determining coronary flow
- Mechanical
- Metabolic
- Neural.

Mechanical

- Phasic flow
- Autoregulation
- Regional variation supply.

Phasic Flow

Finer branches of the coronary arteries run through the myocardium. So during ventricular contraction flow is obstructed.

In the left ventricle: Obstruction very pronounced. Particularly in the phase of isometric contraction. Flow becomes very high in the early phase of diastole. The flow thereafter begins to decline. In the right ventricle the force of contraction is not so greater and some flow occurs during the systole although the diastolic flow is greater than the flow in systole.

Autoregulation

Between 60 and 150 mm Hg of BP the coronary flow remains unchanged. This is due to autoregulation of the coronary circulation which survives even when the nerve supply to coronary vessels are paralyzed or removed.

Regional Variation of Supply

The subepicardial portions of myocardium are better supplied with arterial blood than the subendocardial part (Fig. 10.12). During systole of the left ventricle the subendocardial parts of the myocardium develops hypoxia due to insufficient blood supply. In this portion of myocardium there is an excess of myoglobin which pitches up O_2 flow blood, stores and supplies most readily to the neighboring cells when they need it.

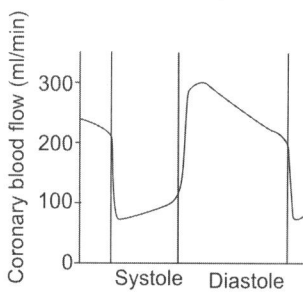
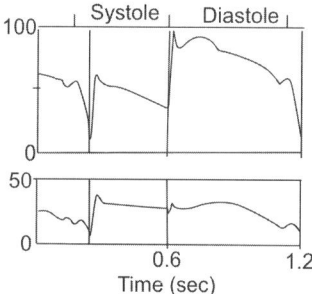

Fig. 10.12: Left coronary artery (LCA) blood flow during systole is 15–16% of diastole

Metabolic Factors

Lack of O_2 in the myocardium is the most powerful coronary vasodilator. Mechanism of the vasodilator action of hypoxia is not clear. Adenosine can cross the cell membrane and appear in the extracellular space where on coming in contact with arterioles it causes a powerful vasodilation.

Neural Factor

Coronary arteries receive motor supply from both sympathetic and parasympathetic system. On the vascular sympathetic muscle of coronary arteries both and β_2 receptors are found. Receptor stimulation cause vascular sympathetic muscle contraction and vasoconstriction. β_2 stimulation lead to vasodilation.

■ CEREBERAL CIRCULATION

The brain receives blood supply from the basilar artery and the two internal carotid arteries.

Factors Determining the Flow

- *Perfusion pressure:* Between 60–150 mm Hg of BP the blood flow is not affected. This is autoregulation of brain blood flow. However, if the systemic BP falls very severely the patient develops the risk of cerebral anoxia greatly as in such cases autoregulation fails to protect.
- *CO_2 concentration:* When the CO_2 concentration of the local brain tissue rises, there is vasodilation leading to increased blood flow. Conversely, if CO_2 is washed out from the body there may be cerebral vasoconstriction leading to cerebral anoxia and visual blackouts.
- *O_2 Tension:* High O_2 tension in the inspired air and brain is protected from O_2 poisoning.
- *Anesthetics:* Majority of the anesthetics reduce the brain blood flow.
- Intracranial pressure
  Monro-Kellie Doctrine: Brain tissue and spinal fluid are essentially incompressible, the volume of blood, spinal fluid and brain in the cranium at any time must be relatively constant. Cerebral vessels are compressed whenever the intracranial pressure rises.
- *Autoregulation:* The flow to many tissues is maintained at relatively constant levels despite variations in perfusion pressure. In the brain autoregulation maintains a normal cerebral blood flow at arterial pressures of 65 to 140 mm Hg.
- *Vasomotor and Sensory Nerves:* Nor adrenergic discharge occurs when the blood pressure is markedly elevated.

So, results in passive increase in blood flow and helps to protect the blood brain barrier from disruption. Thus, vasomotor discharges affect autoregulation.

- *Blood flow in various parts of the Brain:* Blood flow to brain is tightly compelled to brain metabolism. In resting humans the average blood flow to grey matter is 69 mL/100 g/min compared with 28 mL/100 g/min in white matter. A striking feature of cerebral function is the marked variation in local blood flow with changes in brain activity.

In subject who are awake but at rest blood flow is greatest in the premotor and frontal regions. This is the part of brain that concerned with decoding and analyzing afferent input and with intellectual activity. During voluntary activities of the right hand flow is increased in the hand area of left motor cortex and the corresponding sensory areas in the postcentral gyrus. When the movements performed are sequential flow is also increased in the supplementary motor area. Creative speech increases blood flow to Broca's and Wernicke's area. Right handed individuals blood flow to the left hemisphere greater when verbal task is being performed and blood flow to the right hemisphere is greater when a spatial task is being performed.

■ BRAIN METABOLISM AND OXYGEN REQUIREMENTS

Oxygen Consumption: O_2 consumption by the human brain averages approximately 20% of the total body resting O_2 consumption. The brain is extremely sensitive to hypoxia. Basal ganglia use O_2 at a very high rate and symptoms of Parkinson disease as well as intellectual defects can be produced by chronic hypoxia. Thalamus and the inferior colliculus (IC) are also very susceptible to hypoxic damage.

Energy Sources: Glucose is the major ultimate source of energy for the brain 90% of energy needed to maintain ion gradients across cell membranes and transmits electrical impulses comes from this source. Glucose enters the brain via GLUT I in cerebral capillaries. Other transporters then distribute it to neurons and glial cells.

Glucose is taken up from the blood in large amounts and the RQ of cerebral tissue is 0.95–0.99 in normal individuals. Glucose utilization at rest parallels blood flow and O_2 consumption. The substances other than glucose are metabolized for energy during convulsion. Glutamate entering the brain takes up ammonia and leaves as glutamine. The reverse reaction is responsible for production of ammonia which enters the renal tubules. This glutamate—glutamine conversion in the brain serves as a detoxifying mechanism to keep the brain free of ammonia. Ammonia is very toxic to nerve cells. In hepatic coma-ammonia intoxication is responsible for bizarre neurological symptoms.

■ CUTANEOUS CIRCULATION

Special Functions: In addition to general duty of supplying nutrients exchange of O_2 and CO_2 and removing waste products the special duties are:
- Thermal homeostasis
- Circulating readjustment of blood.

Triple Response: If the skin is stroked lightly by a smooth end of a stick or glass rod, along the line described by the stroke a white line develops in a few seconds, which lasts for about 5 mins. The white line develops due to contraction of the precapillary sphincters which contracts as a direct response to stroke. If firmly stroked the characteristic triple response develops particularly in a sensitive subject.
- **Red Reaction:** A red line appears where the stroke is made. This is due to capillary engorgement which in turn

is due to relaxation of the precapillary sphincter. The line appears within about 10 sec.

- *Wheal:* This is followed in a few minutes by local swelling and mottled reddening around the injury. This is called wheal. It is local edema due to increased permeability of capillaries and postcapillary venules, with extravasation of fluid.
- *Flush or Flare:* If the stroke is still firmer flush or flare appears causing reddening. Also skin temperature increase. Cause of flare is arteriolar dilation produced by the axon reflex. Flare develops after about ½ minutes of stroking.

Axon Reflex

When an area of the skin is firmly stroked the sensory nerve fibers arising from the area are stimulated and carry the impulse to the respective spinal cord segment. Along with this due to axon reflex a response in which impulses initiated in sensory nerves by the injury are relayed antidromically down other branches of the sensory nerve fibers. Substance P released at the sensory C fiber ending is the neurotransmitter responsible.

CHAPTER 11

The Mononuclear Phagocytic and Lymphoid Systems

Phagocytes are cells which can engulf and digest or encapsulate foreign material, such as inert particles and microorganisms. The polymorphonuclear leukocytes of the blood can do this but are not included under the mononuclear phagocytic (or macrophage) system. The mononuclear phagocytic cells of which this system consists, and which are distributed throughout the body, are called macrophages. They are of two types, those circulating in the blood and known as monocytes and those which are derived from the peripheral blood monocytes but which are relatively fixed in the tissues and referred to as tissue macrophages. In the connective tissues, the latter cells are called histiocytes and in the thymus, lymph nodes and spleen they are known as sinus-lining macrophages. In the lungs, alveolar macrophages migrate from the connective tissue into the alveoli and may later be found in the sputum, having engulfed dust particles and bacteria which have been inhaled. The importance of macrophages in both innate and acquired immunity, providing first-line and second-line defense against invading microorganisms. Macrophages are also involved in the phagocytosis and destruction of effete red blood cells in the spleen and liver. The name mononuclear phagocytic system is now used in preference to the older term, reticuloendothelial system.

THE LYMPHOID SYSTEM

The principal cells of the immune system, the lymphocytes, operate in close association with phagocytic cells and, like them, are disseminated throughout the body. They may be found singly or in diffuse aggregations or within the lymphoid organs. Separate central and peripheral lymphoid tissues are recognized. The bone marrow, where, B-lymphocytes are produced, and the thymus, where T-lymphocytes are formed, are the central lymphoid organs and the lymph nodes, spleen and lymphoid nodules associated with the gut and bronchial tree are the peripheral lymphoid organs.

The tissues of the body are permeated by a vast network of capillaries containing blood. The walls of the capillaries consist of a single layer of cells and, except for the white cells which at certain times are able to make their way through these walls, the blood does not actually come into direct contact with the tissues. The tissues are, however, bathed in tissue fluid which may be regarded as an intermediary between the blood and the tissues; all interchange of nourishment and waste products between them takes place through the medium of the tissue fluid.

The lymphatic system is a subsidiary or second circulatory system which drains the tissue fluids. From the tissue spaces, the

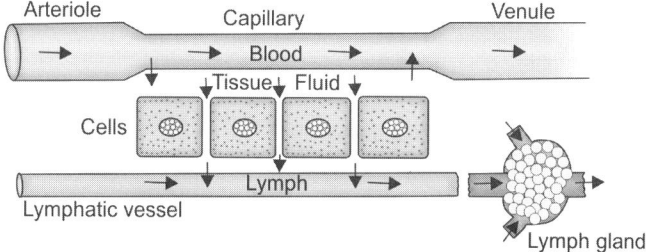

Fig. 11.1: Circulation of tissue fluid and lymph

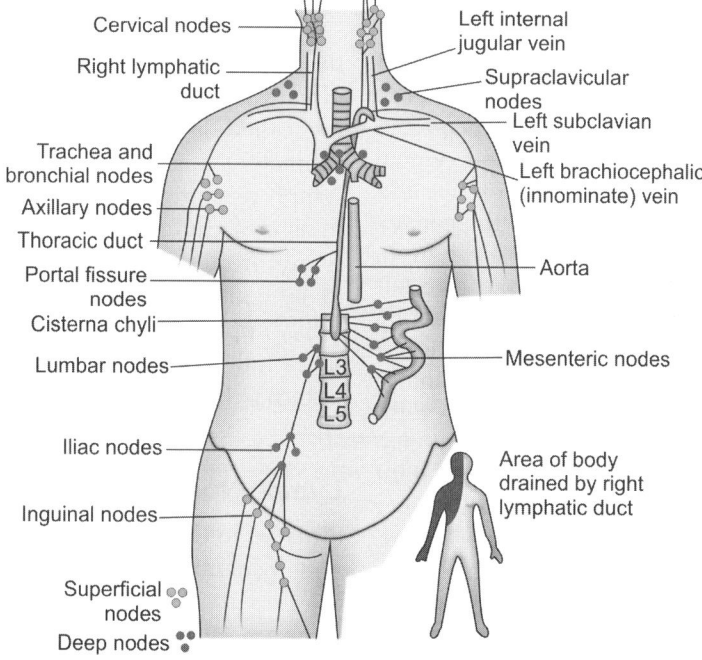

Fig. 11.2: Main lymph nodes and ducts

tissue fluid passes into lymph capillaries which unite to form larger trunks which ultimately re-join the general circulation (Fig. 11.1). Lymph is the name given to the tissue fluid when it has entered the lymphatic vessels and it may be looked upon as a part of the plasma which has filtered through the walls of the blood capillaries. The larger lymphatic vessels resemble small veins and are provided with valves to prevent back flow. A plexus of fine blood vessels accompanies the larger lymph vessels and nourishes them. If the lymph vessels under the skin become inflamed (lymphangitis) the accompanying plexuses of blood vessels become congested and red lines are seen in the skin.

The lymph channels unite to form larger vessels which eventually converge into two large ducts, the thoracic duct and the right lymphatic duct, which empty their lymph into the left and right brachiocephalic veins respectively (Fig. 11.2). The more important of the two ducts, because it conveys the greater quantity of lymph back into the blood, is the thoracic duct. This

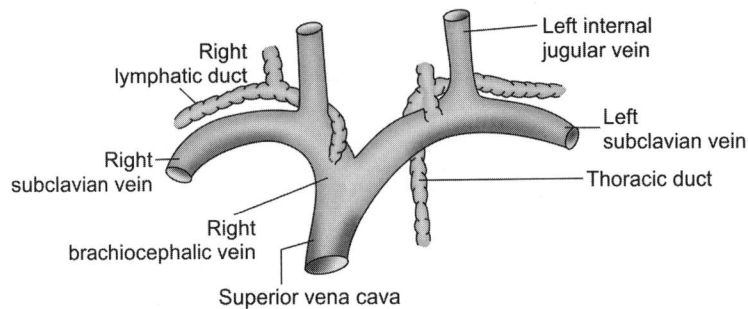

Fig. 11.3: Return of lymph to the great veins

duct is about 40 cm long in the adult and extends from the second lumbar vertebra to the root of the neck. It commences as a dilated sac, the cisterna chyli, into which the lymph vessels from the lower limbs and the abdomen except for part of the convex surface of the liver, empty their lymph. After passing upwards in front of the left side of the thoracic vertebrae, it is joined by the lymphatics from the left arm and the left side of the head and neck before it terminates in the left brachiocephalic vein. The right lymphatic duct, which is about 1 cm in length, conveys lymph from the right side of the head and neck, the right upper limb, the right side of the chest and heart, and part of the convex surface of the liver.

Utilizing the thoracic duct and the right lymphatic duct, all the lymph of the body returns to the blood (Fig. 11.3). There is thus a constant circulation of lymph from the capillaries into the tissue spaces and back again into the blood stream. The lymphocytes are a recirculating population; migrating from blood to spleen and back and from blood to lymph and back. The recirculation of lymphocytes increases the chances that the 'correct' ones will encounter specific antigens and it also ensures the body-wide distribution of memory cells.

The lymph vessels of the small intestine are of special importance because of the digested fat which is absorbed into them. The minute projections, called villi, each contains a small lymph vessel into which the fat, as chylomicra (microscopic fatty globules), is absorbed. These channels are called lacteals and their contents all ultimately pass to the cisterna chyli. The lymph reaching the thoracic duct from the intestines differs from the clear colorless lymph from other parts of the body in that its fat content makes it cloudy or gives it a milky appearance. This fluid draining from the small intestine is called chyle, the term cisterna chyli meaning 'the receiver of the chyle'.

Lymph Nodes

Situated in the course of the lymph vessels and generally occurring in groups are the small and oval or kidney-shaped lymph nodes (Fig. 11.4). These are highly organized structures richly populated with lymphocytes and phagocytes and capable of making a controlled response to antigenic stimulation.

The lymph nodes act as filters for the lymph, trapping particulate matter and microorganisms. The vessels bringing lymph to the node are called the afferent vessels; they enter the gland at points around its periphery and drain into its cortex or outer zone. After percolating through the substance of the node the lymph leaves via the efferent vessel; this emerges directly from the medulla, or inner zone, at the small concavity called the hilum. Lymph

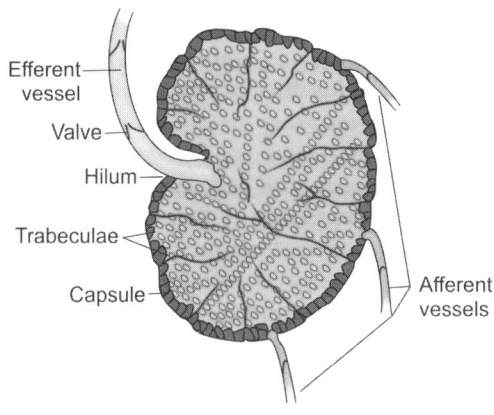

Fig. 11.4: Lymph node

may pass through several groups of glands before it is returned to the bloodstream. A lymph node is covered by its capsule which is largely composed of collagen fibers. From the capsule, trabeculae extend into the node and become continuous with the reticulum or meshwork of fine reticulin fibers, which forms the supporting framework for various cells, particularly lymphocytes and macrophages. Numerous lymph channels (sinuses) run through the lymph node, connecting the afferent vessels entering the cortex to the efferent vessel emerging at the hilum. The hilum is also the portal of entry and exit for the blood vessels of the lymph node.

There are many groups of lymph nodes in the body. Among the most important are those in the accompanying table (Table 11.1).

Lymph nodes may be enlarged as a result of viral infections such as German measles and glandular fever. The lymph nodes draining an area of suppuration are often swollen and tender, the axillary lymph nodes being thus affected in patients with a septic finger. The axillary nodes also receive lymph from the breast and may be enlarged as a result of metastatic spread of cancer from the breast. Similarly the hilar lymph nodes in the thorax may be enlarged due to secondary malignant involvement in cases of lung cancer. In Hodgkin's disease the lymph nodes are primary sites of the malignant process.

Filariasis, due to a tropical worm, or malignant disease may block all or most of the lymphatic pathways in a limb or in parts of the trunk, resulting in gross swelling of the limb (lymphedema, elephantiasis) or fluid in the peritoneal cavity (ascites) or pleural cavity (pleural effusion).

Lymphoid Tissue Elsewhere in the Body

Apart from the lymph nodes, there are a number of other collections of lymphoid tissue, namely:

Table 11.1: The major groups of lymph nodes

Nodes	Location	Region drained
Near the surface		
Cervical (superficial and deep)	Neck	Head and neck
Axillary	Axilla	Upper limbs and breasts
Inguinal	Groin	Lower limbs
Deep		
Iliac	Iliac fossa	Pelvic viscera, etc.
Lumbar	Close to lumbar vertebrae	Abdominal wall and viscera
Mesenteric	mesentery	Alimentary tract
Hepatic	Portal fissure of liver	Liver, gallbladder, etc.
Pre-aortic	Anterior to the abdominal Aorta	Alimentary tract and accessory organs
Thoracic (bronchopulmonary group)	Hilum of lung	Lungs

- Those situated in the walls of the alimentary and respiratory tracts and including the tonsils, nasopharyngeal tissues which when enlarged constitute adenoids, Peyer's patches scattered in the small intestine, and the appendix
- The spleen
- The thymus.

The Tonsils

The tonsils are two ovoid masses of lymphoid tissue embedded in the side walls of the oral part of the pharynx, between the anterior and posterior pillars of the faces. Their size varies but they tend to be relatively larger in children than in adults. The lower pole of each tonsil is continuous with lymphoid tissue situated in the base of the tongue. On the surface of the tonsil can be seen a dozen or more small openings which lead into deep narrow recesses called crypts.

The efferent lymph vessels of the tonsils (which have no afferent lymph vessels) drain into the upper deep cervical lymph nodes, especially the jugulodigastric group situated below the angle of the jaw. The blood supply of the tonsil is derived from branches of the external carotid artery, the tonsillar branch of the facial artery being the chief artery of supply. The nerves supplying the tonsil are the lesser palatine nerves, which are branches of the pterygopalatine ganglion, and the glossopharyngeal (ninth cranial nerve). As the latter nerve, through its tympanic branch, also supplies the mucous membrane lining the tympanic cavity, tonsillar pain due to inflammation or cancer may be referred to the ear.

The tonsils form part of a ring of lymphoid tissue guarding the entrance of the alimentary and respiratory tracts against bacterial invasion. Inflammation of the tonsils—tonsillitis—is common, particularly in young people. An abscess in the bed of the tonsil is called a quinsy.

The Spleen

The spleen is a dark purple-colored organ lying for the most part in the left hypochondriac region of the abdomen, between the fundus of the stomach and the diaphragm. Its long axis lies in the line of the tenth rib. It varies in size and weight during the lifetime of an individual but in an adult it is usually about 12 cm long, 8 cm broad and 3 or 4 cm thick. The normal spleen is not palpable and any spleen which can be palpated is therefore necessarily abnormally large due to disease of some kind, for example glandular fever, Hodgkin's disease or portal hypertension.

The spleen has diaphragmatic and visceral surfaces. The diaphragmatic surface is in contact with the under surface of the diaphragm, which separates it from the left lung. The visceral surface presents gastric, renal, pancreatic and colic impressions (Fig. 11.5). The gastric impression is in contact with the posterior wall of the stomach and presents, near its lower limit, a long fissure, termed the hilum, where the branches of the splenic artery enter the spleen. The major tributaries of the splenic vein emerge from the hilum and this vein eventually joins with the superior mesenteric vein to form the portal vein.

Structure

The spleen has an outer coat of peritoneum which is firmly adherent to the internal fibro-elastic coat or splenic capsule. From the capsule, trabecular pass into the spleen and branch to form a framework which is continuous with a fine reticulum. Closely associated with the reticulum are reticular cells, or fibroblasts, and macrophages. Two kinds of splenic pulp, red pulp and white pulp, occupy the interstices of the reticulum. The white pulp consists of periarteriolar sheaths of lymphatic tissue with enlargements, called splenic lymphatic follicles or Malpighian bodies, containing

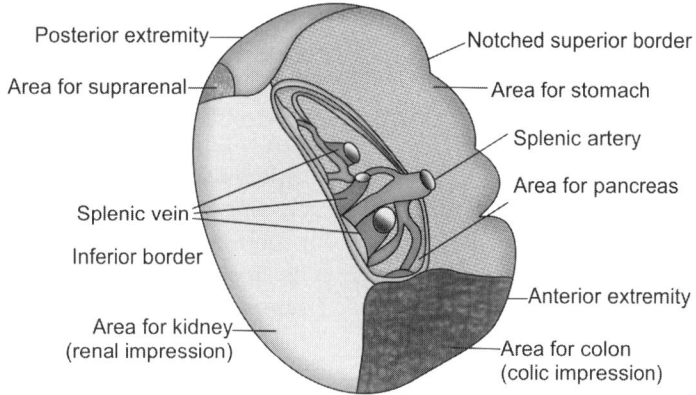

Fig. 11.5: The medial or visceral aspect of the spleen

rounded masses of lymphocytes. These follicles, which are centers of lymphocyte production, are visible to the naked eye as whitish dots against the dark red background of the red pulp on the freshly cut surface of the spleen. The red pulp consists of numerous venous sinusoids, containing blood, separated by a network of perivascular tissue which is referred to as the splenic cords. These so-called cords contain numerous macrophages and are the sites of intense phagocytic activity. They also contain numerous lymphocytes, many of which are derived from the white pulp.

Functions

The spleen is a lymphoid organ which is not essential to life and can safely be removed (splenectomy) but which has several functions.

- *Phagocytosis:* The phagocytes of the spleen, mostly macrophages, remove microorganisms and worn-out red cells, white cells and platelets from the blood. Iron is removed from the hemoglobin of the red cell debris and is conveyed to the bone marrow for re-use in red cell production. From the remaining pigment, the spleen forms bilirubin which, together with that formed in the liver, is secreted in the bile.

- *Immune response:* Just as the spleen shares with the other peripheral lymphoid organs the function of phagocytosis, so it joins with them in the immune response. B-lymphocytes are sited mainly in the follicles and T-lymphocytes are the main cells of the periarteriolar sheaths. These lymphocytes can migrate into other areas of the spleen. B-lymphocytes stimulated by particular antigens, are transformed into plasma cells which produce antibodies (immunoglobulins) which are released into the general circulation, so conferring humoral immunity against specific bacterial infections. Some of the T-lymphocytes cooperate with the B-cells and are known as helper T-cells. Other T-lymphocytes, which are cytotoxic and able to kill infected circulating cells, are called killer T-cells. Cellular immunity, based on T-lymphocytes, provides defense against infection by viruses, fungi and a few bacteria including the tubercle bacillus.

- *Hemopoiesis:* In the fetus, the spleen is an important hemopoietic organ and precursors of red cells, neutrophils and platelets are found in the red pulp. The white pulp of the mature spleen

contributes to the circulating pool of immunocompetent lymphocytes.
- *Red cell storage:* The spleen can act as a reservoir for red cells, which it discharges into the blood stream in an emergency, such as that created by anoxia. This function is probably of relatively minor importance in human beings.

The spleen is a soft organ. A normal spleen may be ruptured by severe external trauma and an enlarged spleen (as in glandular fever) may occasionally be ruptured by even trivial trauma. Rupture of the spleen leads to severe internal hemorrhage and shock. Diagnosis of the condition may be difficult but is essential, if the patient's life is to be saved, because only splenectomy will stop the bleeding.

The Thymus

The thymus is situated superiorly in the anterior mediastinum of the thorax. It lies in front of the heart and pericardium and the aortic arch and its branches and on the front and sides of the trachea. It is a central organ of the lymphoid system. It controls lymphocyte production in both the peripheral and the central lymphoid organs, including the thymus itself, and is essential for the maturation of lymphocytes into the cells responsible for cellular immunity, T-lymphocytes.

The thymus is relatively large at birth and continues to increase in size until puberty, where after it usually gradually diminishes as a result of atrophic changes.

Thymectomy is beneficial in some cases of myasthenia gravis, a rare chronic disease characterized by abnormal fatiguability and weakness of certain muscles; this is due to an autoimmune process affecting the receptor proteins of the neuromuscular junctions, antibodies being formed against these receptors.

CHAPTER 12

The Digestive System

Mouth extends from the lips and cheek to the oropharynx (palatoglossal arch). Palate forms roof of mouth and separates oral cavity from nasal cavity. Floor of mouth is formed by mylohyoid muscle and is occupied by tongue. Lateral wall of mouth is formed by cheeks. Three pairs of major salivary gland and numerous minor salivary glands open into mouth.

Tongue: The tongue is a muscular organ of deglutition. It is partly oral and partly pharyngeal in position and attached to hyoid bone, mandible, styloid process, soft palate, pharyngeal wall by its muscles. Mucosa is pink and moist and attached to underlying muscle. It has an apex, root, curved dorsal surface and a ventral surface. Dorsal surface is covered with papilla. Root of tongue is attached to hyoid bone and mandible. The dorsum of tongue is convex and it is divided into an anterior or pre-sulcal part and a posterior or post-sulcal part by a V-shaped sulcus terminalis. Both the presulcal and postsulcal part differ in their mucosal lining, innervations and development.

Oral (presulcal) part: Presulcal part is located in floor of oral cavity. It has apex, lateral margin and dorsum. On each side there are 4–5 foliate papillae. The dorsal surface is covered by filiform, fungiform and circumvalate papilla. The mucosa on the inferior surface is smooth and purplish and continuous with mucosa of floor. The mucosa is connected to floor of oral cavity by frenulum. Deep lingual veins lie lateral to frenulum.

Pharyngeal (post-sulcal) part: It lies posterior to palatoglossal arch. The mucosa is reflected to epiglottis by a median and two lateral glossoepiglottic fold. The depression between the two folds is called vallecula. Pharyngeal part of tongue is devoid of papilla. It has small projections on its surface which are lymphatic nodules termed lingual tonsils.

Muscles of tongue: There are extrinsic and intrinsic muscles for the tongue. The extrinsic muscles are genioglossus, hyoglossus, styloglossus, palatoglossus. Intrinsic muscles are superior longitudinal, inferior longitudinal, transverse and vertical muscles.

Hyoglossus: It is a thin quadrilateral muscle. It passes vertically upwards from the hyoid bone to the side of the tongue. The hypoglossal nerve and lingual nerve lie on its lateral surface. The lingual artery lies on its medial surface.

Genioglossus: The genioglossus originates from genial tubercle in mandible and extends from tip to root of tongue. This muscle prevents tongue from falling back and obstructing respiration. So it is called safety muscle of tongue. Other muscles of tongue are styloglossus and palatoglossus.

Innervation of tongue: All muscles of tongue are innervated by hypoglossal nerve except palatoglossus which is innervated by cranial accessory nerve. Proprioceptive sensations of tongue may be via lingual, glossopharyngeal and hypoglossal nerve. Sensory innervations of the tongue reflects its embryological development. Anterior

2/3 of tongue is derived from first arch and posterior 1/3 by third arch. Nerve of first arch is mandibular nerve and nerve of third arch is glossopharyngeal nerve. General sensation of anterior 2/3 of tongue is by lingual nerve which is the nerve of first arch and special sensation by chorda tympani which is the trematic branch of first arch. General and special sensations from posterior 1/3 of tongue is by glossopharyngeal nerve.

Vascular supply: It is by dorsal lingual artery, deep lingual artery, and lingual artery.

■ SALIVARY GLANDS

Parotid Gland

It is the largest salivary gland. Each gland is irregular and lobulated mass lying below external acoustic meatus. The gland is pyramidal in shape and has a superior surface (base), superficial surface, anteromedial surface and postero-medial surface. Apex is directed downwards. Concave superior surface is related to external acoustic meatus.

Superficial surface: It is covered by skin, superficial fascia and superficial parotid lymph nodes. It extends from zygomatic arch to mandibular angle.

Anteromedial surface: This surface is grooved by mandibular ramus, related to masseter, medial pterygoid muscle.

Posteromedial surface: This surface is related to mastoid process and muscles attached to it, styloid process and muscles attached to it, and transverse process of atlas. Branches of facial nerve emerge from its anterior margin. Structures within the substance of parotid gland- external carotid artery, retro-mandibular vein, facial nerve.

Parotid capsule: It is an unyielding capsule of deep cervical fascia.

Parotid duct: It is 5 cm long, traverses buccal fat pad, buccopharyngeal fascia and buccinator muscle and opens in mouth opposite upper 2nd molar tooth.

Vascular supply: External carotid artery and its branches.

Submandibular Salivary Gland

Submandibular salivary gland is irregular in shape about the size of a walnut. It consists of a superficial and deep part. It is a seromucous gland.

Superficial part: Situated in digastric triangle (triangle formed by the two bellies of digastrics muscle and lower border of mandible. This part has inferior, lateral and medial surfaces.

Inferior surface is covered by skin and deep fascia.

Lateral surface is related to submandibular fossa situated on medial side of body of mandible. Medial surface is related to muscles like mylohyoid and hyoglossus muscles, hypoglossal nerve and lingual nerve.

Secretomotor supply: It is by submandibular ganglia.

Submandibular duct: It is 5 cm long. It has thinner wall than parotid duct. It opens in the floor of mouth by the side of frenulum of tongue.

■ STOMACH

It is the widest part of alimentary tract and lies between esophagus and duodenum. In newborn the capacity of stomach is 30 mL, at puberty 1000 mL, and in adults 1500 mL.

Parts of stomach: For descriptive purposes, stomach is divided into fundus, body, pyloric antrum and pylorus (Fig. 12.1). The fundus is dome-shaped and lies on the left side of cardiac opening. Body of stomach extends from fundus to pylorus. Pylorus forms pyloric antrum, pyloric canal and pyloric orifice.

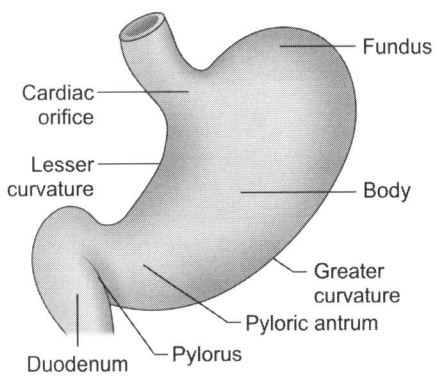

Fig. 12.1: Diagram illustrating parts of the stomach

Gastric Curvatures

Lesser curvature: Extends between cardiac orifice and pyloric orifice and forms the medial border of stomach. The lesser omentum is attached to lesser curvature of stomach and contains right and left gastric vessels.

Greater curvature: It is four to five times longer than lesser curvature. It starts from lateral border of cardiac orifice and arches towards left. It ends at the pylorus. Greater curvature gives attachment to greater omentum and contains the gastroepiploic vessels.

Gastric Surfaces

Antero-superior surface: Lateral part of anterior surface is in contact with diaphragm. Towards the right side of anterior surface is liver. The entire anterior surface is covered with peritoneum.

Postero-inferior surface: Structures related to this surface include diaphragm, left kidney, the pancreas, transverse mesocolon and left suprarenal gland. All these structures form stomach bed. Lying between these structures and stomach is lesser sac. Posterior surface of stomach is also covered by peritoneum.

Gastric Orifices

Cardiac orifice and gastroesophageal junction: The opening of esophagus into stomach is the cardiac orifice. It is situated to the left of midline behind 7th costal cartilage at level of T-11 vertebra. It is located 10 cm deep to anterior abdominal wall and 40 cm from incisor teeth. Right side of cardiac orifice is continuous with lesser curvature and left side is continuous with greater curvature.

Barrett's esophagus: Squamous epithelial lining of lower part of esophagus is replaced by simple columnar epithelium of stomach resulting in reflux of contents of stomach to esophagus.

Pyloric orifice: It is the opening from stomach to duodenum and typically lies 1–2 cm to the right of midline at the level of L-1 vertebra. The pyloric sphincter is a muscular ring, formed from thick circular smooth muscle. The sphincter can be felt on the abdominal wall of infants as a thickening. The prepyloric vein crosses its surface.

Gastric form and internal appearances: Empty stomach is J-shaped. Fundus of stomach contains gas and pylorus lies at level of L-1 vertebra.

Internal appearance (Fig. 12.2): Mucosa of the fundus has folds called rugae. Body of the stomach has more pronounced mucosal folds. These are long mucosal folds extending from fundus to pyloric antrum. They are near lesser curvature and called magenstrasse.

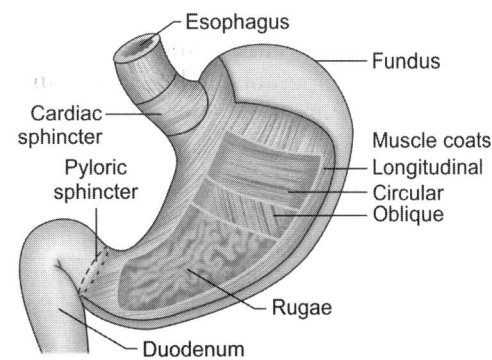

Fig. 12.2: Structure of the stomach

Gastrostomy: It is establishing communication between lumen of stomach and surface of skin.

Vascular supply: Arterial supply of stomach comes from celiac axis. The left gastric artery arises from celiac axis and right gastric artery arises from hepatic artery of celiac trunk. Splenic artery gives origin to short gastric arteries and left gastroepiploic artery. Gastroduodenal artery gives rise to right gastroepiploic artery.

Veins: Veins draining stomach ultimately drain to portal vein.

Nerve supply: Parasympathetic supply is from anterior and posterior branches of vagus nerve.

Small intestine: Small intestine consists of duodenum, jejunum and ileum. It extends from pyloric canal to ileocecal valve. Length of small intestine is 5 m. Duodenum extends up to duodenojejunal junction and remaining small intestine is called small bowel. The proximal 2/5th is jejunum and the distal 3/5th is ileum. The distal 30 cm of ileum is called terminal ileum. Duodenum lies mostly in the upper retroperitoneum. Jejunum and ileum occupy central and lower parts of abdominal cavity and is attached to the posterior abdominal wall by mesentery.

■ DUODENUM

It is 20–25 cm long. It is the smallest and widest part of small intestine. It is only partly covered by peritoneum. The proximal 2.5 cm is intraperitoneal and the rest of it is retro-peritoneal. The duodenum is C-shaped extending between L-1 and L-3 vertebra. Head and uncinate process of pancreas lies in the concavity of duodenum.

Duodenum has four parts:

First (superior) part: It is the most mobile part and about 5 cm long. It is covered by peritoneum. The first 2–3 cm is called duodenal cap and it forms a triangular gas shadow in plain X-ray. The first part of duodenum lies anterior to the gastroduodenal artery and portal vein. Penetrating duodenal ulcer can erode the artery and cause torrential bleeding. At the junction of first and second part is neck of gallbladder which imparts a greenish color to that area.

Second (descending) part: Second part of duodenum is 8–10 cm long and lies on the right side of vertebral column and extends up to L-3 vertebra. It is crossed by transverse colon and lies below right lobe of liver and gallbladder. It lies anterior to inferior vena cava and head of pancreas lies medial to it. Common bile duct and pancreatic duct enter into its medial wall.

Third (horizontal) part: It is approximately 10 cm long. It lies at the level of L-3 vertebra. It lies anterior to right ureter, inferior venacava, right gonadal vessels, abdominal aorta.

Fourth part: It is 2.5 cm long. It lies on the left side of abdominal aorta. It is anterior to left ureter, left kidney, left renal vessels, left gonadal vessels.

Vascular supply: Superior and inferior pancreaticoduodenal arteries supply the duodenum.

■ JEJUNUM

It has an external diameter of 4 cm and an internal diameter of 2.5 cm. It has thicker wall than ileum and an extensive arterial supply that makes it more red in color. Mucosal folds called plica circularis are numerous in small intestine. Lymphoid aggregates are absent in jejunum.

Jejunal feeding: In diseased conditions where oral nutrition becomes difficult, feeding through jejunum is possible by bringing the jejunum into contact with anterior abdominal wall called surgical jejunostomy.

■ ILEUM

Ileum has thinner wall than jejunum. Mucosa of terminal part of ileum is almost flat, with no plica circulars. Lymphoid aggregates in ileum are called payers patches. Ileum ends by opening into ileo-cecal valve.

Meckel's diverticulum: It is ileal diverticulum seen in 3% people. It is present in the anti-mesenteric border of ileum, 50–100 cm from ileo-cecal valve. It is almost 5 cm in length and lumen is similar to ileum. Inflammation mimics appendicitis near umbilical region.

Vascular supply: Branches from superior mesenteric artery supply jejunum and ileum.

Superior mesenteric artery: It originates from aorta 1 cm below celiac trunk at the level of L-1 vertebra. Its branches are—middle colic, right colic, ileocolic, jejunal and ileal branches. Jejunal and ileal branches form arcades in the mesentery of small intestine. Jejunal branches are 5–10 in number whereas ileal branches are more numerous.

Veins: Superior mesenteric veins drains small intestine, cecum, ascending colon and transverse colon. Superior mesenteric vein joins with splenic vein to form portal vein behind neck of pancreas.

CECUM

Cecum is a large blind pouch lying in right iliac fossa. It is continuous with ileum and ascending colon. The vermiform appendix arises from its medial side. Length of cecum is 6 cm and breadth is 7.5 cm. Breadth is more than length. Anterior abdominal wall is the anterior relation. Cecum is intraperitoneal (covered by peritonum). Cecum is broader than longer. Infantile cecum, length is more than breadth. Cecum can store large volumes of semi-liquid chyme and so it is more vulnerable to intracolonic pressure and perforation.

Vermiform appendix: Appendix is a narrow worm like structure arising from cecal wall. Most common position of appendix is behind cecum (retrocecal). Other positions are pelvic, subcecal, preileal, postileal. Lumen of appendix opens into cecum which is guarded by a valve sometimes.

Acute appendicitis: Occurs following obstruction of lumen of appendix. Symptoms include severe pain in right iliac fossa and around umbilicus.

The Ascending Colon

This passes upwards from the cecum through the right lumbar region and is held in position on the posterior abdominal wall by peritoneum. When it reaches the under surface of the liver it turns sharply to the left at the right or **hepatic flexure** to become the transverse colon.

The Transverse Colon

This passes across the abdominal cavity as a loop that may hang well below the umbilicus. It rises as it reaches its left extremity and comes in contact with the spleen, where it turns sharply downwards at the left or **splenic flexure** to continue as the descending colon. The transverse colon lies in a fold of peritoneum which extends downwards from the greater curvature of the stomach called the **greater omentum**. It is therefore freely movable within: the abdominal cavity.

The Descending Colon

This passes downwards in the left lumbar region. It is anchored to the posterior abdominal wall by peritoneum, and like the ascending colon is not movable.

The Pelvic or Sigmoid Colon (Fig. 12.3)

This is the continuation of the descending colon, and it makes an S-shaped curve, the **sigmoid flexure**, to enter the pelvic cavity to become the rectum. It is attached to the left side of the pelvis by a fold of peritoneum called the sigmoid mesacolon.

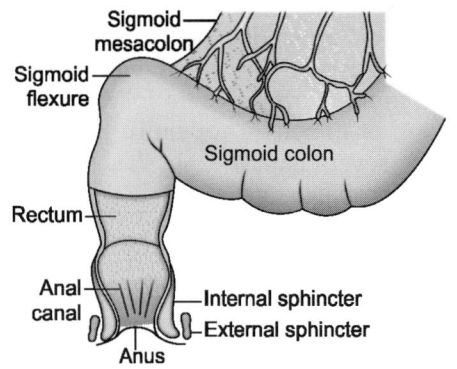

Fig. 12.3: Diagram of sigmoid colon, rectum and anus

The Rectum and Anal Canal

The rectum lies in the pelvic cavity and is situated in the concave hollow formed by the anterior surface of the sacrum. It is about 13 cm (5 in) long and narrows to form the anal canal. This is about 3 cm (1.2 in) length and its lower half is lined with stratified squamous epithelium which is continuous with the mucous membrane lining the rest of the anal canal and the rectum and with the skin where the anus opens to the exterior of the body.

Structure of the Large Intestine

The large intestine, like the small intestine, has four coats; peritoneal or serous, muscular, submucous and mucous.

The characteristic feature, however, is that the longitudinal muscles do not form a continuous layer over the whole gut but are arranged in three separate longitudinal bands, the **taenia coli**. These bands are somewhat shorter than the length of the large intestine, which accounts for its sacculated appearance.

When the longitudinal fibres reach the rectum they spread out over the whole surface. In the upper half of the anal canal the circular smooth muscle fibres are thickened to form the **internal anal sphincter**. The lower half is composed of striated muscles fibers, which form the **external anal sphincter**.

The mucous membrane lining contains no villi and is not thrown into folds like that of the small intestine. The large intestine, like the esophagus, does not take any part in digestion but the whole of its mucosa contains mucous glands that secrete large quantities of mucus to protect it from the effects of the digestive enzymes of the small intestine, and to provide lubrication for the passage of feces.

Blood Supply

The superior mesenteric artery supplies the cecum, the appendix, the ascending colon and most of the transverse colon, whilst the inferior mesenteric artery supplies part of the transverse colon, the descending colon, the sigmoid colon and the upper part of the rectum.

The blood supply of the lower rectum and the anus is from branches of the inferior mesenteric, internal iliac and pudendal arteries. The veins of the anus form dilated vessels within the anal ring called the hemorrhoidal plexus, and this blood is drained into the inferior mesenteric, pudendal and internal iliac veins. Back pressure along the venous system causes enlargement of the veins in the hemorrhoidal plexus which results in the formation of hemorrhoids (piles).

Nerve Supply

This is from the autonomic nervous system. The internal anal sphincter is controlled by the parasympathetic and sympathetic nerve fibers, but the external sphincter receives its nerve supply from the spinal nerves of the sacrum and is under voluntary control.

Functions of the Large Intestine

The functions of the large intestine are the absorption of water and electrolytes from the chyme which enters it from the small intestine, and the storage of fecal material until it is expelled as feces.

By the time the contents of the small intestine reach the cecum the digestive process is completed and most of the products of digestion have been absorbed. However the residue is still in a liquid state, amounting to approximately 800 ml per day. Most of the water and electrolytes are reabsorbed by the first half of the large intestine, leaving only a fecal residue of between 100 and 200 ml each day.

The large intestine also contains a multitude of bacteria living in symbiosis. These synthesize vitamins B and K, which are absorbed into the blood by the mucosa. As long as these bacteria remain within the colon they are harmless to the body, but if they reach other organs they become pathogenic (i.e. disease producing). Destruction of the bacteria by the administration of antibiotic drugs can occasionally lead to vitamin K deficiency within a few days.

The walls of the large intestine are able to excrete an excess of calcium, iron and drugs of the heavy metal type, such as bismuth, into the feces. Iron given by mouth makes the feces black in color.

The Feces

The feces are normally a semi-solid, paste-like mass colored brown by stercobilin, a pigment derived from the bilirubin and biliverdin of the bile. Water, even after the absorption which takes place in the colon, still forms 65 to 70 per cent of the total bulk of the feces. The remainder consists mainly of undecomposed cellulose, some fatty acids, protein residue, bacteria and epithelial cells. The surface of the feces is lubricated by the mucin secreted by the large intestine.

If the feces are passed too rapidly through the intestine insufficient time will be allowed for the absorption of water, and this results in the watery character of the stool in some cases of diarrhea.

Movements of the Large Intestine

Peristaltic movements of the large intestine are generally very sluggish, and consist of mixing movements similar to the segmentation movements of the small intestine, or of mass peristalsis which transfers the fecal material into the descending colon and the pelvic colon. These latter movements occur two or three times a day.

Defecation is the expulsion of feces from the anal canal. The rectum is usually empty until mass peristaltic movements propel fecal matter from the pelvic colon into the rectum. The entry of feces into the rectum distends the walls of the cavity and causes nervous impulses to pass to the lower part of the spinal cord. Reflex signals are transmitted through the sacral parasympathetic nerves causing contraction of the descending colon, sigmoid flexure and rectum, and relaxation of the internal anal sphincter. At the same time impulses are sent to the brain, where they arouse the conscious sensation of the desire to defecate. If the time is appropriate the external sphincter is relaxed by conscious control and defecation takes place.

However, since the external sphincter is under voluntary control it can be tightened and the call to defecate ignored. The rectum accomodates itself to its contents by relaxation of its muscular walls, nerve impulses cease and the desire passes off. The arrival of more fecal material in the rectum causes further distension and initiates the defecation reflex again.

Repeated failure to respond to the defecation reflex is a common cause of constipation. The retention of feces in the rectum allows continued absorption of water and results in a hardened or constipated stool.

Defecation in the infant is by reflex action and cannot be controlled until the nervous system is fully developed.

During defecation the following actions occur:
- The sphincter muscles of the anus relax
- The muscular walls of the rectum contract
- The muscles of the pelvic floor contract
- Intra-abdominal pressure is raised by holding the breath and contracting the diaphragm, and by contracting the muscles of the abdominal wall.

The injection of an enema into the rectum has the effect of rapidly distending its walls and so initiating the defecation reflex. It also helps to softer and break up hard masses of feces.

The Peritoneum

The peritoneum (Fig. 12.4) is a serious membrane, and like the other important serous membranes of the body, the pleura and the pericardium, consists of two separate layers. The **parietal layer** lines the walls of the abdominal cavity and the **visceral layer** partly or completely covers the organs. The membrane secretes a small amount of serous fluid to lubricate the surface of the viscera so that they are free to move without friction within the abdomen.

The detailed arrangement of the peritoneum and its various folds is very complicated, but a general conception can be obtained in the following way. Imagine the peritoneum to be a closed bag having front and back surfaces. Then consider the effect if an organ were pushed into the middle of the back surface in such a way that this surface completely surrounded the organ. It will then be understood that one organ may be completely covered by peritoneum while structures like the pancreas, lying on the posterior abdominal wall will be covered by the membrane only on their anterior surfaces.

Thus the organs completely surrounded by peritoneum will be suspended from the posterior abdominal wall by a double-fold of the membrane. It is in this way that a **mesentery**, or fold of peritoneum, by which the intestine is attached to the posterior abdominal wall is formed. It is between the two layers of this fold that the blood vessels reach the organs, for the abdominal aorta and its branches lie outside the peritoneal cavity.

The stomach, intestines (except for the duodenum and rectum), the liver and spleen are almost completely surrounded by peritoneum, which therefore forms an outer coat for these structures. The duodenum, rectum and pancreas are covered only on their anterior surfaces.

Peritoneal Ligaments

The liver, uterus and other organs are partly maintained in position by means of double folds of peritoneum which form suspensory ligaments.

The Omenta

These are folds of peritoneum connected to the stomach. The **great omentum** hangs from the lower border of the stomach like

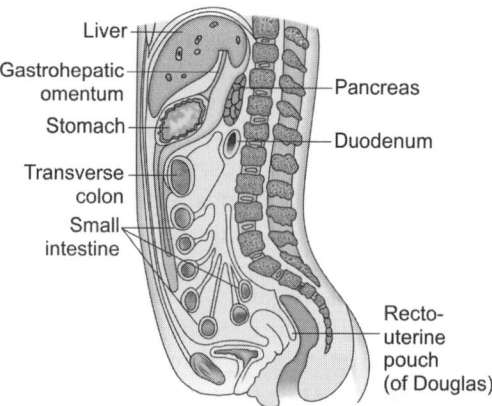

Fig. 12.4: Sagittal section of the abdomen showing disposition of the peritoneum. (The arrow passes through the foramen of Winslow into the lesser sac)

an apron in front of the small intestines; in its posterior portion lies the transverse colon. The **lesser omentum** stretches from the lower border of the liver to the lesser curvature of the stomach.

The Mesentery

This is the fold of peritoneum which encloses the small intestine and anchors it to the posterior abdominal wall. The attachment to the abdominal wall is relatively short, whereas the intestinal part is many feet long, so that the mesentery can be described as a fan-shaped structure.

The Pelvic Peritoneum

The peritoneum in the pelvis is continuous with that of the rest of the abdominal cavity. It covers the front aspect of the rectum. In the male it passes forwards over the posterior and upper surfaces of the bladder to become continuous with that on the anterior abdominal wall. In the female it passes from the rectum over the posterior and anterior surfaces of the uterus before reaching the bladder. The sac between the rectum and the uterus in the female is called the **rectouterine pouch (of Douglas)**. On either side, in the female, the membrane covers the uterine (**Fallopian**) tubes. These tubes have an opening into the peritoneal cavity where their mucous membrane is directly continuous with the peritoneum. It is in this way that the ova are able to pass from the ovaries, which lie within the peritoneal cavity, into the uterus. In the male the peritoneum is a completely closed sac.

Functions of the Peritoneum

- It is a serious membrane which enables the abdominal contents to glide over each other without friction.
- It forms a partial or complete covering for the abdominal organs.
- It forms ligaments and mesenteries which help to keep the organs in position.
- The omenta and mesentery contain a considerable amount of fat, and act as important fat stores for the body.
- The omentum can move about inside the cavity and in the event of inflammation tends to wrap itself round the affected part of the alimentary tract and prevent the infection from spreading to the rest of the peritoneum. It is very common in cases of acute appendicitis to find the appendix totally surrounded by the omentum. On account of its protective mobility it has been called the 'abdominal policeman'. It is shorter and less well-developed in infancy and childhood, so that appendicitis in these cases may be very serious.
- It has the power to absorb fluids in large quantities.

Peritoneal Dialysis

The peritoneum is a membrane through which some electrolytes and simple substances can be exchanged with others in the blood. For example, if a suitable glucose-electrolyte solution is introduced into the peritoneal cavity its strength will equalize with the blood, i.e. urea will pass from the blood into the dialysis fluid which lacks this substance. The fluid is then removed from the peritoneal cavity, the blood urea having been reduced. The procedure is therefore used in the treatment of some cases of renal failure (uremia).

■ THE ACCESSORY ORGANS OF DIGESTION

The liver, biliary system and pancreas form the accessory organs of digestion.

The Liver

The liver is the largest organ in the body; it weighs between 1.0 and 2.5 kg (2.2 and 5.5 lb) and is heavier in the male than the female. It is a wedge-shaped organ lying immediately below the diaphragm in the right hypochondrium and epigastrium.

The liver is described as having right and left lobes, superior and inferior, anterior and posterior surfaces.

The Lobes

The right lobe is much larger than the left; the division between them is marked by the falciform ligament on the anterior surface, and by the ligamenta teres and venosum on the inferior and posterior surfaces. The under surface of the right lobe is further subdivided into the quadrate and caudate lobes.

The Surfaces of the Liver

The **superior surface** is in contact with the under surface of the diaphragm; the potential spaces between the liver and the diaphragm are called the subphrenic spaces (Fig. 12.5).

The **inferior surface** is related to other abdominal viscera, including the kidney and right (hepatic) flexure of the colon on the right and the fundus of the stomach on the left (Fig. 12.6).

The **anterior surface** is separated from the right lower ribs and costal cartilages by the margin of the diaphragm and, in the midline is related to the anterior abdominal wall.

The **posterior surface** crosses the vertebral column in the midline and is also related to the aorta, inferior vena cava and lower end of the oesophagus.

In the center of the inferior surface, lying between the quadrate and caudate lobes, is the hilum or **porta hepatis** (the door of the liver). All the vessels and nerves entering and leaving the liver, with the exception of the hepatic vein, pass through the porta hepatis.

Attached to the under surface of the right lobe is the gallbladder.

Blood Supply (Flowchart 12.1)

The liver receives blood from two sources and is an extremely vascular organ (approximately one-fifth of the liver volume is blood).

The hepatic artery, which is a branch of the celiac axis from the abdominal aorta, conveys oxygenated blood to the liver cells.

The portal vein conveys venous blood, poor in oxygen but rich in nutrients, from the stomach and intestines.

Venous drainage from the liver is by the hepatic veins which empty into the inferior vena cava.

Due to its great vascularity, lacerations of the liver are very dangerous and result in profuse hemorrage.

Structure of the Liver (Fig. 12.7)

The liver is composed of a large number of hexagonal lobules, each about 1 mm in diameter a small branch of the hepatic vein extends through the center of each lobule. The liver cells are arranged in plates or sheets, one cell thick, around the central vein. The plates of cells form an irregular anastomosing system throughout the liver; between the plates of cells lie spaces which contain the sinusoids. The sinusoids are blood vessels with incomplete walls, and are irregular in shape and wider than blood capillaries. They are lined by thin endothelium and Kupffer cells, which are phagocytes and remove cellular debris and bacteria from the blood.

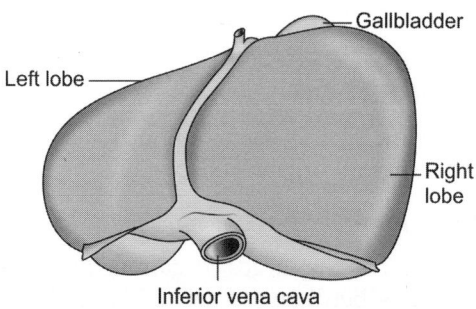

Fig. 12.5: The liver-superior surface

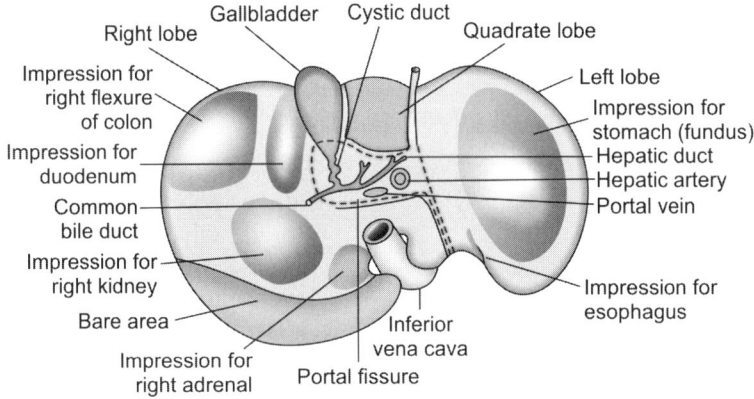

Fig. 12.6: The inferior surface of the liver

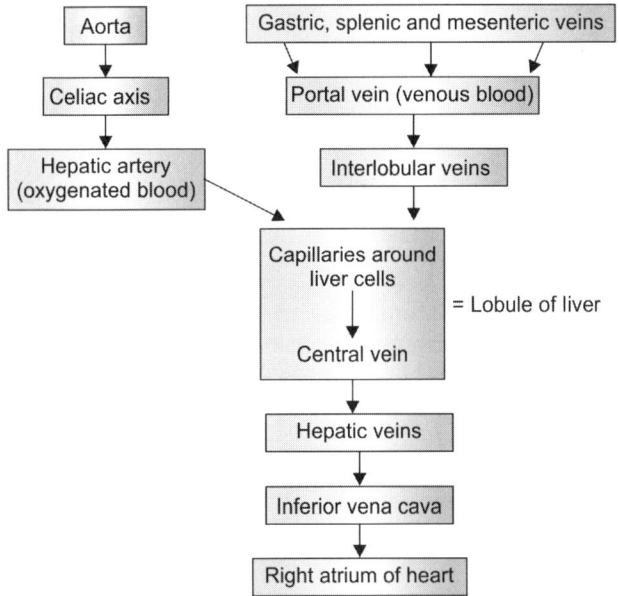

Flowchart 12.1: The blood supply of the liver

Arranged around the periphery of each lobule are branches of the hepatic artery, the portal vein and the hepatic bile ducts. The blood vessels form small branches which pass between the lobules and enter the sinusoids (Fig. 12.8). Thus the sinusoids receive oxygenated blood from the hepatic artery and blood rich in nutrients from the portal vein. The sinusoids drain into the central vein which joins the veins from adjacent lobules to form interlobular veins, these in turn unite to form the hepatic veins, which drain the blood from the liver into the inferior vena cava.

The hepatic cells are polyhedral (have many sides) and perform many metabolic activities. Each cell has two surfaces that face sinusoids, and several surfaces in contact with other cells. As the blood passes through the sinusoids, the liver cells remove

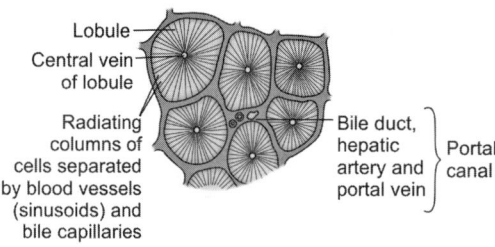

Fig. 12.7: Liver lobules and radial arrangement of the cells

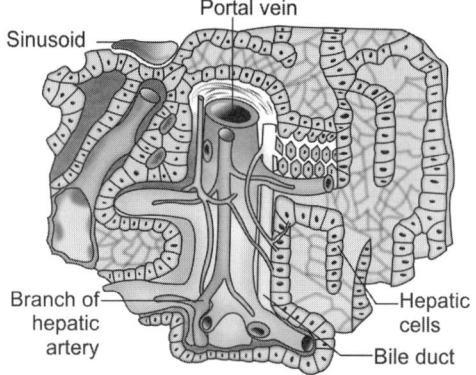

Fig. 12.8: Liver lobule, Illustrating plates of liver cells and sinusoids

absorbed nutrients from the circulation. Bile is secreted by the liver cells and drains into minute **bile canaliculi** which lie between the walls of the cells. The bile canaliculi join to form **intralobular ductules**, which unite to become the right and left **hepatic ducts**.

The liver has a thin fibrous capsule (Glisson's capsule), almost completely covered by peritoneum.

Functions of the Liver

The liver performs a variety of different functions, and in addition to the secretion of bile, plays a vital role in body metabolism.

- *Secretion of bile:* The secretion of bile is an exocrine function. All the liver cells continually form a small amount of bile, which is secreted into the bile canaliculi and passes via the hepatic ducts to the gallbladder for storage until required to assist the digestive processes.

- *Storage of glycogen:* Carbohydrate taken in the food is broken down by the digestive juices into the monosaccharide, glucose, and in this form is absorbed into the tributaries of the portal vein and conveyed to the liver. Here it is converted into a polysaccharide, glycogen, and stored. Glycogen is reconverted into glucose whenever the blood glucose level begins to fall too low.

  The liver is also capable of converting amino acids and glycerol to glucose (the process of gluconeogenesis), should the need arise (p. 222).

- *Metabolism of fats:* Fats are split to fatty acids and glycerol by the lipase of the pancreatic juice in the presence of bile salts, and are absorbed in this form. In the villi of the small intestine these substances are recombined into neutral fats and carried by the thoracic duct to the blood which conveys them to the fat depots of the body. The liver metabolizes fats, whether these reach it from the intestine, or are mobilized from the fat stores, to a form in which it can be used by the tissues of the body. The liver also converts excess carbohydrate and amino acids into fat for storage.

- *Deamination of amino acids:* The end-products of protein digestion are amino acids which are absorbed into the portal circulation through the villi of the small intestine. Many of the amino acids pass through the liver and are used by the tissues for growth, and repair of tissues. Any remaining amino acids are oxidized to provide energy, or converted to carbohydrates and fats. However before they can be used in this way they must be deaminated.

  Deamination is the removal of the nitrogen containing portion of the amino acids and its conversion to ammonia, which in turn combines with carbon dioxide to form urea. The urea is excreted in the urine by the kidneys.

- *Production of the plasma proteins:* The liver forms 90–95% of the plasma proteins, albumin, globulin and fibrinogen. The remaining 5–10% are gamma globulins formed by the plasma cells of the lymphoid tissue.
- *Storage of vitamins:* Large quantities of vitamins A, D and B_{12} are stored in the liver. Sufficient amounts of vitamin A can be stored to prevent deficiency for up to two years, whilst vitamins D and B_{12} can be stored to prevent deficiency for up to four months. The liver is also capable of synthesizing vitamin A from carotene, found in tomatoes, carrots, and other vegetables.
- *Storage of iron:* The liver stores iron in the form of a protein compound called ferritin. The iron is derived from the hemoglobin of worn-out red blood cells which have been destroyed in the spleen, and from iron absorbed by the small intestine. This reserve of iron is re-used for the formation of hemoglobin.
- *Production of clotting factors:* The liver plays an important role in blood coagulation by forming many of the substances involved in the clotting process. These include fibrinogen, prothrombin and factor VII. Vitamin K is needed for the formation of pro-thrombin and factors VII, IX, and X.
- *Production of heat:* The metabolic functions of the liver involve the expenditure of large amounts of energy, which is accompanied by the production of heat. This excess heat is distributed to the body by the blood stream and helps to maintain normal body temperature.
- *Detoxification:* The liver is able to destroy or modify toxic substances in the body. Many drugs are chemically reduced to simpler non-toxic compounds for excretion or are totally destroyed. Several hormones, including thyroxine, estrogen and aldosterone, are either chemically altered or excreted by the liver.

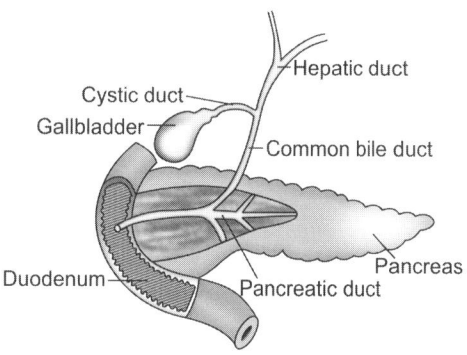

Fig. 12.9: Extrahepatic biliary tract

The Biliary Tract (Fig. 12.9)

The biliary tract is the excretory apparatus of the liver and consists of:
- The common hepatic duct
- The gall-bladder
- The cystic duct
- The common bile duct.

The common **hepatic duct** is formed by the junction of the right and left hepatic ducts which drain bile from the right and left lobes of the liver. It runs downwards from the portal hepatic for about 3 cm, where it is joined at an acute angle by the **cystic duct** from the gallbladder and continues downwards closely related to the hepatic artery and the portal vein as the **common bile duct**. This passes behind the first part of the duodenum and then is buried in the head of the pancreas. It enters the duodenum at a small papilla called the ampulla of Vater, where it is joined by the pancreatic duct.

The Gallbladder (Fig. 12.10)

This is a pear-shaped sac, with a capacity of approximately 60 ml, attached to the under surface of the right lobe of the liver. The rounded end of the sac, the fundus, projects from beneath the inferior border of the liver.

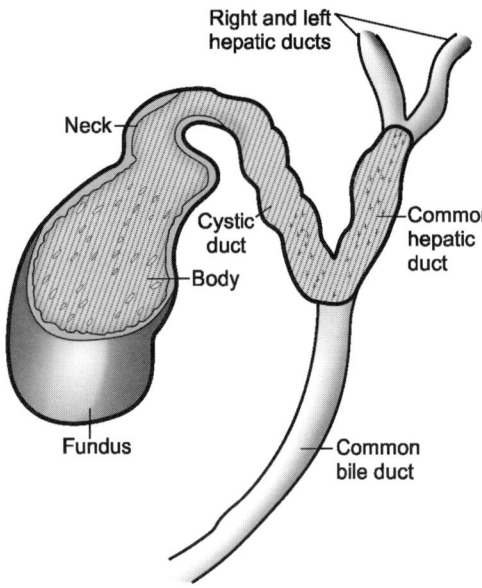

Fig. 12.10: Structure of gallbladder

Structure of the Gallbladder

The gallbladder consists of three coats:
1. An outer peritoneal coat continuous with the peritoneum covering the liver, which binds the gallbladder in position on the under surface of the liver.
2. A muscular coat, which contracts to enable the gallbladder to empty its contents into the common bile duct.
3. An inner coat of mucous membrane of columnar epithelial cells which secrete mucus. The mucous membrane is highly vascular and is thrown into rugae.

The neck of the gallbladder is continuous with the cystic duct. The mucous membrane lining the neck and cystic duct projects into the lumen in oblique folds which form a spiral valve.

Functions of the Gallbladder

The gallbladder acts as a reservoir for the storage of bile, which after leaving the liver by the hepatic duct, passes up the cystic duct to the gallbladder. The liver secretes between 600 and 1000 ml of bile per day, but the mucosal lining of the gallbladder reabsorbs the fluid and electrolytes, thus concentrating the other bile constituents.

When food enters the duodenum, especially fat containing food, the hormone **cholecystokinin** is secreted by the duodenal walls and passes in true blood to the gallbladder, where it causes the muscular walls to contract and expel the bile. At the same time, duodenal peristalsis inhibits the sphincter of Oddi and causes it to relax and allow the bile to enter the duodenum.

Bile

Bile is the external secretion of the liver, and is produced in a dilute form, which is then concentrated by the gallbladder to a viscid, greenish fluid. It is composed of:
- Water
- Bile salts (sodium glycocholate and sodium taurocholate)
- Bile pigment (bilirubin)
- Cholesterol
- Mucus

Bile salts have important functions in assisting the digestive action of the pancreatic enzymes, and in aiding the absorption of fats and fat-soluble vitamins from the small intestine.

These salts, by lowering surface tension, cause fats to break up or emulsify into small droplets, allowing the fat-digesting enzymes to work more efficiently and convert them into fatty acids and glycerol, in which form they are absorbed.

Bile salts do not appear in the feces as they are reabsorbed from the small intestine and returned to the liver.

Bile pigments are derived from the breakdown of the hemoglobin of worn-out red blood cells, and give the bile its characteristic color. The bile pigments are converted in the bowel to urobilinogen by bacterial action. Some urobilinogen is reabsorbed into the blood and is excreted by the kidneys into the urine. Exposure of urine to the air causes urobilinogen to be oxidized to urobilin. In the feces, urobilinogen is altered and oxidized to form stercobilin which gives the feces a dark brown color.

If there is an obstruction to the excretion of bile, the bile pigments accumulate in the blood, giving the skin and mucous membranes a yellow color (jaundice). At the same time they appear in the urine, which is turned a dark brown. Absence of bile pigments from the feces results in pale clay-coloured stools, whilst absence of bile salts leads to an excess of foul-smelling fat in the stools.

The Pancreas

The pancreas is a gland which has both exocrine and endocrine functions. Its exocrine function is the secretion of digestive enzymes. The endocrine secretions of the pancreas are two hormones, **insulin** and **glucagon**.

It is a grayish-pink gland lying transversely across the posterior abdominal wall at the level of the first and second lumbar vertebrae and is situated behind the stomach.

The pancreas is described as having a head, a body and a tail. The **head** is situated to the right and fits into the C-shaped curve of the duodenum. Buried in the substance of the gland is the termination of the common bile duct as it joins the pancreatic duct to form the ampulla of vater, which is guarded by the sphincter of Oddi.

The **body** lies in front of the lumbar vertebrae, behind the stomach; the **tail** of the gland is in contact with the gastric surface of the spleen.

The anterior surface of the pancreas is covered by peritoneum.

Structure of the Pancreas

The pancreas consists of a number of lobules, supported by fine loose connective tissue. Each lobule contains masses of secretory acini (cells arranged in a grape-like formation), lined with columnar epithelium (Fig. 12.11). From the lobules small ducts emerge which unite to form larger ducts until they reach the main pancreatic duct, which extends from left to right in the center of the organ and, in the head of the pancreas, joins the termination of the common bile duct to enter the duodenum at the ampulla of Vater.

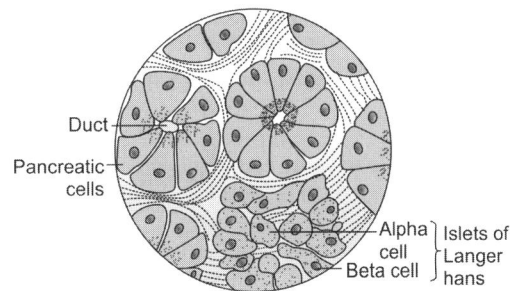

Fig. 12.11: Diagram of pancreatic cells

Embedded between the acinar cells of the pancreas lie clusters of cells differing in character and appearance from those of the secretory epithelium. There are the **islets of Langerhans**, which secrete the hormones insulin and glucagon directly into the blood.

Functions of the Pancreas

Exocrine: The acinar cells of the pancreas secrete digestive enzymes in an inactive form, which only become activated after their release into the pancreatic juice and the small intestine. When chyme enters the duodenum it causes the release of secretin and cholecystokinin into the blood which pass to the pancreas and stimulate the secretion of large quantities of fluids containing sodium bicarbonate and the release of the **digestive enzymes**, amylase, lipase, trypsinogen and chymotrypsinogen (p. 229). The pancreatic juice enters the duodenum by the pancreatic duct at the ampulla of Vater with the bile released from the gallbladder.

The **endocrine** function of the pancreas is the secretion of insulin and glucagon. Insulin is important in the metabolism of carbohydrates, fats and protein (p. 221). Glucagon is concerned with the break down of liver glycogen (glycogenolysis), and with increased gluconeogenesis. It is also lipolytic (breaks down fat) and has numerous other actions.

■ PHYSIOLOGICAL ANATOMY
Enteric Nervous System (ENS)

It lies entirely in the wall of the gut extending from esophagus to anus. ENS controls the Gastrointestinal (GI) movements and secretion. ENS is composed mainly of 2 plexuses:
1. Outer plexus lying between the longitudinal and circular muscle layer called myenteric plexus or Auerbach's plexus.
2. An inner plexus called susmucosal plexus or Meissner's plexus that lies in the submucusa.

Myentric → control mainly gastrointestinal movements. submucosal plexus → GI secretion and local blood flow. The sympathetic and parasympathetic fibers that connect with both the myenteric and the submucosal plexuses. The ENS can function independently of these extrinsic nerves. Stimulation by the parasympathetic and sympathetic system can further activate or inhibit gostrointestinal secretion and local blood flow.

Sensory nerve endings originating in the GI epithelium or gut wall send afferent febers to both plexuses of ENS and:
- Prevertibral ganglia of the symp NS
- To the spinal cord
- In the vagus nerves all the way to brainstem.

Organization of the Wall of Gastrointestinal Tract (GIT)

The wall of GIT is having four layers starting from the lumen outwards (Fig. 12.12). They are:
1. Mucosa
2. Submucosa
3. Muscularis
4. Serosa.

Mucosa is formed of three layers epithelium, lamina propria, and basement membrane. The smooth muscle in mucosa form muscularis mucosa. Submucosa contain the submucous plexus of Meissner inner to the inner circular muscle layer.

The muscularis has outer longitudinal and an inner circular muscle layers. Between circular and longitudinal muscle there is myenteric plexus of Auerbach. The mesothelium outer to muscularis forms serosa.

■ INGESTION OF FOOD

Mastication: The incisors provide a strong cutting action and molars a grinding action. Most of the muscles of chewing are innervated by the motor branch of the fifth cranial nerve and chewing process is controlled by nuclei in the brainstem. The presence of a bolus of food in the mouth at first initiates reflex inhibition of the muscles of mastication, which allow lower jaw to

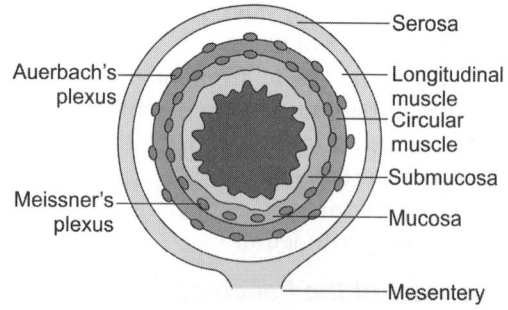

Fig. 12.12: Cross section wall of GIT showing innervation

drop. The drop initiates a stretch reflex of jaw muscles causing rebound contraction chewing of the food is important for digestion of all foods, especially important for most of fruits and raw vegetables because these have indigestible cellulose membranes around their nutrient portions that must be broken before food can be used. Digestive enzymes act only on the surface of food particle.

Secretion of Saliva

The principal glands of salivation are the parotid, submandibular and sublingual glands (Fig. 12.13). There are also buccal glands. Daily secretion of saliva ranges between 800 and 1500 mL. Saliva contains two major types of protein secretion.
1. Serous secretion—containing ptyalin (an a amylase) which is digesting starch.
2. Mucous secretion that contains mucin for lubricating and surface protective purposes. Parotid glands secreted serous submandibular and sublingual glands secrete both serous and mucous type for protective purpose. Buccal glands secrete only mucus. The pH of saliva 6–7 favorable for digestive action of ptyalin. Submadibular gland contains acini and salivary ducts.

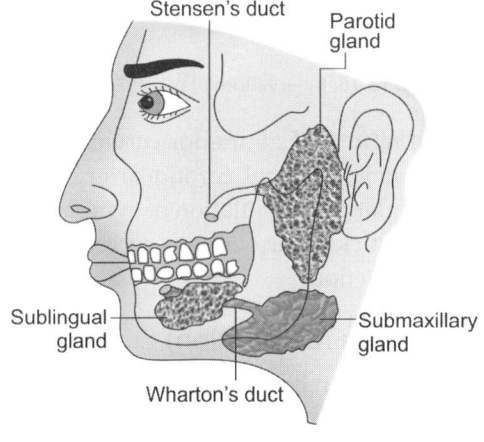

Fig. 12.13: Salivary glands

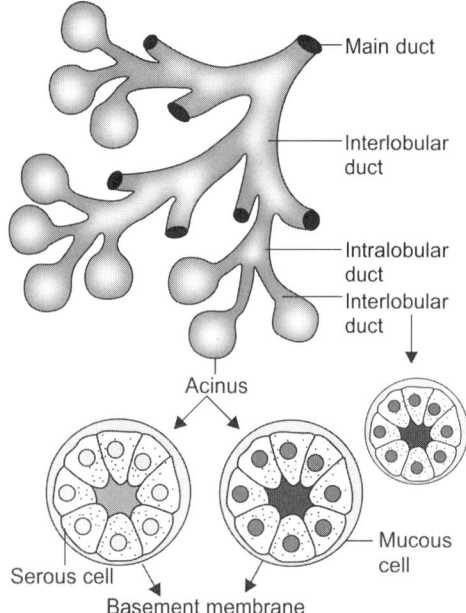

Fig. 12.14: Acini and duct system of parotid gland

Second stages of salivary secretion (Fig. 12.14):
1. Acini
2. Salivary ducts

The acini secrete a primary secretion that contains ptyalin and mucin in a solution of ions almost similar to ECF. As the primary secretion flows through the ducts two major active transport processes takes place that markedly modify the ionic composition of the fluid in the saliva. Na^+ → Actively reabsorbed from all the salivary ducts. K^+ → Actively secreted in exchange for Na^+. K^+ ion concentration become increased. There is excess of Na^+ reabsorption over K^+ secretion and this creates electrical negativity of about –70 mv in the salivary ducts. This causes Cl^- ions to be reabsorbed passively. Therefore Cl^- ion concentration in the salivary fluid falls to a very low level, matching the ductal decrease in Na^+ concentration. Second bicarbonate ions are secreted by the ductal epithelium into the lumen of duct. This is at least partly caused by the exchange of HCO_3 for chloride shift.

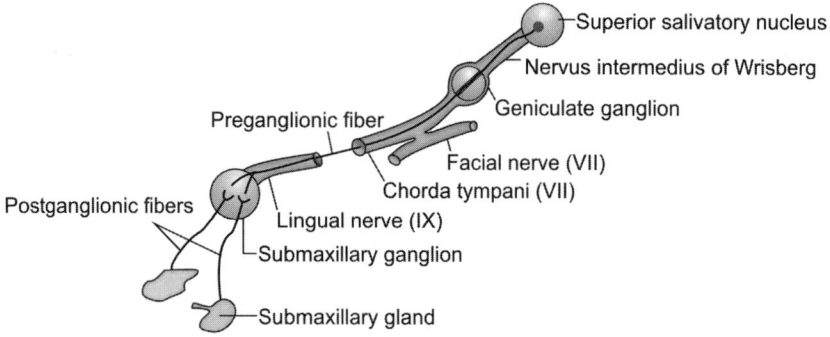

Fig. 12.15: Innervations of submandibular salivary gland

The net result of these transport processes is that under resting conditions the conc. of sodium and Cl⁻ ions in the saliva are only about 15 meq/L each, about one seventh to one tenth their concentration of K^+ ions in plasma. Conversely the concentration is about 30 meq/L, seven times as great as its concentration in plasma and the concentration of HCO_3 ions is 50–70 meq/L about 2–3 times that of plasma.

During maximum the salivation the salivary ionic concentration change considerably because the rate of formation of primary secretion by the acini can increase as much as 20 fold. This acinar secretion then flows through the ducts so rapidly that the ductal reconditioning of the secretion is decreased. So copious quantities of saliva are secreted the Na^+ and Cl^- conc rises to about 1/2–2/3 that of plasma and K^+ conc. falls to only 4 time that of plasma.

Innervations of Submandibular and Parotid Gland (Figs 12.15 and 12.16)

Parasympathetic

SSN → from superior salivatory nucleus → facial nerve → chorda tympani branch → Lingual nerve (branch of 5th nerve) → postganglionic fibers → submaxillary and sublingual.

ISN → from inferior salivatory N → Glossopharyngeal → Tympanic branch → lesser petrosal N → Otic ganglion → Auriculotemporal branch of Vth cranial N → parotid gland.

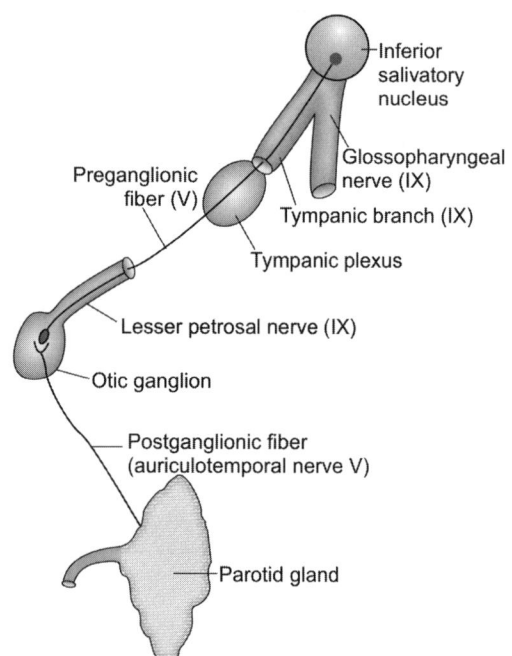

Fig. 12.16: Innervatiom of parotid gland

Sympathetic T_1–T_2: Superior cervical ganglia. → along external carotid artery to all salivary glands. Stimulation of sympathetic produce thick scanty viscous secretion and vasoconstriction.

Swallowing (Deglutition)

Swallowing can be divided into:
- A voluntary stage which initiates the swallowing process
- A pharyngeal stage which is involuntary and constitutes the passage of food

through the pharynx into the esophagus.
- Esophageal stage another involuntary phase that promotes passage of food from pharynx to the stomach.

Voluntary Stage of Swallowing

When the food is ready for swallowing it is voluntarily squeezed or rolled posteriorly into the pharynx by pressure of the tongue upward and backward against the palate. After this stage swallowing becomes almost entirely automatic and cannot be stopped.

Pharyngeal Stage of Swallowing

As the bolus of food enters the posterior mouth and pharynx it stimulates epithelial swallowing receptor areas all around the opening of the pharynx especially on the tonsillar pillars and impulses from these pass to brainstem to initiate a series of pharyngeal muscle contractions:
- Soft palate is pulled upward to close the posterior nares, in this way preventing reflux of food into the nasal cavities.
- Soft palatopharyngeal folds on each side of the pharynx are pulled medially to approximate each other. These folds form a sagittal slit through which the food must pass into the posterior pharynx.
- The vocal cords of the larynx are strongly approximated and the larynx is pulled upwards and anteriorly by the neck muscles. This movement of larynx together with swinging backward of epiglottis over the opening of the larynx prevent passage of food to trachea and nose.
- The upward movement of the larynx also pulls up and enlarges the opening of the esophagus. The upper esophageal sphincter relaxes and food pass from posterior pharynx into upper esophagus between swallows this sphincter remains strongly contracted there by preventing air from going into esophagus during respiration. The upward movement of the larynx lifts the glottis out of the main stream of food flow, so that food passes on each side of epiglottis than over its surface. This prevents passage of food into trachea.
- Then the entire muscular wall of pharynx contracts beginning in the superior part of the pharynx and spreading down as a rapid peristaltic wave over the middle and inferior pharyngeal areas which propels the food into the esophagus.
- At the same time the larynx is raised and pharyngoesophageal sphincter is relaxed muscular wall of pharynx contracts and food is propelled to the esophagus.

Nervous Control of Pharyngeal Stage of Swallowing

The most sensitive tactile areas of the posterior month and pharynx for initiation of the pharyngeal stage of swallowing lie in a ring around the pharyngeal opening with greatest, sensitivity on the tonsillar pillars. Impulses are transmitted from these areas through the sensory portions of the trigeminal and glossopharyngeal nerves into the medulla oblongata either in or closely associated with the tractus solitaries.

The successive stages of the swallowing process is controlled by reticular substance of the medulla, and lower pons. This centers are collectively called deglutition or swallowing center.

The motor impulses from the swallowing center to the pharynx and upper esophagus that cause swallowing are transmitted successively by the 5th, 9th, 10th, and 12th criminal nerves and even a few of the superior cervical nerves. During pharyngeal stage of swallowing the respiratory center is inhibited for a fraction in usual respiratory cycles.

Esophageal stage of swallowing: Two types of peristalsis primary peristalsis and secondary peristalsis. Primary peristalsis is the continuation of the penstalsis during pharyngeal stage of swallowing. Secondary peristaltic waves result from the distention of the esophagus by the retained food and continue until all the food has emptied into the stomach. The musculature of the pharynx and upper one-third of the esophagus is striated muscle. So the peristaltic waves are controlled by skeletal nerve impulses from 9th and 10th N.

In lower two-third of esophagus musculature is smooth muscle, and it is controlled by vagus.

Receptive Relaxation of the Stomach

As the esophageal peristaltic wave passes towards stomach a wave of relaxation precedes the peristalsis. The stomach and duodenum become relaxed as the peristaltic wave reaches the lower end of the esophagus. At the lower and of the esophagus extending 3 cm above its junction with the stomach esophageal circular muscle functions as a lower esophageal sphincter. Tonic constriction of the lower esophageal sphincter helps to prevent reflux of stomach contents, into esophagus.

Motor Functions of the Stomach

- Storage of large quantities of food until it is processed in the duodenum
- Mixing of food with gastric secretions and it is called chyme
- Slow emptying.

Secretions of Stomach

Three types of glands are seen in the stomach. They are oxyntic glands (fundus) and (corpus) of the stomach, cardiac glands, and pyloric glands (Fig. 12.17).

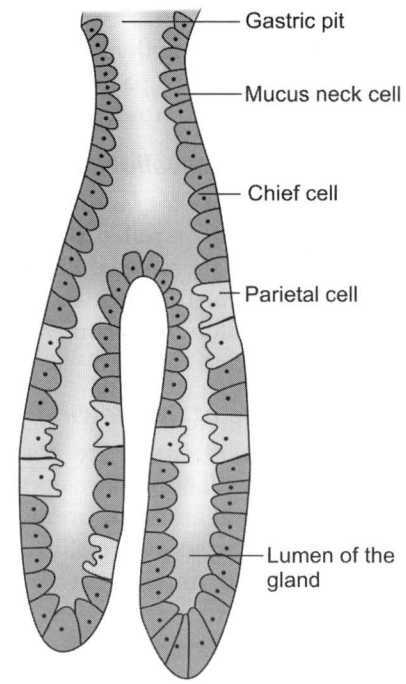

Fig. 12.17: Oxyntic gland

	Peptic (chief)	Oxyntic (parietal)	Mucus	Endo-crine
Cardiac			xx	x
Oxyntic	xx	xx	x	x
Pyloric		x	xx	xx

Enterochromaffine cells: Serotonin
Endocrine cells: Gastrin, somatostatin, VIP, glucagon
    Pancreatic polypeptide
    Bombesin and enkephalins

■ ACID SECRETION

Parietal cells are conical in shape the apex facing the lumen of the gland. Parietal cells have a high energy requirement and has a very large number of mitochondria. Secreting cell show a system of intracellular canaliculi which opens into the lumen. The walls of the canaliculi as well as the apex of the cell show numerous microvilli which increase the surface area enormously. Non-secreting cells contain a system of tubulovesicular membranes. The intracellular canaliculi no longer communicate with the lumen, become distended and loss their microvilli.

Intracellular water is ionized into H+ and OH-ions.

$H_2O \rightarrow H^+ + OH^-$

HCl Secretion (Fig. 12.18)

- Hydrogen ions are actively secreted into the lumen. The H+ pump is activated by a (H+–K+) ATPase. (H+–K+) ATPase is Mg++ dependent and is highly specific to parietal cells. It is not inhibited by oubains but is inhibited by substituted omeprazole. Therefore omeprazole is a highly specific inhibitor of gastric acid secretion.
- OH raise the intracellular pH to lethal levels and need to be neutralized $H_2CO_3 \rightarrow H^+ + HCO_{-3}$

  H+ neutralizes OH−. Since CO_2 is only poorly solvable in water the requisite quantities of H_2CO_3 are generated by catalyzing the reaction by carbonic anhydrase.

  $CO_2 + H_2O \xrightarrow{CA} H_2CO_3 \rightarrow HCO_3^-$
  $+ H^+ \rightarrow H_2O$

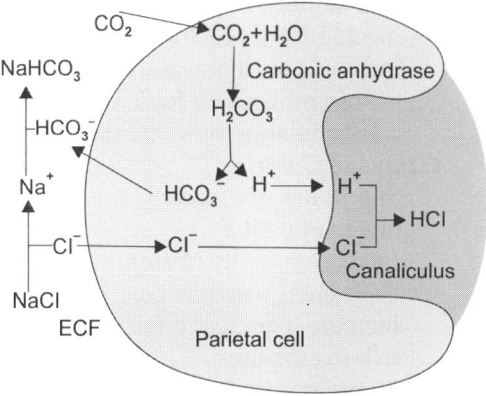

Fig. 12.18: Mechanism of secretion of HCl

- Bicarbonate ions (HCO_3^-) are actively removed from the cell at its basolateral surface by a pump activated by HCO_3^- ATPase HCO_3^- enters the interstitial fluid and diffuses into blood stream. In exchange Cl− diffuse from blood into the interstitial fluid and from there into parietal cell.
- The Cl− that enter the parietal cell in exchange for HCO_3^- are secreted into the lumen. The Cl− accompany the H+ secreted in step (1) to form HCl.

The transport of Cl− at the serosal surface is passive. The secretion of Cl− at the luminal surface is active.

Regulation of Gastric Secretion

The secretion begins when food is about to enter the stomach; and continues till food is present in the stomach. The important constituents of gastric juice are 99.5% water and 0.5% solids. Solids are organic and inorganic substances.

Organic:
- Enzymes
- Mucus
- Intrinsic factor.

Inorganic: HCl, Na+, Ca++, K+, Cl−, HCO_3^-, PO_4^-, SO_4^- concentration of HCl in gastric juice is up to 150 mEq/Liter.

Functions

Digestive Function

Pepsin: Major proteolytic enzyme in gastric juice secreted as pepsinogen enzyme in gastric juice. Secreted as pepsinogen which is inactive. Pepsinogen is formed in zymogen granules in the cytoplasm of chief cells. In pH less than 6 (acidic medium) pepsinogen is converted to pepsin.

Rennin: It is a milk curding enzyme. It is present only in animals and not is man.

Gastric lipase: Gastric lipase is a weak lipolytic enzyme when compared to pancreatic lipase. At pH below 2.5 gastric lipase is inactive. Fatty acids and glycerol are the products lipid digestion.

Hemopoietic Function

The intrinsic factor present in gastric juice plays an important role in erythropoiesis. This is necessary for absorption of Vitamin B_{12} from GIT into the blood. Absence of intrinsic factor in gastric juice causes deficiency of Vitamin B_{12}, leading to pernicious anemia.

Protective Function

The mucus present in the gastric juice is responsible for the protection of wall of the stomach. Mucoprotein secreted by mucous neck cells of gastric glands and surface mucous cells in the fundus body and other parts of stomach.

Functions of Mucus

- The mucus membrane of the stomach is lined by a thick coat of mucus. The mucus lubricates the gastric mucosa and protects it from irritation or mechanical injury by virtue of its high viscosity.
- It prevents the digestive action of pepsin onto wall of the stomach particularly gastric mucosa.
- Because of alkaline nature and its acid combining power mucus protects the gastric mucosa from HCl of gastric juice.
- Function of HCl
  - Activates pepsinogen into pepsin
  - It has bacteriolytic action. It kills some of the bacteria entering the stomach along with food.
  - It cause acidity of the chyme. The acidity of chyme causes release of hormones secretin and cholcystokinin.

Agents that Stimulate Parietal Cells

- *Ach:* It stimulate parietal cells and G cells that produce gastrin
- *Gastrin:* G cells present largely in antral mucosa produce hormone gastrin
- *Histamine:* Stimulate acid secretion
- *Enterogastrone:* Inhibits acid secretion.

Phases of Gastric Secretion

Secretion of gastric juice occurs when the food is taken in the mouth. Neural and hormonal mechanisms are involved in gastric secretion which occurs in three phases.
1. Cephalic
2. Gastric
3. Intestinal.

In human beings a fourth phase called inter digestive phase exists, i.e. secretion of small amount of gastric juice in between meals.

1. *Cephalic phase:* Under nervous control. Even before food enters stomach the secretion of gastric juice starts. This occurs as conditioned and unconditioned reflex. In both pepsinogen and HCl are secreted.
2. *Gastric phase:* This is under both nervous and hormonal control. When food enters stomach, secretion of gastric juice increases which is rich in pepsinogen and HCl.
   - *Local myenteric reflex:* Nervous mechanism
   - *Vasovagal reflex:* Nervous mechanism
   - *Gastric-hormonal mechanism:* The stimuli which activate these mechanisms are the distension of stomach, mechanical stimulation of gastric mucosa by food and chemical stimulation by contents of food.

   Actions of Gastrin:
   - Stimulates the secretion of pepsinogen and HCl
   - Increase motility of stomach
   - Promotes growth of gastric mucosa
   - Increase pancreatic juice secretion rich in enzymes
   - Stimulate production of hormones by pancreas

3. *Intestinal phase:* When the chyme enters intestine from stomach initially secretion of gastric juice is increased and later it is inhibited.
   - Via gastrin
   - Via enterogastrone and VIP and GIP

Interdigestive phase: Secretion of gastric juice in between meals. This is mostly due to the hormones, like gastrin.

Pancreatic Secretion

Composition

- 99.5% of water
- 0.5% of solids. The solids are the organic and inorganic substances.

Proteoytic

Trypsin, chymotrypsin, carboxy peptidase A, carboxy peptidase B, nuclease, elastase, collaginase.

Lipolytic Enzymes

- Pancreatic lipase
- Cholesterol ester hydrolase
- Phospholipase A
- Phospholipase B.

Amilolytic enzyme: Pancreatic amylase.

Other Organic Substances of Pancreatic Juice

Albumin: Globulin.

Inorganic Substances

Sodium, calcium, potassium, magnesium, bicarbonate, chloride, sulfate and PO_4.

Peptidases

Trypsin and chymotrypsin: It is secreted in an inactive from as trypsinogen and activation occurs by enterokinase. The trypsin formed from trypsinogen it self can activate trypsinogen.

$$Trypsinogen \xrightarrow{Enterokinase} Trypsin$$

$$Chymotrypsinogen \xrightarrow{Trypsin} Chymotrypsin$$

Trypsin and chymotrypsin are endopeptidases and act on proteins and convert them to peptidase.

Procarboxy peptidase: It is inactive and converted to carboxy peptidase and converts protein to peptides

Nucleases: Ribonuclease and deoxy ribonuclease. They act on RNA and DNA and convert them to nucleotides.

Lipase: Pancreatic lipase is an important fat digestive enzyme. It requires the presence of bile salts for its action. Lipase converts fat into glycerol, mono and diglycerides in the presence of bile salts.

Phospholipases: They act on phospholipids and convert them to lecithin and lysolecithin.

Amylase: Pancreatic amylase acts on starch and converts it to maltose which is disaccharide.

Trypsin Inhibitor

It is also secreted by the exocrine pancreas and its function is to protect pancreas (Fig. 12.19) from autodigestion by proteases.

■ REGULATION OF PANCREATIC SECRETION

Control in Cephalic Phase

The regulation of pancreatic secretion is mainly from hormones. Although the vagal activity during the cephalic and gastric phases causes pancreatic secretion. It is a low volume secretion in this phase. In cephalic phase, the sight smell, and thought of food causes pancreatic secretion and is mediated through vagal activity.

There is also enteric plexus causing the secretion of pancreatic juice which is mediated through the release of ACh and VIP. ACh acts on acinar cells and VIP controls the secretion of centroacinar cells.

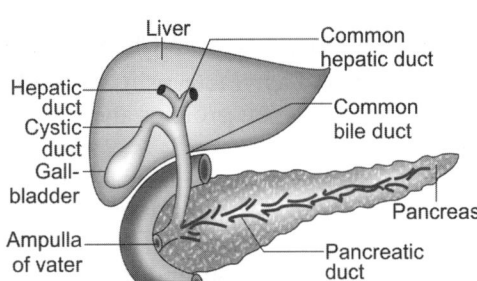

Fig. 12.19: Diagram of biliary tract and pancreas

Regulation in Gastric Phase

In gastric phase the distention of pyloric antrum gives vagovagal reflex which causes low volume secretion. The gastrin that is released will also stimulate the pancreatic secretion, with the high enzyme content but less in volume.

Regulation in Intestinal Phase

The main secretion occurs in this phase and the secretion is regulated by hormones. They are:

Secretin: It is the first hormone discovered. It is a polypeptide produced from the duodenal mucosa. This peptide hormone acts on the centroacinar cells and causes pancreatic secretion rich in water and bicarbonate. The stimulus for the hormone secretion is acid chyme in the duodenum. The secretion of watery fluid rich in bicarbonate helps to neutralize the acid pH. The action of secretin is potentiated by cholecyrtokinin CCK.

CCK: It is a peptide hormone which acts on the acinar cells and causes secretion of pancreatic juice rich in digestive enzymes. CCK also acts on gallbladder. It causes its contraction and expulsion of bile. The hormone is produced more from duodenal mucosa and the stimulus for its release is the products of food digestion entering the duodenum.

Clinical Importance

Acute pancreatitis caused by the inflammation of pancreas results in the release of digestive enzymes into the circulation. Estimation of serum amylase shows significant rise which is of diagnostic importance.

Chronic pancreatitis the digestive enzymes are not sufficiently secreted, fat digestion is affected steatorrhea occurs. Also poor digestion of fat soluble Vitamins leading to malnutrition.

Bile

Bile is secreted from the liver. Liver contains lobules and each lobule shows rows of hepatocytes radiating centrifugally from a central vein. At the other end in the connective tissue a triad is present. It includes portal vein hepatic artery and bile duct.

Portal vein open into sinusoids which drain into central vein. The sinusoids are present at the basolateral surface of hepatocytes. The blood from the central vein is ultimately drained into hepatic vein. Between the rows of hepatocytes at the apical border bile ductules are present which drain bile into the bile duct. They join to form right and left hepatic duct which join cystic duct from gallbladder to form CBD. Pancreatic duct joins with CBD before opening into second part of duodenum where the orifice is guarded by the sphincter of oddi.

Composition of Bile

The volume that is secreted per day is 500–750 mL and secretion occurs when chyme enters the duodenum. Secretion is alkaline in nature (pH 7.6–7.8). Inorganic constituents are Na^+, K^+ Cl^- and HCO_3^-. The organic substances includes, bile salts, bile pigments, cholesterol, phospholipids.

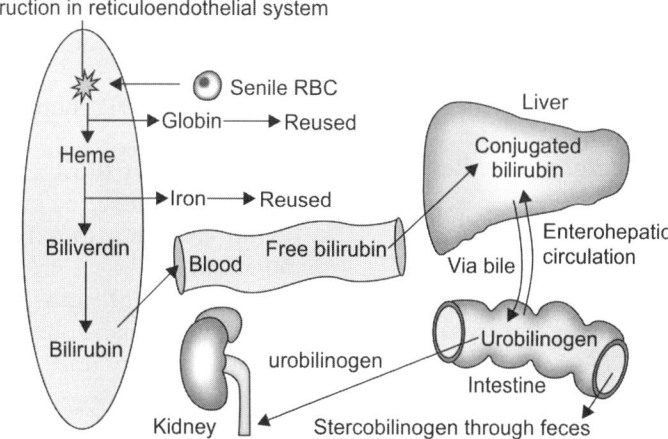

Fig. 12.20: Enterohepatic circulation of bile pigments

Bile salts: Primary bile acids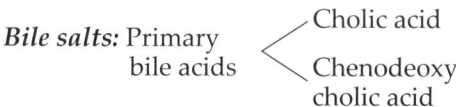

The conjugation with sodium or potassium gives taurocholate and glycocholate. In the small intestine primary bile acids are connected to secondary bile acids by the action of bacteria. Secondary bile acids are deoxycholic and lithocholic acids.

Bile Pigments

The breakdown of Hb gives bilirubin and biliverdin which are the bile pigments. They are the excretory products of liver. The golden yellow color of bile is due to the presence of bile pigments.

Functions of Bile

The bile salts have digestive function. They are necessary for fat digestion and absorption. The digestion and absorption of fat and fat soluble vitamins depend on bile salts presence. Fat is lipid soluble and digestive enzyme lipase is water soluble.

- The bile salts produce emulsification of fat
- They show hydrotropic effect. This action of bile salts enables lipase enzyme to digest fat
- Bile salts reduce surface tension, this effect facilitates the action of lipase enzyme.

The micelles that is formed after fat digestion promotes absorption. The micelles consists of digested glycerides combined with bile salts.

Enterohepatic Circulation of Bile Salts

The bile salts are secreted into duodenum 90% of bile salts that enter the small intestine are absorbed from terminal ileum and enter the liver through portal circulation. From liver they are recirculated into the duodenum. This forms the enterohepatic circulation (Fig. 12.20).

Choleretic effect: Bile salts in bile cause stimulation of liver to secrete bile.

Cholagogue: Action of cholecystokinin (CCK) on the gallbladder (GB) smooth muscle to cause its contraction and expulsion of bile.

Gallbladder

Functions — Storing (Capacity 20–50 mL) / Release of bile

Concentration of bile by the active reabsorption of Na^+, and passive reabsorption of water when fat reaches duodenum.

Hormone CCK produce this effect. The release of bile from GB also occurs by vagal activity.

Gallstones

2 types
- *Cholesterol stones:* Radiolucent
- *Pigment stones:* Ca-bilirubinate
  ↓
  Radiopaque

Metabolic Functions

- *Carbohydrate metabolism:* Liver helps in glucose homeostasis. It shows glucogenesis, gluconeogenesis and glucogenolysis. It is the site for the conversion of galactose to glucose and fructose to glucose.
- *Protein metabolism:* Formation of urea from ammonia deamination and transamination reactions takes place in liver.
- *Fat metabolism:* Lipogenesis, lipolysis, β-oxidation of fatty acids. Synthesis of lipoproteins, synthesis and esterification of cholesterol, formation of bile acids from cholesterol, ketogenesis.
- *Synthetic:* Formation of blood coagulation factors, prothrombin synthesis in presence of vitamin K synthesis of plasma protein, formation of bilesalts.
- *Excretory:* Excretion of bile pigments, drugs, metals and dyes (BSP).
- *Storage:* Liver stores glycogen vitamin A, D, B_{12} and iron.
- *Detoxification:* Inactivation of hormones, drugs, toxic substances
- *Destruction of blood cells:* Kupffer cells and macrophages in the liver destroy blood cells.
- Formation of blood cells.

■ JAUNDICE

It is the yellow coloration of skin and mucous membrane, due to increased bile pigment level in plasma. This condition occurs when bilirubin level in the plasma exceeds 2 mg% depending on the cause 3 types:
1. Hemolytic (Prehepatic)
2. Hepatic
3. Obstructive (Posthepatic)

Hemolytic: Caused by increased destruction of red cells due to extrinsic and intrinsic defects in RBC.
Hepatic: Hepatitis caused by virus
Obstructive: Gallstones in bile ducts and tumors of biliary trace.

Gastric Motility

Gastric motility is initiated by ENS; and the stimulus comes from the distension of the wall by food. The activity of intrinsic nerve plexus can be modified by extrinsic nervous system, which consists of parasympathetic and sympathetic divisions. Parasympathetic stimulation causes increased motility, while the sympathetic stimulation inhibits motility.

Movements of the Stomach

The stomach shows receptive relaxation; accommodating large volume of food. The receptors for this are present in the wall of pharynx and stomach.

Function of fundus and body of the stomach is to store the food (storage function). The afferent and efferent impulses for receptive relaxation are carried by vagus (vagovagal reflex) and causes the myenteric plexus to secrete VIP. This transmitter causes relaxation of the wall of the stomach. Vagotomy decreases the receptive relaxation though not completely abolishes because the intrinsic nerve plexus is responsible for the receptive relaxation.

Mixing of Food (Digestive Peristalsis)

The distal part of the stomach shows digestive peristalsis. The distension of the wall of the distal part of body and antrum stimulates the intrinsic plexus. The smooth muscle in the wall shows slow waves. They are also called BER. The diffusion of the wall or the activity of the vagus causes development of spikes on the peak of slow waves. They are action potentials developed when the slow waves reach the threshold level of firing. The entry of Na^+ and Ca^+ in the cell causes depolarization. Once the AP spikes are developed, it becomes propagatory in the form of peristalsis. Vagal stimulation and acetylcholine, and gastrin cause development of spikes or AP on the peak of slow waves which results in peristalsis. The digestive peristalsis travel towards the pylorus pushing the food forwards. The peristalsis is the wave of contraction followed by relaxation. The frequency of digestive peristalsis in the stomach is 3/min. The food when reaches the pylorus is retropulsed into the antrum due to the closure of pyloric sphincter. The closure of sphincter when peristalsis arrives the pylorus is necessary to prevent the entry of food into the duodenum without thorough mixing and forming acid chyme. The propulsion, mixing, and retropulsion in the pylorus breaks down the food in to smaller particles (chyme) and helps thorough mixing with the gastric juice. Each time the peristalsis arrives at the pylorus only 2–3 mL of chyme is emptied into the duodenum.

Gastric Emptying

Gastric emptying occurs mainly due to the gastroduodenal pressure cycle caused by the digestive peristalsis of the stomach. The digestive peristalsis when reach the pylorus results in rise of duodenal bulb pressure. The pyloric sphincter closes and allows the food to be retropulsed. The peristalsis allows only about 2 mL of chyme to enter the duodenum before the closure of pyloric sphincter. The transit time for the gastric emptying of food is 3–4 hrs.

Enterogastric Reflex

Presence of fat, acid, and hyperosmolar solution in the duodenum inhibits gastric emptying. The inhibition is mediated by both neural and hormonal mechanisms. The neural mechanism involves inhibition of vagus (enterogastric reflex) and hormonal mechanism includes the release of secretin, CCK, GIP. These hormones are called enterogastrones. They cause inhibition of gastric motility and gastric secretion.

Small Intestinal Motility

Small intestine consists of Duodenum, jejunum and ileum. Movements that are seen here are:
- Rhythmical segmental contractions
- Peristaltic contractions
- Pendular contractions
- Villi movement.

Segmental Peristalsis

This type of movement is a frequently occurring type. It occurs as a small segment due to the contraction of circular smooth muscle. The contraction is a result of slow waves developed in the wall of the intestines low wave is formed due to the intrinsic nerve plexus. The frequency and amplitude of the slow wave is used by the parasympathetic stimulation, acetyl choline, gastric juice, and motilin.

Sympathetic stimulation, secretin and glucagon inhibit the slow wave development. The segmental contraction results when slow wave depolarization reaches the threshold level.

The slow wave show a gradient in its frequency with highest rate at the duodenum 12/min and lowest at the ileum 8/min. This helps the bolus to be propelled aborally. This is known as the law of intestine.

The segmental contractions involve ring like regular constrictions along the length of a segment of intestine. The constricted part later relaxes and relaxed part constricts. This process is repeated over and again, and called peristalsis or peristaltic rush.

Sometimes the longitudinal muscle contractions give pendular movements which facilitate mixing of bolus with digestive enzymes. The intestinal villi shows forward and backward movements due to the contractions of the smooth muscle in the villi. The hormone villikinin stimulate the villi movements and they facilitate absorption digested food. Emptying of lymph from central to peripheral lacteal.

Gastroileal Reflex

Distention of stomach by the food, causes relaxation of ileocecal sphincter and allows emptying of ileal contents into the cecum which is the first part of colon. Distention of ileum cause realization of ileocecal sphincter and ileal emptying. The distention of cecum on the other hand results in the contraction of the sphincter and prevents reflux of cecal contents into the ileum. The activity of the ileocecal sphincter is controlled by the myenteric plexus.

Motility of Large Intestine

Functions of large intestine:
- Absorption of water and electrolytes
- Formation of feces
- Secretion of mucus to lubricate feces
- The bacterial flora synthesize B group vitamins and Vitamin K.

Motility

- Haustral shuttling (segmental contractions)
- Peristaltic contractions
- Mass peristalsis.

The wall of colon has ENS. It has inhibitory and excitatory effects on the smooth muscle. But the overall neural effect is inhibitory on colon. If ENS is destroyed colon segments remain contracted due to the reduction in colonic tone (e.g. Hirchsprung's disease).

Haustral Contractions

Similar to small intestinal segmental colon has both parasympathetic and sympathetic controls. The PS innervation of proximal colon is by the vagus and distal colon is innervated by pelvic nerve. The stimulation of parasympathetic nerves to colon increase motility and the sympathetic nerves to colon cause inhibition of motility contractions. In large intestine longitudinal muscle give taenia coli. The enteric nerve plexus below this region is greater. The region adjacent to taenia coli has a thin wall, and so when segmental contractions occur, it give rise to sac-like pouches along the length of segment of colon. They are called haustra the back and forth movements cause the chyme to be exposed for absorption of water and electrolytes. Out of 1500 mL of fluid chyme entering colon per day 50–100 mL are absorbed in the colon. The haustral shuttling also facilitate propulsive movements of feces to distal colon. The transit time in the colon is very slow 5 cm/hr.

Mass Peristalsis

It occurs in a large segment of colon and these contractions are powerful enough to cause the colon to be in contracted state for a long period of time. Intrinsic myenteric plexus activity is responsible for mass peristalsis. The mass peristalsis sweeps feces along long segment of colon to the sigmoid colon. Mass peristalsis occurs 3–4 times in a day and this along with arrival of fecus into rectum gives the desire to defecate. The gastrocolic reflex forms the stimulus for initiating mass peristalsis.

Defecation

The center for this reflex process is $S_{2,3,4}$. The higher centers are in the pons, hypothalamus and cerebral cortex. The distal segments of colon are innervated by the parasympathetic pelvic nerves. The pudendal nerve which is a somatic nerve supplies the external anal sphincter. It is a striated muscle and is under voluntary control.

The activity of pelvic nerve is responsible for the motor activity of distal colon, and relaxation of internal anal sphincter. The stretch receptor of rectum is stimulated when the wall of rectum is distended, the afferent impulses are send through pelvic nerves. If central inhibition is not present, internal anal sphincter is inhibited causing it to relax. Pudendal nerve is also inhibited which relaxes the external anal sphincter. The contraction of abdominal muscles, straining efforts and descend of diaphragm increase intra-abdominal pressure which augments the defecation reflex.

■ DIGESTION AND ABSORPTION OF FOOD

Carbohydrates

In man 50–60% of diet contains carbohydrates which includes starch, sucrose and lactose. The daily intake of carbohydrate in humans varies from 250 to 800 g.

Digestion of Starch

Starch is a polysaccharide. It is hydrolyzed by salivary amylase and pancreatic amylase enzymes. Both hydrolyze the 1–4 α linkages in the starch molecule and convert it to oligosaccharides namely maltose (disaccharide) maltotriose and α limit dextrins. Further digestion of these oligosaccharides takes place in the brush border of villi of SI. The α limit dextrinases hydrolyze limit dextrins, while maltase act on maltose and malto triose to give two molecules of glucose.

Digestion of Sucrose and Fructose

Both are disaccharides and are hydrolyzed by sucrase and lactase present in the brush border of the villi of the small intestinal mucosa. Sucrase act on sucrose and convert it into fructose and glucose, while lactase act on lactose and convert it to glucose and galactose.

Absorption of Glucose and Galactose

The transport of glucose across the intestinal mucosal cell requires a carrier protein $SGLT_1$ which carries both Na^+ and glucose (symport). It is a secondary active transport. The active transport of Na^+ across the lateral intercellular surface supplies energy for the glucose entry into the cell and also creates concentration gradient for Na^+ to move into the cell. If Na^+ entry is facilitated glucose also is transported into the cell. The transport is not dependent on insulin. Transport from the cell into the interstitial fluid occurs through the lateral intercellular border and the carrier protein involved is $GLUT_2$.

Galactose

Similar to glucose. Deficiency of co-transporter into mucosal surface of the villi leads to malabsorption of glucose and galactose.

Fructose

Different from glucose absorption. It is independent of Na^+ absorption. Transport across the brush border of villi occurs by facilitated diffusion with the help of transporter $GLUT_5$. From the cell to the lateral intercellular space the transport is helped by transporter $GLUT_2$. Some amount of fructose is converted to glucose in the mucosal cell itself. Absorption of pentose shows simple diffusion.

Digestion and Absorption of Proteins

Proteins for digestion come from two sources:

1. From diet
2. From digestive secretions and desquamated epithelial cells.

The daily requirement of proteins in adult is 0.5 to 0.7 g/kg of body weight. Digestion of protein begins in the stomach. The enzyme pepsin hydrolyses proteins to peptones and peptides. Pepsin is secreted as inactive pepsinogen and activated by HCl at pH 1–2. In the duodenum the alkaline pH inhibits the action of pepsin.

In small intestine pancreatic juice contains important proteolytic enzymes. Pancreatic secretion contains trypsin, chymotrypsin carboxypeptidase and elastase. Trypsin is secreted as trypsinogen and is activated by enterokinase. Trypsin can activate trypsinogen chymotrypsinogen and procarboxypeptidase and forms peptides.

The peptides undergo further digestion in the small intestinal cell brush border. Tripeptidases and dipeptidases act on tripeptides and dipeptides respectively and forms amino acids. Cytosol of the cell also contains peptidases. Polypeptides (more than three peptides) are poorly absorbed in the intestinal mucosal cell.

Absorption of Amino Acids

Three transporters; one each for basic, neutral and acidic amino acids. They are transported together with Na^+ as co-transport. The entry into cell occurs by secondary active transport similar to glucose. The amino acids from cytosol to the basolateral space are transported by facilitated diffusion or simple diffusions.

Digestion and Absorption of Fat

Dietary intake of fat consists of triglycerides, sterols, sterol esters and phospholipids. The daily intake of fat in man ranges from 25–150 g.

Lipids are absorbed by passive diffusion but they should be made water soluble to enter the cell.

Digestion of Lipids

Three lipases in pancreatic juice:
1. Pancreatic lipase
2. Cholesterol esterase
3. Phospholipase A_1 and A_2.

Pancreatic lipase cleaves, fatty acids from triglycerides from 1 and 1^1 positions and leaves 2 monoglycerides.

Cholesterol esterase cleaves fatty acids from cholesterol ester and gives free cholesterol. Phospholipase A_1 and A_2 cleave fatty acids from phospholipids.

The lipase enzyme is water soluble and to act on the lipids requires the assistance of bile salts. The bile acids and lecithin *emulsify fat* which gives smaller molecules of lipids. This provides large surface area for the enzyme action. The bile salts shows *hydrotropic effect*. Colipase from pancreatic secretion combines with the lipase to activate it. The products of triglycerides digestion are fatty acids and 2 monoglycerides. They combine with the bile salt and form micelles with a diameter of 5 nm. The interior of micelles contains the hydrophobic chains such as 2 monoglycerides, fatty acids, and lysophosphatides while the polar water soluble ends face the exterior. The fat soluble vitamin and cholesterol are present in the interior of micelles. The micelles are formed only if bile salts concentration in the duodenum is above the critical level.

Absorption of Digested Fat

The long chain fatty acids and monoglyceride (MG) are resynthesized into triglycerides (TG) after absorption. Absorption of fat involves simple diffusion but to make it water soluble the digested product of fat form micelles by combining with bile salts. The micelles transports fatty acids, 2 monoglyceride and cholesterol, fat soluble vitamin, etc. across the bush border of the villi and after their transport bile salts comeback to the lumen of the SI. Bile salts are absorbed from the terminal ileum by a Na$^+$ dependent active transport.

In the cytosol of the intestinal mucosal cell, the absorbed products of fat digestion are reconstituted in the smooth ER as follows:
- 2 MG combine with FA and 4 TG
- Lysophosphatides combine with FA and form phospholipid.
- The combination of cholesterol with FAs give cholesterol ester.

The reconstituted TG, PL, and cholesterol ester coalesce to form chylomicrons within the smooth ER. These are small lipid droplets with 1 nm size. The chylomicrons leave the cell by exocytosis. Before the exit the chylomicron is covered by a β lipoprotein coating. These chylomicrones form a large droplet to enter the lacteal of the villi and through the lymphatic circulation enter the systemic circulation. The short chain FA the more soluble in water and hence they diffuse into the mucosal cell of small intestine. From the cell they enter liver through the portal vessel.

CHAPTER 13

Metabolism and Nutrition

Energy is needed for the multitude of activities performed by the body. It is also required for growth, and repair of tissues. This energy is obtained from ingested food, which is first digested and absorbed, and finally metabolized.

Metabolism is the total of the chemical reactions which occur in the whole body. Metabolism consists of two major processes, catabolism and anabolism.

Catabolism is the breaking down of large molecules to smaller units to release energy and heat.

Anabolism is the building or synthesis of new compounds, and this process is energy consuming.

In the healthy adult there is a balance between catabolism and anabolism, which is called the energy-balance, (i.e. energy produced equals energy used). Both processes occur continuously and simultaneously, and consist of a series of precisely regulated chemical reactions.

The principal nutrients of the body are carbohydrates, fats and proteins. During the process of digestion, carbohydrates are converted to glucose, fats are converted to fatty acids and glycerol, and proteins are converted to amino acids. These molecules are able to enter the cells of the body tissues. Inside the cells the nutrients react chemically with oxygen under the influence of enzymes to release energy.

The energy liberated from the nutrients by oxidation is utilized to form a high energy compound, adenosine triphosphate (ATP). This is synthesized and stored in the mitochondria of the cell, and thus provides an energy reserve which is available for cellular metabolism.

Attached to the nucleus of the ATP molecule are three phosphate groups, two of which are connected by high-energy bonds. ATP releases its energy by splitting one or both of these bonds. The splitting of the first bond yields energy and reduces ATP to adenosine diphosphate (ADP). Splitting of the second bond releases further energy and the ADP is degraded to adenosine monophosphate (AMP).

The ADP and AMP are rapidly reconverted to ATP by the mitochondria, using energy obtained from the oxidation of nutrients (Fig. 13.1). This ATP/ADP cycle can be repeated again and again.

The oxidation of the nutrients releases energy and heat. The heat is distributed to the whole body by the bloodstream and helps to maintain normal body temperature. Excess heat is dissipated from the body by the skin, by respiration and in the urine and feces.

The metabolic rate is the rate at which energy is released in the body. A convenient method of estimating the energy requirements of the body is to measure it in terms of heat. The unit of heat used for this purpose is the Calorie (abbreviated to C). A Calorie (or kilocalorie) may be defined as the amount of heat required to raise 1 liter of water through 1°C.

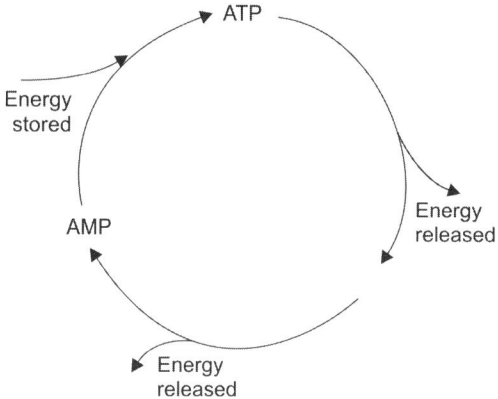

Fig. 13.1: ATP is degraded to ADP and AMP which are rapidly reconverted to ATP in a continuous cycle

The energy value of food is also measured in calories:

1 gram of carbohydrate = 4 calories (16 kJ, or kilojoules)
1 gram of protein = 4 calories (17 kJ)
1 gram of fat = 9 calories (37 kJ)

■ BASAL METABOLIC RATE

The basal metabolic rate (BMR) is the rate of the body's energy expenditure under 'basal conditions'. This means the individual is at rest, mentally and physically, has not eaten for at least 12 hours (i.e. is in the post-absorptive state), and is in a warm comfortable environment. Under these conditions the metabolic needs of the body are at their lowest, energy being used only to sustain vital functions (e.g. breathing, the beating of the heart, maintenance of normal body temperature).

The basal metabolic rate can be calculated by estimating the amount of oxygen consumed in a given time. Since individuals vary greatly in size; the BMR is expressed in calories per square meter of body surface per hour. The body surface area is calculated from measurements of an individual's weight and height.

Men oxidize food faster than women and therefore have a higher basal metabolic rate. For example, a male in his twenties has a BMR of about 40 calories per square meter of body surface per hour, whilst a woman of the same age has a BMR of about 37 calories per square meter of body surface per hour.

Factors Influencing Metabolism (Fig. 13.2)

- *Age:* The metabolic rate of children is relatively greater than that of adults due to high rates of cellular activity and growth. The BMR decreases with increasing age.
- *Exercise:* Requires energy. Strenuous physical exercise can increase the metabolic rate as much as a hundred times that of the BMR of an individual for a few seconds at a time.
- *Body temperature:* An increase in body temperature increases the BMR. A decrease in body temperature results in a decrease in the metabolic rate and in oxygen consumption.
- *Environmental temperature:* The average metabolic rate of individuals living in tropical countries is considerably lower than that of people living in cold climates.
- *Thyroid hormone:* Plays an important part in metabolism. When an excess of

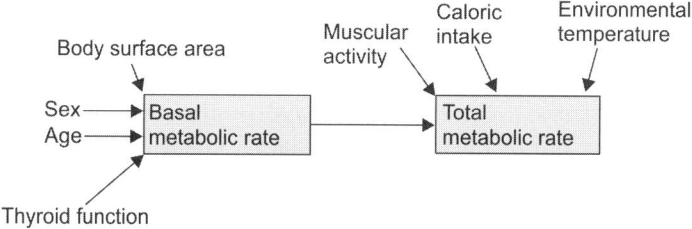

Fig. 13.2: Relationship between basal metabolic rate and total metabolic rate

the hormone is secreted (thyrotoxicosis) the basal metabolism is increased; when there is a deficiency of thyroid hormone (myxedema and cretinism) basal metabolism is slow.

- Stimulation of the sympathetic nervous system as in fright or acute anxiety, causes a temporary increase in the metabolic rate in order that the body may cope with an emergency.
- *Drugs:* Certain drugs, such as the amphetamines, or caffeine, can increase the BMR.

Carbohydrate Metabolism

Carbohydrate is the term used to describe starches and sugars. They are compounds of carbon, hydrogen and oxygen ($C_6H_{12}O_6$). Carbohydrates are absorbed through the villi of the small intestine as glucose, fructose and galactose. They are the primary energy source of the body. The fructose and galactose are converted to glucose by the liver and returned to the bloodstream.

Glucose is used to provide energy for cellular activity. Before glucose can be oxidized in the cells it must be transported across the cell membrane by a process called facilitated diffusion, which requires the use of a carrier substance. The presence of the hormone insulin accelerates this process. Failure of the pancreas to secrete sufficient insulin, as in diabetes mellitus, means that only very small amounts of glucose are able to enter the cells.

The maintenance of the blood glucose concentration at a relatively constant level is essential for the survival and function of brain cells. A fall in the blood glucose level rapidly results in disturbance of the central nervous system and, if uncorrected, leads to loss of consciousness and death within a few hours.

The blood glucose level is regulated by the liver and hormones (Fig. 13.3).

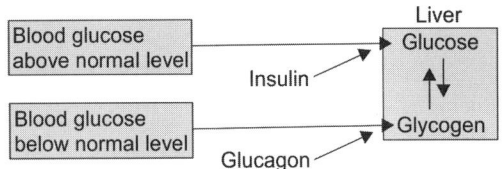

Fig. 13.3: Blood glucose levels are regulated by the liver and hormones

Following a meal, glucose is rapidly absorbed and the blood glucose level rises above normal. As the blood passes through the liver, excess glucose is transported with the aid of insulin into the liver cells, where it is converted to glycogen and stored. This process reduces the blood glucose concentration to normal. A fall in the blood glucose level stimulates the pancreas to secrete the hormone glucagon, which causes the liver to reconvert glycogen to glucose and release it into the blood, thus raising the blood glucose to normal.

Several other hormones are also involved in accelerating the conversion of glycogen to glucose, these include adrenalin, glucocorticoids, ACTH, and thyroxin.

Gluconeogenesis

Glucose is stored mainly in the liver and muscles of the body, but these stores are limited. During periods of starvation the liver converts proteins or glycerol to glucose in order to maintain blood glucose levels at normal concentration.

Catabolism of Glucose

The catabolism of glucose by cells to release energy occurs in two stages, an anaerobic stage called glycolysis (Fig. 13.4), which does not require oxygen, and an aerobic stage for which oxygen is essential.

Glycolysis

Each molecule of glucose is split by a series of cellular enzymes into two molecules of pyruvic acid, with the release of a small amount of energy. This process is specially

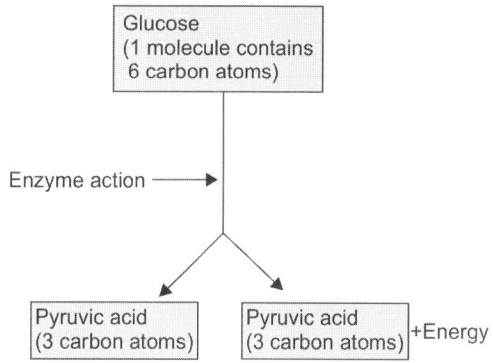

Fig. 13.4: Glycolysis (an anaerobic process) is the first stage of carbohydrate metabolism

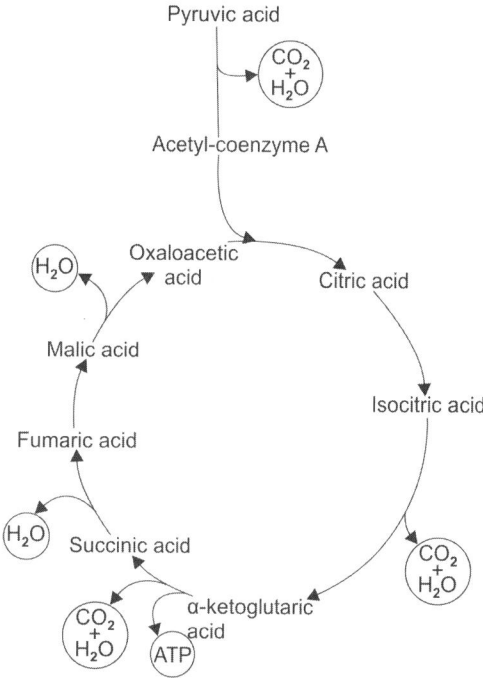

Fig. 13.5: Simplified diagram of citric acid cycle (Krebs cycle)

important when oxygen is in short supply. For example, during strenuous exercise the respiratory and circulatory systems may not be able to deliver sufficient oxygen to the muscle cells for the oxidation of glucose. However, this process can only be used for very limited periods of time because it results in the accumulation of lactic acid, and the muscles incur an 'oxygen debt'. Immediately following such exercise the oxygen debt must be repaid. Respiratory stimulation increases the respiratory rate to provide enough oxygen to reconvert lactic acid to pyruvic acid which is either oxidized to carbon dioxide and water for excretion, or converted back to glucose.

Oxidation of Glucose

When adequate oxygen is available the pyruvic acid is converted to acetyl coenzyme A, which then combines with oxaloacetic acid to enter the citric acid cycle or Krebs cycle (Fig. 13.5). The citric acid cycle completely oxidizes the glucose to carbon dioxide, water and ATP.

The conversion of one molecule of glucose to pyruvic acid (glycolysis) yields four molecules of ATP, whilst the conversion of pyruvic acid to acetyl coenzyme A and the citric acid cycle yield a further thirty-four molecules of ATP. Thus the greatest amount of energy is released from glucose by the oxidative process.

Fat Metabolism

Fats are absorbed as fatty acids and glycerol into the lacteals of the villi in the small intestine, where they are recombined to neutral fats and transported to the bloodstream by the lymphatic vessels. Fats are compounds containing carbon and hydrogen with very little oxygen. They constitute a more concentrated energy source than carbohydrates since catabolism of 1 gram of fat yields 9 calories of heat and energy, whilst 1 gram of carbohydrate yields only 4 calories.

Catabolism of Fats (Fig. 13.6)

Neutral fats are split by the liver to glycerol and fatty acids. Glycerol is similar to the breakdown products of glucose, and can be converted to a compound that enters the glycolytic pathway. Fatty acids are oxidized to acetyl coenzyme A and, provided that carbohydrates are being metabolized,

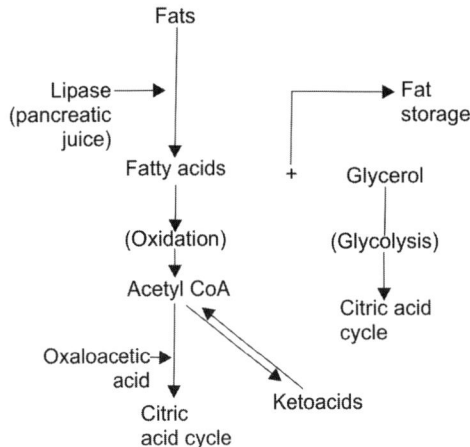

Fig. 13.6: Fat catabolism

can enter the citric acid cycle. Both carbohydrates and fats enter the citric acid cycle by combining with oxaloacetic acid, which is manufactured from carbohydrate. Thus carbohydrates can supply their own oxaloacetic acid, but fats cannot, and must use that produced by carbohydrates to be fully oxidized.

If no carbohydrate is available, as in starvation, or when carbohydrate cannot be metabolized as in diabetes mellitus, then the acetyl coenzyme A molecules from fatty acids accumulate in the body. The liver cells condense the acetyl coenzyime A molecules to form acetoacetic acid, some of which is converted to beta-hydroxybutyric acid and acetone. These three substances are collectively known as ketone bodies or ketoacids. Accumulation of ketone bodies in the blood is called ketosis, and when severe can cause coma and death. The presence of ketone bodies can be detected on the breath and in the urine as acetone.

Any fat which is not immediately required for heat and energy is stored in the fat depots of the body. The fat depots are the body's largest energy reserve source, and are found under the skin, in the folds of the omentum, between the muscles and around various organs such as the kidneys. This adipose tissue also provides heat insulation for the body.

Excess glucose and amino acids are converted by the liver to fat, which is also stored in the fat depots. Thus, when an individual takes in more calories than are required for metabolic needs, the excess is stored as fat regardless of whether the food was carbohydrate, fat or protein.

When fat is required to provide energy, it is withdrawn from the fat depots and carried to the liver to be desaturated and split to glycerol and fatty acids.

Phospholipids and Cholesterol

These two substances are present in large quantities in the body, and are synthesized in all the cells of the body. Both are fat-soluble and only slightly water-soluble.

Phospholipids are complex compounds which appear to be important in the transport of fats in the blood, and in the formation of cell membranes and the structure of the myelin sheaths of the nerve fibers.

Cholesterol is composed mainly of a sterol nucleus synthesized from acetic acid. Cholesterol is found in cell membranes, and is also used by the adrenal glands in the formation of adrenocortical hormones, by the ovaries to form estrogen and progesterone, and by the testes to form testosterone.

A large amount of cholesterol is present in the horny layer of the epidermis, where, with other lipids, it contributes to the 'water tightness' of the skin.

Atherosclerosis is a disease of the arteries in which fatty deposits containing large quantities of cholesterol and other lipids develop in the arterial walls. Fibrous tissue grows into the deposits and they become calcified, leading to narrowing of the lumen and 'hardening of the arteries'.

Protein Metabolism

Proteins are complex organic compounds containing carbon, hydrogen and oxygen with the addition of nitrogen, sulfur and phosphorus. Large protein molecules consist of many amino acids linked together to form chains known as peptides. The links between the chains are called peptide bonds.

Proteins are essential to the body, for they provide most of the structural elements of the cells and the enzymes which are necessary for all biochemical reactions.

Twenty-one amino acids have been identified and named (Table 13.1). Some of these are known as essential amino acids because they cannot be synthesized in the human body and therefore must be supplied in food. The other amino acids are known as nonessential because, although they are vital to life, they do not need to be supplied in food, but can be synthesized by the body itself.

Every cell in the body is capable of manufacturing the proteins it needs, and this process is controlled by the genes in the

Table 13.1: List of essential and non-essential amino acids

Essential amino acids (those which must be supplied in food)	Non-essential amino acids (those which do not need to be supplied in food since they can be synthesized in the body)
Arginine	Alanine
Histidine	Aspartic acid
Leucine	Cystine
Isoleucine	Glutamic acid
Lysine	Glycine
Methionine	Hydroxyproline
Phenylalanine	Proline
Threonine	Serine
Tryptophan	Tryosine
Valine	Cysteine
	Hydroxylysine

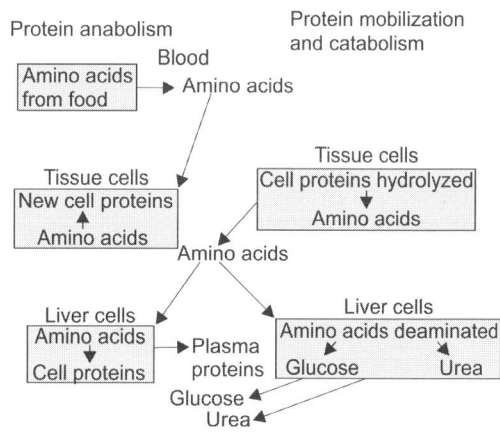

Fig. 13.7: Main features of protein metabolism

cell nucleus (Fig. 13.7). Protein anabolism thus produces many substances necessary for healthy body function. Among these are the plasma proteins synthesized by the liver, which are essential for the maintenance of fluid balance and osmotic pressure. The plasma proteins prothrombin and fibrinogen play vital roles in blood coagulation. Protein synthesis is also important for the production of the gamma globulin of antibodies essential in the defense of the body against infection and for growth and the replacement of cells destroyed by daily wear and tear.

When the blood concentration of amino acids is high, some are absorbed into the liver cells and stored. As the amino acid concentration of the blood falls to below normal the stored amino acids are released from the liver back into the blood. To some extent most of the other body cells can also store amino acids. The amino acids stored in this way are referred to as the amino acid pool.

Surplus amino acids are utilized for heat and energy. The first stage of protein catabolism is deamination, and takes place in the liver. The nitrogen portion is split off from the amino acid molecule to form ammonia, which in turn combines with carbon dioxide to form urea in the liver.

The urea is excreted by the kidneys into the urine.

The deaminized amino acids can be directly oxidized to form carbon dioxide and water with the release of heat and energy, or they may be converted to fat or carbohydrate.

Normally a state of nitrogen balance exists in the healthy adult body, i.e. the rate of protein intake equals the rate of protein utilization. A negative nitrogen balance occurs when protein utilization is greater than the protein intake, and results in a state of 'tissue wasting'. Malnutrition and debilitating diseases such as thyrotoxicosis may cause a negative nitrogen balance.

A positive nitrogen balance occurs when protein intake is greater than protein utilization. This happens during growth, pregnancy, and recovery from a debilitating illness.

Protein metabolism is controlled by hormones. Growth hormone and testosterone have a stimulating effect on protein synthesis and are sometimes known as anabolic hormones. Glucocorticoids have a profound effect on protein catabolism. Thyroid hormone is also necessary for protein anabolism, but excessive thyroxine secretion stimulates protein mobilization and catabolism.

Mineral Metabolism

A number of mineral salts play an important part in the vital processes of metabolism. Some are present in relatively large amounts, whilst others are needed only in minute quantities, and are known as trace elements. These inorganic compounds must be derived from food.

Calcium is found mainly in dairy products and green vegetables. In the UK, calcium carbonate is added to flour and is therefore also present in bread and cakes.

Growing children need more calcium than adults, and deficiency results in poor growth, rickets and badly formed teeth. Pregnant women also require extra calcium to form the developing bones and teeth of the fetus.

Calcium is most plentiful in the body in the form of calcium phosphate in the bones (Fig. 13.8). A small constant concentration of calcium is maintained in the blood and plays an important role in blood coagulation and normal muscle function. The bones act as a reservoir for calcium so that when the blood level falls below normal, calcium is withdrawn from the bones.

The presence of vitamin D is necessary for the absorption of calcium from the intestine. Large amounts of undigested fats in the intestine inhibit calcium absorption because the calcium forms salts with the fat which cannot be absorbed.

The metabolism of calcium is controlled by parathormone from the parathyroid glands and the thyroid hormone calcitonin. Damage to the parathyroid glands may lead to low blood levels of calcium which

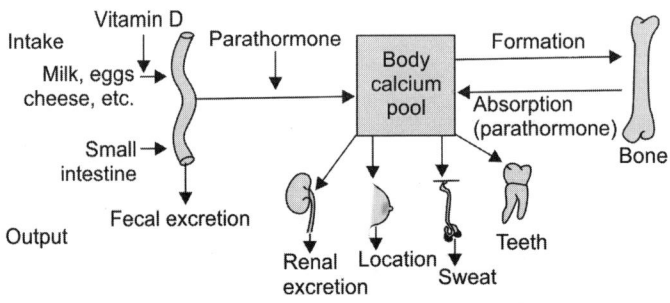

Fig. 13.8: Main features of calcium metabolism

increase the excitability of nerve fibers and result in a condition called tetany.

Phosphorus is present in many foods, specially dairy products, liver and kidney. Phosphate is extremely important in the body, for not only is it combined with calcium in the formation of bones and teeth, it is the principal anion of intracellular fluid and is essential in a large number of chemical reactions in the body (e.g. in adenosine triphosphate).

Magnesium is present in many foods, specially those of vegetable origin. It is an essential constituent of all cells but most of the body's magnesium is in the bones. It is required for the functioning of some of the enzymes involved in the utilization of energy. Deficiency of magnesium is rare but may result from losses in the stools, in patients with diarrhea or, together with potassium, in the urine of patients taking diuretics.

Sodium is present in most foods, and is also added to food as salt (sodium chloride) during cooking and at the table. Sodium is the principal extracellular cation in the body and maintenance of normal concentrations are essential to life, for it is involved in the electrolyte and fluid balance of the body, in the transmission of nerve impulses and muscular contraction.

Sodium is lost from the body in urine and sweat. Excretion of sodium in the urine is controlled by hormones from the pituitary gland and the adrenal glands, but there is less control over the loss of sodium in sweat. Thus extra salt intake may be needed in conditions which cause increased sweating (e.g. in strenuous physical exercise, high environmental temperatures).

Potassium is the principal intracellular cation, and is present in most foods. It is required for the chemical activities of cells and, like sodium, is needed for the maintenance of electrolyte and fluid balance, transmission of nerve impulses and muscular contraction. Potassium is

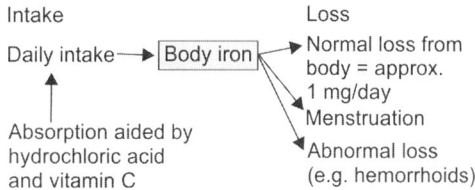

Fig. 13.9: Intake and loss of iron

excreted in urine but, unlike sodium, is not lost in sweat.

Iron is found in foods of animal origin (especially liver, kidney and beef), in egg yolks, potatoes, green vegetables and carrots. In the UK flour and white bread are fortified with iron.

Iron is essential for the manufacture of hemoglobin in the red blood cells, and is needed by all body cells in small amounts (Fig. 13.9). The body is very economical in its use of iron, for when red blood cells are destroyed the iron is extracted and recycled for use in new erythrocytes. Iron is lost from the body in cells which are shed from the skin, mucous membranes and gastrointestinal tract, and the loss amounts to about 1 mg per day. It is also lost when bleeding occurs, and women in the child-bearing years have a greater loss of iron than men due to menstrual blood loss, pregnancy and childbirth.

Absorption of iron occurs mainly in the duodenum and jejunum, and is aided by hydrochloric acid and the presence of vitamin C (ascorbic acid).

Iodine is a trace element, needed only in minute quantities but essential for the formation of thyroid hormones, which in turn are essential for normal metabolism. Iodine is found mainly in sea fish and shellfish, and in vegetables grown in soil containing iodine. In areas where soil and water are deficient in iodine it is added to table salt to prevent goiter.

Fluorine is a trace element found in bones and teeth, where it helps to prevent dental caries (dental decay). The only important nutritional sources are drinking water, tea and fish, especially those fish of which the bones are eaten. The natural content of fluorine in water is often below the optimal level of 1 part per million (1 mg per liter) and some water authorities bring it up to this level by adding fluoride as a dental health measure, teeth apart, increasing evidence suggests that fluorine is essential for life and health.

Some other trace elements are essential for human metabolism and include copper, zinc, manganese, cobalt and chromium. These elements and needed only in minute amounts.

VITAMINS

Vitamins, or accessory food factors, are organic compounds which are needed in small quantities for normal metabolism. They are not oxidized to supply energy and do not form part of the body structure. Although some vitamins can be manufactured in the body, the amounts are insufficient and these vitamins must be supplemented by the vitamins taken in the diet.

Vitamins A, D, E and K are fat-soluble, whilst vitamins of the B group and vitamin C are water-soluble (Table 13.2).

Vitamin A (Retinol)

This is found in animal foods such as liver, dairy product, eggs and fish-oils. Yellow and green vegetables contain substances called carotenes; which can be converted by the liver to vitamin A.

Vitamin A is used to synthesize the light-sensitive pigments of the retina, and is necessary for normal growth of most cells of the body, especially epithelial cells.

Lack of vitamin A manifests in (a) night blindness; (b) dry, scaly skin which becomes susceptible to infection; (c) hardening or keratinization of the cornea which may result in blindness; (d) atrophy of the germinal epithelium of the gonads.

Table 13.2: Types of vitamins and its source

Vitamin	Source
1. Fat soluble	
A (retinol)	Liver, dairy produce, eggs and fish-oils
D	Fish, margarine, butter and eggs, sunshine
E (tocopherols)	Wheat germ, vegetable oils, peanuts and dairy products
K	Present in many foods; synthesized by bacteria in large intestine
2. Water soluble	
B_1 (thiamine)	Cereals, whole meal flour, yeast, peas and beans
B_2 (riboflavin)	Meat, milk arid whole meal flour
B_3 (nicotinamide)	Meat, liver and whole meal flour
B_6 (pyridoxine)	Present in many foods
B_{12} (cyanocobalamin)	Liver, meat and animal products
Folic acid	Present in many foods; synthesized by bacteria in large intestine
Pantothenic acid	Liver, meat, eggs and milk
C (ascorbic acid)	Fresh fruit and vegetables

Vitamin D

This increases calcium absorption from the gastrointestinal tract and is concerned with the deposition of calcium and phosphorus in bones. It is particularly important in infants and children for development and growth of bones and in the pregnant woman for development of the bones and teeth of the fetus.

Several vitamin D compounds exist. Vitamin D_2 (ergocalciferol) and vitamin D_3 (cholecalciferol) are closely related a substance called 7-dehydroxycholesterol, present in the skin, is converted in the skin to vitamin D_3 on exposure to the ultraviolet rays of sunlight. Foods containing vitamin

D include fatty fish, margarine, butter and eggs. The vitamin D compounds must be altered to 1,25-dihydroxycholecalciferol by a complicated process that involves first the liver and then the kidneys, under the influence of parathormone. 1,25-dihydroxycholecalciferol is the active form of vitamin D. In the absence of the kidneys the active form of the vitamin is not produced.

Lack of vitamin D results in rickets in children and osteomalacia in adults.

Vitamin E (Tocopherols)

This includes several related compounds, found mainly in wheat germ, vegetable oils, peanuts, milk, butter and eggs. In animals, lack of vitamin E causes muscle weakness and paralysis (especially of the hind quarters), anemia and infertility in both sexes. The effects of this vitamin in the human body are not yet clear, but deficiency prevents normal growth.

Vitamin K

This is necessary for synthesis of clotting factors by the liver (including prothrombin, and factors VII, IX and X). Vitamin K consists of a number of naturally occurring substances, which are present in many foods, and are synthesized by bacteria in the large intestine.

Absorption of vitamin K requires the assistance of bile salts, and any obstruction which prevents bile from being produced or entering the duodenum leads to deficiency of the vitamin within a few days. Administration of oral antibiotics may destroy the bacteria in the gut and may lead to vitamin K deficiency.

Vitamin B Complex

This comprises a number of chemically distinct compounds, which are often but not always present in the same foods (see Table 13.2). Some of these vitamins act as coenzymes in the body (i.e. they work closely with an enzyme and are vital to its function).

Thiamine (vitamin B_1) is essential for many biochemical reactions, but is especially important for the conversion of pyruvic acid to acetyl coenzyme A. Without thiamine the oxidative processes in the metabolism of carbohydrate and fats become deficient. This results in widespread abnormalities in the body which particularly affect the nervous system, the gastrointestinal tract and cardiac function.

Riboflavin (vitamin B_2) is required for the oxidation of foodstuffs. Lack of this vitamin is associated with soreness of the lips and keratitis (inflammation of the cornea).

Nicotinamide (vitamin B_3), sometimes also called niacin, is essential for carbohydrate oxidation and the citric acid cycle. The body is able to manufacture nicotinamide from the amino acid tryptophan. Deficiency causes a disease called pellagra, which is characterized by gastrointestinal disturbances, lesions in the central nervous system with mental changes, and scaly, pigmented skin in areas exposed to sunlight or mechanical irritation.

Pyridoxine (vitamin B_6) functions as a coenzymes for many chemical reactions in amino acid and protein metabolism.

Cyanocobalamin (Vitamin B_{12})

Unlike other vitamins, cyanocobalamin (vitamin B_{12}) contains a metal, cobalt. Vitamin B_{12} performs several metabolic functions, acting as a coenzyme. It is essential for the maturation of red blood cells, and deficiency of the vitamin leads to pernicious anemia and demyelination of the nerve fibers of the spinal cord (a condition known as subacute degeneration of the spinal cord).

The cause of vitamin B_{12} deficiency is rarely lack of the vitamin in the diet, but often lack of a substance called intrinsic factor produced by the mucosal cells of the stomach, which combines with vitamin B_{12} in the food. Intrinsic factor combined with the vitamin is bound to the wall of the small intestine and the vitamin is then absorbed.

Folic Acid

Folic acid is essential for the synthesis of nucleoproteins and for cell division. It is widely distributed in food, and is also produced by bacteria in the large intestine.

Pantothenic Acid

This is used by the body to form acetyl coenzyme A, thus deficiency of this vitamin leads to depressed metabolism of carbohydrates and fats.

Vitamin C (Ascorbic Acid)

Vitamin C is essential for many oxidative reactions of metabolism, and maintains normal intercellular substances in the body, including the formation of connective tissue, and the intercellular matrix of bones and teeth.

Deficiency of vitamin C leads to a disease called scurvy. Wounds fail to heal because connective and fibrous tissue are not formed. Bone growth ceases, and blood capillaries become fragile, resulting in bleeding into the gums, skin and joints.

Vitamin C is also required for the absorption of iron, and the normal function of folic acid; thus anemia is another feature of deficiency of this vitamin.

WATER

Water forms approximately 60% of the body weight and forms the basis of the body fluids (blood plasma, lymph and tissue fluids). Water is an essential constituent of all the body tissues and cells. Many chemicals are dissolved in water, while others are in suspension, and thus can be transported between the blood plasma and the tissue fluids, and then between the tissue fluids and the cells.

Water is a very important part of the diet, because, although it has no nutritional value, a lack of water can lead to dehydration and death within a few days. Many foods consist largely of water, but in addition 1.5 Liters of fluids a day are necessary to ensure an adequate fluid intake.

Water passes readily through the walls of the stomach and intestines by diffusion and osmosis. During metabolism, the oxidation of nutrients results in the production of carbon dioxide and water, and in the healthy adult this amounts to about 1–1.5 Liters of water a day.

The control of body temperature is assisted by the evaporation of water as sweat. Water is also excreted by the kidneys as urine, by the large intestine in feces and by the lungs as water vapor.

FIBER

Adequate peristalsis in the bowel only occurs when there is a sufficient food residue for the muscle in its walls to act upon. This is because the normal stimulus to peristaltic action is the stretching of the walls by the bowel contents. The undigested fecal residue which performs this function consists of fiber and in the normal diet it is mainly provided by the cellulose found in vegetables, salads, fruit and whole meal bread. Insufficient fiber leads to sluggish peristalsis and a tendency to constipation.

NUTRITION

Nutrition is the supply of food to the tissues and its absorption and metabolism for growth, energy, maintenance and repair of the living body.

For maintenance of a healthy body, food must include carbohydrates and fats, which can be oxidized to provide heat and energy, in sufficient quantities to suit an individual's metabolic needs.

Proteins are required to supply essential amino acids to provide materials for growth and repair of body tissues. Minerals and vitamins are needed to provide the special compounds required for the chemical reactions of metabolism.

The nutrients described above are present in varying proportions in different foods, and to be satisfactory any diet must contain adequate proportions of all the nutrients required by the body. Thus the requirements of a balanced diet will vary throughout an individual's life-cycle. A child grows most rapidly in the early years of life and growth can only occur if the organs and tissues receive the nutrients needed for synthesis of their protein and cellular structures. A new born infant needs about five times as much protein as the adult per unit of body weight. As the child grows older the rate of growth slows down, and after puberty the need for nutrients gradually changes, although a greater protein intake is needed until growth ceases. An inadequate supply of energy and protein are the commonest causes of failure to grow.

Each individual requires food to supply sufficient calories to maintain the basal metabolic rate and to supply energy for the activities of everyday life. The average adult needs about 25 calories per kilogram of body weight per 24 hours for basal metabolism, i.e. a man weighing 63 kg (10 stone) needs 1575 calories per day (63 kg × 25 C = 1575 C). Additional Calories are needed for his daily activities, the amount of which will depend on his occupation and physical activity; thus if he has a sedentary job he will need a total of approximately 2700 Calories per day, but if his occupation is moderately active this would increase to 3000 C, and if very active to 3600 C per day.

Women, because they have a lower basal metabolic rate than men, need between 2200 and 2500 Calories depending on their physical activity.

The energy requirements of the individual are thus dependent on body size and composition, age, sex, physical activity, climate and environment.

The nutritional value of a protein depends on the amino acids that it contains. Proteins which contain all the essential amino acids are called complete or first class proteins, whilst those that lack one or more of the essential amino acids are called incomplete, or second, class proteins. First class proteins are mainly those derived from foods of animal origin such as meat, fish, milk and eggs. Second class proteins are mainly derived from vegetables.

Fats are the most concentrated source of energy in the diet, providing more than twice as much as proteins or carbohydrates. Fats are of animal or vegetable origin. Animal fats are found in dairy products, meat and oily fish. Vegetable fats are found in olive oil, vegetable oils and margarine. Carbohydrates represent the cheapest and most commonly occurring class of food in the diet. They are widely distributed in vegetable foods and fruit and include sugars, starches and cellulose.

Dietary intake of food varies widely, due partly to the availability of some foodstuffs. For example, in the UK protein forms approximately 15% of food intake, with approximately 30% fats and 55 % carbohydrates. However in the underdeveloped areas of the world the intake of protein and fats may be as little as half these values.

Religious, cultural and traditional practices also affect the diet of many people throughout the world.

■ CONTROL OF FOOD INTAKE

Within the lateral hypothalamus are a group of neurons that function as an appetite center, and stimulation of these cells results in sensations of hunger. Hunger means a craving for food. When a person has not eaten for some hours the stomach is stimulated to contract rhythmically, causing 'gnawing' sensations, which are called hunger pangs. These are relieved when food is eaten.

Appetite is the term used when there is a desire for specific types of food.

A cluster of neurons in the medial hypothalamus is thought to function as a satiety center, and stimulation of these cells inhibits food intake.

Both centers may be affected by blood levels of nutrients and by hormones.

Obesity

Obesity results from an imbalance between energy intake and energy output. When more energy, in the form of food, is taken into the body than is used in energy expenditure the surplus energy is converted to fat and stored as adipose tissue (for each 9 Calories of excess energy 1 gram of fat is stored). Thus most cases of obesity are caused by overeating. This may be due to habit rather than hunger, but rarely may also arise due to an abnormality of the appetite center in the hypothalamus.

Starvation

During a period when very little or no food is being taken into the body, stores of carbohydrate (i.e. the glycogen stored in the liver and muscles) are used up within the first 24 hours. After this the individual starts to break down stored fats to provide the energy necessary for cellular function. When the store of fats is almost depleted, the body begins to use protein to supply energy. However, proteins are needed for cellular structure and chemical activities, and continued depletion of protein for use as energy results in death when the proteins of the body have been reduced to one-half their normal level.

CHAPTER 14

The Endocrine System

■ INTRODUCTION

Many of the activities of the body are controlled by the nervous system and one of the characteristics of this system is the rapidity of its response to various kinds of stimuli. There is, however, a second major system which exercises control over the body's activities, especially those of a slower character, such as growth, which are manifest over long periods. The organs of this second system are called the endocrine or ductless glands. They produce special chemical substances called hormones which they secrete directly into the bloodstream. They are, therefore, sometimes referred as the organs of internal secretion.

A hormone may be defined as a chemical messenger, secreted by a ductless gland, which is transported by the circulation to its target cells in distant organs, which it is thereby able to influence. An alternative, simpler definition of a hormone, is that it is a circulating substance which acts on organs distant from its site of origin.

In some instances an organ may have both an internal secretion which enters the blood directly and an external secretion which leaves it by a duct. The pancreas is an example. The internal secretions of the pancreas, insulin and glucagon, pass into the blood while the pancreatic juice reaches the duodenum via the pancreatic duct. The pancreas is therefore said to have both endocrine and exocrine functions.

Numerous hormones have been isolated and their chemical structure elucidated. An increasing number can be prepared artificially in the laboratory either by direct chemical synthesis or by recombinant DNA technology, which is already used commercially to produce human insulin on a large scale.

Some hormones, such as adrenalin, have an immediate action. Others, especially the pituitary growth hormone, exercise their influence over many years.

The function of the ductless glands has been studied in a number of ways. Before any hormones were isolated, some knowledge of their action was gained by observing the effects of disease. It was found that two sets of symptoms existed, namely those produced by excessive activity of the gland and oversecretion (hypersecretion) of hormones and those resulting from under activity and under secretion (hyposecretion). Clearly, therefore, the action of a gland in health is to maintain a balance between these effects.

Another method of study is to obtain the hormone itself either by recovering it from the gland or manufacturing it in the laboratory and to consider the effects produced by its administration both in health and in disease.

A third method is to study the results of the destruction or removal of the gland in animals.

The major endocrine glands may be arranged in two groups:
1. (a) The anterior pituitary gland
   (b) The adrenal cortex

(c) The thyroid gland
  (d) The sex glands or gonads.
2. (a) The posterior pituitary gland
  (b) The adrenal medulla
  (c) The parathyroid glands
  (d) The pancreas.

The anterior pituitary gland controls the other members of the first group via the intermediary of trophic hormones (such as adrenocorticotropic hormone [ACTH] or corticotropin), which it secretes. The anterior pituitary gland is itself under the control of the hypothalamus which secretes releasing and inhibiting hormones (e.g. corticotropin releasing factor).

The glands of the second group are controlled by other stimuli, both chemical and neural.

The gastrointestinal tract also produces certain internal secretions, all of which are peptides and some of which, such as gastrin and secretin, fulfil the criteria necessary for their inclusion as hormones. Some of them are present in both the gastrointestinal tract and within the nervous system, where they appear to act as neurotransmitters. These are known as the 'brain-gut peptides' and include enkephalins, somatization and vasoactive intestinal peptide (VIP).

Disorders of the thyroid gland are common and relatively easy to understand; this gland is therefore considered first.

■ CLASSIFICATION OF HORMONES

- According to the mode of secretion and site of action:
  - *Endocrine:* Transmit molecular signal from a classic endocrinal cell through blood stream to a distant target cell.
  - *Neurocrine hormones:* Peptides secreted to blood from neurosecretary neuron, e.g. oxytocin, vasopressin.
  - *Paracrine hormones:* Chemical messengers secreted by a cell carried over short distance by diffusion through the interstitial spaces (extracellular fluid) to act on the neighboring different cell types.
  - *Autocrine hormones:* Chemical messengers which regulate the activity of neighboring similar type of cells, e.g. prostaglandins.
- According to the chemical structure:
  - Amines or amino acid derivatives. These include catecholamines (epinephrine norepinephrine) Thyroxine (T4) and Triiodo-thyronine (T3).
  - *Proteins and polypeptides:* Include posterior pituitary hormones. ADH, oxytocin, insulin, glucagon, parathormone, other anterior pituitary hormones.
  - *Steroid hormones:* Include glucocorticoids, mineralocorticoids, sex steroids and vitamin D.
- Group I and Group II hormones according to the mechanism of action:
  Group I: They act by binding to intracellular receptor and mediate their actions via formation of a hormone receptor complex, e.g. retinoid, and thyroid hormones.
  Group II: These involve second messenger to mediate their effect. Group II hormones further subdivided according to the nature of second messenger.
  Mechanism of action:
  Group I: Open or close ion channels in cell membrane, e.g. (1) ACh on nicotinic cholinergic receptor, (2). Norepinephrine on K^+ channel in the heart.
  Group II: Cytoplasmic or nuclear receptors to increase transcription of selected mRNAs, e.g. thyroid hormones, retinoic acid, steroid hormone.
- Depending on the chemical nature of second messenger
  - Activate phospholipase C with intracellular production of DAG,

IP3 and other inositol phosphates, e.g. angiotensin II, norepinephrine via α1 adrenergic receptors, vasopressin via V1 receptors.
- Activate or inhibit adenylyl cyclase causing increased or decreased production of cAMP, e.g. Norepinephrine via β1 adrenergic receptor (↑cAMP), norepinephrine via α2 adrenergic receptor.
- Increase cGMP in the cell, e.g. ANP, Nitric oxide (NO), EDRF.
- Increase tyrosine kinase activity of cytoplasmic portions of transmembrane receptors, e.g. insulin, EGF, PDGF, MCSF.
- Increase serine or threonine kinase activity, e.g. TGFβ, MAP K3.

PITUITARY GLAND

Small gland 0.5–1 gm in weight. Connected to hypothalamus by pituitary stalk.
- Anterior pituitary: Adenohypophysis
- Posterior pituitary: Neurohypophysis
- Pars intermedia.

Cell Types and Hormones in the Anterior Pituitary

- Chromophobes → inactive with few secretary granules
- Chromophils
  - Acidophils
  - Basophils

Five types of chromophils:

1. Somatotropes → GH (30–40%) } Acidophil
2. Lactotropes (mammotropes) → prolactin
3. Corticotropes - ACTH and βLPH (20%)
   Others-3–5%
4. Thyrotropes - TSH } Basophils
5. Gonadotropes

Posterior Pituitary

- Supraoptic - Oxytocin
- Paraventricular - Vasopressin.

THE PITUITARY GLAND (HYPOPHYSIS)

This is a gland about 1 cm (0.4 in) in diameter, situated at the base of the brain in the saddle shaped depression in the sphenoid bone known as sella turcica. Its attachment to the brain is by a short stalk placed just behind the optic chiasma where the optic nerves from each eye meet.

The pituitary gland consists of two parts, the anterior and posterior lobes, which have different modes of development and entirely different functions. Both are under the control of the hypothalamus but by different mechanisms. A neural mechanism between the hypothalamus and pituitary controls the secretion of hormones by the posterior lobe. The secretion of anterior pituitary hormones is controlled by stimulatory and inhibitory factors or hormones which are secreted by the hypothalamus. These factors are secreted into the blood of the portal venous system which runs in the pituitary stalk and they are thereby carried to the anterior pituitary gland. The control of secretion of hypothalamic, anterior pituitary and dependent peripheral glands is by feedback loops which 'turn off' the trophic hormone when the peripheral gland has secreted enough hormone to achieve normal plasma levels (Figs 14.1 and 14.2).

ANTERIOR PITUITARY HORMONES

Functions of the Anterior Pituitary (Adenohypophysis)

Six hormones are produced by the anterior lobe of the pituitary gland. They are the thyroid stimulating hormone (TSH), corticotropin or adrenocorticotropic hormone (ACTH), growth hormone (GH), follicle stimulating hormone (FSH), luteinizing hormone (LH) and prolactin (PRL).

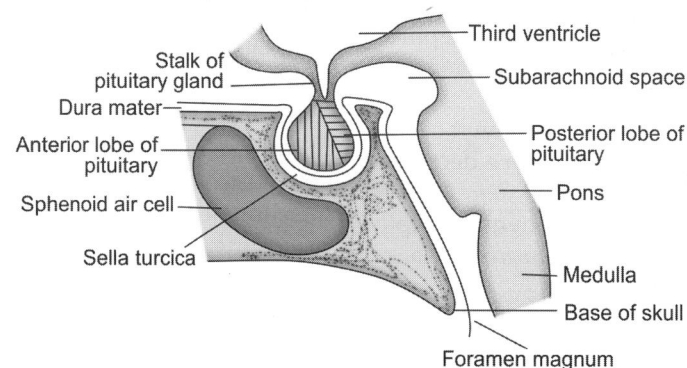

Fig. 14.1: Pituitary gland

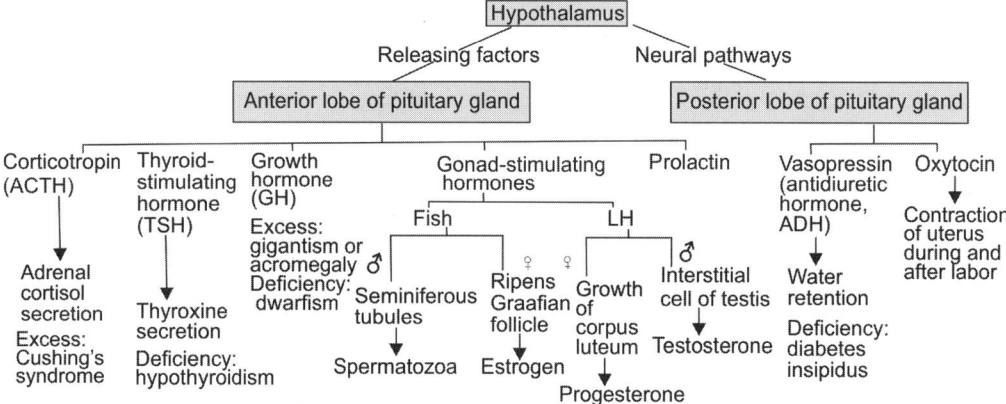

Fig. 14.2: Functions of the pituitary gland

Thyroid Stimulating Hormone

This stimulates the growth and activity of the thyroid gland. The release of TSH into the circulation is stimulated by thyrotropin-releasing hormone (TRH) from the hypothalamus. Its production is inhibited by a high circulating triiodothyronine (T_3) level.

Corticotropin

Adrenocorticotropic hormone (ACTH) promotes the production of steroid hormones, especially cortisol, in the suprarenal cortex. The circulating level of cortisol provides feedback to the pituitary and to the hypothalamus, which controls the anterior pituitary by its secretion of corticotropin-releasing factor (CRF). There is diurnal variation in the secretion of ACTH; resulting in plasma cortisol levels being at their peak at about 6 am and at their lowest at about midnight. This fact forms the basis of a screening test for Cushing's disease, in which there is hypersecretion of cortisol and the diurnal variation is lost.

Melanocyte pigmentation is also under the control of ACTH and patients with Addison's disease, in whom there is adrenal insufficiency (hypofunction), are abnormally pigmented as a result of loss of the negative feedback normally provided by cortisol.

Growth Hormone (GH) (Somatotropin)

This influences the synthesis by the liver of a group of proteins known as somatomedins and thereby exerts its effect on growth. The release of GH from the anterior pituitary is inhibited by somatostatin, which occurs in the hypothalamus and in the pancreatic islets.

Growth hormone promotes protein synthesis and antagonizes the actions of insulin on carbohydrate metabolism. Oversecretion of growth hormone in childhood leads to excessive growth in the length of bones and the condition known as gigantism. Hypersecretion of growth hormone in adult life, when the length-wise growth of long bones has ceased, results in enlargement of bone and soft tissues, producing a condition known as acromegaly, in which the bones of the face, hands and feet enlarge while the lips become thick and the facial features become coarse. Under-secretion of GH, in children results in failure of growth, with normal proportionment and normal mental development. As soon as the diagnosis is made, injections of growth hormone are begun with the aim of achieving as much normal growth as possible before the epiphyses fuse under the influence of the sex hormones.

The Gonadotropins (FSH and LH)

Follicle-stimulating hormone (FSH) brings about the ripening of ovarian follicles, with attendant estrogen production, in the female, and stimulates spermatogenesis in the male.

Luteinizing hormone (LH) causes ovulation and formation of the corpus luteum, which secretes progesterone, in women, and stimulates the testis to produce testosterone in men.

The release of gonadotropic (gonad-stimulating) hormones from the anterior pituitary is stimulated by the gonadotropin-releasing hormone (GnRH). Production of the latter is inhibited by estrogens and to a lesser extent by progestogens (progesterone-like substances), a fact upon which the effectiveness of the contraceptive pill depends.

Prolactin

This hormone promotes lactation. Its secretion is under the control of the hypothalamus, TRH acting as a prolactin-releasing factor and prolactin inhibiting factor (PIF) inhibiting the secretion of prolactin.

The serum prolactin level rises normally during pregnancy and is very high during lactation. Infertility is the principal effect of pathologically elevated serum prolactin levels which may result from any one of a number of causes, including a pituitary tumor and certain drugs, including phenothiazines.

The actions of the various hormones have been individually described but in health they all work together and in disease there may be multiple deficiencies, as in Simmond disease (panhypopituitarism).

Functions of the Posterior Pituitary (Neurohypophysis)

The hormones of the posterior lobe of the pituitary gland are vasopressin and oxytocin. They are synthesized in the hypothalamus and use neural pathways to reach the posterior pituitary, where they are stored prior to release into the circulation.

Vasopressin (Antidiuretic Hormone, ADH)

This causes the reabsorption of water into the blood from the collecting ducts of the kidneys, thereby concentrating the urine and reducing its volume. The function of vasopressin is to maintain a normal plasma osmolality (270–290 mOsm/kg) and plasma volume. Its release depends upon signals from osmoreceptors in the hypothalamus and volume (stretch) receptors in the walls of the atria of the heart and in the great veins. A rise in plasma osmolality and a low plasma volume both result in an increase in vasopressin release, which causes retention of water by the kidney until the osmotic pressure and volume of the plasma are again within the normal range. Vasopressin release is also affected by pain, emotional stress, alcohol and certain drugs.

Oxytocin

This is released from the posterior pituitary by a neural mechanism and causes contraction of the smooth muscle of the uterus and breast. Suckling stimulates neural pathways and the consequent release of oxytocin from the pituitary causes ejection of milk from the lactating breast.

Oxytocin is used only in obstetrics. Vasopressin is used in the treatment of diabetes insipidus of pituitary type, in which large volumes of dilute urine are passed.

Hypothalamus produce hypothalamic releasing and inhibiting hormones. Hypothalamus control and pituitary through hypothalamic hypo physical portal vessels.

The anterior pituitary is a highly vascular gland. The capillary sinuses among the glandular cells are connected with capillary bed at the lower hypothalamus through small hypothalamic hypophysical portal vessels. Small arteries penetrate into the substance of median eminence and small vessels return to its surface forming hyphothalamic-hypophyseal portal vessels. The hypothalamic releasing and inhibitory hormones are secreted by special nervous originating in various parts of hypothalamus and sending nerve fibers to median eminence and tuber cinereum which is an extension of hypothalamic tissue into pituitary stalk. These hormones are absorbed into hypothalamo-hypophyseal portal system and carried to anterior pituitary sinuses. Most of the anterior pituitary hormones are controlled by releasing hormones except prolactin which is controlled by hypothalamic inhibitory hormone.

- *Thyrotropin releasing hormone:* Control TSH.
- *Corticotropin releasing hormone:* Control ACTH
- Growth hormone releasing hormone (Somatostatin)
  - GHRH
  - GHIH
- *Gonadotropin releasing hormone:* GHRH. Cause release of 2 gonadotropic hormones, LH and FSH.
- Prolactin inhibitory hormone PIH inhibit prolactin secretion.

■ GROWTH HORMONE (GH)

Growth hormone (somatotropic hormone) or somatotropin. It is a small protein molecule that contains 191 AA in a single chain and has molecular weight of 22,005.

Metabolic Effects of GH

- ↑ Protein synthesis
  - Enhanced AA transport through cell membrane
  - Enhanced RNA translation to cause protein synthesis
  - Increased transcription of DNA to form RNA
  - Decreased catabolism of protein and amino acids.
  So act as a protein sparer for energy purpose.
- ↑ Fat utilization for energy
  - Release of FFA from adipose tissue increase
  - FA → acetyl CoA (for utilization for energy)
  - Formation of more aceto acetic acid by liver causing ketosis and fatty liver.
- Decrease carbohydrate utilization
  - Decrease glucose uptake in skeletal muscle and fat.
  - Increase glucose produced by liver
  - Increase insulin secretion due to insulin resistance. (So decrease utilization of glucose) Diabetogenic effect

- Stimulate cartilage and bone growth.
  - Increased deposition of protein by chondrocyte and osteogenic cells, increased reproduction of these cells. Increase new bone formation.
- Increase in plasma phosphorus, decrease B-UN and AA levels. Gastrointestinal absorption of Ca^{++} is increased. K^+, Na^+ excretion reduced.

■ SOMATOMEDINS OR INSULIN LIKE GROWTH FACTORS

Growth hormone causes the liver to form several small proteins called somatomedins that in turn have the potent effect of increasing all aspects of bone growth. These effects are similar to insulin and so somatomedins are also called IGF4. Somatomedins have been isolated and the most important of these is somatomedin C (IGFI). Mol.wt – 7500. Pygmies of Africa have congenital inability to synthesize significant amount of somatomedin C and they are of small stature even though their plasma concentration of growth hormone are normal or high. Levi-Lorains dwarfs also have the same problem. GH attaches only weekly to the plasma proteins in the blood. Therefore, rapidly released into tissues (½ life < 20 min). Somatomedin C attaches strongly to a carrier protein in blood and is released only slowly from blood to tissues (½ life 20 hrs). This prolongs the growth promoting effects of the bursts of GH secretion.

Physiological Stimuli that Increase GH Secretion (Fig. 14.3)

- Starvation
- Hypoglycemia
- Exercise
- Excitement
- Trauma
  It increases during first 2 hours of deep sleep. Normal plasma level of GH.

Adult: 1.6–3 ng/mL
Adolescent: 6 ng/mL

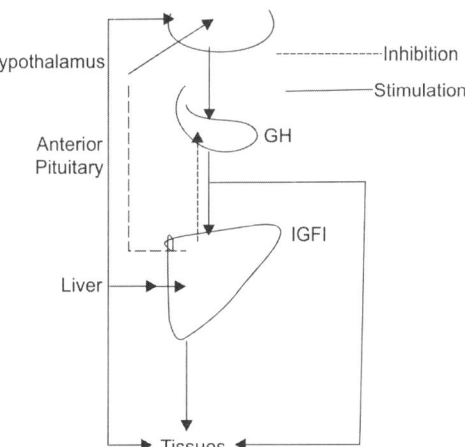

Fig. 14.3: Feedback control of growth hormone secretion

GHRH: Secreted by ventromedial nucleus. (satiety center—sensitive to blood glucose concentration).

Regulation of Growth Hormone Secretion (Table 14.1)

The growth hormone secretion deceases only slowly with aging falling to 25% of adolescent level in very old age. Several factors related to person's state of nutrition or stress stimulate secretion.

Table 14.1: Factors affecting GH secretion

Stimuli that increase secretion	Decrease secretion
1. Deficiency of energy substrate	
Hypoglycemia	REM sleep
Deoxy glucose	Glucose
Exercise	Cortisol
Fasting	FFA
2. Increase in circulating levels of AA	
Protein meal	Medroxy progesterone
Infusion of arginine	Growth hormone
Glucagen	
3. Stress full stimulation	
Pyrogen	
Lysine vasopressin	
Psychological stress	
4. Sleep, L-dopa and adrenergic	
Agents, Apomorphine	
Estrogen, Androgens	

Table 14.2: Short-term and long-term effect of GH

Short-term effect	Long-term effect
Increase Ca^{++} ion transport into cell → exocytosis of GH secretory genes vesicles synthesis. ↓ Release of GH into blood	Increase transcription in the nucleus by the to cause new GH

For example, it increases during the first 2 hrs of deep sleep. Normal plasma level of GH of adult - 1.6–3 mg/mL under severe conditions of protein malnutrition adequate calories alone are not sufficient to correct the excess production of GH. Instead the protein deficiency must be corrected before the growth hormone concentration will return to normal (Table 14.2).

GHRH → attaches to GH cells in pituitary gland → adenyl cyclase cAMP

GH receptors → 620AA protein with 3 subunits.
1. Large extracellular portion
2. Transmembrane domain
3. Large cytoplasmic portion

GH has 2 binding sites for receptors which attaches to 2 subunits of receptors producing a homodimer (Flowchart 14.1).

Ghrelin: Mainly synthesized in stomach and also by hypothalamus stimulate GH and regulate food intake.

Flowchart 14.1: Mechanism of receptor activation

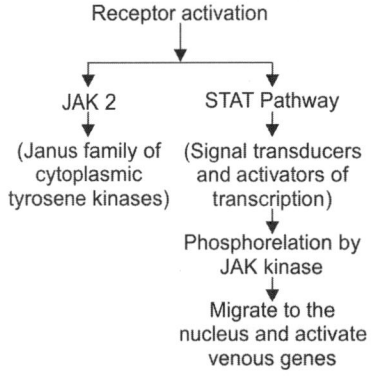

Abnormalities of Growth Hormone Secretion

Dwarfism: Here the dwarfism is proportionate. Short stature can be due to GRH deficiency, growth hormone deficiency deficient secretion of IGF-I or other causes. Isolated GH deficiency is often due to GRH deficiency and in this instance the GH response to GRH is normal.

In another groups of dwarfed children, the plasma GH concentration is normal or elevated but GH receptors are unresponsive due to loss of function mutations of gene for the receptors. The resulting condition is known growth hormone insensitivity or Laron dwarfism. IGF-I and IGF BP I is markedly reduced. African pygmies have normal plasma GH levels and a modest reduction in the plasma level of GH BP (growth hormone binding protein). Their plasma IGF-I concentration fails to increase at the time of puberty. Less growth in prepubertal period also.

Other Causes of Short Stature

Short stature is characteristic of cretinism and occurs in patients with precocious puberty. It is also part of the syndrome of gonadal dysgenesis seen in patients with XO chromosomal pattern instead of XX or XY pattern. Various bone and metabolic diseases also cause stunted growth (constitutional delayed growth).

Chronic abuse and neglect can also cause dwarfism in children. This is known as psychosocial dwarfism or the Kasper Hauser syndrome.

Achondroplasia the most common form of dwarfism in humans is characterized by short limbs with normal trunk. It is an autosomal dominant condition caused by a mutation in the gene that codes for fibroblast growth factor receptor 3 (FGFR3).

Pituitary dwarfism: Treatment is GH developed by recombinant DNA technology.

■ PITUITARY INSUFFICIENCY IN HUMANS

- Tumors of the anterior pituitary.
- Suprasellar cysts remnants of Rathke's pouch that enlarge and compress the pituitary.
- In women shock due to postpartum hemorrhage causing pituitary infarction and postpartum necrosis (Sheehan's syndrome)
- Hemorrhagic fever in Korea causes diffuse vasculitis causing pituitary enlargement as a result of edema.

Features

- Related to changes in other endocrine glands.
  - Atrophy of adrenal cortex result in fall in adrenal glucocorticoids and sex hormones.
  - No mineralocorticoid deficiency. Stress induced secretion of aldosterone are absent.
  - No increase in glucocorticoid secretion in stress. So patients with pituitary insufficiency are sensitive to stress.
  - Decrease growth, cold intolerance, low thyroid function.
  - Atrophy of gonads, stoppage of sexual cycles some secondary sex-characters disappear.
  - The hypoglycemic effect of insulin increase partly due to deficiency of adrenal cortical hormones and also due to lack of anti-insulin effect GH.
  - *Water metabolism:* Transient polyurea ACTH deficiency → decrease protein catabolism
  TSH deficiency → decrease metabolic rate, decreased filtration osmotically active products. So urine volume declines.
  GH deficiency → decrease GFR, decrease RPF.

■ PANHYPOPITUITARISM IN THE ADULT

Causes

- Craniopharyngioma
- Chromophobe tumors compressing pituitary
- Thrombosis of pituitary blood vessels.

Effects

- Hypothyroidism
- Depressed production of glucocorticoids by adrenal
- Suppressed gonadotropins and sexual functions lost.
- Weight gain due to lack of fat metabolism by GH, ACTH, adrenocortical and thyroid hormones.

Treatment

Administer adrenocortical and thyroid hormones.

■ PITUITARY HYPERFUNCTION

- Gigantism in children
- Acromegaly in adults

Gigantism

Acidophilic GH secreting cells of anterior pituitary gland become excessively active or acidophilic tumors develop in the gland. Large quantities of GH produced lead to rapid growth of body tissues including bones. If the condition occurs before fusion of epiphysis of long bones height increase. So that the person becomes a giant as tall as 8 feet. Giants ordinarily has hyperglycemia. Islets of Langerhan's β cells are prone to degenerate because they become overactive due to hyperglycemia. Giants 10% develop full blown DM.

Rx microsurgical removal of the tumor.

Acromegaly

Hyper secretion of GH is accompanied by hyper secretion of prolactin in 20–40% of patients with acromegaly. Acromegaly can be caused by extra pituitary as well as intra pituitary GH secreting tumors and by hypothalamic tumors that secrete GRH.

Findings

- Local effects tumor-enlargement of the sella turcica, headache, visual disturbances
- *GH secretion:* There is enlargement of heads and feet (acral parts)
- Protrusion of the lower jaw
- Over growth of the (prognathism) malar, frontal and facial bones combines with prognathism to produce coarse facial features called acromegalic facies
- Body hair increased in amount
- Skeletal changes predispose to osteoarthritis
- 25% patients have abnormal GTT and 4% develop lactation in the absence of pregnancy.

Cushing's Syndrome

Bilaterally hyperplastic adrenals have small ACTH secreting pituitary tumors (micro adenomas) that are difficult to detect.

Some develop rapidly developing ACTH secreting pituitary tumors (Nelson's syndrome). It cause hyper pigmentation of skin, neurological signs due to pressure on structures in the sellar region. Some are malignant. Blood ACTH levels extremely high. Intrinsic MSH activity accounts for skin pigmentation.

Hypothalamic Releasing and Inhibitory Hormones are Secreted into the Median Eminence

Special neurons in the hypothalamus synthesize and secrete the hypothalamic releasing and inhibitory hormones that control secretion of anterior pituitary hormones. These neurons originate in various parts of the hypothalamus and send nerve fibers to the median eminence and tuber cinereum an extension of hypothalamic tissue into the pituitary stalk. The endings of these fibers are different from most endings in the CNS in that their function is not to transmit signals from one neuron to another but rather to secrete the hypothalamic releasing and inhibitory hormones into the tissue fluids. These hormones are immediately absorbed into the hypothalamic-hypophyseal portal system and carried directly into the sinuses of the anterior pituitary gland.

Hypothalamic Releasing and Inhibitory Hormones Control Anterior Pituitary Secretion

For most of the anterior pituitary hormones, it is the releasing hormones that are important but for prolactin a hypothalamic inhibitory hormone probably exerts most control. The major hypothalamic releasing and inhibitory hormones are the following:

- Thyrotropin-releasing hormone, which causes release of thyroid stimulating hormone.
- Corticotropin releasing hormone which causes release of adreno corticotropin.
- *Growth hormone:* Releasing hormone, which causes release of GH and GHIH and also called somatostation, which inhibits release of growth hormone.
- Gonadotropin releasing hormone (GnRH), which causes release of the two gonadotropic hormones, luteinizing hormones and follicle stimulating hormone.
- Prolactin inhibitory hormone (PIH) which causes inhibition of prolactin secretion.

Specific Areas in the Hypothalamus Control Secretion of Specific Hypothalamic Releasing and Inhibitory Hormones

All or most of the hypothalamic hormones are secreted at nerve endings in the median eminence before being transported to the anterior pituitary gland. Electrical stimulation of this region excites these nerve endings and causes release of essentially all the hypothalamic hormones. However, the neuronal cell bodies that give rise to these median eminence nerve endings are located in other discrete areas of the hypothalamus or closely related areas of the basal brain. The specific loci of the neuronal cell bodies that form the different hypothalamic releasing or inhibitory hormones are still unknown.

Bone Growth Takes Place by Two Mechanism

One in response to GH stimulation, the long bones grow in length at the epiphyseal cartilage where epiphysis at the ends of the bone is separated from the shaft. These epiphyses are pushed further apart and the epiphyseal cartilage is progressively used up. So by late adolescence, no additional epiphyseal cartilage remains to provide for the long bone growth and bony fusion between shaft and epiphysis takes place at each end. Second, osteoblasts in the bone periosteum and in some bone cavities deposit new bone on the surface of older bone, at the same time osteoclasts removing the old bone. When the rate of deposition is greater than resorption thickness of bone increases. GH strongly stimulate the osteoblasts. This growth in thickness occurs even after adolescence in mainly membranous bones namely jaw bones causing protrusion of the chin and lower teeth. Bone grows in thickness to give rise to bony protrusions over the eyes.

Catabolism is decreased in hypophysectomized animals. Because of TSH deficiency metabolic rate is low consequently former osmotically active products of catabolism are filtered and urine volume declines even in the absence of vasopressin. GH deficiency contributes to the depression of the GFR in hypophysectomised animals and GH increases the GFR and renal plasma flow in humans. Due to glucocorticoid deficiency there is some defective excretion of a water load. The climatic activity of anterior pituitary can thus be explained in terms of creations of ACTH, TSH and GH.

Most of the patients with GH deficiency developing in adulthood have deficiencies of anterior pituitary hormones. Deficiency of ACTH and other pituitary hormone with MSH activity may be responsible for pallor of the skin in patients with hypopituitarism.

■ POSTERIOR PITUITARY

Posterior pituitary consists of nerve ending and pituicytes. Pituicytes are supporting cells and do not secrete any hormone. Nerves originate in the supraoptic and paraventricular nucleus of nervous system. Nerve fibers pass through pituitary stalk, reach postpituitary. Nerve endings are bulbous ending and called herring bodies. They secrete hormones.

Antidiuretic hormone and oxytocin: These hormones are synthesized in cell bodies packed into secretary granules, transported by axoplasmic transport, secreted in response to appropriate stimuli. Antidiuretic hormone and oxytocin secreted by separate neurons. Both neurons present in supraoptic and paraventricular nucleus. Supraoptic contains more of neurons secreting ADH. Oxytocin mainly secreted by paraventricular nucleus. Oxytocin are typical neural hormone secreted into blood by nerve cells.

ADH or vasopressin: Precursor prepropressophysin.

Signal peptide: ADH, Neurophysin II, Glycopeptide.

Oxytocin

Signal peptide oxytocin: Neurophysin I
Secretary granules (herring bodies) are released on appropriate stimuli.

Both the hormones contain 9AA

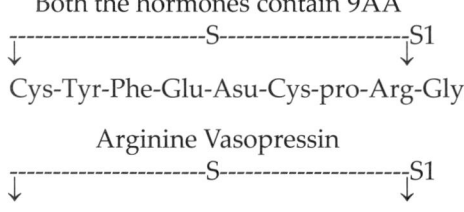

Cys-Tyr-Phe-Glu-Asu-Cys-pro-Arg-Gly

Arginine Vasopressin

Cys-Tyr-leu-Glu-Asu-Cys-pro-Leu-Gly

Oxytocin

Circulatory half-life 80 mins, both metabolized in liver and kidney.

ADH (AVP)

ADH receptors are of 3 types V1A, V1B, V2. V1A and V1B act by increasing intracellular Ca^{++} concentration.

Actions

- *Antidiuretic Action:*
  - Acts on collecting ducts
  - Increase permeability of collecting duct to water thus conserve water.
  - ADH +V2 receptor of principle cells of collecting duct
  - Increase cAMP increases permeability of CD
  - Water reabsorption
- *Urine volume decrease:* Inside the cell ADH causes their rapid translocation into the luminal membrane. This translocation occurs in 5–8 min, when ADH secretion stops. Water enters into hypertonic renal interstitium leading to water retention and effective osmotic pressure of body fluid will be reduced.
- *Vasopressure action:* Very high concentrations ADH combine with V1A receptors present in vascular smooth muscle
  - Increase intracellular Ca^{++}
  - Increase arterial BP.

Regulation of ADH Secretion

Osmotic Stimuli: Principle stimuli that regulate ADH secretion. The normal plasma osmolality is 285 million osmols/kg. When plasma osmolality increases, this increase is sensed by osmoreceptors present in or near the hypothalamus. These osmoreceptor sent in signals to SO and PV nuclei (mainly SO).

- Increase ADH
- Increase permeability of CD
- Increase water reabsorption
- Plasma concentrations become normal.

Plasma concentration increase → osmoreceptor ⟨ ADH → ↓ output / Thirst → ↑ intake ⟩

Plasma concentration normal

Plasma osmolality 285 mOsmol/kg is the threshold for thirst.

Osmoreceptor that mediate thirst are the same and threshhold for thirst may be almost higher, when fluid is pulled out of osmoreceptor.

Volume Effects

This is the second major effects of ADH.

Changes circulating blood volume = decrease blood volume → decrease BP → decrease stimulation of stretch receptors → increase ADH → decrease renal excretion of H_2O → blood volume and BP normal.

Severe hypertension → high concentration of ADH → vasoconstriction → increase BP.

Stimuli that Increase ADH Secretion

- Increase plasma osmolality
- Decrease ECF volume
- Nausea and vomiting
- Pain emotion - stress exercises
- Angeotensin II.

Stimuli that Decrease ADH Secretion

- Decrease plasma osmolality
- Increase ECF volume
- Alcohol.

Abnormalities of ADH Secretion

Syndrome of inappropriate hypersecretion of ADH (SIADH).
Causes: Cerebral, pulmonary, heart, liver, kidney disease.
Features: Decrease water excretion, hypo-osmolality hyponatremia.
   Hyponatremia due to dilutional hyponatremia and also due to suppression of aldosterone leading to loss of salt in urine.
Treatment: Restrict water intake
   Demeclocycline → reduces renal response to ADH.

Posterior Pituitary: Abnormalities

Hyposecretion of ADH: Diabetes insipidus decrease renal response to ADH.
   Neoplasmic lesion, systemic lesions
   Nephrogenic → deficiency of V2 receptor, or aquaporin 2.
Clinical features: Polyuria, polydipsia severe dehydration.
Rx: Arginine vasopressin, desmopressin, Synthetic AVP
Mechanism: High antidiuretic action. Pressor action is less.

Function of Oxytocin

Milk Ejection

Oxytocin receptor present in breast and uterus. These are coupled with G protein. It triggers increase in intracellular calcium. It is a neuroendocrine reflex. In this case afferent is neural, efferent pathway is endocrine.
   Sucking of nipple; touch receptor in nipple and areola stimulated, through somatic touch pathway reach brainstem, supraoptic and paraventricular nuclei, center is stimulated oxytocin release enter blood reach breast effector organ is myoepithelial cells surrounding mammary alveoli.
Synthesis of milk: Prolactin from anterior pituitary and secretion into mammary alveoli contraction of myoepithelial cell milk is squeezed into mammary alveoli. All this occurs in 30 sec to 1 min.
Milk let down: When mother hears baby's cry or poddles baby, impulse reach hypothalamus, oxytocin release causes milk ejection. Mother worried, mother will not be able to nurse the baby.
Alcohol: Inhibit milk ejection reflex.

Effect on Pregnant Uterus

Expelling fetus and placenta during labor causes contraction of uterine smooth muscle. It will contract. Sensitivity of myometrium to oxytocin increase by estrogen, and inhibited by progesterone.
   Number of oxytocin receptors increase during pregnancy and reach peak during labor. Estrogens increase the number of oxytocin receptor in the myometrium. Oxytocin levels are not increased during early labor. But marked increase in oxytocin receptor will cause increased action during labor. Once uterine contraction occur, uterus has to contract and cervix has to dilate and distension of vagina, stimuli from cervix and vagina reach hypothalamus and oxytocin released. It is a positive feedback reaction, until fetus and placenta expelled.
   Oxytocin can cause increase PG synthesis which in turn can cause uterine contraction.

Postpartum Contraction of Uterus

Action on Non-pregnant uterus: Helps in sperm transport and genital stimulation will lead to increased oxytocin secretion cause uterine contraction to propel sperm into fallopian tube.

During ejaculation increased oxytocin help contraction of SM of vas deference and propel sperm into the urethra.

Disorders

Excess: Not reported
Deficiency: Failure to nurse the baby.
Use: Induction of labor when uterine contractions are poor and impaired ejection.

■ THE THYROID GLAND

The thyroid gland (Fig. 14.4) is situated in the lower part of the neck and when enlarged it forms the once familiar goiter. It consists of two lobes, one on either side of the trachea, joined together by an isthmus which passes in from of the trachea just below the cricoid cartilage. The lobes are conical and have upper and lower poles, the upper pole extending to the side or wing of the thyroid cartilage. It receives its plentiful blood supply from the superior and inferior thyroid arteries which are respectively branches of the external carotid and subclavian arteries. In the groove between the trachea and esophagus on each side of the neck, the recurrent laryngeal nerve lies in close relationship to the thyroid gland and may be damaged by a carcinoma of the gland or by thyroid surgery, resulting in a change in the voice.

Microscopically, the thyroid contains two types of hormone-producing cell, the follicular cells which produce thyroid hormones and the C (clear) cells which produce calcitonin. The shape of the follicular cells depends upon whether or not they are being stimulated by thyrotrophic (thyroid stimulating hormone, TSH), derived from the pituitary and circulating in the blood.

The thyroid gland stores large amounts of thyroid hormones in an inactive form, called colloid, within compartments called follicles, which are lined by follicular cells. The colloid consists of thyroglobulin and is produced by the follicular cells. These cells are also responsible for converting it into the thyroid hormones, triiodothyronine (T_3) and thyroxine (T_4) and releasing them into the bloodstream. Thyroxine is the main hormone secreted by the thyroid but itself relatively inactive. The active hormone is triiodothyronine and, by its action on cells, it regulates the basal metabolic rate and influences growth and maturation, particularly of nerve tissue.

Both thyroid hormones contain a high proportion of iodine which the thyroid gland 'traps' from the blood. It is particularly this stage (the trapping of iodide) of thyroid hormone production that is influenced by TSH. In turn the release of TSH from

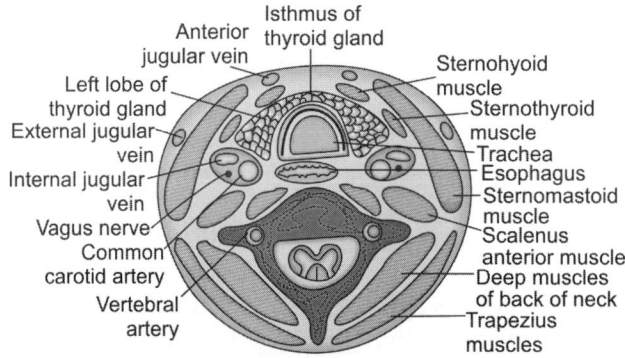

Fig. 14.4: Transverse section of the neck at the level of the seventh cervical vertebra showing the position of important structures

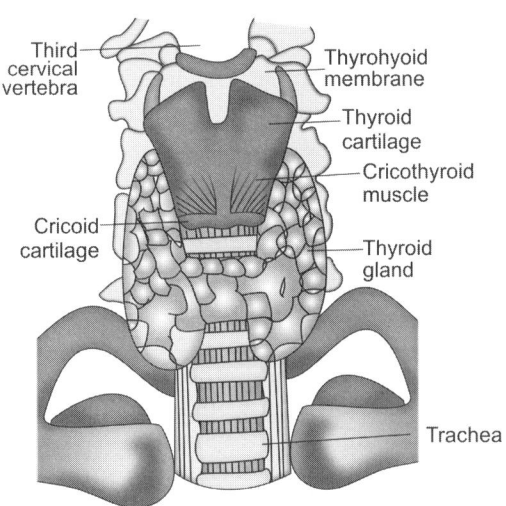

Fig. 14.5: The larynx, the thyroid gland and the cervical portion of the trachea

the anterior pituitary is stimulated by thyrotrophin-releasing hormone (TRH) secreted by the hypothalamus. There are feedback mechanisms to inhibit the secretion of TSH and TRH (Fig. 14.5).

The iodine required for thyroid hormone synthesis is obtained from foods, especially sea foods, and drinking water. In all continents, there are regions in which the soil is deficient in iodine. If these are inland regions, in which sea fish are rarely eaten and the population lives mainly on local foods, the iodine deficiency will manifest itself among the inhabitants by enlargement of the thyroid gland to form a goiter. At one time, this was prevalent in the Peak District of England and was known as 'Derbyshire Neck.' Such 'endemic' goiters may still be found in the Andes and the Himalayas.

A goiter may also be found in some patients who have no dietary deficiency of iodine but who have thyroid disease. It is most often found with hypersecretion of the gland, which causes thyrotoxicosis, in which there is loss of weight despite a good appetite, indicating that the rate of general metabolism is increased. Other clinical features are nervousness and restlessness, increased sweating, hot moist hands, a rapid pulse, a tremor, and protrusion of the eyeballs (exophthalmos).

Under activity (hyposecretion) of the thyroid gland produces cretinism in infants and myxedema in adults. In contrast with the appearance of extreme nervousness seen in hyperthyroidism, the patient often has a mentally dull appearance and there is slowness of speech and movement. The skin is dry and thick and the pulse is slow. The body temperature tends to be subnormal and these patients are at risk from hypothermia. The metabolism of the body is slowed down and this is reflected in the reduced level of bodily activity. Myxedema and cretinism are both treated by administering thyroxin by mouth, thereby supplying the missing factor; this is called substitution therapy.

The C cells, or parafollicular cells of the thyroid gland produce the hormone calcitonin which lowers blood calcium levels. Its secretion is controlled solely by the level of calcium in the blood, providing another example of a feedback mechanism.

■ THE THYROID

Thyroid means shield like. Weighs between 15–20 gm in adults. Microscopically, the glands contain about 3 million follicles. Each follicle is lined by a single row of epithelial cells called follicular cells. Follicle is filled up by a structure less material called colloid. Parafollicular or C cells are found between the lining follicular epithelium and the basement membrane of the follicle. Follicular epithelial cells synthesis the T3, T4 while C cells produces calcitonin.

Biosynthesis

Iodine containing foods are taken → food iodine reduced to KI in GIT → KI reaches the thyroid gland through blood.

- From blood KI is taken by follicular cells and it is called iodide trapping. The iodide trapping takes place against electrochemical gradient and requires energy expenditure and extra O_2 usage. Na^+/K^+-ATPase is required for iodide trapping.
- *Oxidation of iodide:* KI is oxidized to atomic iodine (I) by the help of enzyme thyroperoxidase. H_2O_2 is required for this oxidation.
- *Organification:* Follicular cells also synthesize thyroglobulin. Thyroglobulin contains many tyrosenes in its polypeptide chains. Iodine atoms get attached with these tyrosene to form MIT (monoiodotyrosene) or DIT (diiodotyrosine) molecules. This is organification of iodine. MIT and DIT still remain attached with the thyroglobulin and the whole molecule is within the follicular cell. TSH facilitates organification, while propyl thiouracil inhibit it. Thyroperoxidase catalyzes organification.
- *Coupling:* Two DIT molecules are coupled with each other. T4 is produced. 1MIT and 1DIT couples to form T3. This T3 or T4 is still attached to thyroglobulin and is within the follicular cells. Thyroperoxidase catalyzes the reaction. TSH facilitates iodine source, auto regulation.
  Sea food contains plenty coupling: Colloid expands and the follicular cells extrudes little thyroglobulin containing (T3 and T4).
- *Release:* When necessary, the apical portion of the follicular cell engulfs (endocytosis) a little thyroglobulin from food is the ultimate source of iodine to the body. Daily iodine requirement is 200 µgm.
  Colloid of the follicular spaces: Where it is digested by protease enzyme T3 and T4 released into the blood, of iodine. The iodine deficiency is common in hilly areas and sub-Himalayan regions of India. The iodide trapping mechanism become inefficient if food contains excess iodine.

Functions

Metamorphosis—Metabolism—Growth Development

Addition of thyroxine in the watery environment of tadpole accelerate metamorphosis—the tadpole becomes frog. T3 causes growth of CNS in the fetus and postnatal infants. Absence of thyroxine leads to cretinism (deficiency of growth in every aspect, mental, musculoskeletal and sexual).

Metabolism

Oxidative metabolism: Except brain and testis metabolism of all tissues are increased by thyroid hormones. T3 and T4 causes calorigenesis because higher consumption of O_2 means higher expenditure of calories (BMR increases in hyperthyroidism). Explanation for thyroid induced calorigenesis is:
- Na^+/K^+-ATPase stimulation + O_2 consumption
- Overworking of Ca^{++} pump in muscles.

Carbohydrate Metabolism

- T3 increases:
  - *Gluconeogenesis:* Production of glycogen from amino acids, lactic acid, and glycene
  - Glycogenolysis (glycogen breaking down to glucose) T3 enhances the efficiency of adrenalin to cause glycogenolysis.
- *T3 enhances the peripheral utilization of glucose:* Explanation is the demand of the tissues increases because of T3 induced calorigenesis. In hyperthyroidism, blood sugar level usually rises. The resistance of the target cells of insulin

rises due to excess T3. This may be a major factor contributing to the hyperglycemia of hyperthyrodism.

Lipid Metabolism

Hypothyroidism causes high cholesterol level. Thyroxine will raise the FFA level. T3 increases the number of LDL receptors so that more LDL can bind with the hepatocytes. → LDL contains cholesterol and cholesterol metabolism is increased → reduction of serum cholesterol level.

Adrenalin increases lipolysis and FFA is released from triglycerides. T3 potentiates adrenalin.

Protein Metabolism

- T3 enhances both anabolism and catabolism of protein. However, under physiological conditions anabolism supervenes. In hyperthyroidism muscle wasting (reduction of body weight) and increased gluconeogenesis (increase availability of AA) are common features.
- In hypothyroidism a protein + hyalaronic acid + chondroitin sulfate together form a complex. This complex attracts water and it stays in the skin and subcutaneous tissue. It causes local retention of water (non-pitting) edema. Thus hypothyroidism is otherwise called myxedema.

Mineral

T3 causes loss of calcium via urine, osteoporosis can develop in hyperthyroidism. In cretin (congenital thyroid deficiency) (Flowchart 14.2).
- Skeletal and muscular growth inhibited. So short stature, muscle weakness. But visceral growth is less restricted. Result:
  - Weak abdominal muscles but abdominal viscera of near normal volume—pot belly
  - Small mouth cavity but nearly normal sized tongue protruding tongue and dribbling of saliva.

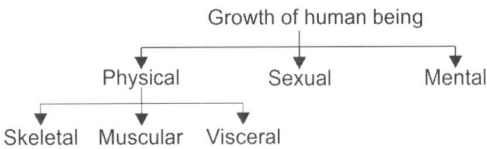

Flowchart 14.2: Growth of human being suffering from congenital thyroid deficiency

- *Sexual growth is stopped:* Small penis, small testes, no pubic hair, no axillary or chest hair and no libido.

  In females also infantile sex in girls no axillary or pubic hair, no breast development, no growth of vulva, vagina and uterus, no menstruation.
- *Mentally:* The child is an idiot (IQ below 70) or imbecile.

  Skeletal System: T3 potentiates the effects of GH, and IGF on bone growth and maturation.

  CNS: T3 required for growth and development of brain during fetal and postnatal periods. Lack of T3 causes lack of myelination of nerve fibers in the brain, number of nerve fibers in brain reduced and brain becomes smaller.

  Result: Child is an idiot, reflexes sluggish.

  CVS - ANS: Myocardial cells supplied by sympathetic nerves and have 1 receptors. 1 receptor increases in response to T3, so tachycardia and palpitation with slightest provocation occurs in hyperthyroidism. Gs protein show increased activity under the influence of T3, i.e. after adrenalin or noradrenalin binds with its receptor on cardiomyocyte signal transduction become more vigorous.
- *Temperature regulation:* Increased calorigenesis by T3, increased heat production. Sympathetic induced thermogenesis is potentiated by T3.
- *Blood:* Normocytic, hypochromic anemia.

Mechanism of Action

All cells of our body are target cells. Thyroid hormones enter cells and T3 binds to thyroid receptors (TR) in the nucleus. T4 can bind less avidly to nuclear receptors. HRC binds to DNA via zinc fingers to produce gene expression and production of hormone sensitive nuclear transcription factors.

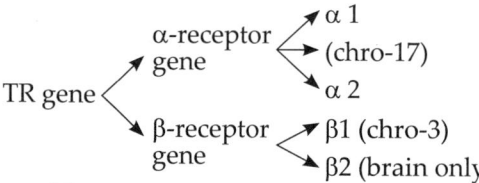

This gene expression lead to transcription of more specific proteins (enzymes) (e.g. Na^+K^+-ATPase).

Attention deficient hyperactivity disorder (ADHD) associated with TR resistance due to mutation of gene that code for TRβ. High T3, T4 levels children, who are overactive and impulsive.

Effect on CVS

- Tachycardia, increase force of contraction of myocardium → due to combined activity of T4 and catecholamines.
- Increase temperature, vasodilatation, decrease peripheral resistance, decrease diastolic BP, increase systolic BP, increase pulse pressure and mild decrease in mean BP.
- Decrease circulation time, increase velocity of blood flow causing inadequate tissue perfusion. High output cardiac failure. Shortness of breath on exertion.
- Increased myocardial O_2 utilization more than increase in coronary blood flow precipitate cardiac arrhythmias.

Effect on CNS

In Fetus or up to 2 Years of Age

Myelination, synapse formation abnormal. Vascular development in brain affected, causing infantile brain, mental retardation.

In Adults

- Loss of all intellectual functions.
- Memory loss.
- Slow speech due to hoarse slow voice.
- Mental and physical lethargy.
- α-wave in EEG not recordable.

Regulation of Thyroid Secretion

Hypothalam-pituitary-thyroid axis: The released T4 causes elevation of S. T4–T3 level → T3 inhibits.

- Primarily the thyrotropes
- Hypothalamus to a less extend by negative feedback, T4–T3 level remain normal (Fig. 14.6).

Cold: In young human infants and experimental animals exposure to cold increase TRH secretion → rise of T4–T3 level.

Somatostatin: Of HT, inhibits thyroid secretion.

Autoregulation: Excess supply of food iodine inhibits iodide trapping.

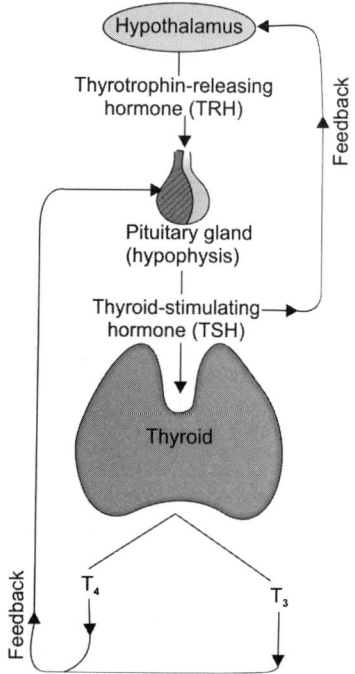

Fig. 14.6: The hypothalamus-hypophyseal control of thyroid function

ANTITHYROID DRUGS

Drugs that suppress secretion of thyroid gland are called antithyroid substances. For example, thiocyanate, propylthiouracil, High concentration of inorganic iodides.

Thiocyanate ions decrease iodide trapping. The active pump that transports iodide ions into the thyroid cells can also pump thiocyanate ions, perchlorate ions and nitrate ions. So thiocyanate in high concentration can cause competitive inhibition of iodide transport into the cell.

Propylthiouracil Decreases Thyoid Hormone Formation

Propylthiouracil, methimazole, carbinazole, etc. prevent formation of thyroid hormone from iodide and tyrosine. Mechanism is by blocking the peroxidase enzyme required for iodination of tyrosine and partly to block the coupling of 2 iodinated tyrosines to form T4 and T3.

Propylthiouracil does not prevent formation of thyroglobulin.

Iodides in High Concentrations Decrease Thyroid Activity and Thyroid Gland Size

When iodides are present in the blood in high concentration (100 times) most activities of thyroid gland are decreased, iodide trapping and iodination of tyrosine to form thyroid hormones are also decreased. The endocytosis of colloid from the follicles by the thyroid glandular cells is paralyzed by high iodide concentrations. So there is immediate shut down of thyroid hormone secretion into the blood.

Iodides in high concentration decrease all phases of thyroid activity, decrease the size of thyroid gland, and decrease blood supply. Iodides are administered to patients 2–3 weeks by surgical removal of thyroid gland to decrease the necessary amount of surgery and decrease amount of bleeding.

Hypothyroidism

Adult hypothyroidism is called myxedema
- May be secondary to pituitary failure
- Hypothalamic failure

In these two conditions thyroid respond to a test doze of TSH.

Hypothalamic hypothyroidism can be distinguished from pituitary hypothyroidism by the presence of a rise in plasma TSH following test doze of TRH in the case of pituitary hypothyroidism. TSH response to TRH is normal in hypothalamic hypothyroidism.

It is increased in hypothyroidism caused by thyroid disease.

It is decreased in hyperthyroidism because of the feedback of thyroid hormones on the pituitary gland.

Features of Hypothyroidism (Myxedema)

- BMR falls to about -40. Hair is coarse and sparse. Skin is dry yellowish. Cold is poorly tolerated musky, slow voice, slow apathy, mentation, memory is poor, mental symptoms are present. Plasma cholesterol is elevated. Pulse is slow, BP low, COP reduced, circulation time slowed. Heart may be Dilated. T wave in ECG inverted.
- Thyroid gland may be enlarged or atrophied, slow cerebration, lethargy, muscular weakness and dull appearance, anemia, serum cholesterol high.

Bagginess under the eyes and swelling of the face. There is increased quantities of hyaluronic acid and chondroitin sulfate bound with protein form excessive tissue gel in the interstitial spaces and this causes the total quantity of interstitial fluid to increase. Because of the gel nature of excess fluid the edema is immobile and edema is of non-pitting type.

Diagnosis

Free thyroxine in the blood is low. BMR ranges between -30 and -50. Secretion of

TSH by anterior pituitary when a test dose of TRH is administered is usually greatly increased.

Treatment: Thyroxine in tablet form.

Cretinism

Cretinism is caused by extreme hypothyroidism during fetal life, infancy or childhood. It is characterized by failure of body growth and by mental retardation.
- Congenital
- Genetic defect
- Iodine lack (endemic)

Milestones delayed holding the head up, crawling, sitting, standing, waking, speech all are delayed – due to late myelination.

Rx: Thyroxine of nerve fibers, mental retardation, iodine pubertal sexual development is arrested. BMR decrease. High S. cholesterol.

  Normal BMR→ –20 to +20%
  Toxic goiter → 80–90%
  Myxedema→ –45%

Skeletal growth in cretinism is more inhibited than soft tissue growth. So obese, stocky and short appearance for the child. Tongue becomes so large in relation to skeletal growth and so obstructs swallowing and breathing.

Screening tests like RIA of TSH in first week after birth is useful.

Hyperthyroidism

Characterized by nervousness, weight loss, hyperphagia heat intolerance increase pulse pressure, fine tremor of the outstretched fingers. A warm soft skin pulse rate 100 – 160/min, palpitation, sleeping pulse rate is high.

Sweating and a BMR from +10 to +100. Commonest cause of hyperthyroidism is Grave's disease - 60–80% cases. It is common in women and etiology is autoimmune in which antibodies to TSH receptor stimulate the receptor. This produces marked T4 and T3 secretion and enlargement of thyroid gland (Goiter). Due to feedback effect plasma TSH is low. Another feature is Grave's disease is the swelling of tissues in the orbits producing protrusion of eyeballs (exophthalmos) occurs in 50% patients. When TSH receptor stimulating antibodies in the circulation stimulate these cells releasing cytokines that promote inflammation and edema. (Diminished libido in men, oligomenorrhea and amenorrhea in women) COP and velocity of blood flow increased heart may hypertrophy, lead to high output failure. Rapids bounding carotid pulse, muscle weakness in spite of increased appetite and food intake.

Iodine Deficiency

When dietary iodine intake falls below 50 µg/dL, thyroid hormone synthesis is inadequate and secretion declines. As a result of increased TSH secretion the thyroid hypertrophies producing iodine deficiency goiter.

Diagnosis of Hyperthyroidism

- Free T3 and T4 in the plasma by RIA, PB1 increase.
- BMR – increased to +30 to +60 in severe case.
- *Concentration of TSH in plasma:* TSH secretion is completely suppressed by the large amount of T4 and T3 in circulation.
- Concentration of TSH measured by RIA is usually high in thyrotoxicosis but low in thyroid adenoma

Thyroid adenoma: Not associated with autoimmune disease. It secretes large amount of thyroid hormone and secretary function in the remainder of thyroid gland is inhibited because adenoma depresses the production of TSH by the pituitary gland.

Physiology of treatment in hyperthyroidism: Surgical removal of gland.

Administer propyl thirouracil for several weeks until BMR of patient has returned to normal. Then high concentration of iodide for 1–2 weeks before operation so that size and blood supply of gland diminish.

Treatment of hyperplastic thyroid gland with radioactive iodine: 80–90% of an injected dose of iodide is absorbed by the hyperplastic toxic thyroid gland within 1 day after injection. The radioactive iodine destroy most of secretary cells of the gland. 5 millicuries of radioactive iodine is given to the patient 1st then additional doses are administered until normal thyroid status is reached.

Endemic colloid goiter: Caused by dietary iodide deficiency, 50 mg iodine/year for thyroid hormone production. Lack of iodine prevents production of both T4 and T3. So no hormone is available to inhibit TSH by anterior pituitary. So pituitary secretes large quantities of TSH which stimulate thyroid cells to secrete tremendous amounts of thyroglobulin colloid into follicles and gland grows larger and larger. But due to lack of Iodine T4 and T3 production does not occur in the thyroglobulin molecule and so there is no normal suppression of TSH production by anterior pituitary. Follicles become tremendous in size and thyroid gland may increase to 10–20 times normal size.

Idiopathic Non-toxic Colloid Goiter

Enlarged thyroid glands similar to that of endemic colloid goiter occur in people who do not have iodine deficiency. Thyroid hormone secretion may be normal or depressed. Cause of enlarged thyroid gland is not known but most of the patients show signs of thyroiditis which produce hypothyroidism. So increase in TSH secretion and progressive growth of non-inflamed portions of the gland. So glands become nodular and portions of gland growing while other portions are destroyed by thyroiditis.

Etiology

- Deficient iodide—trapping mechanism
- Deficient peroxidase system
- Deficient coupling of iodinated tyrosines in thyroglobulin molecule, so that the final thyroid hormones cannot be formed.
- Deficiency of the deiodinase enzyme
- Food containing goitrogens like turnips and cabbages.

Thyrotoxic Crisis or Thyroid Storm

Rapid aggravation of signs and symptoms with high fever, severe tachycardia, restlessness, low BP, vomiting and diarrhea. It may brought on by stress, infection or surgery especially in inadequately treated patient.

Rx: Antithyroid drugs
- Iodine
- Glucocorticoids
- β-achenergic blockers like propranolol.

■ CALCIUM METABOLISM

Physiology of Bone

Bone is a connective tissue composed of organic matrix in which mineral salts are impregnated. Bone consists of 20% organic matrix, 35% mineral salts and 45% water. 90% of organic substance is formed of collagen fibers. Rest forms the ground substance which consists of ECF and proteoglycans namely chondroitin sulfate and hyaluronic acid. Mineral salts are hydroxyapatite ($CaPO_4$ and $CaCO_3^-$).

Function: mechanical support
   Act as reservoir of Ca^{++}, Mg^{2+} and PO_4.

Deposition and Resorption of Bone

Bone building cells are called osteoblasts. Calcification is the process by which mineral salts are deposited around collagen fibers of the matrix where they crystallize. These are 4 types of cells:
1. Osteogenic cells
2. Osteoblasts

3. Osteocytes
4. Osteoclasts

Osteogenic cells: Stem cells derived from mesenchyme which are able to divide. Their daughter cells develop into osteoblasts.

Osteoblasts: Bone building cells. New bone formation and mineralizing bone. They secrete alkaline phosphatase and PO_4 ions are released locally. $Ca^{++} \times PO_4$ = constant. These slats remain saturated.

Osteocytes: Osteoblasts mature to form osteocytes and they maintain the bone tissue. Found on the bone surface or within lacunae. Osteocytes send their processes through the canaliculi of bone and make contact with other osteocytes and osteoblasts.

Osteoclasts: One multinucleated giant cells, formed by the fusion of many monocytes. These cells are concentrated in the endosteum. Main function is bone resorption. They secrete lysosomal enzymes like acid phosphatase and acids. They phagocytose bone fragments and release calcium. Bone breakdown is essential for bone remodeling and also helps to release Ca^{++} and PO_4 at times of need.

Applied Aspect

Sex Steroids: Slow down bone resorption and promote calcification of bone. Estrogen promotes apoptosis of osteoclasts thus reducing bone resorption. It increases osteoblast activity. Osteoporosis after menopause due to estrogen deficiency. In males testosterone starts declining only after age 60 yrs. Only 3% of bone mass lost every 10 yrs in males after this age.

Body Calcium

Total body calcium in 70 kg adult man is 1100 gm.
- 99% – in skeleton
- 4–5 gm – in soft tissues
- 1 gm – ECF (mainly in plasma)

2 forms
- Diffusible form
- Non-diffusible form or bound form

Calcium is loosely bound to albumin mainly and to a small extend to globulin. Protein bound Ca^{++} is physiologically inactive.

Diffusible calcium is in 2 forms:
1. Ionized calcium which constitute 50%
2. Complex Ca^{++} – Ca^{++} bind to diffusible anions like citrate and HCO_3^-. This form is also physiologically inactive.

Functions of Ionic Calcium in the Body

- Helps in the formation of bone and teeth.
- Necessary for blood coagulation.
- *For excitation:* Contraction coupling in muscles.
- Necessary for secretion from glands.
- For formation of milk.
- Acts as intercellular cementing substance.
- Acts as second messenger.
- Activate enzymes like amylase, lipase, thromboplastin, etc.
- Help in release of neurotransmitters.
- Affects excitability of excitable tissue and help stabilization of cell membrane.

■ PHOSPHORUS METABOLISM

Total body phosphorus: 500–800 gm and 2/3rd of it is organic, 1/3rd is inorganic. 90% incorporated in bone. It is also present in ATP, ADP, CP 2, 3 diphosphoglycerate, etc.

Plasma phosphate level, 12 mg/dL

3 gm P moves into and out of bone each day. 90% of this is reabsorbed back. This reabsorption is inhibited by PTH. Intestine absorption is stimulated by PTH.

Functions of Phosphorus in the Body

- Essential component of cell membrane
- It plays important role in intracellular, energy generation

- PO_4 is useful to buffer Ca^{2+}, Mg^{2+}, etc.
- PO_4 is a major cytoplasmic buffer.
- Maintain pH of blood by buffering H^+ in blood and urine.
- Necessary for the formation of ATP, ADP, phospholipase adenine and guanine nucleotides.
- Necessary for enzymatic activities like glycolysis.

Product of Ca^{++} and phosphate concentration is called solubility product. When this value exceed normal limit salts get precipitated and form $CaPO_4$. This mechanism is involved in the calcification process of bone.

The Hormones

- Parathormone
- Calcitonin
- 1,25, Dihydroxycholecalciferol

THE PARATHYROID GLANDS

These are small ovoid glands, smaller than peas, which lie on the posterior surface of the thyroid gland. Usually there are two pairs of parathyroid glands, a superior pair and an inferior pair. The chief cells of the parathyroid glands secrete a hormone called parathormone, which raises serum calcium levels. The activity of the parathyroid gland is controlled by alterations in the level of calcium in the blood. A raised blood calcium level inhibits the secretion of parathormone and a low blood calcium level stimulates secretion of the hormone. This is the main feedback mechanism for the regulation of blood calcium levels, thyroid calcitonin secretion playing a lesser role. The maintenance of blood calcium levels within narrow limits is essential for the normal function of cells, most obviously those of the heart, skeletal muscles and nerves.

Decreased activity of the parathyroid glands (hypoparathyroidism) results in a low blood calcium level and the condition known as tetany. This is characterized by muscular spasms and increased irritability of the nervous system. Increased activity of the glands (hyperparathyroidism) causes an increase in the levels of calcium in the blood and urine and results in renal calculi and bone disease (otitis fibrosis).

Parathyroid Glands

4 parathyroid glands—2 types of cells
- Chief cells – secrete parathormone
- Oxyphil cells

Parathyroid Hormone (PTH)

Action on Bone

- Bone resorption thus plasma Ca^+ level increase
- Increase permeability of osteoblasts and osteoclasts to calcium.
- Stimulate the precursor of osteoclasts in the bone marrow and increases the number of osteoclasts.
- It increases the release of lysosomal enzymes which in turn increase breakdown of collagen. At the same time it stimulates osteoblastic activity and increases collagen synthesis.

Action on Kidney

- Increase PO_4 excretion and plasma PO_4 levels falls. Thus, phosphaturic action is due to inhibition of reabsorption of PO_4 in the PCT of nephron.
- Increase exrection of Na^+, K^+, HCO_3^- and cAMP.
- It increases reabsorption of Ca^{2+} and H^+ from distal nephron. Hyperparathyroidism increases filtered load of calcium. Ca^{++} excretion is increased.
- PTH stimulates conversion of 25 hydroxycholecalciferol to 1, 25 dihydroxycholecalciferol in kidney.

Action on Intestine

Stimulates the formation of calcitriol. It stimulates reabsorption of Ca^{2+} from intestine.

Mechanism of Action of PTH

cAMP with the help of adenylate cyclase.

Regulation of Secretion of PTH

- Level of Ca⁺ in plasma. When plasma level of Ca^{++} falls, PTH secretion increases more Ca^{2+} is mobilized from bone to plasma.
- Plasma Mg^{2+} level has a direct effect on PTH secretion. An acute decrease in Mg^{2+} stimulates PTH secretion.
- 1, 25, Dihydroxycholecalciferol or calcitriol acts directly on parathyroid and inhibits secretion of PTH.
- Plasma PO_4^- has indirect effect on PTH secretion when PO_4^- level increases, ionic calcium level decreases and this stimulates PTH secretion.

ABNORMALITIES

Hypoparathyroidism

- Surgical removal along with thyroidectomy, Radiation, Auto antibodies
- *Congenital absence:* DiGeorge syndrome symptoms are due to decreased plasma Ca^{++}

1. Accoucher's hand or obstetric gland: The hands in carpopedal spasm adapt a peculiar posture in which there is flexion at metacorpophalangeal joints, extension at interphalangeal and flexion at MP joints and opposition of thumb. Pedal spasm is less frequent. In it the toes are plantal flexed feet are drawn up.
2. *Troussean's sign:* On occluding blood supply to a limb for about 3 min by inflating BP cuff produces a carpal spasm.
3. *Laryngeal stridor:* Produced by spasm of laryngeal muscles. It may produce asphyxia and cyanosis.
4. *Paraesthesias* tingling sensations in peripheral parts of limbs or around the mouth.
5. *Chvostek's sign:* Twitching of facial muscles produced by tapping the facial nerve at the angle of jaw.
6. Numbness and tingling of extremities
7. Intestinal colic, biliary colic bronchospasm.
8. Profuse sweating
9. *ECG:* Prolonged ST segment abnormal T.

Latent Tetany

- Chvostek's sign
- Trousseau's sign
- *Erb's sign:* Stimulation of motor nerves with galvanic current contraction of muscle supplied.

Hyperparathyroidism

- Diffuse enlargement of gland
- Adenoma of parathyroid
- Carcinoma of parathyroid—rare cause.

Blood Ca^{++} rises, symptoms are due to hypercalcemia

- Renal stones
- Pathological fracture and Bone cysts
- Muscle weakness, lassitude, anorexia, nausea, vomiting, constipation, polyuria, decreased thirst and mental symptoms.

Calcitonin

Calcium lowering hormone secreted by parafollicular cells or C cells of thyroid gland.

Actions

- Inhibits bone resorption by inhibiting osteoclasts.
- Enhance excretion of Ca^{++} by kidney.
- Increase PO_4 excretion and lower plasma PO_4.
- Increase Na^+ excretion from renal tubule.
- It inhibits PTH effects on bone.
- Calcitonin plays a very important role in maintaining normal blood Ca^{++} level when blood Ca^{2+} is increased.
- Bone remodeling.

Regulation

Stimulus: Increase in plasma ionic calcium level. Calcitonin is not secreted until the plasma Ca^{++} is more than 9.5 mg%. Above this level calcitonin secretion is proportional to increase in blood calcium.

Dopamine, estrogen, gastrin, cholecystokinin (CCK), secretin and glucagon stimulate calcitonin secretion.

Abnormalities

Medullary carcinoma of thyroid—increase in calcitonin. No clinical symptoms.

1, 25 Dihydroxycholecalciferol (Calcitriol)

7 Dehydrocholesterol from diet
↓
UV light
Cholecalciferol (Vit D$_3$)
↓
Slow diffusion with help of D$_3$ carrier protein to blood
↓
Liver (25OH cholecalciferol)
↓
1 α hydroxylase
Kidney (PCT – 1,25, Dihydroxycholcalciferol)
Normal blood level – 0.03 ng/mL

Actions

Receptors for calcitriol present in:
- Intestine → increase absorption of Ca^{++} from intestine
- Bone → Mobilize Ca^{++} and PO$_4^-$ by increasing permeability of membrane of osteroblasts to Ca^{++}
- Ca^{++} pumped into ECF.
- Kidney → Increase reabsorption of Ca^{++}. So increase blood Ca^{++} level.

Regulation

Plasma Ca^{++} and PO$_4$ level:
- PTH → Increase in blood calcium level so high blood Ca^{++} inhibit PTH and calcitriol thus bringing blood calcium back to normal.
- Renal 1 α hydrozylase decreases to unstimulated levels within 24 hrs of parathyroidectomy.
- Plasma PO$_4$ levels also influences the secretion of calcitriol. PO$_4$ mechanism acts directly through 1 α hydroxylase enzyme.

Deficiency: Rickets (failure of mineralization), Osteomalacia (adults).

■ THE PINEAL GLAND

The pineal gland is a small reddish-grey structure, about the size of a pea, situated in the midline of the brain immediately behind the third ventricle and under the posterior end of the corpus callosum. In adults it may be calcified and identifiable on skull X-ray films, in which its displacement to one side would indicate the presence of a space-occupying lesion within the cranium.

The pineal gland was considered by Descartes to be the seat of the soul and more recently it was considered to be an evolutionary relic. There is now evidence that it is an active endocrine gland and, although its function is poorly understood, it is thought to have a regulatory role in modulating the activity of the pituitary and other glands. Its secretions generally have an inhibitory effect and there is evidence that a pineal hormone inhibits the growth and maturation of the gonads until puberty. The pineal has a circadian rhythm of endocrine activity and may have an extensive role in co-ordinating circadian and diurnal rhythms throughout the body, acting via the hypothalamus and pituitary gland.

■ THE SEX GLANDS OR GONADS

See Chapter 19 on the Reproductive System.

■ THE SUPRARENAL GLANDS

The suprarenal or adrenal glands are two small flattened yellowish bodies situated on the upper pole of each kidney (Fig. 14.7). Each is about 5 cm (2 in) high, 3 cm

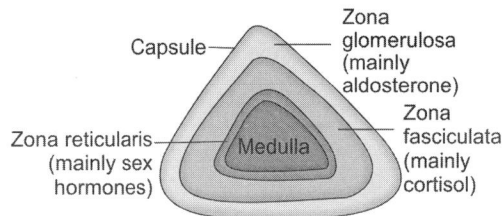

Fig. 14.7: The suprarenal gland—general structure and function

(1.2 in) wide and 1 cm (0.4 in) thick and is plentifully supplied with blood by three arteries, derived from the aorta, the renal artery and the inferior phrenic artery. The profuse sympathetic nerve supply from the coeliac plexus goes almost entirely to the medulla, which is the dark interior of the adrenal gland. The outer part of the gland, the cortex, is yellowish, because it is rich in lipids, and has entirely separate functions from the medulla.

Functions of the Suprarenal Cortex

The hormones of the suprarenal cortex are derived from cholesterol and belong to a class of fatty or wax-like substances called steroids. They fall into three main groups corresponding to their main effects:

1. *The mineralocorticoids:* These regulate the body sodium and potassium ion levels and therefore help to maintain the fluid and electrolyte balance of the body. The principal mineralocorticoid is aldosterone and of lesser importance is corticosterone. They act on the collecting tubules of the kidney in such a way that sodium is retained in the body and any excess of potassium is excreted.
2. *The glucocorticoids:* These derive their name from their influence on carbohydrate metabolism. The principal glucocorticoid is cortisol (hydrocortisone) and others, of lesser importance, are corticosterone and 11-deoxycortisol. Among their main effects are:
   (a) increased output of glucose from the liver into the blood;
   (b) increased breakdown (catabolism) of protein;
   (c) liberation of lipid from tissue stores and redistribution of adipose tissue;
   (d) suppression of growth hormone release and activity;
   (e) diminution of eosinophil's and lymphocytes in the blood;
   (f) immunosuppression;
   (g) suppression of inflammation;
   (h) enhancement of water diuresis.
   Cortisone (which is converted to hydrocortisone in the body) and many similar synthetic substances (analogues), such as prednisone and prednisolone, are used in clinical medicine for many different purposes but mostly to suppress inflammation not due to infective agents. In high dosage they may have many side-effects including a mineralocorticoid effect which causes a disturbance of salt and water balance.
3. *Sex hormones:* Small quantities of sex hormones, androgens and estrogens, are produced by the suprarenal gland. These influence sexual development and growth. In females, the suprarenal glands are the principal source of androgens, which are required by both sexes for normal pubertal and skeletal development.

Unlike the secretions of the adrenal medulla, those of the cortex are not regulated by nervous impulses. The adrenal production of glucocorticoids and sex hormones is controlled by pituitary adrenocorticotropic hormone (ACTH) or corticotropin. The pituitary secretion of this hormone is, in turn, stimulated by corticotropin releasing factor (corticotropin-RF). The whole control structure is known as the hypothalamic pituitary-adrenal (HPA) axis. Large doses of cortisone

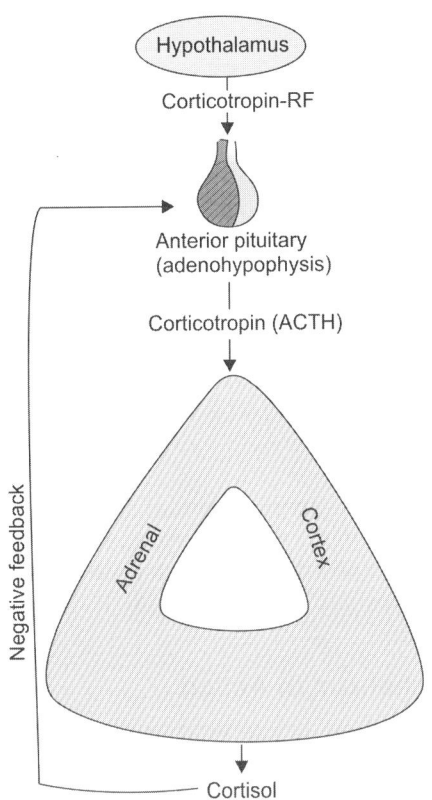

Fig. 14.8: The secretion of cortisol—the HPA axis

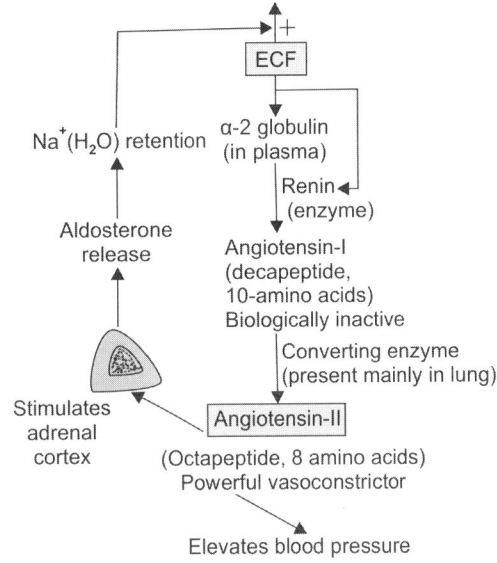

Fig. 14.9: The renin-angiotensin-aldosterone mechanism

will suppress the pituitary secretion of corticotropin by a negative feedback mechanism (Fig. 14.8). This effect may be very persistent in patients after steroid therapy has been discontinued. Such patients, with partial suppression of pituitary activity, have a diminished ability to respond to stress such as that of an infection, an accident, or a surgical operation. Booster doses of corticosteroids are necessary for these patients at such times to prevent a hypoadrenal crisis, which could be fatal.

Hypoadrenalism may also result from destructive disease of the adrenal glands by an autoimmune process or tuberculosis, e.g. the condition is known as Addison's disease and is characterized by a low blood pressure (hypotension), brown pigmentation of the skin and mucous membranes, and excessive loss of sodium from the body, with hypernatremia (a low serum sodium level) and often dehydration.

Over secretion of cortisol occurs in Cushing's syndrome, which is characterized by rounding ('mooning') of the face, obesity with a 'lemon on tooth-picks' distribution and a 'buffalo-hump', hypertension, diabetes and osteoporosis.

Aldosterone secretion is largely independent of ACTH but is influenced by changes in the volume of extracellular fluid, a decrease in the latter causing greater aldosterone secretion and vice versa. Aldosterone also plays a part in blood pressure regulation through the renin-angiotensin mechanism controlled by the juxtaglomerular apparatus of the kidney (Fig. 14.9).

Functions of the Suprarenal Medulla

The medulla secretes adrenalin and noradrenalin. The secretion of these catecholamines is not controlled by the anterior pituitary gland but by the sympathetic nervous system. They cause a constriction of the arterioles of the body, resulting in a rise of blood pressure, and also an increase in the rate and force of the heartbeat. They also relax the involuntary muscle of the bronchi and stimulate the liver to convert glycogen into glucose, which is liberated into the bloodstream.

Adrenal secretion of catecholamine's constitutes a reserve mechanism that comes into action at times of stress. These hormones are poured into the bloodstream during fear or anger and they are responsible for many of the changes which accompany these emotions. Blanching of the skin due to constriction of the arterioles favors diversion of the blood to the muscles, where it is most needed. The increased blood pressure and force of the heartbeat result in better circulation both in the muscles and the brain, while the liberation of glucose supplies the muscles with the necessary fuel for increased activity.

A tumor of the adrenal medulla, known as a pheochromocytoma, is a rare but important cause of hypertension.

ADRENAL CORTEX

Suprarenal gland situated on the upper pole of each kidney has two parts:
1. Adrenal cortex
2. Adrenal medulla

The outer part is called cortex and inner part medulla.

The outer cortex has three zones:
1. *Outer most zone:* Zone glomerulosa—secrete aldosterone.
2. *Middle zone:* Zone fasciculata—secrete cortisol.
3. *Inner most zone:* Zone reticularis—weak androgens.

Mineralo Cortico Steroids

For example, aldosterone and DOC (Desoxycorticosterone)

Functions: Target cells of aldosterone are present in the (1) kidney (2) GIT (3) sweat glands and (4) brain.

Kidney

- Epithelial cells of DCT
- Principal cells of collecting tubules are the target cells.

Aldosterone

Causes

- Facilitation of Na^+ reabsorption
- Facilitation of K^+ extrusion

Drugs opposing aldosterone, e.g. spironolactone.

Produce hyponatremia

Aldosterone therapy—produce hypertension and edema. Aldosterone causes Na conservation + K excretion by its action on kidney.

Mechanism of Action

Aldosterone being lipid soluble together with cortisol enters the cytosol. In the cystosol, there are aldosterone receptors identical with glucocorticoid receptors. In the target cells of aldosterone, there is 11-β-hydroxysteroid dehydrogenase which destroy the glucocorticosteroids.

Aldosterone combines with receptor. New proteins synthesized which are responsible for the biological effects of aldosterone.

Action on GIT, Sweat Glands and Brain

GIT: Target cells are present in the ileum and colon. Aldosterone causes more reabsorption of Na^+ from the fluid in GIT lumen.

Sweat gland: More sodium is reabsorbed from the sweat. So sweat with very low Na^+ concentration is secreted.

Brain: Aldosterone by acting on hypothalamus increases thirst. Also concerned with memory.

Regulation of Aldosterone Secretion

- Renin
- Serum K⁺ concentration
- Serum Na⁺ concentration
- ACTH

The stimuli that increase rennin secretion
- BP Falls
- Blood volume perfusing kidney falls sharply.
- Serum K rises even little
- Serum Na⁺ falls moderately
- Sympathetic stimulation.

Renin acts on
Angeotensinogen $\xrightarrow{Renin}$ Angeotensin I
$\downarrow$ACE

Angeotension II (produced by liver)
Vasoconstrictor action
Aldosterone secretion

ACTH injection causes a mild to moderate but temporary rise of aldosterone secretion.

Glucocorticosteroids

- Physiological
- Pharmacological
- Permissive actions.

Physiological Actions

- Metablolic actions
  - Glucose
  - Fat
  - Protein
  - Ca, Na, K
- Actions during stress.

■ ACTIONS OF GLUCOCORTICOIDS

Mechanism of Action

By binding to glucocorticoid receptors and the steroid receptor complexes act as transcription factors that promote the transcription of certain segments of DNA. This leads via in RNAs to synthesis of enzymes that alter cell function. In addition glucocorticoids have non-genomic actions.

Actions

1. *Effects on intermediary metablolism:*
   (a) Increased protein catabolism and increased hepatic glycogenesis and gluconeogenesis.

   Glucose 6 phosphatase activity is increased and the plasma glucose level rises. Glucocorticoids exert on anti-insulin action in peripheral tissues and make diabetes worse. But brain and heart are spared so the increase in plasma glucose provides extra glucose to these vital organs. In DM, glucocorticoids raise plasma lipid levels and ketone body formation. But in normal individuals increased insulin levels provoked by rise in plasma glucose obscure this action. In adrenal insufficiency, plasma glucose level is normal as long as adequate calories intake is maintained but fasting causes hypoglycemia. The adrenal cortex is not essential for the ketogenic response to fasting.

2. *Permissive action:* Small amounts of glucocorticoids must be present for a number of metabolic reactions to occur. This effect is called their permissive action, e.g. requirement for glucocorticoids to be presented for glucagon and catecholamines to exert their calorigenic effects and for catecholamines to exert their lipolytic effects and for catecholamines to produce presser responses and bronchodilation.

3. *Effects on ACTH secretion:* Glucocorticoids inhibit ACTH secretion and ACTH secretion is increased in adrenalectomized animals. The consequences of the feedback action of cortisol on ACTH secretion is also important.

4. *Vascular reactivity:* In adrenally insufficient animals, vascular smooth muscle becomes unresponsive to NE,

EN. The capillaries dilate and terminally become permeable to colloidal dyes. Failure to respond to NE liberated at NE nerve endings impairs vascular compensation for the hypovolemia of adrenal insufficiency and promote vascular collapse. Glucocorticoids restore vascular reactivity.

5. *Effects on nervous system:* Appearance of electroencephalographic waves slower than normal proportional to personality changes. It includes irritability apprehension and inability to concentrate.

6. *Effects on water metabolism:* Adrenal insufficiency leads to water intoxication. Only glucocorticoids repair this deficit. In patients with adrenal insufficiency, who have not received glucocorticoids, glucose infusion may cause high fever followed by collapse and death. Glucose is metabolized, the water dilutes the plasma and the cells cause the cells of the thermoregulatory centers in the hypothalamus to swell so that their function is dispersed.

   Plasma vasopressin levels are elevated in adrenal insufficiency and reduced by glucocorticoid treatment. The glomerular filtration rate is low and it contributes to reduction in water excretion. The selective effect of glucocorticoids on abnormal water excretion is consistent with this possibility, because even though the mineralocorticoids improve filtration by restoring plasma volume, the glucocorticoids raise GFR to much greater degree.

7. *Effects on the blood cells and lymphatic organs:* Glucocorticoids decrease the number of circulating eosinophils by increasing their sequestration in the spleen and lungs. Glucocorticoids also lower the number of basophils in circulation and increase the number of neutrophils, platelets and RBCs.

   Glucocorticoids decrease the circulating lymphocyte count and size of the lymph nodes and thymus by inhibiting lymphocyte mitotic activity. They reduce the secretion of cytokines and lead to reduced proliferation lymphocytes which undergo apoptosis.

8. *Resistance to stress:* Most of the stressful stimuli that increase ACTH secretion also activate the sympathetic nervous system. Part of the function of circulating glucocorticoids may be maintenance of vascular reactivity of catecholamines. Glucocorticoids are also necessary for the catecholamines to exert their full FFA mobilizing action. FFA are important emergency energy supply. Stress causes increase in plasma glucocorticoids to high pharmacologic levels that in the short run are lifesaving.

   Increase in ACTH is beneficial in the short-term, becomes harmful and disruptive in the long-term and produce abnormalities of Cushing syndrome.

9. *Anti-inflammatory effects of glucocorticoids:* Glucocorticoids inhibit the inflammatory response to tissue injury. It also suppresses manifestation of allergic diseases that are due to histamine release from tissues. Both of these effects require high levels of circulating glucocorticoids and cannot be produced by administering steroids without producing the other manifestations of glucocorticoids excess.

   Large doses of exogenous glucocorticoids inhibit ACTH secretion to the point that severe adrenal insufficiency can be also a dangerous problem when therapy is stopped. But local glucocorticoid administration by injection into inflamed joint or near an irritated nerve produces a high local concentration of the steroid without serious side effects.

10. *Anti-allergic effects:* Actions of glucocorticoids in patients with bacterial infections are dramatic and dangerous. In pneumococcal pneumonia or active

tuberculosis—febrile reaction, the toxicity and lung symptoms disappear. But the bacteria spread through the body unless at the same time antibiotics are given.

When these symptoms are masked by treatment with glucocorticoids there may be delay in diagnosis and institution of treatment with antimicrobial drugs.

The role of NF-KB in the anti-inflamatory and anti-allergic effects of glucocorticoids is important. Local inflammation is caused by inhibition of phospholipase A2. This increases release of arachidonic acid from tissues phospholipids and consequently reduces the formation of leukotrienes, thromboxanes, PGs, Prostacyclin, etc.

11. *Other effects:* Large doses of glucocorticoids inhibit growth decrease GH secretion.

During fetal life, glucocorticoids accelerate the maturation of surfactant in the lungs.

The medulla is exposed to high levels of adrenal cortical hormones which is of great significance especially in stressful situations.

■ HORMONES OF ADRENAL MEDULLA

The hormones of adrenal medulla are collectively called catecholamines. They are:
- Epinephrine (Adrenalin)
- Norepinephrine (Noradrenaline)
- Dopamine.

Epinephrine is the predominated catecholamine, synthesized, stored and secreted by adrenal medulla. Norepinephrine is mainly synthesized and stored in the sympathetic nerve endings.

Small amounts of opioid peptides like encephalin (met-encephalin, leu-encephalin) are also present in adrenal medulla. Stress induced analgesia is due to the action of these opioid peptides released from adrenal medulla.

Epinephrine: Secreting neurons are also present in the medulla oblongata that project to the thalamus, periaqueductal grey matter, hypothalamus and spinal cord.

Biosynthesis

PNMT absent in postganglionic sympathetic nerve endings. So epinephrine is not produced in postganglionic sympathetic nerve endings.

Applied Physiology

Phenylketonuria: It is a condition where there is accumulation of phenylalanine and it's keto acid derivatives in blood, tissue and urine.

Deficiency: Phenylalanine hydroxylase due to mutation of gene coding for that. Here catecholamine are synthesized from tyrosine.

Tetrahydrobiopterine deficiency: Phenyl ketonuria + failure of synthesis of catecholamines. Since tetrahydrobiopterine is a cofactor for phenylalanine hydroxylase as well as tyrosene hydroxylase.

Storage: Chromaffin granules epinephrine comprises 80% of chromaffin granules. Rest by NE, and DOPA

NE → stimulates mainly receptors

EN → stimulate both α and β receptors equally. β2 receptors respond more to epinephrine (Table 14.3).

Table 14.3: Adrenergic receptors

α Effect	β1 Effect	β2 Effect
Vasoconstriction	Increase HR	vasodilation calorigenesis
Pupillary dilatation piloeruction	increase force of contraction of myocardium	Uterine relaxation
	Glycogenolysis	intestinal relaxation
Constriction of	Lipolysis	Relaxation of bladder
Intestinal sphincter and bladder sphincters contraction		Bronchiolar dilatation Intestinal relaxation

Actions of Catecholamines
1. Metabolic effect
2. Calorigenic effect
3. Systemic effects

Metabolic Effect: Mechanism of Action (Flowchart 14.3)
- β-cAMP
- Phosphorylase
- α-increased intracellular Ca^{++}
- *Carbohydrate metabolism:* Diabetogenic, blood glucose level increases. Causes glycogenolysis in muscle and liver, increase plasma lactate, stimulate metabolic rate, increase insulin and oxidation of lactate in liver, increase temperature, cutaneous vasoconstriction, increased muscular activity.
- *Lipid metabolism:* Lipolytic effect increase FFA level by stimulating hormone sensitive lipase.
- *Mineral metabolism:* Distribution of intracellular and extracellular K^+. Release of K^+ from liver. So increase plasma level, lactate entry to skeletal muscle increase. So later decrease plasma lactate.

Calorigenic Effect
Adrenaline increases tissue metabolism leading to increased O_2 consumption and increased CO_2 production. This cause increase BMR and temperature. This calorigenic effect will be absent in the absence of thyroid and adrenal cortical hormones.

Systemic Actions
- *Action of adrenalin on skeletal muscle:* Increase the contractility and excitability of skeletal muscle. Postpones fatigue, lowers chronaxie value, and prevents loss of intracellular potassium.
- On adipose tissue causes release FFA from adipose tissue.
- *On blood:* Increase blood glucose and blood lactic acid level. It increases RBC count Hb concentration and plasma protein content. Produce hemoconcentration. Decreases eosinophil and lymphocyte count. Coagulation time is shortened.
- *On spleen:* Adrenalin causes contraction of splenic capsule, but produces relaxation of plain muscles of spleen.
- *Action on CNS:* Lowers threshold of ARAS and stimulate it by producing alert and arousal phenomenon. Large closes of adrenalin inhibit spinal reflexes. In humans epinephrine evokes more anxiety and fear.
- *Action on other endocrine glands:* Adrenalin stimulates anterior pituitary via hypothalamus which in turn stimulates adrenal cortex to increase secretion of glucocorticoids. It inhibits ADH secretion and insulin secretion from pancreas. Stimulates glucagon secretion.
α effect – Inhibit insulin and glucagon, β effect – stimulate secretion of insulin and glucagon.

Flowchart 14.3: Dopamine metabolism steps

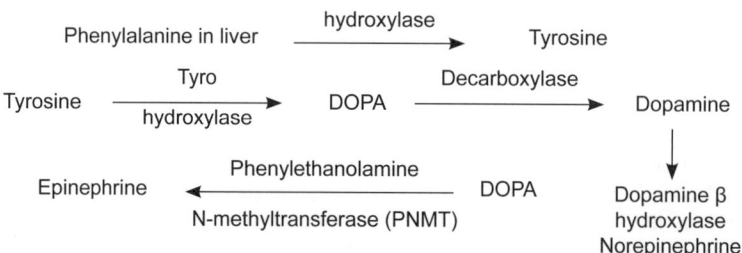

- *Effects on CVS*

Epinephrine	Norepinephrine
Isolated heart (β1 receptor)	
Increase force and rate of cardiac contraction	Increased rate and force of cardiac contraction
Increase myocardial excitability • extra systoles are produced • serious cardiac arrhythmias	Vasoconstriction in most organs (α1)
Dilates the blood vessels in	Skeletal Muscle and liver
(β2 receptor) This over balances	
The Vaso constriction produced by Epinephrine elsewhere.	[EN—affinity for α1, β1, β2] [NE—High affinity for Low affinity of β1 No affinity for β2]
So total peripheral resistance	

Intact Animal and Humans
Widening of pulse (Systolic Pressure, Diastolic Pressure) BP increase
(Systolic pressure increase) So reflex bradycardia
(force and rate of cardiac contraction increase-)
(Baroreceptor) which
overrides direct cardio
Acceleratery effect of norepinephrine
(Diastolic pressure decrease peripheral resistance ↓)
COP↑ HR↑ COP/min - falls
(reflex baroreceptor
Stimulation insufficient
to obscure direct
effect on heart)

Effects of Dopamine

Injected dopamine produces renal vasodilation probably by acting on a specific dopaminergic receptor. It also produces vasodilation in the mesentery. Elsewhere it produces vasoconstriction probably by releasing nor epinephrine. It has positive ionotropic effect on heart (β receptor).

Dopamine: Moderate Rate

- Increase Sy. Pressure
- No change Dia. Pressure

Useful in traumatic and cardiogenic shock. Dopamine is made in the renal cortex. It causes natriuresis and may exert this effect by inhibiting renal $Na^+ K^+$-ATPase.

Regulation of Adrenal Medullary Secretion

Neural (increase secretion due to symp. discharges provoked in emergency)
[Sympathoadrenal system] – by cannon
Selective secretion
Familiar emotional stress NE ↑
Unfamiliar situations of stress
in which individual does not know what to expect. Epinephrine ↑

Adrenomedullin: A vasodepressor polypeptide sound in adrenal medulla.

■ PHEOCHROMOCYTOMA

Most adrenal medullary tumors secrete NE or EN or both and produce sustained hypertension. However 15% of EN secreting tumors secrete epinephrine episodically, producing intermittent bouts of palpitations, headache glycosuria and extreme systolic hypertension.

■ THE PANCREAS

This organ and its secretions are described in Chapter 12 on the Digestive System. The endocrine tissue of the pancreas is in the form of clumps of secretory cells known as the islets of Langerhans. The islet cells are of three-types, alpha, beta and delta. Insulin is secreted by the beta cells and, like the other hormones, passes directly into the blood stream. Insulin acts on a cell membrane receptor and enhances the entry of glucose into most cells, thereby diminishing the plasma glucose concentration. With of the cell, insulin promotes the conversion of glucose to glycogen (glycogenosis), promotes protein synthesis and inhibits fat breakdown (lipolysis). Insulin deficiency results in breakdown of glycogen, protein and fat, leading to a raised plasma glucose level (hyperglycemia) and ketoacidosis. The ketone bodies are acetoacetic acid, beta-hydroxybutyric acid and acetone, which are derived from the free fatty acids released during fat breakdown or lipolysis.

Normally the blood glucose level remains within a certain range. Any excess of glucose is stored in the liver and muscles as glycogen. If the blood glucose rises above its normal or 'threshold' level the excess of glucose is excreted by the kidneys and glucose appears in the urine (glycosuria). Some people, however, have a low renal threshold, so that they have glycosuria while their blood glucose level is within the accepted limits of normal.

Deficiency of insulin due to disease of the islets of Langerhans results in diabetes mellitus, a condition in which the blood glucose is high and glucose is passed in the urine. In severe cases the disturbed metabolism of fat results in ketoacidosis and the presence of ketone bodies in the urine.

The alpha cells of the pancreas secrete glucagon, the metabolic effects of which are the opposite of those of insulin. It causes the breakdown of liver glycogen, thereby releasing glucose into the blood stream, and promotes lipolysis.

The third hormone of the pancreas is somatization, which is secreted by the delta cells of the islets of Langerhans. It is able to inhibit the secretion of many hormones and other substances and is one of the 'brain-gut peptides', which act as neurotransmitters. Somatization is also secreted by the hypothalamus and, because it inhibits the pituitary release of growth hormone, is also known as growth hormone release inhibiting hormone (GHRIH).

■ THE ENDOCRINE PANCREAS

The endocrine part consists of islets of Langerhans. There are between 1 and 2 million islets in a pancreas accounting for 1–2% of weight of the pancreas. Each islet consists of four kinds of cells.

(i) α (or A) (ii) β (or B) (iii) $ (or D) (iv) F (or PP)

α *cells:* Constitute 25% of islet cells secrete glucagon

β cells: Constitute 60% of the islets cells. Secrete insulin.

$ *cells:* 10% of the islet cells. Secrete somatostation

F *cells:* 5% of the islet cells. Secrete pancreatic polypeptide.

Islet cells are very vascular. The blood from the islets is ultimately drained by splenic vein → portal vein → liver.

The pancreatic hormones (insulin-glucagon) are directly poured into the splenic vein. So liver is fed by a blood which is highly concentrated in insulin – glucagon.

So exogenous insulin in a larger dose has to be administered than what could have been achieved by endogenous insulin in case of DM. Glucagon can enter the β cells via gap junction. Situated between α and β cells, that is without being borne by blood. Similarly insulin can enter by blood via gap junctions. This route is called the paracrine effect. By paracrine effect insulin influences glucagon secretion and glucagon influences insulin secretion.

■ INSULIN

Insulin contains 51 amino acids, arranged in two chains. Chain A containing 21 amino acids and Chain B containing 30 amino acids. The two chains are connected by S-S (disulfide) linkages.

β cells of the islets synthesize a big chain of amino acids called preproinsulin
↓
Signal sequence is removed
↓
Proinsulin
↓
C peptide removed
↓
Insulin

Insulin formed and stored in β cells. For every mole of insulin there is one mole of C-peptide stored and released into the blood. But C-peptide has no biological activity. Fasting blood insulin concentration is about 10 μ/mL and after taking a meal the level shoots up to values like 50–70 μ/mL.

Action of Insulin

Insulin is an anabolic hormone, that is it causes anabolism of carbohydrates – fat and proteins.

The major target organs of insulin are:
(1) Liver (2) muscle and (3) adipocytes (fat cells in adipose tissue).

Effects of Insulin on Target Organs

1. *Liver:* (i) Glycogenesis↑ (ii) Gluconeogenesis ↓ (iii) Protein synthesis ↑ (iv) Ketogenesis ↓ (v) Glucose energy ↑
2. *Skeletal Muscle:* (i) Glucose entry ↑ (ii) Amino acid uptake increase (iii) Muscle glycogenesis ↑ (iv) K+ uptake ↑
3. *Adipocytes:* (i) Glucose entry ↑ (ii) Fatty acid synthesis ↑ (iii) Triglyceride formation ↑ (iv) Lipolysis ↑ (v) K+ uptake ↑

Glucose Entry

Cell membrane as such is impermeable to glucose. GLUT molecules when appear in the cell membrane glucose can cross the cell membrane from ECF to ICF. Once glucose is inside the cell the glucose is metabolized, thus there is no accumulation of glucose inside the cell.

GLUT is a abbreviated form of glucose transporter. GLUT is a protein structure, that stays in the cytosol of hepatocyte—adipocyte—myocyte. In presence of insulin, the GLUT is transported to the cell membrane. GLUT contains channels that produce direct communication between ECF and ICF. There as GLUT 1,2,3,4,5,6,7, isoforms.

The metabolic activities of insulin are produced by altering the state of activities of some enzymes.

Insulin stimulates: (i) Hexokinase (ii) Glycogen synthase (iii) Phosphofructokinase.

Insulin inhibits: (i) Phosphorylase (ii) Glucose 6 phosphatase

Mechanism of Action of Insulin

Insulin combines with its receptor at target cell → Formation of insulin - receptor complex at cell membrane →
The complex Internalized (enters cytoplasm) → Insulin released in the cytosol.

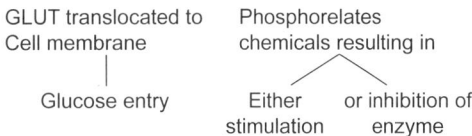

Insulin Receptor

Insulin receptors are present in the cell membrane of target cells. The receptor is a protein structure containing 2 α subunits and 2 β subunits. The β subunit is partly intramembranes. It contains an enzyme tyrosine kinase.

After combining with the insulin the receptor insulin complex is internalized. After internalization most of the receptors are degraded but a few are recycled.

Control of Insulin Secretion

- Substrate
- Hormonal
- Neural

Substrate Control

Most fundamental control, the substrates are (i) Glucose (ii) Amino acids. The rise in blood level of substrates increases the insulin secretion. When blood glucose level is < 70 mg% no insulin is secreted. When blood glucose level becomes more than 70 mg% the secretion intensifies till BGL reaches 300 mg%. When blood amino acid

level rises, provided the blood glucose level is not too low, the insulin secretion rises.
Mechanism of control of BGL: More glucose molecules enter the β cells secretion of insulin.

Hormonal Control

Glucagon from cells of the islets by paracrine effect suppresses insulin secretion. GI hormones, e.g. GIP promotes insulin secretion.

Neural Control

Islet cells receive both sympathetic and parasympathetic supply. α Adrenergic stimulation causes inhibition and β2 adrenergic stimulation which causes stimulation of insulin secretion.

■ APPLIED PHYSIOLOGY

Fasting blood sugar level at health is between 70–110 mg%. But only when FBS level is > 140 mg% according to WHO a person is diabetic. The intermediate zone is between 111–139 mg% is impaired fasting glucose level.

The postprandial (2 hrs after 75 gm glucose mg) blood sugar level at health < 140 mg% according to WHO, the postprandial blood sugar level in a frank diabetic has to be > 200 mg%. The intermediate zone, 141–199 mg% has thus impaired glucose tolerance test.

■ DIABETES MELLITUS

Decrease is characterized by hypoglycemia: Glycosuria, atherosclerosis, microangiopathy, neuropathy infections and diabetic ketoacidosis.

Cut off Level for Hyperglycemia

- Normal fasting level of blood glucose is maximum up to 6.1 mmol/L (110 mg/100 mL)
- Postprandial (postmeal) that is exactly two hours after a meal of 75 gm of glucose is maximum up to 8.9 mmol/L (160 mg/100 mL)

According to WHO a person is diabetic if her/his plasma blood glucose level is (i) fasting > 7–8 mmol/L (=140 mg per 100 mL) (ii) Postprandial > 11.1 mmol/L (= 200 mg/100 mL).

Classical Features

- *Polyurea:* Hyperglycemia exceeding renal threshold result in glycosuria sugar molecules in the renal tubules increase the osmolality of tubular fluid and act as osmotic diuretic diuresis = polyuria.
- *Polyphagia:* Glucose is being lost via urine this causes a demand of more fuel in the body polyphagia.
- *Polydypsia:* Polyuria result in water loss, dehydration.
   Thirst develops → polydypsia.
- *Wasting:* To meet the challenge of rising demands of fuel, endogenous proteins (muscle proteins) are catabolized substrates for gluconeogenesis produced, also causes loss of muscle mass.

Complications

- *Big blood vessels:* Atherosclerosis common in diabetics causes—serum cholesterol and LDL tend to be high, proneness to develop atherosclerosis increases—LDL molecules are oxidized and glycosylated. Such molecules are deposited in subintimal layers of big vessels causing atherosclerosis. Due to atherosclerosis diabetics are prone to angina pectoris/myocardial infarction/cerebrovascular accidents.
- *Microangiopathy:* In this condition, capillary wall is thickened leading to obliteration of blood flow through the affected capillaries.
   Anoxic damage of tissues supplied by capillaries. Thickening of capillaries due to formation of Sorbitol (Oxidized

product of glucose) in the blood. Renal arterial capillaries develop micro-angiopathy the clinical condition is diabetic nephropathy. When retinal vessels are affected it is called diabetes retinopathy.
- *Neuropathy:* Degeneration of both autonomic and somatic nerves. Nerves are damaged. There can be impotence, in continence, gastroparesis, constipation (ANS damage) or loss of tendon reflexes/weakness of skeletal muscles (somatic nerve damage, etc.). Brain is not affected.
- *Diabetic ketoacidosis:* Lack of insulin leads to unsatisfactory combustion of glucose. To meet demands of fuel, there is excessive adipose tissue lipolysis. Also lack of insulin causes adipose tissue lipolysis. As a result massive amounts of FFA become available. β oxidation in liver leads to massive amount of acetyl CoA. Acetyl CoA conjugates to form 4C structures like acetoacetic acid and β hydroxybutyric acid and a 3C structure acetone. They are collectively called ketone bodies. First two ketone bodies accumulate in blood and cause (1) lowering of blood PH and (2) Hyper osmolality of plasma both of which are lethal. Acetone is formed in the urinary bladder.

Classification of Diabetes

IDDM (insulin dependent diabetes mellitus): No β cells and endogenous insulin is absent. This is because β cells are destroyed by some disease (autoimmune disease following a viral infection). IDDM cases usually develop while the patient is still young. They must be treated with insulin.

NIDDM (Non-insulin dependent diabetes mellitus): Here the victims are usually middle aged (hence the older name maturity onset diabetes) often obese and physically under active, and have a positive family history of DM. Here the insulin secretion is alright, also the receptors in the target cell are present but there is some fault beyond the receptor. Receptor insulin complex formation occurs as usual but after that further events (transduction of signal) in the target cell are faulty, the biological effects do not develop. NIDDM can be treated with insulin but instead of insulin they can be treated with oral hypoglycemic agents (like sulfonylurea, metformin).

■ GLUCAGON

Glucagon is produced by the cells of the islets of Langerhans of pancreas. Upper part of small intestine also produces glucagon. Glucagon is a polypeptide hormone containing 29 amino acids with mol weight of 3500 Dalton. It is produced from a precursor proglucagon.

Functions

Target cells of glucagon are (1) hepatocytes (2) β cells of the islets. At high doses glucagon can influence (3) adipocytes also.

Effects on Hepatocytes

Major effects are:
- Promotion of hepatic glycogenolysis – that is hepatic glycogen broken down to glucose—released in the blood—glucose level rises.
- Promote gluconeogenesis that is production of glucose from substrates which are not carbohydrates (e.g. amino acid).
- A third effect of glucagon is ureogenesis. For gluconeogenesis – NH_2 free portion of the amino acid is required. The NH_2 radicle is utilized as urea.

Control of Glucagon Secretion

On the whole
Blood glucose level: High blood glucose level inhibits glucagon secretion. Glucose

level of 200 mg per 100 mL or more inhibits maximally whereas all inhibitory effects of glucose are withdrawn at around 60 mg/100 mL level or so.

Hypoglycemia

This is a condition when blood sugar level falls below the physiological limits. Clinical signs appear when the glucose level of blood falls below 55 mg/100 mL. The symptom includes giddiness, palpitation, sweating, hypertension, anginal pain, mental confusion convulsion, coma leading to death.

Pathogenesis

Brain normally depends only on glucose supplied by blood. Low blood glucose level damages brain and immediately compensatory mechanisms develop. They are:
- Stimulation of sympathetic
  - Release of adrenalin from adrenal medulla both these help to restore blood sugar level immediately
  - But sympathetic stimulation and release of adrenalin help glycogenolysis in the liver
- *Sympathetic stimulation:* Lead to glucagon secretion. Hypoglycemia sympathetic stimulation glycogenolysis—stimulation of glucagon secretion leading to correction of hypoglycemia.
- *Amino acid level in blood:* When blood level of amino acid rises glucagon secretion stimulated.
- *Insulin and somatostatin:* Inhibit glucagon. Two routes of insulin to reach the cells of the islets (i) Blood circulation (ii) Paracrine effect.

Applied Physiology

In large doses, glucagon relaxes bowel muscles so can be used in radiological examination of bowel.

■ SOMATOSTATIN

Secreted by $ cells of the islets. It inhibits insulin and glucagon both somatostatin secretion is stimulated by glucose—amino acid meals. Due to paracrine effect of somatostatin inhibitory effect of and β cells are enhanced.

■ PANCREATIC POLYPEPTIDE (PP)

F cells of the islets produce PP. Pancreatic polypeptide contains 36 amino acids. Fasting and hypoglycemia increase the secretion of PP.

CHAPTER 15

The Skin and Regulation of Body Temperature

■ THE SKIN

The skin is the outer covering of the body and is continuous with the mucous membrane lining the body orifices. It is an extensive and diverse organ, with functions which are vital for survival, including protection, excretion, sensation and temperature regulation. The skin consists of two layers: the epidermis and the dermis.

The Epidermis (Fig. 15.1)

The epidermis is the most superficial layer of the skin and is derived from the embryonic ectoderm. It is composed of many layers of stratified squamous epithelium.

The basal or germinative layer is the deepest, and consists of a single layer of columnar cells firmly attached by a basement membrane to the underlying dermis. These cells are constantly dividing to produce new prickle cells which push the older cells upwards towards the surface. Prickle cells derive their name from minute intercellular bridges which hold the cells together. As they approach the surface of the epidermis these cells become flattened to compose the stratum granulosum (granular layer). The nuclei of cells in the granular layer contain granules of keratohyalin, which is a precursor of keratin, a tough fibrous protein. Under the influence of enzymes the nuclei disintegrate and the keratohyalin is converted to keratin.

In the thickest areas of skin over the palms of the hands and the soles of the feet the granular layer transforms into the stratum lucidum (or clear layer), but elsewhere it transforms directly into the stratum corneum or horny layer. The cells of the horny layer are thin, flat non-nucleated cells composed mainly of keratin. They are bound together to form a strong, pliable membrane which is relatively impermeable to water and prevents loss of tissue fluids from the body. The cells of the horny layer are constantly being shed and replaced by cells from the deeper layers.

The life of an epidermal cell, from its formation as a prickle cell by the germinative layer until it is shed from the surface of the skin is between 28 and 30 days, approximately 14 days being spent in the stratum corneum. In some skin diseases, cell division in the germinative layer is greatly increased and in psoriasis the time taken for new cells to be produced and shed is reduced to 7–10 days. Disease or trauma which destroys the intercellular bridges of the prickle cells results in the separation of the cell layers and the formation of blisters.

Between the cells of the basal layer are melanocytes. These are specialized cells, derived from embryonic nervous tissue, which secrete the pigment melanin. Melanin is produced from tyrosine under the influence of the enzyme tyrosinase. This pigment is secreted into the cells of the epidermis and protects the deeper layers of the skin from the effects of the ultra-violet rays in sunlight. Production of melanin is partly controlled by genetic inheritance and partly by the melanocyte-stimulating

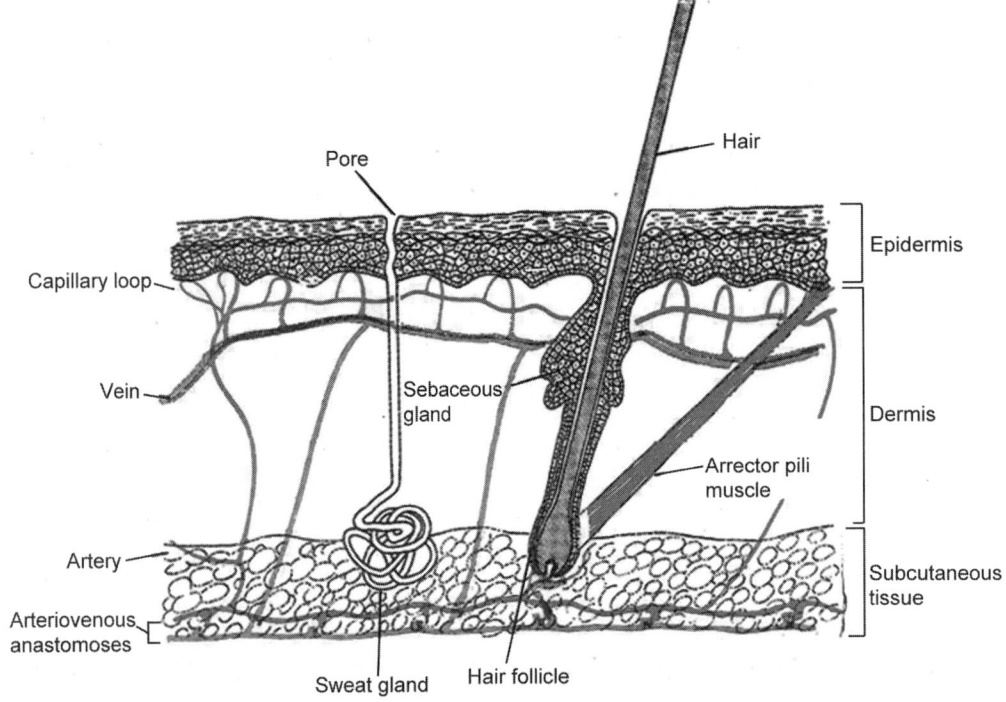

Fig. 15.1: Section through the skin (diagrammatic)

hormone (MSH) secreted by the anterior pituitary gland. Adrenocorticotrophic hormone (ACTH) has a similar structure to MSH and in excess can cause an increase in melanin secretion. Prolonged exposure of the skin to sunlight also stimulates increased pigment production.

Negroes have no more melanocytes than fair-skinned people, but the negro melanocyte produces far greater quantities of melanin.

The Dermis

The dermis, or corium, is composed of dense connective tissue containing collagen fibers which strengthen the skin, and some elastic, fibers that give the skin its resilience and pliability.

The surface of the dermis is thrown into ridges, or papillae, which interlock with the epidermis. The configuration of the papillae are responsible for the skin patterns of the palmar aspects of the hands and fingers, and the soles of the feet and toes. The patterns formed by the papillae are so characteristic for each individual that they can be used as a means of identification.

The under surface of the dermis merges into the subcutaneous tissues which contain a varying number of fat cells and white and yellow connective tissue. The adipose tissue acts as an insulating layer between the skin and the deeper underlying structures of the body.

The dermis contains blood vessels, lymphatics, nerves and some specialized structures derived from the epidermis known as skin appendages. These are the sweat glands, hair, sebaceous glands and nails.

Blood Vessels

The circulation of blood through the dermis nourishes the skin and plays an important role in the regulation of body temperature.

The dermis contains an extensive network of blood capillaries arising from arteries in the subcutaneous layers. Each papilla of the dermis is supplied with a loop of capillaries which provides nourishment to the germinative layer of the epidermis and the structures of the dermis. These capillaries drain into veins which join to form venous plexuses a few millimeters below the skin surface; the venous plexuses of the skin contain large quantities of blood that can heat the surface of the skin.

The rate of blood flow through the skin is regulated according to body temperature, the cutaneous arterioles are supplied with sympathetic nerve fibers which are under the control of the heat regulating center in the hypothalamus. When body temperature is low the arterioles constrict, blood flow through the skin is reduced and heat loss from the skin is minimal. When body temperature is high the arterioles dilate, blood flow through the skin is increased and heat carried in the blood from the internal organs is lost from the skin surface.

In some areas of the body, such as the hands, feet, lips and ears, large vascular connections are found between the arteries and the venous plexuses, called arteriovenous anastomoses; these contain powerful muscle fibers which, when relaxed, allow blood to pass from the arteries to the veins without entering the capillary loops and thus help in the conservation of heat by the body.

Lymphatics

The dermis has a rich network of lymphatic vessels. They begin as lymph spaces at the tip of each papilla and pass between the connective tissue fibers to form lymph capillaries in the subcutaneous tissue.

Nerves

The skin supplies much of the body's sensory information and is provided with both sensory nerves and sympathetic nerve fibers. The sensory nerve endings are widely distributed in a fine network of myelinated and unmyelinated fibers throughout the skin and respond to touch, pressure, pain and temperature. Recent evidence suggests that itching should also be regarded as a specific skin sensation, and may be invoked by a variety of physical stimuli. Exogenous chemicals, such as weak acids or alkalis, are thought to cause itching by releasing histamine, while substances containing proteolytic enzymes (e.g. biological washing powders) probably act directly on the nerve endings of the skin.

Nerve impulses from the cutaneous nerves are relayed via the sensory tracts of the spinal cord to the sensory centers in the cerebrum.

Sympathetic nerve fibers are supplied to the blood vessels, the smooth muscle of the hair follicles and the secretory cells of the sweat glands.

Sweat Glands

Sweat glands develop as down growths from the epidermis. In humans there are two varieties: the eccrine and the apocrine. Eccrine glands are found over the entire skin surface, but are not present in mucous membrane. They are most numerous on the palms of the hands and soles of the feet.

The sweat glands have a glomerulus, or secreting coil, buried deep in the dermis, and a duct which conveys the sweat on to the surface of the skin through a minute opening known as a sweat pore.

The glands are formed of cubical epithelium, and the glomerulus is surrounded by a layer of smooth muscle enclosed in a thin fibrous capsule. Sweat glands are supplied with blood capillaries that form a network around the secreting coils. They are also profusely supplied with sympathetic nerve fibers.

Sweat is a clear watery fluid containing 0.5% of solids. These include sodium chloride, small amounts of other mineral salts and urea.

Sweating is one of the mechanisms by which humans regulate their body temperature. The secretion of sweat is controlled by the heat-regulating center in the hypothalamus via the sympathetic nervous system.

At normal body temperature water is lost continuously through the skin as insensible perspiration; this water loss is not sweat, but is related to evaporation of water passing through the tissue spaces of the epidermis. A rise in body temperature such as occurs in a warm environment or during strenuous exercise leads rapidly to stimulation of the sweat glands and the appearance of sweat over the entire body surface.

Sweating may also be induced by emotional stress such as anxiety or fear, and occurs mainly in the palms, soles and axillae. Excessive production of sweat is called hyperhidrosis.

Apocrine Glands

These are large sweat glands whose ducts open into the hair follicles above the sebaceous glands. They are found in the genital and anal regions, the axillae, nipples and areolae, and only begin to function at puberty.

The apocrine glands produce a viscid, milky secretion which is odorless until contaminated with bacteria. Apocrine secretion is stimulated by stress, pain, fear or sexual activity.

The wax-secreting ceruminous glands found in the external acoustic meatus are modified apocrine glands.

Hair (Fig. 15.2)

Each hair consists of a free shaft extending above the skin surface and a root embedded in the skin. The hair root is enclosed in a hair follicle which is formed by an invagination of the epidermal cells into the dermis. The lower end of the follicle expands to form the hair-bulb. At the base of the hair-bulb is a small projection of cells derived from the dermis called the papilla, which contains blood vessels, nerve endings and melanocytes.

The surface of the papilla is covered by a layer of epidermal cells, the germinal matrix. Hair is formed by proliferation of these cells, which as they are pushed further and further away from the papilla die and become keratinized.

A hair consists of three layers:
1. A cuticle of thin flattened horny cells
2. A cortex of pigmented spindle-shaped cells
3. A medulla of cells which lose their nuclei as they are pushed upwards away from the papilla.

Inserted into the walls of the hair follicle is a minute bundle of smooth muscle fibers, the arrector pilorum, which is innervated by sympathetic nerve fibers. Contraction

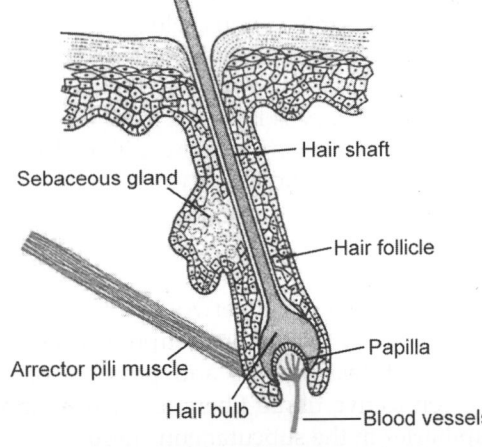

Fig. 15.2: Diagram of hair follicle

of the arrector pilorum causes the hair to 'stand on end' (gooseflesh).

Hair growth occurs in alternating cycles of growth and rest. The growth phase of the human scalp is between 2 and 4 years, while the rest phase lasts about 3 months. Neighboring hair follicles are at different stages in the cycle.

At the end of a growth cycle the hair becomes detached from the papilla and the hair-bulb passes into a rest phase. When growth is resumed the new hair pushes out the old dead hair.

Loss of hair or balding may occur as a result of mechanical trauma (e.g. excessive brushing or the application of very tight curlers), autoimmunity or the systemic administration of certain anticancer drugs. The common male type baldness, also known as androgenetic alopecia, is the result of a dominant hereditary trait in which the hair follicles are excessively sensitive to androgens.

Sebaceous Glands

The sebaceous glands are found all over the body except for the palms of the hands and soles of the feet. They are most numerous on the scalp, forehead, cheeks and chin. The glands are small saccular structures composed of epidermal cells which open into the hair follicles, to form a pilosebaceous unit.

Sebaceous glands secrete sebum, which is formed by the disintegration of large nucleated cells within the gland. Sebum contains fatty acids, cholesterol and other substances, and is discharged through the sebaceous duct into the hair follicle.

Sebum is a natural lubricant, which keeps the hair supple, and the skin soft and pliant, protecting it from the effects of moisture and heat.

Modified sebaceous glands, such as those of the areolae and labia minor, and the Meibomian glands of the eyelids, open directly on to the skin surface.

The activity of sebaceous glands is low until puberty, when it increases rapidly due to the effects of the sex hormones.

Hypersecretion of sebum is involved in the etiology of acne vulgaris, a skin condition occurring in adolescents and young adults.

Nails (Fig. 15.3)

The nails are solid plates of modified horny cells, and form a protective covering on the dorsal surfaces of the fingers and toes, corresponding to the claws arid hoofs of animals.

The nail plate or body is firmly attached to the underlying nail bed, which consists of modified epidermal cells. Each nail has a root embedded in a fold of skin called the nail groove, and is flanked by the nail wall which extends to form the cuticle. The body of the nail plate is semi-translucent and derives its pink color from the blood vessels of the nail bed, while in the region of the lunula (half moon) at the root the nail is more opaque. The nail plate is free at its distal border.

Fingernails grow more rapidly than toenails, taking between 5 and 6 months to grow from the nail matrix to the fingertip. Nail growth accelerates in summertime, and is increased by nail-biting. Growth may be inhibited by disease or malnutrition.

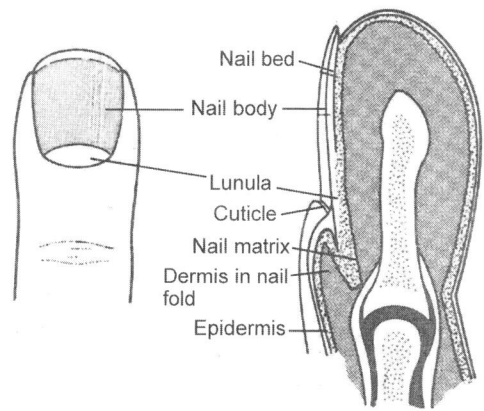

Fig. 15.3: Diagram of nail and nail bed

■ FUNCTIONS OF THE SKIN

Protection

The skin forms a protective covering for the internal structures of the body. It acts as a barrier preventing the entry of microorganisms and other harmful agents. It helps to maintain a stable internal environment by preventing excessive loss of water, electrolytes, proteins and other substances.

Sensation

The sensory nerve endings of the skin constantly convey information about the external environment to the brain, and serve as an important protective mechanism for the body, besides giving an awareness of immediate surroundings and acting as an organ of expression. The skin is able to express fear by its pallor, anxiety by sweating and embarrassment by blushing.

Storage

The skin and subcutaneous tissues act as a store for water and fat. Approximately 15% of the total water content of the body is contained in the skin, while the subcutaneous tissue serves as one of the main fat depots of the body.

Secretion

The secretion of sebum by the sebaceous glands helps to maintain the integrity and suppleness of the skin.

Sweat produced by the eccrine and apocrine gland plays an important part in the regulation of body temperature and aids in the excretion of metabolic waste products.

Formation of Vitamin D

Vitamin D is formed by the action of sunlight on 7-dehydrocholesterol, a fatty substance widely distributed in the skin (p. 246).

Absorption

Substances can be absorbed through the intact skin into the bloodstream and advantage is taken of this fact in the percutaneous administration of certain drugs. An example is trinitrin, a nitrate used in the treatment of angina. This drug is most commonly taken under the tongue (sublingually) because it is quickly absorbed through the mucous membrane of the mouth to bring rapid relief from the chest pain. Its effect is brief, however, and if continuous action is required the percutaneous route may be used. The drug may be incorporated into an ointment (e.g. percutol) or into a 'patch' (e.g. transiderm-nitro) which presents a steady dose to the skin through a rate-limiting membrane.

The Skin and Systemic Disease

There are many diseases of the skin alone but often skin lesions represent only one manifestation of a more generalized (systemic) disease. Measles, for example, is not regarded as a skin disease although the rash may be its most obvious feature. It is an example of an exanthem, a condition with eruptions on the skin. Many infectious febrile illnesses, especially the 'childhood fevers', are characterized by a rash and a variety of other systemic diseases also have a skin component. Skin lesions associated with deep-seated cancer are known as dermal markers of malignancy.

■ REGULATION OF BODY TEMPERATURE

Man is a warm-blooded animal and is capable of maintaining a relatively constant central body temperature which is independent of the surrounding environment.

The central, or core, temperature is the temperature of the internal organs and, in health, is maintained at an almost constant level, while the temperature of the skin and subcutaneous tissues is variable, depending on environmental temperature.

The average normal body temperature is 36.8 °C (98.2 °F) when measured in the closed mouth and approximately 0.5 °C (1.0 °F) higher when measured in the rectum. The normal body temperature varies during each 24 hour period, being at its highest in the early evening and at its lowest in the early morning.

The constant level of the body temperature is maintained by a balance between the heat produced and the heat lost by the body. Failure to maintain this balance results in a rise or fall in the body temperature.

Heat Production

All body tissues produce heat as a by-product of the chemical processes of metabolism, but the greatest heat production is from the most active tissues such as the liver, endocrine glands and muscles.

Muscular activity accounts for about 30% of the body's heat production even at rest. During physical exercise the amount of heat produced is greatly increased. When insufficient heat is produced or when the body is exposed to extreme cold shivering occurs. Shivering is the involuntary contraction of skeletal muscles and is a very powerful means of increasing heat production.

Heat may also be gained by the body when the environmental temperature exceeds body temperature.

Heat Loss

Heat is lost from the body principally through the skin by radiation, conduction, convection and evaporation. A small amount of heat is lost in expired air, urine and feces.

Radiation

Heat is transferred from the body surface to nearby objects that are cooler than the skin, and is transferred to the skin by objects which are warmer than the skin.

Heat is conveyed from the internal organs to the skin by the bloodstream, and radiation of heat from the skin surface can be greatly increased by dilatation of the cutaneous blood vessels.

When the environmental temperature is higher than that of the body, heat cannot be dissipated by radiation.

Conduction

Heat is transferred to any object or substance in direct contact with the body. A rapid loss of heat occurs to an object which is a good conductor of heat, such as metal or light cotton clothing. Heat loss may be minimized by wearing clothing made of wool or fur, which are poor conductors of heat.

Convection

Heat is transferred away from the body surface by movement of air. The air close to the skin is warmed and, as this warm air becomes less dense it rises, allowing cold air to take its place next to the skin.

Evaporation

Heat must be expended to change water into water vapor on the skin surface. There is a small continuous loss of heat from the body in this way due to insensible perspiration. This process cannot be controlled for the purpose of temperature regulation but, when body temperature rises, larger amounts of heat can be lost by sweating. The evaporation of sweat is a very efficient way of cooling the body, and is particularly important when environmental temperature is higher than 37 °C (98.6 °F), since under these conditions the body will gain heat by radiation, conduction and convection. Sweat which drips off the body is ineffective as part of the cooling process. However, if the humidity of the surrounding air is high, sweat cannot evaporate and even environmental temperatures of 27 °C (80.6 °F) become physically uncomfortable.

Control of Temperature Regulation

Body temperature is controlled by the temperature regulating centers of the hypothalamus. These contain two groups of neurons; one group is hot-sensitive, while the other is cold-sensitive. The temperature regulating centers behave like a thermostat, operating in response to the information received through nervous feedback mechanisms from temperature receptors in the body.

A fall in body temperature causes the temperature regulating centers to conserve heat by increasing sympathetic nerve impulses, resulting in constriction of cutaneous blood vessels, and to stimulate heat production by shivering.

A rise in body temperature causes the temperature regulating centers to inhibit sympathetic nerve impulses to cutaneous blood vessels resulting in dilatation of the blood vessels and increased blood flow through the skin. Sweat glands are stimulated to secrete sweat which is evaporated from the skin surface with consequent loss of heat. Skeletal muscle tone is reduced to slow down the rate of heat production (Flowchart 15.1).

Pyrexia

Pyrexia means a body temperature higher than normal and may be caused by toxins produced by infecting organisms or by protein breakdown products from rapid tissue destruction. These substances act on the temperature regulating centers, causing the thermostatic control to be reset at a higher level. As a result, the body is stimulated to produce more heat until the body temperature equals that of the new level, and is then maintained at this level as

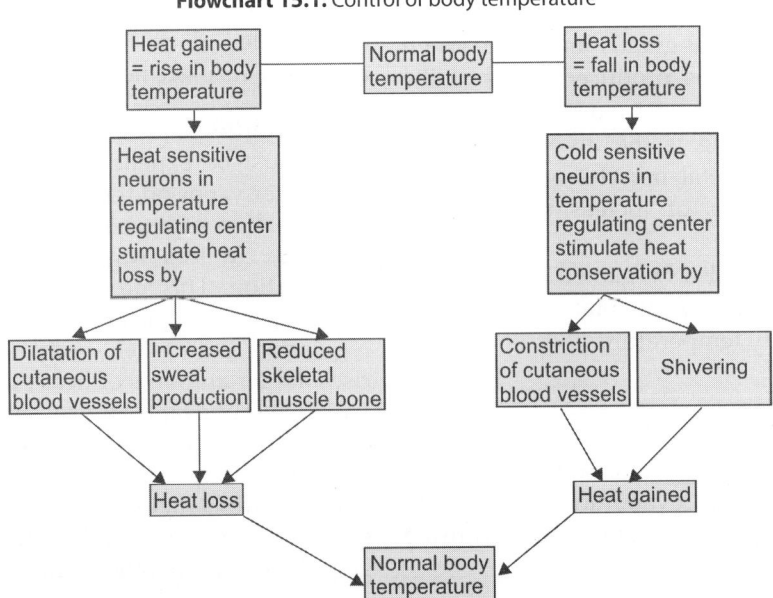

Flowchart 15.1: Control of body temperature

long as the abnormal substance is present in the body.

Substances which affect the temperature regulating system in this way are called pyrogens.

Hyperpyrexia

A body temperature of 40.5 °C (105 °F) or more is called hyperpyrexia, and is extremely dangerous as cellular metabolism is increased so much and so rapidly that the temperature regulating mechanisms are unable to dissipate heat rapidly enough to overcome the rate of heat production. Hyperpyrexia causes degeneration of many body cells (because they literally 'burn themselves out'), and a rectal temperature exceeding 42 °C (108 °F) causes irreversible brain damage.

Hypothermia

A fall in body temperature below 35 °C (95 °F) is called hypothermia. Hypothermia causes a slowing in the chemical reactions of metabolism and reduces the blood flow and oxygen requirements of the tissues. If the condition remains untreated, and the body temperature continues to fall, the temperature regulating mechanisms are lost. The individual becomes increasingly drowsy, and then comatose due to cerebral ischemia; heart and respiratory rates become slower as metabolism is progressively reduced. Death may occur when body temperature falls below 26 °C (78.8 °F), usually from ventricular fibrillation.

Newborn babies and the elderly are particularly susceptible to hypothermia.

CHAPTER 16

Excretory System

The function of the urinary system is the formation and excretion of urine, thereby eliminating waste products, substances (e.g. drugs) which would be toxic if allowed to accumulate in the body, and excess water. The urinary system consists of the following structures (Fig. 16.1):
- The kidneys—the excretory organs
- The ureters—the ducts draining the kidneys
- The urinary bladder—the urinary reservoir
- The urethra—the channel to the exterior.

■ THE KIDNEYS

The kidneys are a pair of organs, each of which is about 11 cm (4½ in) long, 6 cm (2½ in) wide and 3 cm (1¼ in) thick. They lie obliquely rather than vertically with their upper poles nearer than their lower poles to the midline, behind the peritoneum of the posterior abdominal wall. The right kidney is about 1.25 cm (½ in) lower than the left and its lower pole may sometimes be felt on examination of normal subjects during full inspiration. The kidneys move up and down with respiration and are about 2.5 cm (1 in) lower in the standing position than in the recumbent position. The average weight of the adult kidney is about 150 g (5 oz) in the male and 135 g (4½ oz) in the female. The kidneys are dark red in color. Although they may be described as bean-shaped, their shape is so characteristic that the term kidney-shaped is frequently used to describe other objects.

Each kidney has anterior and posterior surfaces, superior and inferior poles, and a lateral convex and a medial concave border. In the center of the medial border is a notch known as hilum, which contains the renal blood vessels and nerves and the renal pelvis, which is the funnel-shaped upper end of the ureter. The center of the hilum is opposite the lower border of the spine of the first lumbar vertebra, about 5 cm from the median plane. The suprarenal glands are sited one on the upper pole of each kidney.

Relations

The kidneys lie embedded in fat (the perrenal or perinephric fat) retroperitoneally on the posterior abdominal wall. Posteriorly

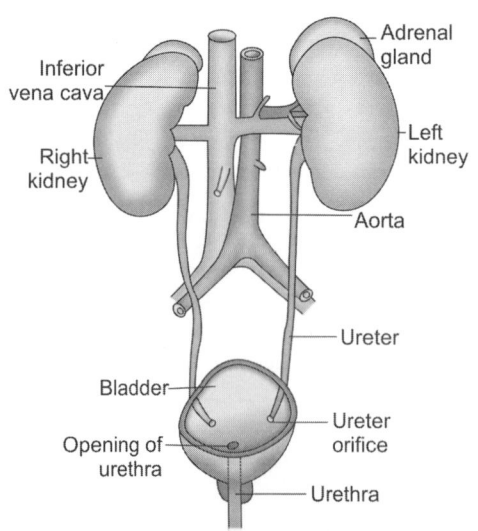

Fig. 16.1: Urinary tract

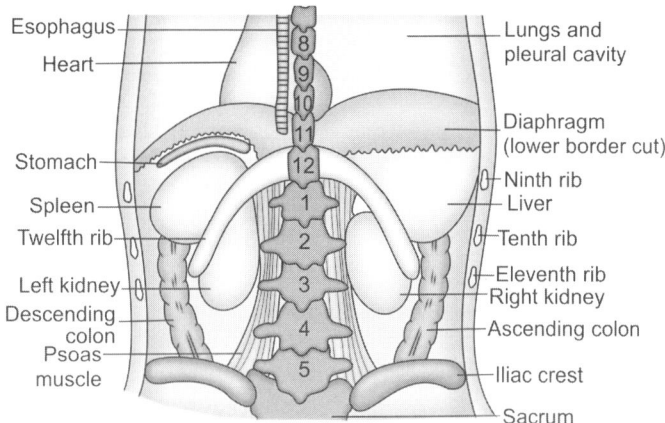

Fig. 16.2: Position of kidneys, liver and spleen from behind

the kidneys are related to the diaphragm (which separates it from the pleura), the psoas major and quadrates lumborum muscles and three nerves (Fig. 16.2). Anteriorly the right kidney is related to the liver, the duodenum, the small intestine and the right or hepatic flexure of the colon. In front of the left kidney lie the stomach, the pancreas, the spleen, the jejunum, the left or splenic flexure of the colon and the commencement of the descending colon. The medial border of the right kidney is related to the inferior vena cava and the right ureter. The medial border of the left kidney is related to the aorta and the left ureter. It is not necessarily intended that the student should learn these relations by rote but rather that, with the aid of diagrams or an anatomical model, a mental picture may be obtained,

■ STRUCTURE

Surrounding each kidney is a thin smooth fibrous capsule. When the kidney is cut in half lengthways by a knife passing through its medial and lateral borders, it is seen to consist of two layers, an outer cortex and an inner medulla. The pelvis of the ureter is seen to divide into two or three major calyces, each of which subdivides into a number of minor calyces. The renal medulla is arranged in conical masses called renal pyramids, the apices of which end in nipple-like papillae which project into the minor calyces. The terminal uriniferous ducts open on the papillae and discharge urine into the ureter (Fig. 16.3).

Microscopically the kidney substance is seen to be composed of:
- Renal corpuscles (Malpighian bodies)
- Renal tubules
- Blood vessels and supporting tissue.

The Renal Corpuscle

Each tubule begins in the cortex in a blind expanded end, known as the glomerular capsule or Bowman's capsule, which is indented by a lobulated tuft of convoluted capillary blood vessels called a glomerulus. The two parts together constitute the renal corpuscle or Malpighian body (Fig. 16.4). Its function is filtration of the plasma. The glomerular filtrate passes down the tubules, in which its composition is modified by processes of reabsorption and secretion so that urine is finally formed. Water is conserved in the body by its reabsorption from the renal tubules; amongst solutes which are selectively reabsorbed are electrolytes, glucose and amino acids.

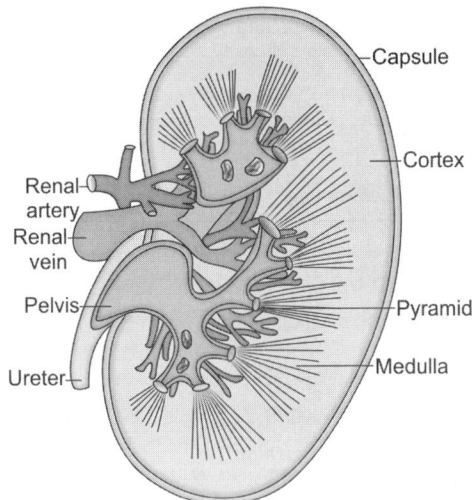

Fig. 16.3: Section through the kidney

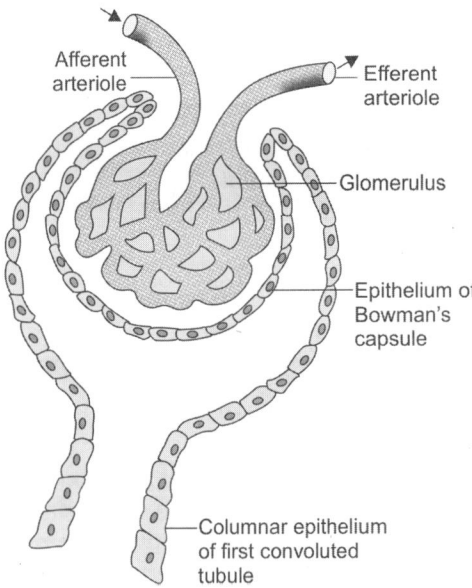

Fig. 16.4: A renal corpuscle, highly magnified

The Renal Tubule (Fig. 16.5)

This consists of:
- The glomerular (Bowman's) capsule
- The proximal convoluted tubule, situated in the cortex
- The loop of Henley in the medulla, with a descending limb, a 'U' bend and an ascending limb

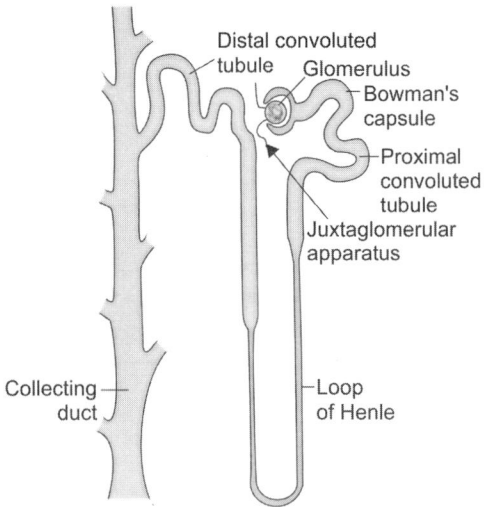

Fig. 16.5: A renal tubule

- The distal convoluted tubule
- The junctional tubule
- The collecting duct.

The collecting ducts commence in the cortex and unite with one another to finally open into the terminal uriniferous ducts or papillary ducts, known as the ducts of Bellini, which open on the papillae of the renal pyramids.

Selective reabsorption of solutes occurs mainly in the proximal convoluted tubule. Sodium and chloride are selectively absorbed in the ascending limb of the loop of Henley and in the distal convoluted tubule under the influence of aldosterone. Because of this, the filtrate reaching the end of the distal convoluted tubule is hypotonic in comparison with the blood. However, the filtrate is finally concentrated in the collecting duct, the walls of which have a variable permeability to water under the influence of the antidiuretic hormone (ADH). Up to 95% of the water in the glomerular filtrate is reabsorbed in the renal tubules so that the end product, the urine, is hypertonic to the blood. The concentrations of osmotically active particles are expressed in milliosmoles (mOsm) per liter or per kilogram and human urine can contain 1400 mOsm/L, achieving almost five times the osmolality of plasma, which is normally 270–300 mOsm/kg of plasma water.

The normal osmolality of the urine varies with diet and fluid intake between 300 and 1000 mOsm/kg of water. Measurement of the urine and plasma osmolality's is often performed in cases of acute renal failure, where a urine/plasma ratio of more than 1.4 indicates a personal cause and a ratio of 1.1 or less indicates acute tubular necrosis.

Selective reabsorption is not the only function of the tubules. There is secretion of various substances into the lumens of the tubules. The secretion of hydrogen ion (H^+) by the cells of the proximal and distal convoluted tubules is important in the maintenance of acid base balance.

Each unit of a renal corpuscle and its renal tubule is called a nephron. Each kidney contains between one and two million nephrons, the number diminishing with increasing age. All of the tubules of the kidney are lined by a single layer of cuboidal epithelium and are surrounded by capillary blood vessels.

Near the glomerulus of each nephron, is the juxtaglomerular apparatus which is formed principally by cells of the distal convoluted tubule and neighboring arterioles. The juxtaglomerular cells secrete an enzyme called renin into the bloodstream. Working in a feedback mechanism, renin helps to maintain the constancy of the extracellular fluid volume through regulation of the secretion of aldosterone by the cortex of the suprarenal gland. A variety of stimuli, such as sodium depletion and dehydration, increase renin secretion. Some patients with hypertension have high renin levels in their blood.

Apart from being an enzyme, renin may be regarded as a hormone and its secretion is one of the endocrine activities of the kidney. Its other endocrine function is the production of a factor which leads to the formation of erythropoietin in the blood. This hormone stimulates erythropoiesis, the production and release of red blood cells from the bone marrow.

■ BLOOD SUPPLY

The kidneys are plentifully supplied with blood from the renal arteries, which are branches of the abdominal aorta. The vascular architecture of the kidneys is complicated but the blood eventually leaves the organs via the renal veins, which enter the inferior vena cava.

Constriction of a renal artery causes increased renin secretion with consequent angiotensin II formation which may account, in part, for the hypertension found in some patients with renal artery stenosis.

■ FUNCTIONS OF KIDNEYS

- Primary function of the kidneys is acting as excretory organ for removal of dissolved waste products of metabolism, urea, uric acid creatine, creatinine, etc. Also removes dyes and drugs introduced into the body. Excess water and solutes are also excreted.
- *Maintenance of homeostasis:* maintaining a constant internal environment, maintaining electrolyte balance, regulating water content, acid–base balance and regulation of BP. It is also important in regulating temperature.
- Role as an endocrine organ in the body.
  - Erythropoietin is secreted by kidney which stimulates erythropoiesis.
  - Secretes renin.

  Angiotensinogen $\xrightarrow{\text{Renin}}$ Angiotensin I

  Angiotensin I $\xrightarrow{\text{ACE}}$ Angiotensin II
- 25-hydroxycholecalciferol → 1, 25-dihydroxycholecalciferol
- Kidney also forms local hormones like kinin, prostaglandin, etc.
- Regulation of blood pressure.

Composition of Urine

Inorganic
Na⁺ — 6 gm/day
K⁺ — 2 g/day
Ca⁺⁺ — 0.2 g/day
Phosphate — 1.7 g/day

Organic
Urea — 20.3 gm/day
Uric acid — 0.6 g/day
Creatinine — 1.2 gm/day

Volume
1 — 2.5 L/day
pH — 4.5 – 8

Mechanism of Urine Formation

Four processes are involved in the mechanism of formation of urine.
1. Glomerular filtration
2. Tubular reabsorption
3. Tubular secretion (Table 16.1)
4. Concentration and acidification of urine.

Glomerular Filtration

Glomerular filtration occurs across the glomerular membrane. Mechanism is similar to tissue fluid formation, i.e. according to starling's hypothesis. Since the pressure in the glomerular capillary is very high, water and solutes which are less than 4 nm are forced through the glomerular membrane into the capsular space. This filtration is the ultrafiltration of plasma. About 180 L of filtrate enter capsular space each day. Out of this 178 to 179 L return to circulation by tubular reabsorption. Only 1–2 L is excreted as urine.

Factors Favoring Filtration

- Glomerular capillaries are 50 times more permeable than capillaries elsewhere in the body. Glomerular filtrate contains all the materials present in blood except formed elements and most of the plasma proteins.
- Glomerular capillaries present a large surface area
- Glomerular capillary blood pressure is high. This is because efferent arteriole is smaller in diameter than afferent arteriole. So, highly resistant to outflow of blood from glomerulus. Since plasma is filtered out from the glomerular capillary, the blood in the efferent arteriole become very viscous and thus also contributes to the increased resistance to flow.

Glomerular Filtration Rate (GFR)

GFR is defined as the amount of filtrate formed in all the nephrons of both kidneys in one minute. It is normally 125 mL/min.

Factors Influencing GFR

(a) Net filtration pressure
(b) Permeability of glomerular membrane
(c) Surface area of filtering membrane
(d) Age

Net Filtration Pressure

Filtration across the glomerular membrane depend on three main pressures.
1. Glomerular blood hydrostatic pressure (GBHP)
   This pressure promotes filtration. Hydrostatic pressure is the force that a fluid under pressure exerts against the wall of its container.
2. Capsular hydrostatic pressure (CHP) oppose filtration.

Table 16.1: Tubular secretion substances

Substances secreted	Endogenous substances secreted by the tubule
PAH	Ethereal sulfates
Phenol red	Steroid
Sulfonephthalein dye	Glucose
Penicillin	5H1AA-metabolite of serotonin
Iodinated dyes	

3. Blood colloidal osmotic pressure (BCOP) opposes filtration. The greater the solute concentration greater will be the osmotic pressure.
GBHP = 55 mm Hg. CHP = 15 mm Hg
BCOP = 30 mm Hg.
Tubular COP = Negligible
Net filtration pressure = (GBHP + TCOP)
− (CHP + BCOP)
= 55 − 45
= 10 mm Hg.

Thus a pressure of 10 mm Hg cause plasma to be filtered from the glomerular into the capsular space.
GFR = KF × NFP
KF – ultra filtration coefficient.

Factors Affecting GFR

- Changes in renal blood flow
- Changes in the glomerular capillary hydrostatic pressure
- Changes in the systemic pressure
- Afferent or efferent arteriolar constriction
- Changes in hydrostatic pressure in Bowman's capsule
- Ureteral obstruction
- Edema of kidney inside tight renal capsule.
- Changes in concentration of plasma proteins (dehydration, hypoproteinemia, etc.)
- Changes in KF
- Changes in glomerular capillary permeability
- Changes in effective filtration surface area.

Glomerular Ultrafiltration Coefficient

KF is the product of glomerular capillary permeability and effective filtration surface area.
KF = 15.5 mL/min/m^2/mm Hg × 0.8 m^2
= 12.5 mL/min/mm Hg
$$KF = \frac{GFR}{NFP} = \frac{125 \text{ mL/min}}{10 \text{ mm Hg}}$$
= 12.5 mL/min/mm Hg

Regulation of GFR

Autoregulation
Renal blood flow and GFR remains nearly constant even in the presence of large changes in near systemic arterial pressure.

Hormonal Regulation
- *Renin:* Angiotensin aldosterone mechanism
- Atrial Natriuretic peptide.

Renin Angiotensin Aldosterone Mechanism in Regulation of GFR
When there is a reduction in the GFR, the juxtaglomerular cells of juxtaglomerular apparatus (JGA) are stimulated to secrete renin

Angiotensinogen $\xrightarrow{\text{Renin}}$ angiotensin I

Angiotensin I $\xrightarrow[\text{By lungs}]{\text{Renin}}$ Angiotensin II

Atrial Natriuretic Peptide (ANP)
ANP secreted by cells of atria.
Action: Diuresis and natriuresis.
Importance of ANP: In patients with hypertension and renal failure, administration of ANP is of great benefit since it increases GFR decrease in water retention and edema. It thus decrease BP.

Neural Regulation
Moderate sympathetic stimulation causes constriction of both afferent and efferent arteriole and so GFR remains unaltered. With maximum sympathetic stimulation as in exercise, hemorrhage, stress, etc. vasoconstriction of afferent arteriole predominates leading to decrease in GFR. Sympathetic stimulation also cause release of adrenalin from adrenal medulla which cause vasoconstriction of afferent arteriole leading to decreased hydrostatic pressure of glomerulus which decreases GFR.

Measurement of Renal Blood Flow
Using para aminohippuric acid (PAH) applying Fick's principle.

PAH is actively secreted.
C PAH = Effective Renal plasma flow
$= \dfrac{UPAH \cdot V}{PPAH}$
UPAH = 14 mg/mL
Volume = 0.9 mg/min
PPAH = 0.02 mg/mL
ERPF $= \dfrac{14 \times .9}{0.02} = 630$ mL/min
PAH extraction ratio
= 0.9
Actual renal plasma flow
$= \dfrac{630}{0.9} = 700$ mL/min
Extraction ratio
= 0.9
PCV = 45%
700 mL is 55% of blood flowing
Renal blood flow
$= \dfrac{700 \times 100}{55} = 1273$ mL/min

Measuring GFR—Using Inulin

Concentration of inulin in urine = 35 mg/mL
Volume of urine = 0.9 mL/min
Plasma concentration of inulin = 0.25 mg/mL
C in $= \dfrac{35 \times 0.9}{0.25} = 126$ mL/min.

Special Features of Renal Blood Flow

- Enormous volume of blood flow – 1200 mL/min
- Differential distribution of blood flow – to cortex and medulla.
- Low O_2 consumption.
- Similarity to portal circulation.
- Hydrostatic pressure high in glomerular capillaries.
- Shows autoregulation (constant blood flow and constant GFR).

■ FUNCTIONAL ANATOMY

The Nephron

Each individual renal tubule and its glomerulus is a unit called nephron. Each human kidney has approximately 1.3 million nephrons. There are two types of nephrons in kidney.

1. *Juxtamedullary nephrons:* The main feature is the loops of Henle are very long and thin and extend to the medulla of the kidney. Here, the glomeruli are in the juxtamedullary portions of the cortex.
2. *Cortical nephron:* The nephrons with glomeruli in the outer portion of renal cortex have short loops of Henle.

Diagram of Nephron

The parts of nephron includes:
- Glomerulus and Bowman's capsule
- Proximal convoluted tubule
- Distal convoluted tubule
- Collecting duct.

Glomerulus: It is 200 µm in diameter is formed by the invagination of a tuft of capillaries into the dilated, blind end of the nephron (Bowman's capsule). The capillaries are supplied by an afferent arteriole and drained by a slightly smaller efferent arteriole.

Bowman's capsule: Two cellular layers separate the blood from the glomerular filtrate in the Bowman's capsule; the capillary endothelium and the specialized epithelium of the capsule. Basal lamina separates these two layers. Podocytes form epithelium of the capsule. Stellate cells called mesangial cells are located between the basal lamina and the endothelium. Mesangial cells are contractile and play a role in the regulation of glomerular filtration.

The endothelium is fenestrated with pores 70–90 nm in diameter. The epithelial cells made of podocytes form filtration slits along the capillary wall. Slits are approximately 25 nm wide and each is closed by a thin membrane.

Glomerular membrane allows the passage of neutral substances up to 4 nm diameter and excludes those with diameter more than 8 nm.

Proximal Convoluted Tubule: Formed by a single layer of cells that interdigitate with one another and are united by apical tight junctions. Between bases of the cells are extension of extracellular space called lateral intercellular spaces. There are microvilli in the luminal edges forming brush border.

Loop of Henle: The descending portion of the loop and proximal portion of the ascending limb is made of thin permeable cells. The thick portion of the ascending limb is made of thick cells containing many mitochondria. Fifteen percent of nephrons have long loop of Henle and glomeruli are located in the juxtamedullary portions of the cortex and is called juxtamedullary nephrons. Their loop of Henle extend down to medullary pyramids.

Juxtaglomerular Apparatus (Fig. 16.6)

The thick end of the ascending limb of loop of Henle reaches the glomerulus of the nephron from which tubule arose and remain between its afferent and efferent arterioles. Specialized cells at the end form the macula densa which is close to the efferent and particularly the afferent arteriole. The macula, the neighboring lacis cells and the renin secreting juxtaglomerular cells in the afferent arteriole form the JGA.

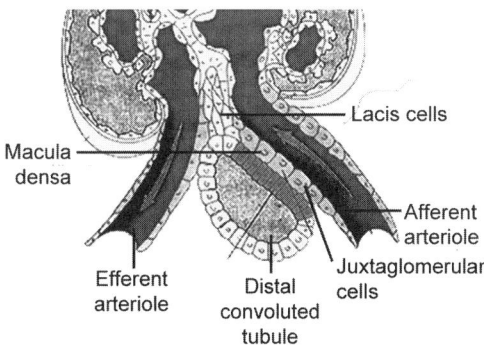

Fig. 16.6: Juxtaglomerular apparatus

Distal Convoluted Tubule (DCT)

It starts at the macula densa is about 5 mm long and, its epithelium is lower than that of proximal convoluted tubules (PCT). A few microvilli are present, but no distinct brush border.

Collecting Duct

DCTs coalesce to form collecting ducts that are about 20 mm long and pass through the cortex and medulla to empty into pelvis of the kidney at the apexes of the medullary pyramids. The epithelium of collecting ducts is made of principal cells and intercalated cells. P (Principal) cells predominate are relatively tall with few organelle. They are involved in sodium reabsorption and vasopressin stimulates water reabsorption. These cells are concerned with acid secretion and HCO_3 transport. Also there are cells secreting prostaglandins.

Filtration Fraction (FF)

The ratio of GFR to renal plasma flow filtration fraction is normally 0.16 to 0.2. The GFR varies less than renal plasma flow (RPF). When there is a fall in systemic BP, the GFR falls less than the RPF because of the efferent arteriolar constriction and consequently the FF rises.

■ TUBULAR FUNCTION

Filtered load: The amount of solute transported across the glomerular membranes per unit time.

Filtered load = GFR × plasma concentration of the solute
= mL/min × mg/min = mg/min.

Renal Tubular Transport Maximum (TM): It refers to the maximal amount of a given solute that can be transported (reabsorbed or secreted) per minute by renal tubules.

The highest attainable rate of reabsorption is called the maximum tubular reabsorptive capacity and is designated Tr (Tm). Substances that are reabsorbed by an active carrier medicated process and that have a Tm include—phosphate ion (HPO_4), Sulfate (SO_4), glucose, amino acids, uric acid, albumin, hydroxy butarate and α keto glutarate.

The amount reabsorbed is proportionate to the amount filtered and hence to the plasma level of glucose times the GFR up to the transport maximum (TmG). When TmG is exceeded; amount of glucose in urine rises. TmG is 375 mg/min in men and 300 mg/min in women.

Tubular secretary capacity Ts (Tm) of substances that are secreted by the kidney such as penicillin certain diuretics, salicylate, PAH, thiamine, etc. exceeds the GFR. Transport maximum is the difference between filtered load and excretion rate.

Excretion Rate: It is the amount of a substance that appears in urine per unit time. Excretion rate = Urine flow rate (V) × urine concentration (U_x) = mL/min × mg/mL = mg/min.

Glucose Reabsorption

Glucose is filtered at a rate of approximately 100 mg/min.

Resting plasma level of glucose × GFR = 80 mg/dL × 125 mL/min is the filtered load of glucose. Hundred percent of the glucose is actively transported into the PCT provided its concentration in the plasma is normal.

The glucose reabsorption and excretion process are function of the plasma glucose concentration (PG).

- Increasing the PG results in progressive linear increase in the filtered load of glucose.
- At low PG the absorbed rate of glucose is complete. Hence, no glucose is excreted in urine.
- When PG increases above 180–200 mg/dL the glucose reabsorption is not complete and it passes through the urine (Glucosuria). This plasma glucose level at which glucose first appears in urine is called renal Threshold for glucose. The actual renal threshold is 200 mg/dL of arterial plasma, and 180 mg/dL of venous plasma.
- As the reabsorptive limit is approached, the urinary excretion rate increases linearly with increase by PG
  - When the reabsorptive limit of tubule is reached the amount of glucose rate per minute remain constant and independent of PG.
  - When the reabsorption limit of tubule is exceeded, the amount of glucose that passes in the urine increases linearly with PG. The limit is referred to as TmG.
- The TmG is approx. 375 mg/minute in men and 300 mg/minute in women. Thus renal threshold, i.e. PG above which glucosuria occurs can be predicted from TmG.

Normally when glucose is filtered at the rate of 100 mg/min, PG will be 80 mg/dL. If glucose is filtered at the rate of 375 gm/min and GFR is 125 mL/min the expected value of renal threshold will be

$$\frac{375 \text{ mg/min}}{125 \text{ mL/min}} = 300 \text{ mg/dL}$$

Therefore, the predicted renal threshold for glucose would be approx 300 mg/dL. However, the actual renal threshold for glucose is 200 mg/dL of arterial plasma or 180 mg/dL of venous plasma. This is so because the relation between PG and TG (glucose reabsorbed) is different, e.g. when we plot PG on X axis and TG on Y axis actual curve obtained is rounded rather than sharply angulated and deviates considerably from the ideal curve. This deviation is called splay. The ideal curve would have been obtained if

- TmG in all the tubules were identical, i.e. 375 mg/min and
- All glucose were removed from each tubule when the amount filtered was below the TmG.

Causes

- Not all the 2.6 million nephrons in the kidney have exactly the same TmG or filtration rate.
- Some glucose escapes reabsorption when the amount filtered is below the TmG because the reactions involved in glucose transport are not completely irreversible.

Mechanism of Glucose Reabsorption

It is similar to its absorption as in the GIT. Glucose and Na^+ bind to a common carrier (SGLT2) in the luminal membrane, and glucose is carried into the cells as Na+ moves down its electrical and chemical gradient. The Na^+ is then pumped out of the cell into the lateral intercellular spaces and the glucose moves into peritubular capillaries.

Glucose transport via GLUT-2 is by simple diffusion. Thus glucose transport across PCT cells is an example of secondary active transport, the energy for the active transport is provided by the Na^+ K^+ ATPase that pumps Na^+ out the cell.

Glucose transport in the kidney is inhibited by plant glucoside phlorizin which completes with D glucose for binding to the carrier. Rate of transport of D glucose is greater than that of L glucose.

Other Examples of Secondary Active Transport

Amino acid (AA) reabsorption in PCT. Main carriers in the luminal membrane cotransport Na^+ whereas carriers in the basolateral membrane are not Na^+ dependent. Na^+ is pumped out of the cells by Na^+K^+ ATPase and the AA leave by passive or facilitated diffusion to the interstitial fluid. Some chloride is reabsorbed with Na^+ and K^+ in the thick ascending limb of the loop of Henle. In addition two members of family of Cl channels are present in kidney.

Dent disease: Mutations of gene for one of Cl channels associated with Ca^{2+} containing kidney stones and hypercalciurea.

Glomerulo Tubular Balance

It is the mechanism of regulation of Na^+ excretion. Total amount of Na^+ reabsorption is directly proportional to GFR, i.e. total amount of Na^+ reabsorbed rises when GFR rises and vice-versa. Most of this change occurs in PCT. The tubule tends to reabsorb a constant fraction of amount filtered, rather than a constant amount. This proportionality is referred to as glomerulo tubular balance.

High GFR → increase oncotic pressure of plasma by the time it reaches the efferent arteriole → increase sodium reabsorption from the renal tubul

Glomerulo – tubular balance
reabsorption in PCT
↓
Fluid delivery to loop of Henle and first part of DCT
↓
Solute reabsorption in thick Ascending limb of loop of Henle.

Applied Aspect

- Patients with kidney disease return excessive amount of Na^+ and become edematous due to
  - ↑ Amount of Na^+ filtered
  - ↑ In aldosterone secretion
  - ↓ In plasma protein → edema →
  - ↓ Plasma volume → aldosterone secretion via Renin-Angiotensin system.
- In hypokalemic alkalosis (c/c vomiting, or hyper aldosteronemia)
  Exchange of H^+ for Na^+ is greater than exchange of K^+ for Na^+. Urine becomes more acidic, i.e. and plasma becomes more alkaline.
- *In hypoaldosteronism:* Decrease Na^+ reabsorption from DCT decrease

secretion of K⁺ and H⁺ causing hyperkalemia and acidosis.

Fate of Na⁺ Inside the Tubular Cell

Na⁺–K⁺ ATPase is present in the basolateral membrane of the tubular epithelium. This pumps Na⁺ actively from the tubular cell into lateral intercellular space and the peritubular space and pumps in K⁺ from interstitial space into the cell. The Na⁺ in the interstitial and lateral intercellular space enters the peritubular capillaries. Low hydrostatic pressure and high colloid osmotic pressure of peritubular capillaries help in the movement of Na⁺ into the peritubular capillaries. The osmotic pressure of blood in the peritubular capillaries is high because fluid has been filtered across the glomeruli into the renal tubule leading to an increase in the concentration of plasma proteins. Reabsorption of Na⁺ promotes the reabsorption of water by osmosis from renal tubules into peritubular space. As water leaves the filtrate the concentration of the remaining solutes in the filtrate increases. This creates a concentration difference for substances like K⁺, Cl⁻, HCO_3^-, urea, etc. and these will be absorbed by simple diffusion into the tubular cell and from there to the peritubular capillaries.

Importance of Na⁺ Reabsorption

Na⁺ is the most abundant cation in the ECF and is the main determinant of ECF volume. When there is hyponatremia, there will be a fall in the ECF volume followed by a fall in the blood pressure.

Factors Affecting Na⁺ Reabsorption

GFR

A constant fraction of the filtered load is reabsorbed → load dependent reabsorption or glomerulo tubular balance. Percentage of solute reabsorbed is held constant. Two third of filtered Na⁺ reabsorbed from PCT.

GFR   Absorption in PCT

125 mL/min   65% GFR → 81 mL/min
    ↓
150 mL/min → 65% of GFR → 98 mL/min.

Mechanism
- Oncotic pressure in peritubular capillary increase
- Surface area of proximal tubule is high—brush border
- Leaky tight junctions in luminal epithelium of PCT.

Significance: Over loading of DCT when GFR increases.

Neural Factors
- Sympathetic stimulation occurs when decrease ECF Volume. → Stimulate Na⁺ reabsorption in PCT, also stimulate Renin secretion.
- ↑ Plasma volume → Baroreceptor stimulation
- → Sympathetic tone → inhibit Na⁺ reabsorption and renin secretion
  Thus blood volume brought to normal.

Hormonal Factors

RAA mechanism operates when plasma Na⁺ decreases and plasma K⁺ increases

Angiostensin II ⟨ Directly stimulate Na⁺ reabsorption in PCT
                  Stimulate aldosterone from adrenal cortex

↑ Plasma Volume →↑ Na⁺ reabsorption in DCT

↓ Renin from JGA →↓ formation of Angiotesin II

Inhibit Na⁺
Reabsorption from PCT
Decrease angiotensin II →↓ Na⁺ reabsorption from DCT.

Actions of Aldosterone
- Increase the permeability of luminal membrane to Na⁺
- Stimulate Na⁺ K⁺ ATPase so that ICF, NA⁺ is decreased in the renal tubular cell and more Na⁺ reabsorbed from the tubule.

ANP

An increase plasma volume increase secretion of ANP from heart (stimulate–arterial stretch).

Actions of ANP
- Dilate afferent arteriole
- *Relax mesangial cell:* Increase total surface area
- *Direct action:* On adrenal cortex → decrease aldosterone secretion → inhibit Na⁺ reabsorption in collecting duct
- Inhibit renin secretion
- Inhibit renal sympathetic nerves.

Starling's Forces

↑ PTC hydrostatic pressure or
↓ PTC oncotic pressure
} Referred reabsorption of fluid into capillaries

→↑ hydrostatic pressure of interstitial space
→↓ reabsorption of water and solutes from tubular lumen – especially PCT →↑ excretion of Na⁺ and water.

Drugs
- *Xanthines:* Caffeine, theophyllin ↓ tubular reabsorption of Na⁺ and GFR.
- *Carbonic Anhydrase Inhibitors:* → Acetezolamide H⁺ secretion ↑ Na⁺ and K⁺ excretion.
- *Thiazides:* Inhibit Na⁺ Cl⁻ cotransporter in the distal tubule.
- *Loop:* Diuretics furosemide inhibit Na⁺ K⁺ 2Cl⁻ cotransporter in thick ascending limb of loop of Henle.

Reabsorption of Amino Acids

Filtered AA are completely reabsorbed in the proximal tubule by secondary active transport by sodium-amino acid symporter. Once inside the cell AA is transported to the peritubular space by simple diffusion or facilitated diffusion.

Reabsorption of Uric Acid

Ninety eight percent of filtered uric acid is reabsorbed by the renal tubules. Eighty per cent of uric acid in urine is due to tubular secretion. Normal plasma uric acid concentration—3–6 mg/100 mL. Normal uric acid excretion—1 gm/day. Increase in plasma uric acid may be due to:
- Decreased excretion, e.g. treatment with thiazide diuretics.
- Increased production of uric acid, e.g. leukemia, pneumonia, etc. increased breakdown of uric acid rich white blood cells. Reabsorption of uric acid by renal tubules can be inhibited by drugs like.
  - Probenecid
  - Phenylbutazone, etc. Thus, renal excretion of uric acid can be increased. These drugs are used in the treatment of gout. Gout included a group of disorders like arthritis renal stones, etc. due to hyperuricemia. Other drugs used in the treatment of gout:
    - Colchicines inhibit uric acid crystal phagocytosis by WBC and decrease joint manifestations.
    - Allopurinol which inhibits xanthine oxidase acts by decreasing uric acid production.

Chloride Reabsorption

- By passive diffusion along with Na+ into the cell.
- It diffuses passively through the inter cellular tight junctions in the proximal tubule.

Ca²⁺ and Pi Reabsorption

Ninety-nine percent of filtered Ca^{++} is reabsorbed by the nephron. One percent is excreted through urine. Urinary Ca^{2+}

excretion is 200 mg/day. Eighty percent of Ca^{2+} channels, in the renal tubule. From the cell Ca^{2+} reaches the interstitial space by Ca^{2+} pump which is an active process. Ca^{2+} reabsorption is regulated by parathyroid hormone, calcitonin and calcitriol.

HCO_3 Reabsorption

HCO_3 reabsorption occurs throughout the nephron except in the descending limb of loop of Henle.

Reabsorption from PCT

- Approx 90% of the filtered HCO_3 is reabsorbed into the PCT by secondary active transport (antiport) via the Na+ H^+ exchanger, this represents more than 4000 mEq/day.
- The secreted H^+ reacts with filtered HCO_3 to form carbonic acid (H_2CO_3). The presence of carbonic anhydrase on the microvillus of the luminal border of the PCT catalyzes the rapid dehydration of H_2CO_3 to form CO_2 and water.
- Both CO_2 and H_2O diffuse back into PCT cells which together with CO_2 derived from cell metabolism is rehydrated by intracellular CA into H_2CO_3 which dissociates to form H^+ and HCO_3^-. Thus HCO_3^- is formed as newly synthesized HCO_3^- by renal tubular cells.
  - This newly synthesized HCO_3^- is reabsorbed across
  - The basolateral membrane by a secondary active transport system into the peritubular blood along with equimolar amounts of Na^1
  - The H^+ is secreted again by H^+ pump into the lumen.

Reabsorption from the DCT and CT

- The remaining 10–15% of the filtered HCO_3^- is reabsorbed by the DCT and CT via a mechanism that involves the exchange of Na^+ for K^+ or H^+ (as in PCT).
- Unlike the PCT the DCT and CT have H^+ K^+ ATPase or Na^+ K^+ ATPase pumps

at the luminal membrane and the lack of CA from that site.

K^+ Reabsorption

Whole of the filtered load of K^+ is reabsorbed from the renal tubules. About 2 gm of K^+ is excreted/day and this is due to secretion of K^+ by renal tubules. Distal tubules secrete K^+, in exchange for Na^+ under the influence of aldosterone.

Urea Absorption

The amount of urea excreted depends on the amount of urea formed which in turn depends on the amount of protein ingested. Breakdown product of protein metabolism urea is also secreted into the tubular lumen in the thin ascending limb of loop of Henle. *Normal blood urea:* 20–40 mg/100 mL of blood. Amount excreted = 25 g/day.

Increase in the blood urea level is known as Uremia or azotemia.

K^+ Transport

K^+ is completely filtered at the glomerulus and it is the only plasma electrolyte that is both reabsorbed and secreted into the renal tubercles.

Water Reabsorption

GFR is 180 L/day. Only 1–15 L is excreted as urine. The rest is reabsorbed by renal tubular cells. Percent of water reabsorbed in the different segments of nephron.

Proximal tubule	– 65%
Loop of Henle	– 15%
DCT	– 5%

Collecting tubule:
Cortical collecting tubule – 10%
Medullary collecting tubule – 4.7%.

Ninety percent of water reabsorption occurs by osmosis together with the reabsorption of solutes such as Na^+, Cl^- and glucose. Solutes reabsorbed accumulate in the peritubular and lateral intercellular spaces leading to an increase in the tonicity of this area. So, water moves from tubular lumen to these areas by osmosis through two routes.

1. Transcellular route
2. Pericellular route.

The increase in hydrostatic pressure in the peritubular space drives water and solutes into peritubular capillary. This is termed obligatory water reabortion because water is obliged to follow the solutes. This type of water reabsorption occurs in the PCT and descending limb of loop of Henle because these structures are always permeable to water.

The remaining 10% of water reabsorption occurs in the distal nephron, i.e. the last part of DCT and collecting tubule under the influence of ADH. This is termed facultative water reabsorption, since this reabsorption of water is facilitated by ADH. Homeostasis is maintained by this portion of renal water reabsorption. A negative feedback system regulates ADH—stimulated water reabsorption. When osmotic pressure of blood is high osmoreceptors in the hypothalamus are stimulated. They send impulses to the supraoptic and para ventricular nuclei of hypothalamus and also to the posterior pituitary gland leading to the release of ADH into blood stream. ADH acts on the collecting duct causing increased reabsorption of water from the distal tubule bringing the blood osmotic pressure back to normal.

■ AQUAPORINS

Diffusion of water across cell membrane depends on protein water channels called aquaporins. There are four types aquaporins in humans:

1. Aquaporin 1
2. Aquaporin 2
3. Aquaporin 5
4. Aquaporin 9.

Most of the aquaporins are found in the kidneys. They are also found in liver, lungs, spleen, salivary and lacrimal glands. Aquaporin 1 is localized in the proximal tubule. Aquaporin 2 is present in the collecting ducts. Unlike other aquaporins this aquaporin is stored in vesicles in the cytoplasm of principal cells. These aquaporins get inserted on the cell membrane of collecting duct only in the presence of ADH. The effect is mediated via V2 receptors.

Diabetes insipidus is a condition caused by ADH deficiency where the urine becomes hypotonic to plasma and urine volume is increased.

In nephrogenic diabetes insipidus, the collecting ducts fail to respond to ADH. This can be due to mutation of gene coding for V2 receptors, making the receptors unresponsive or may be due to mutation of the gene for aquaporin 2.

Normal osmolality of urine is 1200 with osmoles/kg of water. It varies with urine flow rate.

In diabetes insipidus it becomes 30 mOsm/kg of water.

■ WATER INTOXICATION

Normal urine flow rate is 2 mL/min. Maximum urine flow that can be achieved is 16 mL/min. If water is ingested at a higher rate than this, swelling of the cells become severe due to hypotonic ECF. This leads to symptoms of water intoxication like convulsions, coma, etc. due to swelling of cells in the brain that may even lead to death.

■ TUBULAR SECRETION

Tubular secretion is the movement of materials from blood into tubular fluid, i.e. tubular secretion removes materials from blood into the renal tubules across the renal tubular cells. It secreted substances include

H^+, K^+ NH_3, creatinine steroids, drugs like penicillin, salicylates, etc.

K^+ Secretion

Normally almost all the K^+ that is filtered is reabsorbed by the renal tubules. To maintain K^+ homeostasis (concentration of K^+ in body fluids constant). DCT and collecting duct secrete variable amounts of K^+. The rate of flow of tubular fluid through the distal portions of the nephron because with rapid flow there is less opportunity for the tubular K^+ concentration to rise to a valve that stops further secretion of K^+. So, when urine flow rate is increase there will be increased secretion of K^+.

Regulation of K^+ Secretion

- Aldosterone increases K^+ secretion.
- When plasma K^+ concentration increases K^+ secretion also increases.
- In the distal tubules Na^+ is reabsorbed and K^+ secreted into the tubular lumen. When concentration of Na^+ in the DCT is high, there will be increased Na^+ reaborption and K^+ will be secreted into the lumen in exchange for Na^+. This is because reabsorption of Na^+ lowers the potential difference across the tubular cell and there will be passive movement of K^+ out of the cell. It is also secreted by an antiport mechanism in exchange for Na^+.
- When urine flow rate is increased K^+ secretion is also increased.
- When H^+ ion secretion is increased in the renal tubules K^+ secretion is decreased due to competition with Na^+ for the carrier protein.

Importance of K^+ Secretion

The amount of K^+ secreted is approximately equal to the K^+ intake and K^+ balance is thus maintained in the body. High plasma K^+ referred to as hyperkalemia is a serious situation and it may even lead to cardiac arrest. It occurs only in cases of impaired renal function.

Normal K^+ excretion = 2–3 g/day.

■ HYPOKALEMIA

Decrease in plasma K^+ is known as hypokalemia and is a common condition.

Causes of Hypokalemia

- Excessive loss of K^+ from the body as in severe vomiting, diarrhea, polyuria, etc.
- Decreased dietary intake of K^+
- Drugs like:
  - Steroids
  - Insulin shifts K^+ intracellularly
  - Adrenergic agonists
  - Loop diuretics inhibit Na^+ K^+ $2Cl^-$
  - Carbonic anhydrase inhibitors.

H^+ Secretion

H^+ secretion occurs by two mechanisms in the proximal and distal tubules.
- By secondary active transport.

  Extrusion of Na^+ into the lateral intercellular space by Na^+ K^+ ATPase decreases intracellular Na^+ and Na^+ enters the cell from the tubular lumen in exchange for H^+ (antiport). Thus for each H^+ secreted, one Na^+ and one HCO_3^- enter the interstitial fluid.
- By aldosterone

  Aldosterone acts on H^+ K^+ ATPase and increases the secretion of H^+.

NH_3 Secretion

In the tubular cell the following reaction occur:

$$\text{Glutamine} \xrightarrow{\text{Glutaminase}} \text{Glutamate} + NH_3$$

$$\text{Glutamate} \xrightarrow{\text{Glutamic Dehydrogena}} \text{Ketoglutarate} + NH_3$$

$$NH_4 \longleftrightarrow NH_3 + H^+$$

The NH_3 formed inside the tubular cell is secreted into the tubular fluid and is excreted.

CONCENTRATION AND DILUTION OF URINE

Even though the fluid intake varies, the total volume of body fluid remains constant. This is accomplished by the ability of the kidney to regulate the rate of loss of water through urine. Urine osmolarity can vary from 50–1200 mOsm/L of water.

When there is a large excess of water in the body the kidney can excrete as much as 20 L/day of dilute urine, with a concentration as low as 50 mOsm/L (Fig. 16.7). The kidney continues to reabsorb large amounts of water in the distal parts of nephron, including the late distal tubule and the collecting duct.

After ingestion of excess water the kidney rids the body of the excess water but does not excrete excess amounts of solutes.

When the glomerular filtrate is initially formed its osmolarity is about the same as that of plasma (300 mOsm/L). To excrete excess water, it is necessary to dilute the filtrate as it passes along the tubule. This is achieved by reabsorbing solutes to a greater extent than water. But it occurs in certain segments of the tubular system.

Tubular fluid remains isosmotic in the proximal tubule. As fluid flows through the proximal tubule solutes and water are reabsorbed in equal proportions, so that little change in osmolarity occurs. That is the proximal tubule fluid remains isosmotic to the plasma, with an osmolarity of about 300 mOsm/L. As fluid passes down the tubule NH_4^+ is formed, thus maintaining the concentration gradient for the diffusion of more NH_3 into urine. This is called non-ionic diffusion.

In the descending loop of Henle, water is reabsorbed by osmosis from the tubular interstitial fluid of the renal medulla, which is very hypertonic (2–4 times the osmolarity of original glomerular filtrate). Therefore, the tubular fluid becomes more concentrated as it flows into the inner medulla.

Tubular fluid becomes dilute in the ascending loop of Henle. In the ascending limb of loop of Henle, especially the thick segment sodium, potassium and chloride

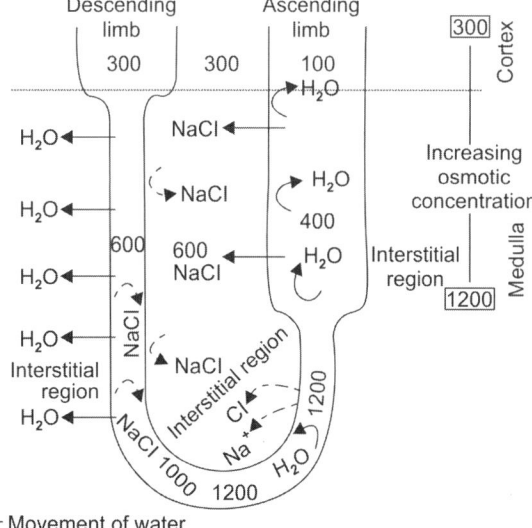

Fig. 16.7: Renal mechanisms for excreting a dilute urine

are reabsorbed. However, this portion of the tubular segment is impermeable to water even in the presence of large amount of ADH. So, the tubular fluid becomes more dilute as it flows up the ascending loop of Henle into the early distal tubule, with the osmolarity decreasing progressively to about 100 mOsm/L by the time the fluid enters the early distal tubule. Thus, regardless of whether ADH is present or absent fluid leaving the early distal tubular segment is hypo-osmotic, with an osmolarity of only about one third the osmolarity of plasma.

Tubular Fluid in Distal and Collecting Tubules is Further Diluted in the Absence of ADH

As the dilute fluid in the early distal tubule passes into late distal convoluted tubule, there is cortical additional reabsorption of sodium chloride. In the absence of ADH, this portion of the tubule is also impermeable to water, and the additional reabsorption of solutes causes the tubular fluid to become even more dilute, decreasing its osmolarity to 50 mOsm/L. The inability to reabsorb water and the continued reabsorption of solutes lead to a large volume of dilute urine.

Mechanism to Conserve Water by Excreting a Concentrated Urine

When water is in a short supply these mechanism are important to maintain homeostasis. When water is deficient in the body, the kidney forms a concentrated urine by continuing to excrete solutes while increasing water reabsorption and decreasing the volume of urine formed. The human kidney can produce a maximal urine concentration of 1200 to 1400 mOsm/L, four to five times the osmolarity of plasma.

Obligatory Urine Volume

It is the maximal concentrating ability of the kidney by which the volume of urine that must be excreted per day to rid the body of waste products of metabolism and ions ingested. A normal 70 kg human must excrete about 600 mOsm of solute each day. Maximal urine concentrating ability is 1200 mOsm/L. The obligatory urine volume can be calculated as:

$$\frac{600 \text{ mOsm/day}}{1200 \text{ mOsm/L}} = 0.5 \text{ L/day}$$

This minimal loss of volume in the urine contributes to dehydration, along with water loss from skin respiratory tract, GIT when water is not available to drink. Drinking sea water produce dehydration, because kidney must excrete other solutes especially urea which contributes about 600 mOsm/L when urine is maximally concentrated. Sea water has osmolarity 1000–1200 mOsm/L, so 1 L sea water when ingested, provide intake of 1200 mOsmoles. There for maximum concentration of NaCl that can be excreted by the kidneys is about 600 mOsm/L. Thus for every liter of sea water drunk 2 liter of urine volume would be required to rid the body of 1200 mOsm. Sodium chloride ingested also contributes in addition to other solutes such as urea. Net loss of fluid for every liter sea water drunk is 2–1 = 1 L.

Requirements for Excreting a Concentrated Urine

- *High level of ADH:* It increases the permeability of the distal tubules and collecting ducts to water, thus increases reabsorption of water.
- A high osmolarity of the renal medullary interstitial fluid provide osmotic gradient necessary for water reabsorption in presence of ADH.
- Renal medullary interstitium surrounding the collecting ducts is hyperosmotic, so with high levels of ADH water moves through tubular membrane by osmosis into renal interstitium. From

there water is carried away by vasa recta back into blood. It is the counter current mechanism which makes renal medullary interstitium hyperosmotic. This mechanism depends on special anatomical arrangement of the loop of Henle and the vasa recta, along with the specialized peritubular capillaries of the renal medulla. Twenty five percent of nephrons are juxtamedullary nephrons with loop of Henle and vasa recta going deep into medulla before returning to the cortex. The collecting ducts which carry urine through the hyper osmotic renal medulla before it is excreted, also play a critical role in the counter current mechanism.

Counter Current Mechanism

The osmolarity if interstitial fluid in almost all parts of the body is about 300 mOsm/L which is similar to the plasma osmolarity. The osmolarity of the interstitial fluid in the medulla of the kidney is much higher increasing progressively to about 1200 to 1400 mOsm/L in the pelvic tip of medulla. This high solute concentration in the medulla is achieved and maintained by a balanced inflow and outflow of solutes and water in the medulla.

Build of solute concentration in renal medulla by:
- Active transport of sodium ions and co-transport of potassium, chloride and other ions out the thick portion of ascending limb of the loop of Henle into medullary interstitium.
- Active transport of ions from the collecting ducts into the medullary interstitium.
- Facilitated diffusion of large amounts of urea from the inner medullary collecting ducts into the medullary interstitium.
- Diffusion of only small amounts of water from the medullary tubules in the medullary interstitium which is less than the reabsorption of solutes into medullary interstitium.
- Passive reabsorption of NaCl from thin ascending limb which is impermeable to water.

Characteristics of Loop of Henle that Cause Solutes to be Trapped in the Renal Medulla

- Thick ascending limb and thin ascending limb of loop of Henle is impermeable to water.
- Descending limb of Henle's loop is very permeable to water and the tubular fluid osmolarity quickly becomes equal to the renal medullary osmolarity. Therefore, water diffuses out of the descending limb of Henle's loop into interstitium and tubular fluid osmolarity quickly becomes equal to the renal medullary osmolarity. Due to this tubular fluid osmotic pressure becomes 1200 mOsm/L. The reabsorption NaCl from ascending limb of loop of Henle's is called the counter current multiplier.

Role of Distal Tubule and Collecting Ducts in Excreting a Concentrate Urine

When the tubular fluid leaves the loop of Henle's and flow into the distal convoluted tubule in the renal cortex the fluid is dilute with an osmolarity 100 mOsm/L. Early distal tubule dilutes the tubular fluid because of active transport of NaCl out of the tubule, but it is relatively impermeable to water.

As fluid flows into cortical collecting tubule, the amount of water reabsorption is dependent on ADH level in blood. In the absence of ADH, it is impermeable to water, but continue to reabsorb solutes making the urine dilute.

When there is a high concentration of ADH, cortical collecting tubule becomes highly permeable to water which is reabsorbed into cortical interstitium and is swept away by rapidly flowing peritubular capillaries (Not to medulla—hence produce the high medullary interstitial fluid osmolarity).

When high ADH levels are present collecting ducts become permeable to water, so that fluid at the end of collecting ducts has the same (1200 mOsm/L) osmolarity. Thus by reabsorbing as much water as possible kidneys form highly concentrated urine.

ROLE OF UREA

Urea contributes to about 40 to 50% of the osmolarity of the renal medullary interstitium, when kidney is forming a maximally concentrated urine. The mechanism of reabsorption of urea into the renal medullary interstium is as follows:

As water flows up the ascending loop of Henle, and into the distal and cortical collecting tubules, little urea is reabsorbed. (Impermeable). In presence of high concentration of ADH water is reabsorbed rapidly from the cortical collecting tubule and urea concentration increased rapidly because urea is not very permeable in this part. As the tubular fluid flows into inner medullary collecting duct, more water reabsorbed, causing even higher conc. of urea in the fluid. High concentration of urea in inner medullary collecting duct, causes urea to diffuse out of the tubule in the renal interstitium helped by specific urea transporters.

Re-circulation of urea from collecting duct to loop of Henle contributes to hyper osmotic renal medulla. In proximal tubule 40–50% of filtered urea is reabsorbed, but tubular fluid urea concentration increases because urea is not nearly as permeable as water. So secretion of urea into this loop of Henle from medullary interstitium. The thick limb of loop of Henle, distal tubule and cortical collecting tubule are relatively impermeable to urea. Re-circulation of urea from these parts to thin limb of loop of Henle.

Counter current exchange in the vasa recta preserves the hyper osmolarity of the renal medulla
- Medullary blood flow is low—so metabolic needs are met but helps to minimize solute loss from medullary interstitium.
- The vasa recta serve as counter current exchanges minimizing washout of solutes from the medullary interstitium. Vasa recta do not create the medullary hyper osmolarity but prevent it from being washed out.

The V-shaped structure of vessels minimizes loss of solute from interstitium but does not prevent the bulk flow of fluid and solute into the blood through the usual cortical osmotic and hydrostatic pressures that favor reabsorption in these capillaries. Plasma flowing down the descending limb of VR becomes more hyper osmotic because of diffusion of water out of blood and diffusion of solutes from renal interstitial fluid into the blood. In the ascending limb of VR solutes diffuse back into the interstitial fluid and water diffuse back to VR. Large amounts of solutes would be lost from renal medulla without V-shape of the VR capillaries.

ACIDIFICATION OF URINE

Role of kidney in acid-base balance limiting pH for secretion of H⁺ is 4.5.

Buffer Systems in Tubular Fluid
- HCO_3^-
- HPO_4^-
- NH_3

Acidosis increases H⁺ secretion—acid urine.

Alkalosis decreases H⁺ secretion—alkaline urine.

■ DIURETICS

- Decrease antidiuretic hormone (water diuresis)
  - Water
  - Alcohol
  - Vasopressin antagonists
- Osmotic diuretics
  - Glucose
  - Mannitol
- Loop diuretics
  - Furosemide
- Acting on initial part of distal tubule—thiazide
- Aldosterone—antagonist—spironolactone
- Carbonic anhydrase inhibiting drugs—diamox.

Dialysis

Two Types

1. Hemodialysis
2. Peritoneal dialysis.

Indications

- A/c and c/c renal failure
- Snake bite
- Poisoning.

Dialysis: Becomes essential when S. creatinine level is more than 6 mg%.

Hemodialysis

Diffusion of substances across a semipermeable membrane with blood of the patient on one side and a cleansing solution called dialysate on the other side of the membrane. The waste materials from the blood diffuse into the dialysate while desirable components from dialysate diffuse into the blood across the membrane.

Another name: Artificial kidney.

Peritoneal Dialysis

An indwelling catheter is introduced into the peritoneal cavity and 2 L of dialysate is introduced into peritoneal cavity. The dialysate remains in the peritoneal cavity and waste products and excess ECF diffuses into the dialysis solution. Every 4–6 hrs empty the peritoneal cavity and replace the dialysate. Hence, the peritoneal membrane acts as the dialysis membrane.

Advantage: It can avoid heparinization and vascular surgery.

Complication: Peritonitis.

Renal transplantation: Most effective treatment for advanced renal failure.

Complication: Rejection.

■ URINARY BLADDER

Urinary bladder is mainly made up of smooth muscle. It is a hollow vesicle and is composed of:

- *The body:* Detrusor muscle.
- *The trigone:* Triangular area near the mouth of urinary bladder, through which both ureters and urethra pass.
- *Internal sphincter:* Main function is maintaining tonic closure of urethral opening.
- *The external sphincter:* It is a voluntary skeletal muscle.

Normally, it remains tonically contracted which prevents constant dribbling of urine. But it can be reflexly or voluntarily relaxed at the time of micturition.

Urinary bladder is innervated by efferent and afferent nerves (Fig. 16.8 and Table 16.2).

Afferent Nerve Supply

- From the external sphincter and posterior urethra, afferent fibers pass along the pudendal nerves into the dorsal nerve root of S2, 3, 4.
- From the body, trigone and internal sphincter afferent fibers take a double route.

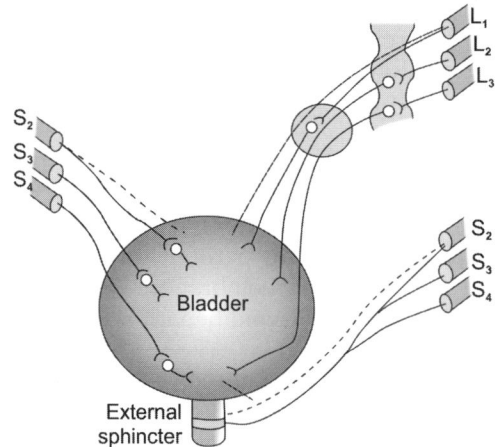

Fig. 16.8: Innervation of bladder

- Along sympathetic nerve into the dorsal nerve roots of L1, 2 and the lower thoracic segment
- Along the sacral parasympathetic nerves into the sacral dorsal nerve roots.

Function

- Indicate the degree of distension (stretch) of urinary bladder.
- Convey pain sensibility.

■ MICTURITION REFLEX

As the urinary bladder fills with urine, the wall stretches, impulses are initiated by stretch receptors in the bladder wall causing sensory signals to convey to spinal cord and then back again to the urinary bladder through parasympathetic fibers in the same nerves. This constitutes the micturition reflex. During this reflex sympathetic efferents are reflexly inhibited.

Higher Control of Micturition Reflex

In brainstem by two areas:
1. Facilitatory area located in the pontine region and posterior hypothalamus.
2. Inhibitory area located in the mid brain. Fundamentally micturition reflex is a spinal reflex facilitated and inhibited by higher brain centers.

Mechanism of Voluntary Micturition

In response to desire to micturite, urinary bladder can be voluntarily emptied. Impulses from the top of motor area in cerebral cortex pass down to sacral segments causing stimulation of efferent parasympathetic fibers. Then impulses pass along pelvic nerves (Nervi irigentes) to cause contraction of body of urinary bladder wall and relaxation of trigone and internal sphincter. The center in the brain controlling the external sphincter is reflexely inhibited, finally resulting in emptying of bladder.

- First urge to pass urine is felt as a urinary bladder volume of approx 150 mL.

Table 16.2: Efferent nerve supply

	Origin	Parts innervated	Effect of stimulation
A	Sympathetic	The body detrusor) Trigone and Internal sphincter	Relaxation of detrusor muscle contraction of trigon and internal sphincter and result in extension of urine
B	Parasympathetic from S2, 3, 4 Segment of spinal cord	Body (detrusor) Trigone Internal sphincter	Contraction of detrusor muscle, Relaxation of trigone and Internal Sphincter result in emptying of bladder
C	Somatic Anterior horn cells of S2, 3, 4	Posterior urethra External sphincter	Parts innervated are under higher control therefore can be reflexly and voluntarily relaxed at the time of micturition

- A marked sense of fullness or discomfort is felt at about 400 mL, which normally results in initiation of micturition reflex.
- If inconvenient to micturite or desire to hold urine impulses from cerebral cortex relaxes the detrusor muscle.

Spinal center → develop in the 5th month of IUL.

Abnormalities of Bladder Function

- Atonic bladder (Tabetic bladder)
- Autonomous bladder (Damage of both afferent and efferent nerves usually seen in tumors of cauda equina). Bladder becomes filled with fluid and distended. Gradually muscles become active and urine is voided in drops. Later bladder becomes shrunken and distended. Another name (Decentralized bladder).
- *Automatic bladder:* Transaction of spinal cord.
- *Spastic neurogenic bladder:* Lesion may be in the brain stem or spinal cord. All inhibitory signals are absent. Micturition becomes uncontrollable and bladder is hyperactive.
- *Nocturnal enuresis:* Poorly developed nervous control of bladder. In children it is normal. In adults due to disease of several spinal segments.

CHAPTER 17

The Nervous System

Overview of nervous system: Human nervous system is the most complex product of biological evolution. The functional capabilities of the nervous system are a product of vast population of intercommunicating nerve cells or neurons estimated to be 10 times 10. Most neurons consist of a central mass of cytoplasm within a limiting cell membrane, cell body or soma from which extend a number of branched processes or neuritis. One of the cell process (axon) is usually longer than the other and conducts information away from cell body. The other processes are dendrites which carry information towards the cell body. The axon terminals form synapses and information are passed from one cell to other. Synapses are called axodendritic, axosomatic, axoaxonic or neuromuscular junctions.

■ NERVOUS SYSTEM

Organization of Nervous System

The nervous system is the most complex and highly developed to all the systems of the body. It makes possible a range of adaptive responses to changes (stimuli) in the environment in the interests of survival of the individual and of the race. Such responses are central to the behavior of all living organisms and are known as homeostatic responses. Simple organisms are simply structured and organized but a large animal with a complex structure requires a nervous system to overcome the problems of recognition of stimuli, storage of information (memory), communication between the various parts of its body, and the execution of effective responses.

The nervous system may be divided into three main portions.
1. The central nervous system, consisting of the brain and spinal cord.
2. The peripheral nervous system, consisting of the nerves between the central nervous system and the muscles and various organs.
3. The autonomic nervous system, which is subdivided into sympathetic and parasympathetic systems.

The brain is the most complex and important part of the nervous system. This is the sites of consciousness, thought, memory, creativity, speech, vision, hearing, smell, control of endocrine glandular secretions and autonomic (involuntary) functions, and the will to carry out purposeful actions. It is only because of the brain (his or hers and our own) that we know anything of the personality of an individual.

The brain receives impulses or sensations which are interpreted and stored in the mind. The accumulation of these stored impulses forms the basis of memory. Parts of the brain particularly concerned with memory are the temporal lobes and the hippocampus and its connections. Bilateral destruction of the ventral hippocampus results in loss of recent memory whilst remote memory remains intact (but cannot be added to).

It is thought that memory might be stored as a biochemical change in the neurons. Protein synthesis seems to be involved in some way. It is suggested that the learning process causes a stable alteration in the ribonucleic acid (RNA) in the neurons.

The brain receives impulses from various parts of the body; they are called sensory or afferent impulses and are said to travel towards the brain along afferent pathways. Impulses travelling away from the brain and destined to result in movement or action of some sort are termed motor or efferent impulses.

The tissue of which the nervous system is constructed has already been described.

■ THE MENINGES (FIG. 17.1)

The central nervous system lies within the skull and vertebral column. In addition to the hard bony protection afforded by the axial skeleton, the brain and spinal cord have the following coverings, called meninges:

- The dura mater or outer layer
- The arachnoid mater or middle layer
- The pia mater or inner layer.

Between the arachnoid mater and pia mater is a fluid called the cerebrospinal fluid which supports the brain and spinal cord and ensures that the pressure upon them is evenly distributed.

The dura mater is a strong, thick fibrous membrane consisting largely of white collagen fibers. It lines the interior of the cranium and the vertebral canal, its outer layer actually forming the periosteum at these sites. Two large rigid folds of the inner layer of the dura mater project into the cranial cavity and help to support the brain and to maintain it in position.

- The falx cerebri is a sickle-shaped fold lying vertically in the mid-line and separating the right and left cerebral hemispheres.
- The tentorium cerebelli is a crescentic arched sheet which lies horizontally and forms a tent-like roof for the posterior cranial fossa, thereby separating the cerebrum above from the cerebellum below.

The venous sinuses, for example the sagittal, transverse and cavernous sinuses are contained between layers of the dura mater. The arachnoid mater (arachnoid = spider-like) is a delicate transparent membrane situated between the dura mater and pia mater. It is closely applied to the dura mater but is separated from the pia mater by the subarachnoid space, a narrow but extensive space which contains the cerebrospinal fluid. Between the under surface of the cerebellum and medulla oblongata this space is enlarged to form the cisterna magna, of importance because a needle is sometimes passed between the occiput and atlas vertebra into this great cistern in order to withdraw cerebrospinal fluid (cisternal puncture). Great care must be taken not to insert the needle too far as it will damage the medulla oblongata, possibly with fatal results.

The pia mater is the innermost of the meninges and is closely applied to the brain and spinal cord. It is a very delicate membrane and carries numerous small blood vessels which supply the surface of the brain and spinal cord. It closely follows the surface of the brain and dips into all the fissures between the convolutions, whereas the arachnoid mater forms only a bag-like covering for the central nervous system. The pia mater is invaginated to form the tela choroidea and choroid plexuses of the third and fourth ventricles and the choroid plexuses of the lateral ventricles.

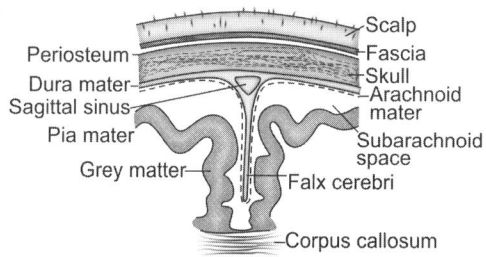

Fig. 17.1: Scalp and meninges

It is the choroid plexuses which secrete the cerebrospinal fluid.

At the lower end of the spinal cord, below the conus medullaris, the pia mater continues downwards as a long slender filament, the filum terminale, to become attached to the dorsum of the coccyx. The subarachnoid space is particularly capacious around the filum terminale, making this the site of election for needling (lumbar puncture) and withdrawal of cerebrospinal fluid.

Most activities of the nervous system are originated by sensory experience, emanating from sensory receptors, whether these be visual receptors, auditory receptors, tactile receptors on the surface of the body or other kinds of receptors.

The Three Major Levels of Nervous System Function

According to evolution there are three major levels of nervous system that have special functional significance.
1. Spinal cord
2. *The lower brain level:* Most of the subconscious activities of the body are controlled in the lower areas of the brain in the medulla, pons, mesencephalon, hypothalamus, thalamus, cerebellum and basal ganglia. Subconscious control of arterial blood pressure and respiration achieved primarily in the reticular substance of the medulla and pons. Control of equilibrium is a combined function of the older portions of the cerebellum and the reticular substance of medulla pons and mesencephalon. Feeding reflexes, such as salivation in response to taste of food and licking of the lips are controlled by areas in the medulla pons, mesencephalon, amygdale and hypothalamus. Emotional patterns, sexual activities, etc. can occur in lower animals without use of cerebral cortex.
3. *Higher brain or cortical level:* Three quarters of all the neuronal cell bodies of the entire nervous system are located in the cerebral cortex. For each area of the cerebral cortex there is a corresponding and connecting area of the thalamus. Also activation of mesencephalon transmits diffuse signals to the cerebral cortex, particularly through the thalamus directly to activate the entire cortex. This process is called wakefulness. On the other hand when these areas of the mesencephalon become inactive the thalamic and cortical regions also become inactive. This process is called sleep.

■ CEREBROSPINAL FLUID

- CNS is enveloped by the meninges from outside to inside the layers of meninges are termed dura, arachnoids and pia.
  - Dura ends at the lower border of 2nd sacral spine, spinal cord end, at the lower border of 1st lumbar spine.
  - The arachnoid is separated from the pia by subarachnoid space, which contains CSF. Arachnoid invests the spinal cord quite loosely. There are definite dilatations of subarachnoid space called cisterna
    - Cisterna magna (In the space between medulla and undersurface of cerebellum)
    - Cisterna pontis and cisterna basalis.
      Cisterna pontis, i.e. on the central aspect of the pons and contains the basiler artery.
      Cisterna basalis formed by the arachnoid bridging across tip of temporal lobes, and contains circle of willis.
  - Pia invests the nervous substance very closely. Pia is loosely adherent to blood vessels. The perivasculer

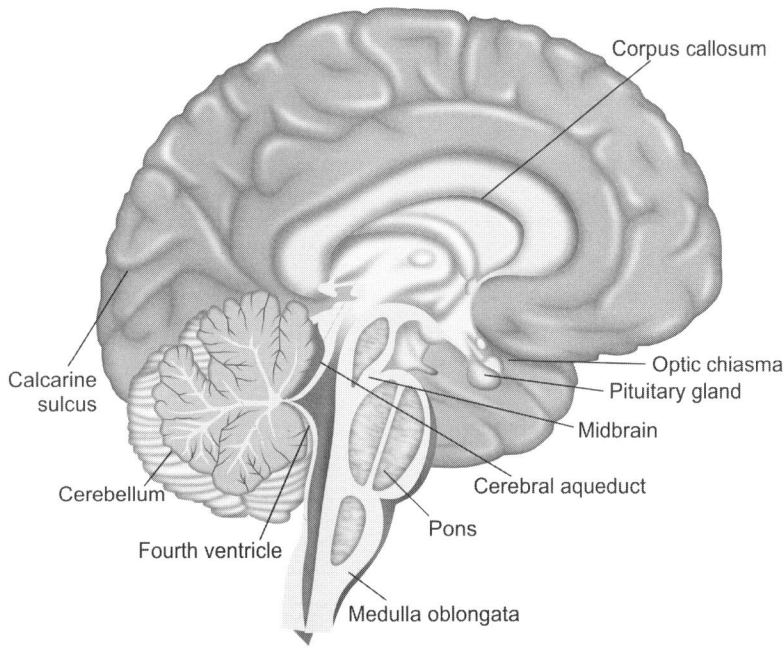

Fig. 17.2: Medial surface of the left cerebral hemisphere

space is modified lymphatic system for brain. They help to transport find protons, waste products and extraneous particulate matter from brain to subarachnoid space.
- *Ventricles:* Interconnecting chambers within the brain
    - *Lateral ventricle:* Chamber in central hemisphere (Fig. 17.2)
    - *IIIrd ventricle:* Narrow chamber in midbrain. Communicates with lateral ventricle above by foramen of monro and below to IVth ventricle by aqueduct of sylvius.
    - *IVth ventricle:* Between pons and medulla oblongata. Surface of ventricles are lined by thin cuboidal epithelium called ependyma.
- *Choroid plexus:* Some arteries pass through the brain substance to reach lining ependymal layer in ventricles, break up to complex blood vessel. The modified lining of blood vessels constitute choroid plexuses. It contributes to formation of CSF.
- *Arachnoid villi:* Small finger like projections of arachnoid trabeculae lined by flat epithelium. The villi project into venous sinuses and allow free flow of CSF, proteins and particles less than 1 µm size into the blood.

■ CSF COMPOSITION

Clear, colorless alkaline fluid with a specific. Gravity 1005–1008. It is almost protein free (20–30 mg%) and almost cell free (lymphocytes 0–5/mm^3). It contains less glucose (50 mg%) than plasma. Also contains some urea and creatinine. Hence, it is similar to blood plasma but it does not that.
Volume: 130–150 mL of which 30 mL is in ventricular system and remainder in subarachnoids space.

CSF Pressure: 130 mm H_2O in lateral lying position.

    pH – 7.33
    Glucose – 64 mg%
    Proteins – 25 mg%
    Cl – 113 meq/L
    HCO_3 – 25.1 mEq/L
    Na^+ – 147 mEq/L
    K – 2.9 mEq/L.

Formation of CSF

- Fifty percent by choroid plexus in the ventricles
- Forty percent by blood vessels of meningeal and ependymal lining of ventricles
- Ten percent by blood vessels of brain and spinal cord.

Absorption

- Eighty percent by arachnoid villi into venous sinuses.
- Twenty percent along sheath of cranial nerves into cervical lymphatics and to perivascular spaces.

CSF formed in the lateral ventricles via foramen of Monro reaches IIIrd ventricle then via aqueduct of sylvius enters into cisterna magna (Dilation in the subarachnoid space.) The CSF from other ventricles flows through the foramen of Magendie and Luschka also to subarachnoid space, towards cerebrum where all arachnoid villi are located.

[Hydrocephalus] CSF pressure < 70% CSF absorption stops and it starts accumulating in excessive amounts within brain spaces.

Functions of CSF

- Buffer
- *Protective function:* Brain floats in CSF
- Reservoir to regulate the contents of cranium
- *Monro-Kellie doctrine:* Because brain tissue and CSF are essentially in compressible, the volume of blood, CSF, and brain in the cranium at any time must be relatively constant.
- It helps transfer of waste products (metabolite exchanges of brain into the blood.
- It may serve as a medium for nutrient exchanges in the nervous system.

Measurement of CSF Pressure

- Subject lie in the lateral position
- A spinal needle is inserted into spinal canal between L4 and L5 and is connected to glass tube.
- Spinal fluid is allowed to rise in the tube as high as it will
- CSF level height in the tube (in mm) above the level of the needle will give CSF pressure is mm H_2O.

Clinical Aspects

Increase in CSF Pressure: Causes

- *Physiological:*
  - *Increased venous pressure:* Following coughing crying or compression of internal jugular vein.
  - *Queckenstedt's sign:* Compression of internal jugular vein decreases absorption of CSF. So Pressure increases.
- *Pathological:*
  - Increased fluid formation, e.g. inflammation of meninges
  - Increased resistance to absorption through arachnoid Villi, e.g. brain tumors, hemorrhage, infection.

Decrease in CSF Pressure: Causes

- Decrease in venous pressure
- Decrease in rate of fluid formation.

■ THE SPINAL CORD

The spinal cord is a part of the central nervous system which lies in the vertebral canal. It commences above at the level of the foramen magnum where it is continuous

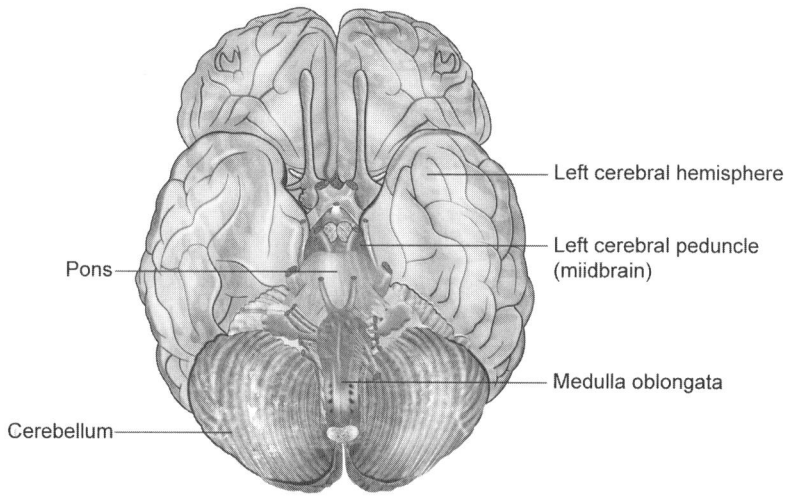

Fig. 17.3: The inferior surface of the brain

with the medulla oblongata (Fig. 17.3). In the adult, it is about 45 cm (18 in) long and tapers into the conus medullaris to end at the lower level of the first lumbar vertebra; it therefore does not completely fill the lower part of the vertebral canal. In childhood, the cord extends to a lower level than the first lumbar vertebra. Surrounding the spinal cord are the meninges. The dura mater and arachnoid mater form a sac which encloses the cord and extends downwards to the lowest part of the vertebral canal, while the pia mater closely covers the surface of the cord in the same way as it adheres to surface of the brain. A prolongation of the pia mater, the filum terminale, descends from the conus medullaris to be attached to the back of the coccyx. Cerebrospinal fluid fills the subarachnoid space between the arachnoid mater and pia mater.

The spinal cord which is oval in cross-section (Fig. 17.4), is increased in circumference in two areas, namely the cervical and lumbar enlargements. From these enlargements the important nerves to the arms and legs arise (see Fig. 17.5).

The spinal nerves arise from the sides of the spinal cord by two roots, anterior and posterior, which unite as they leave the vertebral column to form the spinal nerve trunk.

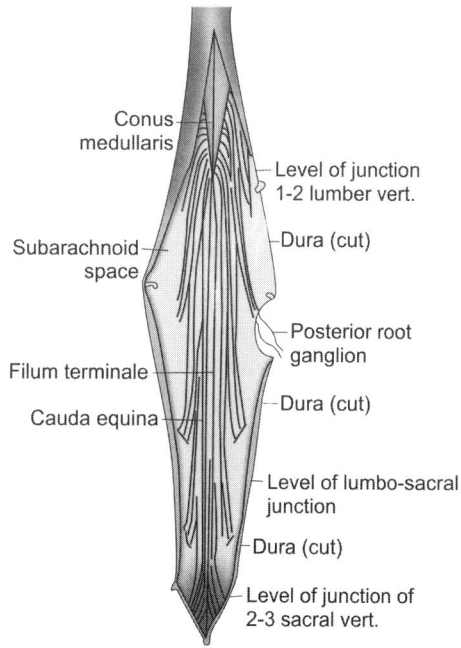

Fig. 17.4: Lower end of the dura and arachnoid laid open to show the cauda equina

There are, in all, thirty-one pairs of spinal nerves corresponding to the segments of the vertebral column, namely:

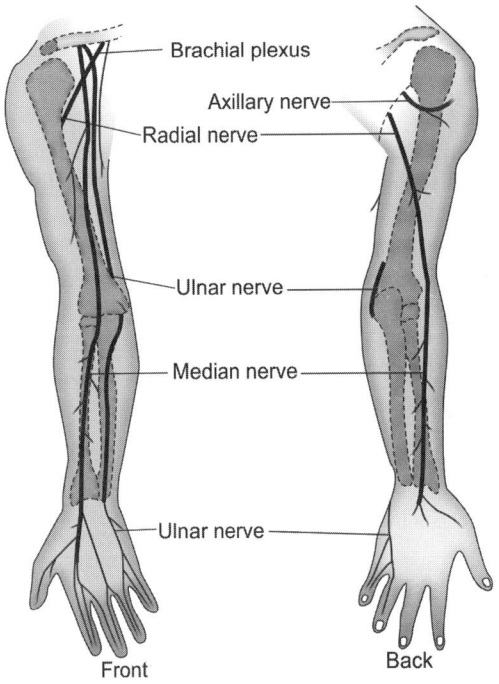

Fig. 17.5: The important nerves of the right upper limb

8 cervical,
12 thoracic or dorsal,
5 lumbar, 5 sacral,
1 coccygeal.

The nerve roots from the lumbar, sacral and coccygeal regions occupy the space in the lower part of the vertebral canal below the termination of the spinal cord, before passing between their corresponding vertebrae. This leash of nerve roots is called the cauda equina (like a horse's tail).

STRUCTURE OF SPINAL CORD

The structure of the spinal cord is best understood by study of transverse cross-sections. It has been noted that the grey matter of the brain is situated on the surface and the white matter in the interior. In the spinal cord this arrangement is reversed, the white matter being on the surface while the grey matter is arranged in an H-shaped manner in its interior.

It will be seen (Fig. 17.4) that the cord is oval in transverse cross-section and that the H-shaped grey matter divides the white matter into ventral (anterior), lateral and posterior columns or funiculi. The ventral columns of the two sides are separated from one another by the anterior median fissure. In the center of the spinal cord is a minute canal, the central canal, which is continuous above with the fourth ventricle in the medulla oblongata and contains cerebrospinal fluid. Most of the latter fluid is, however, contained in the subarachnoid space.

The Grey Matter of the Spinal Cord

The H-shaped grey matter is commonly described as having anterior and posterior horns which represent the anterior and posterior grey columns. There is also a lateral grey column on each side, appearing as a lateral horn in cross-sections of the thoracic and upper lumbar segments of the cord. The lateral grey columns contain the cells from which the preganglionic fibers of the sympathetic nervous system originate.

The ventral or anterior grey columns contain the motor cells (anterior horn cells) from which arise the nerve fibers forming the ventral or anterior roots of the spinal nerves.

The posterior horns are capped by the substantia gelatinosa, a crescentic mass of small nerve cells and fibers intimately concerned with the connections of incoming afferent nerve fibers. The dorsal or posterior root of the spinal nerve, its sensory root, enters the posterior horn of grey matter.

The White Matter of the Spinal Cord

The white matter of the spinal cord is white because of the high proportion of myelinated fibers in it. Sensory fibers ascend in the white matter to the brain and motor fibers descend from the brain. The motor fibers are situated in the lateral columns of white matter in a special tract, the lateral corticospinal tract or pyramidal tract. Its fibers are the axons of the pyramidal cells (upper motor neurons) of the motor cortex. They cross over (decussate) in the medulla and descend in the lateral corticospinal tract of the contralateral side of the cord. The fibers terminate in the anterior columns of grey matter, where they synapse with motor cells (anterior horn cells, lower motor neurons) in successive spinal segments.

Injury or disease causing complete transection of the lower part of the spinal cord results in paralysis of both lower limbs—paraplegia. If the lesion is higher in the cord, all four limbs may be affected—quadriplegia. These conditions present many nursing and social problems, such as care of the bladder, prevention of bedsores and provision of a suitable invalid carriage.

The sensory fibers enter the cord in the posterior roots of the spinal nerves. Fibers conveying sensations of fine touch (tactile discrimination), pressure, vibration and proprioception (position and movement) ascend in the posterior tracts (dorsal columns) of white matter to the medulla oblongata. There are synapse with neurons in the gracile and cuneate nuclei. From these, most of the axons of the second set of neurons cross the midline and ascend, in a band known as medial lemniscus, to the thalamus. From this relay center, fibers convey sensory impulses to the cerebral cortex (postcentral gyrus). Some of the axons of the second neurons, in the gracile and cuneate nuclei, pass to the cerebellum, which also receives the fibers of the spinocerebellar tracts. Unconscious adjustments of muscular tone can therefore be made in response to proprioceptive information received.

Fibers conveying pain and temperature sensation synapse with neurons in the posterior grey columns (posterior horns). Most of the axons from the secondary neurons cross the midline, decussating with the corresponding fibers from the opposite side, to ascend in the anterolateral portion of the spinal cord. These ascending pathways are known as the anterior and lateral spinothalamic tracts.

There are many other ascending and descending tracts in the spinal cord. Fibers also ascend and descend to and from the brainstem reticular system and these are known as spinoreticular and reticulospinal fibers.

■ THE SPINAL NERVES (FIG. 17.6)

It has been seen that there are thirty-one pairs of spinal nerves, each arising from the spinal cord by two roots, ventral (anterior) and dorsal (posterior). The latter unite to form the main nerve trunk as it leaves the vertebral column. On each dorsal nerve root there is a collection of nerve cells called spinal ganglion (posterior root ganglion).

It has also been pointed out that all sensory nerve fibers reach the spinal cord by the posterior root and all motor nerve fibers leave by the anterior root. It follows that the peripheral nerve trunk is a mixed nerve containing both sensory and motor fibers.

The individual nerve trunks arising from certain regions of the spinal cord join-up together to form what is called plexus from which they emerge rearranged as the individual peripheral nerves. Two plexuses are formed by the cervical nerves and two by the lumbar and sacral nerves.

Cervical Plexus

The upper four cervical nerve trunks unite to form a plexus lying deeply in the upper part of the neck from which peripheral nerves are distributed mainly to the skin and muscles of the head and neck.

The most important branch of the cervical plexus is the phrenic nerve which passes down in the neck to enter the thorax, where it is closely related to the side of the

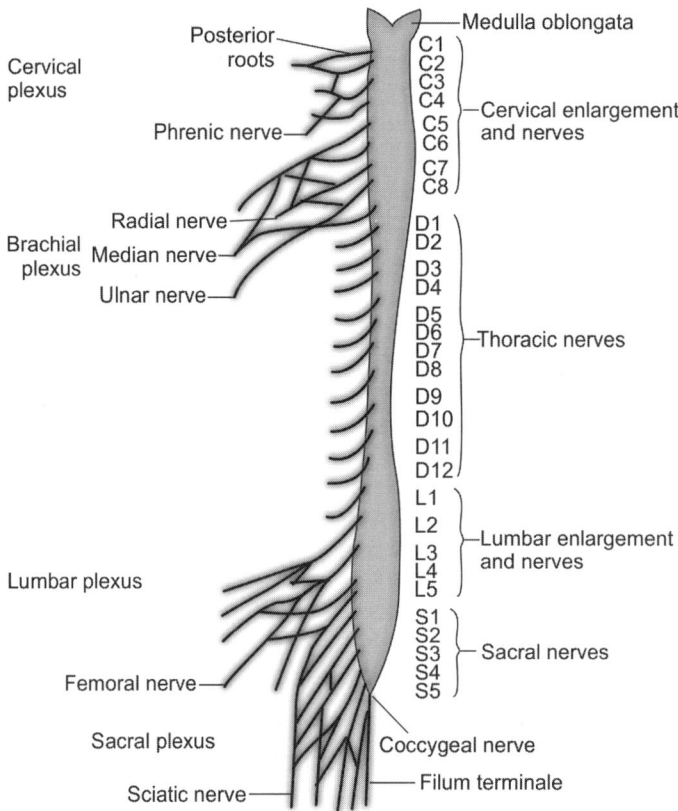

Fig. 17.6: Spinal nerves

pericardium. It terminates in the diaphragm of which it is the motor nerve. Paralysis of the diaphragm may result from a lesion in the neck or thorax. Thus, it may be due to entrapment of the phrenic nerve in the mediastinum by a bronchial carcinoma. The affected side of the diaphragm is then displaced upwards and moves paradoxically; it is seen to move upwards instead of downwards, on fluoroscopy, when the patient takes a vigorous sniff.

Brachial Plexus

This is formed from the lower four cervical and the first thoracic nerves, and is situated deeply in the lower part of the neck behind the clavicle. From this plexus the important nerves of the arm are derived. These nerves enter the axilla where they are closely related to the axillary artery.

Among the more important branches of the brachial plexus are as follows:

- The axillary (circumflex) nerve, which is related to the surgical neck of the humerus and supplies the deltoid muscle. In this region, it may be injured by a fracture of the bone or in dislocations of the shoulder joint.
- The radial nerve, which after leaving the axilla, winds round the posterior aspect of the shaft of the humerus in the spiral groove and supplies branches to the skin, the triceps muscle and the extensor muscles in the back of the forearm. It is liable to injury in the upper part of its course and when

paralysed produces the characteristic deformity known as 'wrist drop', in which the patient is unable to extend the wrist or fingers. The nerve is liable to crutch pressure in the axilla.

- The ulnar nerve, which is at first related to the axillary artery and then accompanies the brachial artery in the arm. It passes down behind the medial epicondyle of the humerus to reach the ulnar side of the forearm. In addition to supplying muscles in the forearm, it gives branches to the skin of the ring and little fingers and small muscles in the hand.

  It is the close relationship with the medial epicondyle of the humerus, where the nerve is relatively superficial, which has given rise to the popular name 'funny bone' for this part of the elbow. A severe knock in this region stimulates the ulnar nerve and produces pain together with a tingling sensation in the ring and little fingers, which clearly demonstrates the distribution of the nerve. The nerve is most commonly injured at this site, behind the medial epicondyle, and the resulting paralysis is characteristic. The hand assumes a claw shape, in which the metacarpophalangeal joints, especially of the ring and little fingers, are extended and the interphalangeal joints are flexed, owing to the unopposed action of opposing muscles.

- The median nerve which also lies close to the brachial artery in the arm. Thereafter it passes down in the midline of the front of the forearm to the hand. It supplies muscles in the forearm and hand. It gives cutaneous branches to the thenar eminence and central part of the palm and to the first three arid one-half digits.

  Injury to the median nerve usually occurs just above the wrist, resulting in inability to oppose the thumb and loss of sensation on the palmar surfaces of the thumb, index and middle fingers and the radial-half of the ring finger. If the nerve is damaged higher in the forearm, there will be many other effects, including weakness in the action of pronation.

  At the wrist, the median nerve lies in a restricted space, between the flexor retinaculum and the carpal bones, called the carpal tunnel. If this space is compromised by bony injury or arthritis, or by soft tissue swelling in some patients with pregnancy, myxedema or acromegaly, the carpal tunnel syndrome results. In many cases the compression is 'spontaneous', meaning that it is incompletely understood. There is weakness and wasting of the outer thenar muscles (short muscles of the thumb). Pain and tingling are felt and sensation is impaired in the digits supplied by the nerve but not in the palm because this is supplied by the palmar cutaneous branch of the nerve, which arises above and lies superficial to the retinaculum.

The Thoracic Nerves

These are twelve in number and one passes to each intercostal space. They run forwards between the ribs, supply branches to the intercostal muscles and muscles of the anterior abdominal wall, and are finally distributed to the skin of the thorax and front of the abdomen.

The Lumbar Plexus (Fig. 17.7)

This plexus originates from the first four lumbar nerves and lies within the psoas major muscle in front of the transverse processes of the lumbar vertebrae. Its principal branches are the femoral and obturator nerves.

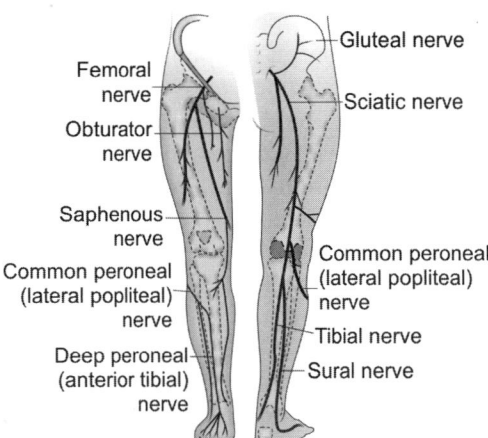

Fig. 17.7: The important nerves of the right lower limb: (a) front of limb, (b) back of limb.

The femoral nerve is the largest branch of the lumbar plexus. It passes behind the inguinal (Poupart's) ligament to enter the femoral (Scarpa's) triangle in the front of the thigh. It supplies the muscles of the front of the thigh (principally quadriceps), the hip and knee joints (sensory fibers) and skin on the front of the thigh and medial side of the leg, ankle, and foot.

The skin of the lateral aspect of the thigh is supplied not by branches of the femoral nerve but by the lateral cutaneous nerve of the thigh, which arises directly from the lumbar plexus. It enters the thigh after passing behind or through the inguinal ligament, usually about a centimeter medial to the anterior superior iliac spine. Entrapment of this nerve results in the condition known as meralgia paresthetica (from the Greek 'meros', thigh, and 'algos', pain), with pain, numbness and paresthesia referred to the lateral aspect of the thigh. The condition may remit spontaneously; if not, it is speedily relieved by surgical division of the fibrous tissue compressing the nerve.

The obturator nerve runs downwards and forwards to leave the pelvis through the obturator foramen in the innominate bone, there upon entering the thigh. It supplies the adductor muscles of the thigh, the hip and knee joints, and an area of skin over the medial aspect of the thigh. In case of spastic paraplegia, spasm of the adductor muscles can be relieved by division of the obturator nerve.

The Sacral Plexus

This originates from the fourth and fifth lumbar and first four sacral nerves. Its branches supply the muscles of the pelvis and hip and the skin of the buttock and back of the thigh. The plexus terminates as the pudendal nerve and the much larger sciatic nerve.

The pudendal nerve provides the principle motor and sensory innervation of the perineum. Pudendal nerve block, with a local anesthetic injected through a long needle, has been used in obstetrics prior to forceps delivery, to relax the pelvic floor muscles and abolish sensation in the lower vagina and vulva.

The sciatic nerve is the largest nerve in the body. It passes out of the pelvis through the greater sciatic foramen of the innominate bone into the gluteal region (Fig. 17.8). Thence, it descends down the back of the thigh, the hamstring muscles of which it supplies, to about its lower one-third, where it terminates by branching into the tibial and common peroneal nerves. The

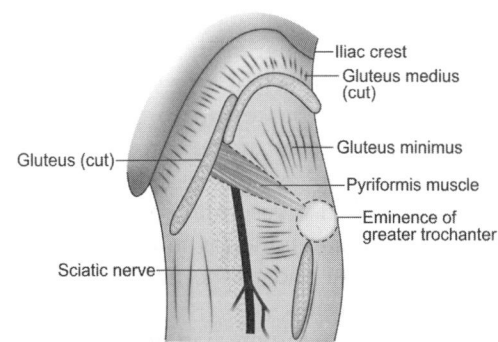

Fig. 17.8: Position of the sciatic nerve

sciatic nerve can be represented on the back of the thigh by a broad line. First, a line is drawn between the ischial tuberosity and the apex of the greater trochanter, both of which bony landmarks can easily be felt through the skin. From just medial to the midpoint of this line, another line is drawn down to meet the popliteal fossa just medially to its apex. A knowledge of this anatomy will prevent intramuscular injections being given too medially and misplaced into the sciatic nerve, causing severe pain and weakness of dorsiflexion and plantar flexion of the foot.

In the buttock, the sciatic nerve may also be damaged by penetrating injuries and by posterior dislocations or fracture dislocations of the hip joint. Higher up, in the pelvis, the sciatic nerve may be compressed in the later stages of pregnancy or damaged by the direct extension of a pelvic neoplasm.

A complete sciatic nerve lesion causes paralysis of the hamstrings and of all the muscles below the knee, with a foot drop deformity. All cutaneous sensibility below the knee is also lost except for the area, medially, innervated by the saphenous nerve, which is a branch of the femoral nerve.

The term 'sciatica' has been used for a syndrome, characterized especially by pain, due to compression of lumbar spinal nerves by one or more protruding intervertebral discs. However, it must be realized that sciatica is a symptom (pain in the lower limb), and not a disease, and that it may occasionally be due to serious intrapelvic disease.

■ SENSATION AND THE SENSORY PATH

Two types of sensation may be considered; special sensation and general sensation (see also Chapter 18).

Special sensations are those which can only be detected by specialized organs, i.e. smell, sight, hearing and taste. Sensory impulses received from these organs are conveyed to the brain by the appropriate cranial nerve. General sensations are the feelings which are appreciated by all parts of the body. They include the superficial sensations detected by the skin and the deep sensations felt in the muscles, joints and other organs.

Superficial Sensation

The important superficial sensations are appreciated by 'the sensory nerve endings in the skin and include:
- Pain
- Touch
- Temperature (heat and cold).

Deep Sensation

In addition to pressure and deep pain, the most important deep sensation is that of the position of muscles and joints. We are always aware of the exact position in space of any limb or part of a limb. This may be demonstrated by closing the eyes and bringing the tip of the index finger to the end of the nose. This can only be done accurately because we know exactly where the respective parts are by muscle and joint sense, without the aid of vision. Vibration is also a deep sensation.

The Sensory Path (Fig. 17.9)

Both superficial and deep sensations travel in the peripheral nerve from the skin, joint or muscle towards the spinal cord. After reaching the trunk of the nerve, the sensory fibers enter the posterior horn of grey matter in the spinal cord via the posterior nerve root. The two types of nerve fiber then take separate courses.

The fibers conveying sensations of position, pressure, vibration and light touch pass upwards in the posterior columns.

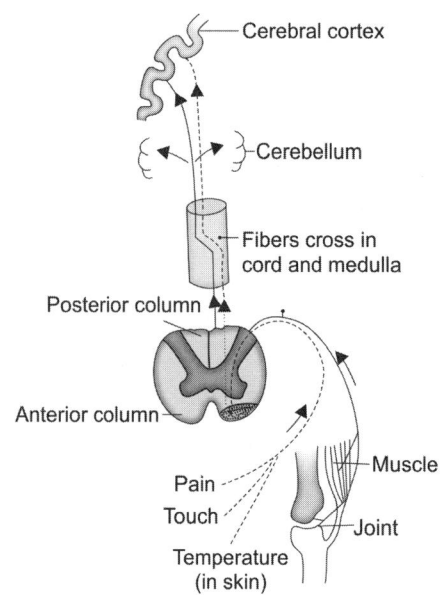

Fig. 17.9: The sensory path

Those taking the superficial sensations of pain and temperature go to the anterior columns.

Both sets of fibers cross to the opposite side of the cord either before or when they reach the medulla oblongata. Thence, they are conveyed via the brainstem, thalamus and white matter of the brain to the parietal and other sensory areas of the cerebral cortex. The sensory impulses of one side of the body are, therefore, like the motor impulses, dealt with by the opposite side of the brain.

■ NEUROTRANSMITTERS

The receiving processes extending from neurons are called dendrites and the efferent processes are called axons. The axon, of which there is normally one per cell, branches near its termination into several fine axon terminals. These end in close proximity to other cells. When the other cell is also a neuron, the junction is known as synapse. When the other cell is a muscle cell, a neuromuscular junction is formed. The axon terminals may also end in glands or other structures.

Transmission of information from one neuron to another at a synapse is in most cases neurochemical, although there are also electrically acting synapses similar to the electrical junctions in cardiac and unstriated muscle. Neurochemical transmission depends on the ability of axon terminals to synthesize, store and release the chemical transmitter. In some cases the axons also reabsorb the transmitter, a process called reuptake, and store it for subsequent use.

Many substances have been identified as neurotransmitters. Among the major ones are acetylcholine, catecholamines noradrenalin and dopamine, serotonin and the amino acid gamma aminobutyric acid (GABA). The transmitter substance binds with special protein molecules called receptors on the surface of the cell to which information is being transmitted. The effect on that cell may be either facilitatory (excitatory) or inhibitory according to whether the transmitter raises or lowers the resting potential of the cell. The effect is required only for a limited time and this limitation is achieved either by reuptake of the transmitter into the axon terminals, as in the case of the catecholamines, or by enzymatic destruction of the transmitter. An example of the latter is the destruction of acetylcholine by the action of cholinesterase, which is present in the synaptic gap. In the muscle disease known as myasthenia gravis anticholinesterase drugs, such as prostigmine, are used to inhibit the enzyme and thereby enhance the action of acetylcholine.

Nerve fibers which secrete acetylcholine are called cholinergic whilst those which secrete noradrenalin, dopamine and serotonin are respectively termed noradrenergic, dopaminergic and serotonergic.

Acetylcholine is the transmitter at synapses in the autonomic ganglia and at the terminals of parasympathetic and somatic motor nerve fibers, i.e. in the latter case, at neuromuscular junctions. Acetylcholine also acts as a transmitter in virtually all parts of the brain including the corpus striatum. Depletion of dopamine at this site in cases of Parkinson's disease may cause an unbalanced state in which the action of acetylcholine is largely unopposed. Anticholinergic drugs, such as benztropine, are therefore useful in Parkinsonism.

Histochemical techniques are used to map out the distribution of groups of neurons which secrete a particular neurotransmitter substance. Thus cholinergic, noradrenergic, dopaminergic and serotonergic neuron groups have all been identified in the reticular formation.

Apart from its presence in parts of the central nervous system, noradrenalin is the transmitter at peripheral (post-synaptic) sympathetic nerve endings. Its action depends upon the type of receptor present in the innervated cell surface. Alpha-adrenergic (α) receptors are stimulated to cause contraction of vascular smooth muscle and hence vasoconstriction. An alpha-adrenergic blocking drug such as phentolamine will prevent this constriction of blood vessels. Beta-1 ($\beta1$) receptors in cardiac muscle respond to adrenalin and noradrenalin by increasing the rate and force of contraction of the heart; effects which can be prevented by administering a beta-adrenergic blocking drug such as propranolol. Beta-2 ($\beta2$) receptors in the bronchi show an inhibitory response to adrenalin and noradrenalin and bronchodilation results from the relaxation of bronchial smooth muscle. In this case, a non-selective beta-adrenergic blocking agent like propranolol will encourage bronchoconstriction. Propranolol is therefore contraindicated in asthmatic patients.

Another class of neurotransmitters is characterized by having polypeptide chains of five or more amino acid residues. These include substance P and the opioid peptides, of which the enkephalins, dynorphins and endorphins seem to be the most important. The opioid peptides bind to opiate receptors and function as either short-acting neurotransmitters or long-acting neurohormones. They are found mainly in the sensory and autonomic systems, limbic system and neuroendocrine systems. They are still being investigated but because they have analgesic activity, the endorphins have been described as the body's own naturally occurring morphine-like substances.

■ THE CRANIAL NERVES

There are 12 pairs of cranial nerves, which arise from the brain and brainstem. Some of them are **sensory**, or afferent, bringing impulses to the brain; others are **motor**, or efferent, carrying impulses from the brain to the periphery, while a few are mixed and contain both motor and sensory fibers.

The cranial nerves are arranged from above downwards as follows:

I	Olfactory
II	Optic
III	Oculomotor
IV	Trochlear
V	Trigeminal
VI	Abducent
VII	Facial
VIII	Vestibulocochlear
IX	Glossopharyngeal
X	Vagal
XI	Accessory
XII	Hypoglossal

The Olfactory Nerves

These are sensory and serve the sense of smell. Their fibers arise from olfactory cells in the mucous membrane of the upper part of the nose. These fibers ascend through foramina in the cribiform plate of the ethmoid bone and synapse with cells in the **olfactory bulb**. In turn, the axons of these cells pass back in the olfactory tract to the primary olfactory cortex in the undersurface of the temporal lobe.

Loss of the sense of smell, **anosmia**, may result from conditions such as the common cold affecting the nasal mucosa, frontal lobe tumors and head injuries. In addition to anosmia, fractures involving the anterior cranial fossa may cause cerebrospinal fluid to leak into the nose, from which it may drip, a condition known as CSF rhinorrhea.

The Optic Nerve

This is the nerve of sight and is entirely sensory. Its fibers commence in the retina of the eye as the axons of ganglion cells. These axons converge from all parts of the retina to form the optic disc, which may be viewed in living subjects using an instrument called an ophthalmoscope. Behind the optic disc, the fibers pierce the sclera (outer coat of the eye) to form the optic nerve.

The optic nerve (and retina) is an extension of the brain and is sheathed with extensions of the meninges. Raised intracranial pressure is therefore transmitted along the extension of the subarachnoid space around the optic nerve, resulting in swelling of the nerve 'head', or optic disc, a condition which is known as **papilloedema**. This may be detected by ophthalmoscopy and may provide a valuable clue to the presence of a space-occupying lesion such as a tumor.

A lesion affecting one optic nerve causes unilateral loss of vision. Inflammation of the nerve (optic neuritis) may be responsible; if it involves the optic disc (papillitis) it may be detected by ophthalmoscopy but often the disc is spared and the nerve is affected behind the eye (retrobulbar neuritis).

The optic nerve passes backwards through the optic foramen and meets its fellow nerve on the undersurface of the brain at the **optic chiasma** where the medial fibers of each nerve cross to the optic tract of the opposite side. These are the fibers from the medial half of the retina, concerned with the temporal half of the visual field. A large adenoma of the pituitary gland, or a suprasellar tumor (above the sella turcica) may press on the optic chiasma and cause loss of vision in both temporal fields, i.e. a **bitemporal hemianopia**.

The fibers from the lateral half of the retina, serving the nasal portion of the visual field, pass backwards in the optic tract of the same side, together with the fibers which have crossed from the other side. Most of them relay in the lateral geniculate body, from which fibres pass to the visual cortex in the occipital lobe. Because the optic tract is composed of crossed and uncrossed fibers, lesions cause visual loss in the temporal half of one visual field and in the nasal half of the other, resulting in **homonymous hemianopia**, i.e. blindness to one side, the side opposite to that of the lesion.

(Oculomotor), (trochlear) and (abducent)

The oculomotor, trochlear and abducent nerves may be considered together because they are all motor nerves of the eyeball. They supply the extrinsic muscles which move the eye and injury to any one of them results in double vision (diplopia) and a squint (strabismus). The **third cranial nerve** also conveys parasympathetic fibers which synapse in the ciliary ganglion, a small ganglion situated in the apex of the orbit. The efferent (post-ganglionic) fibers from this ganglion supply the ciliary body, which effects accommodation of the lens, and the iris muscles which constrict the pupil. A complete third nerve lesion therefore causes not only a diplopia and a divergent squint but also dilatation of the pupil, due to the unopposed action of sympathetic dilator pupillae nerve fibers. Pupillary reflexes (accommodation-convergence and reaction to light) are lost because of paralysis of the constrictor pupillae fibers. As the third nerve also supplies the muscle which suspends the upper eyelid, a complete third nerve lesion also causes drooping of the lid, or **ptosis**.

The **trochlear nerve** supplies only one eye muscle, the superior oblique. A lesion of the fourth cranial nerve results in paralysis of this muscle and diplopia so that the patient is unable to turn the eye downwards and laterally. Attempts to do so cause the eye to be rotated medially, resulting in diplopia.

The **abducent nerve** supplies only the lateral rectus muscle. Paralysis of this nerve results in diplopia and convergent squint. The sixth cranial nerve has a long intracranial course and is vulnerable to injury at the same time as fractures of the base of the skull are sustained. Lateral squint may also be a **false localizing sign** of an intracranial lesion as a result of the abducent nerve, in its long course, being stretched in patients with raised intracranial pressure. The reader will note that two possible signs of raised intracranial tension have now been mentioned, the first being papilloedema.

The Trigeminal Nerve (Fig. 17.10)

This is the largest cranial nerve and is the sensory nerve of the face and anterior part of the scalp. It also has a small motor portion which supplies the muscles of mastication and is therefore a nerve of mixed type. As its name suggests, it has three divisions:
1. The **ophthalmic division**, which supplies the forehead, a large part of the scalp, the upper eyelid, the conjunctiva of the eye and most of the nose
2. The **maxillary division**, which supplies the cheek and upper jaw, including its teeth, the nasal septum, the palate, nasopharynx, uvula and tonsils
3. The **mandibular division** distributed to the temple, parts of the ear and lower face the lower jaw and its teeth, the anterior two-thirds of the tongue and the floor of the mouth. The mandibular nerve also conveys the small motor root to the muscles of mastication and secretomotor fibers to the parotid salivary gland.

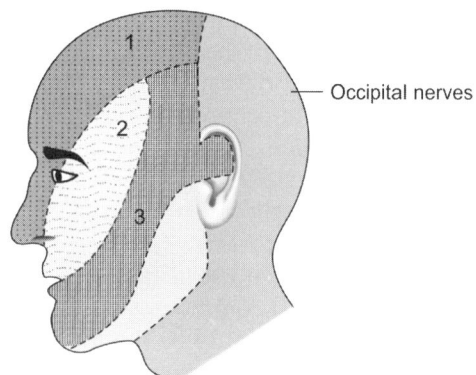

Fig. 17.10: Distribution of the branches of the trigeminal nerve. 1. Opthalmic branch, 2. Maxillary branch, 3. Mandibular branch

The **trigeminal ganglion**, which lies near the apex of the petrous temporal bone, is the first cell station for the sensory fibers of the fifth cranial nerve. It is the equivalent of the dorsal sensory ganglion of a spinal nerve. Controlled heat-coagulation of the trigeminal ganglion is one of the surgical procedures used in cases of trigeminal neuralgia in which drug therapy has proved ineffective.

The Facial Nerve

The seventh cranial nerve is predominantly a motor nerve supplying the muscles of facial expression. It also conveys secretomotor fibers from the parasympathetic system to the sublingual and submandibular salivary glands and the lacrimal gland. In addition, it carries sensory fibers of taste from the anterior two-thirds of the tongue, other types of sensation being conveyed by the mandibular branch of the fifth cranial nerve. The motor fibers originate in the pons and the sensory fibers originate in cells in the genicular ganglion, within the temporal bone.

A lesion of the seventh nerve or its nucleus causes paresis (weakness) or paralysis of all the muscles of the face on that side. The most common cause is Bell's palsy which is thought to be due to a viral infection; the swollen nerve is compressed within the facial canal of the temporal bone and corticosteroids may be used to reduce the swelling and decompress the nerve. The patient with Bell's palsy may at first be thought to have had a 'small stroke'. However, upper facial movements are preserved after a stroke (an upper motor neuron lesion) because they are represented in the cortex of both cerebral hemispheres. Consequently, the patient can still close the eye on the affected side as well as on the unaffected side. The patient with Bell's palsy (a lower motor neuron lesion) cannot do this because it is the final common pathway, in the seventh nerve trunk, which is affected.

The Vestibulocochlear Nerve

The eighth cranial nerve is a sensory nerve consisting of two sets of fibers which convey impulses from the internal ear to the brain. One set of fibers forms the vestibular nerve, which is concerned with equilibrium. The other set forms the cochlear nerve, which is the nerve of hearing.

The **vestibular nerve** is composed of fibers arising from the cells of the **vestibular ganglion** which is situated in the internal acoustic meatus. Impulses from the semicircular ducts are conveyed along the nerve, which lies in the internal acoustic meatus, to the vestibular nuclei in the medulla. From these nuclei, efferent fibers pass via the inferior cerebellar peduncle to the cerebellum, mostly to the flocculus and nodule. The inferior cerebellar peduncle also conveys some vestibular nerve fibers which bypass the vestibular nuclei and pass directly to the cerebellum. Other fibers in the inferior cerebellar peduncle convey impulses in the opposite direction, i.e. from cerebellum to vestibular nuclei. Other connections of the vestibular nuclei are to the motor nuclei of the cranial nerves (III, IV and VI) supplying the eye muscles and to motor nuclei of muscles of the neck. Efferent fibers from the lateral vestibular nucleus descend to form the vestibulospinal tract. The connections of the vestibular system enable it to influence the muscles of the eyes, neck, trunk and limbs so as to preserve balance.

The fibres of the **cochlear nerve**, or nerve of hearing, originate in the spinal ganglion of the cochlea. They pass along the internal acoustic meatus to the medulla and terminate in the ventral and dorsal cochlear nuclei.

The vestibulocochlear and facial nerves are near to each other as they leave the brain stem and they enter the internal acoustic meatus together. An acoustic neuroma in the cerebellopontine angle therefore soon compresses the facial nerve and causes unilateral facial paralysis of lower motor neuron type. Fractures of the base of the skull may cause loss of taste in the anterior two-thirds of the tongue (VIIth nerve) and loss of hearing (VIIIth nerve) on the same side.

The Glossopharyngeal Nerve

The ninth cranial nerve is a mixed nerve. It contains sensory fibers which supply the pharynx, tonsil and posterior one-third of the tongue, including its taste buds. A branch named the carotid nerve serves the carotid sinus and carotid body. It provides the afferent pathways for the baroreceptor and chemoreceptor reflexes associated with these structures.

The motor fibers of the glossopharyngeal nerve supply the stylopharyngeus muscle which helps to elevate the pharynx in swallowing and speaking. Secretomotor fibers are supplied to the parotid salivary gland.

The Vagus Nerve

The vagus nerve is also mixed. It has the most extensive course and distribution of all the cranial nerves. It arises from the medulla oblongata, passes through the jugular foramen in the base of the skull and continues downwards in the neck to the thorax, where it accompanies the esophagus before passing through the diaphragm and into the abdomen. It is distributed to the pharynx, larynx, trachea, bronchi, lungs, heart, esophagus, stomach, upper intestine and kidneys.

The recurrent laryngeal branch of the vagus nerve has a different origin and course on the two sides. On the right side it arises in front of the subclavian artery behind which it passes and ascends obliquely to the side of the trachea. It is intimately related to the inferior thyroid artery. The left recurrent laryngeal branch arises as the vagus nerve crosses the arch of the aorta. It winds below the ligamentum anteriosum, under the arch, and passes upwards in the groove between the trachea and esophagus. Both recurrent laryngeal nerves give branches to the muscles and mucous membrane of the larynx.

Damage to one of the recurrent laryngeal nerves may result in paralysis of the ipsilateral vocal cord and hoarseness of the voice. The nerve may be damaged in the neck by malignant lymph nodes or a carcinoma of the thyroid gland. The left recurrent laryngeal nerve may be affected in the thorax by a bronchial or esophageal carcinoma, a mass of enlarged mediastinal lymph nodes, or an aneurysm of the aortic arch. Rarely, an enlarged left atrium, in a patient with mitral stenosis, causes a recurrent laryngeal nerve palsy by pushing the left pulmonary artery upwards so that it compresses the nerve against the aortic arch.

The superior and inferior **cardiac branches** of the vagus nerve are inhibitory to the heart, which is slowed when they are stimulated. The vagus nerve may be stimulated reflexly by applying external pressure to the carotid sinus in the neck. This is sometimes done to stop a fast abnormal cardiac rhythm but is potentially dangerous and should be performed only by a physician. In a minority of people with a very sensitive carotid sinus, mild stimulation, such as the pressure of a shirt collar when the neck is turned, may be sufficient to cause loss of consciousness (carotid sinus syncope) due to vagal inhibition of the heart.

A little above the diaphragm the vagus nerves form **anterior and posterior vagal trunks** in front of the esophagus and behind it, respectively. These enter the abdomen with the esophagus, through the esophageal opening in the diaphragm, and supply **gastric branches** to the stomach. The surgeon divides the two vagal trunks in the operation of truncal vagotomy in order to reduce the acid-pepsin secretion of the stomach in patients with a duodenal ulcer. However, total **truncal vagotomy** denervates not only the stomach but also the liver, gallbladder, pancreas and most of the intestines. As this widespread denervation is a possible cause of diarrhea and other postvagotomy complications, some surgeons divide only the gastric branches of the vagus nerve (**selective vagotomy**) or only those supplying the parietal cell mass (proximal gastric or **highly selective vagotomy**).

Amongst the other branches of the vagus nerve the auricular branch is of interest when there is a need to syringe wax out of ears. The distribution of this branch includes the posterior wall and floor of the external acoustic meatus and stimulation of this area may reflexly cause coughing, vomiting or cardiac syncope.

The Accessory Nerve

This is a motor nerve possessing cranial and spinal roots. The cranial root is distributed in branches of the vagus nerve to the muscles of the palate, pharynx and larynx. Paresis of these muscles results in dysphagia and dysphonia.

The spinal root of the accessory nerve supplies the sternomastoid and trapezius muscles in the neck. Central irritation causes clonic spasm of these muscles, a condition known as spasmodic torticollis.

The Hypoglossal Nerve

The twelfth cranial nerve is the motor nerve of the tongue. A lesion of this nerve, or its nucleus in the medulla, causes paralysis, or weakness (paresis), and wasting of the muscles of the tongue on the same side and deviation of the protruded tongue towards that side. In contrast to this lower motor neuron lesion, an upper motor neuron lesion (e.g. as part of a stroke) causes paresis without any wasting of the tongue muscles.

■ PAIN

Although pain receptors are specific, the stimulus which cause pain sensation are not as specific as other receptors. The receptors for pain can respond to any type of strong stimulus; mechanical, electrical, thermal or chemical. All these stimuli threaten injury and pain nerve ending respond to it.

Difference between Somatic and Visceral Pain

While somatic structures, skin and subcutaneous tissues and muscles have receptors which subserve sensory functions of touch, temperature, pressure and pain and proprioceptors of muscles concerned with sense of position and movement, the viscera have no proprioceptors, very few tactile and thermal receptors and sparsely distributed pain receptors. The somatic pain travel along with the somatic pathways in the spinothalamic tracts to thalamus and sensory area of the cerebral cortex (Fig. 17.11).

Visceral Pain

Normally the viscera are insensitive to various forms of stimuli. However, pain is an important manifestation of disease of internal organs and discarded viscera is sensitive to pain. The characteristic of visceral pain is—it is diffused and dull, poorly localized though severe, has unpleasant affective component, is associated with autonomic symptoms like vension, and often radiates and referred to other areas.

Stimuli for Visceral Pain

1. Ischemia (Obstruction to blood flow)
2. Overdistension of hollow viscus
3. Obstruction in a hollow viscus, e.g. intestinal obstruction. It produces colicky pain
4. Spasm of hollow viscus or ducts—cramping pain
5. Chemical stimuli, e.g. ruptured gastric or duodenal ulcer causes leakage of proteolytic acid contents into peritoneal cavity and chemical damage and pain.

The pain arise in the discarded viscera can be transmitted via autonomic afferents or it may spread to associated peritoneum, pleura or pericardium which have extensive pain innervation, and pain sensations are transmitted through somatic nerves.

Reffered Pain

When there is a lesion in a viscus, pain may be felt in the viscus or the overlying somatic structure in the vicinity, e.g. pain

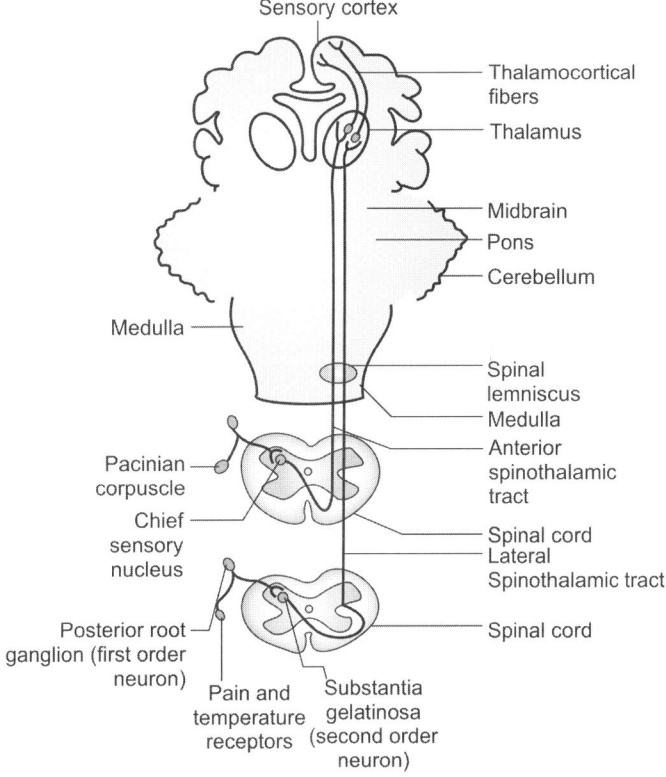

Fig. 17.11: Pain pathway

of appendicitis felt in the right iliac fossa. But quite frequently pain is felt in somatic structures which are at a considerable distance from the diseased organ. This is called reffered pain arriving at the somatic spinothalamic neurons are ineffective and die out. But when strong pain impulses arrive via visceral afferents, they cause the activation of the somatic spinothalamic neurons, by subliminal fringe via collateral fibers.

Ascending and Descending Tracts (Fig. 17.12)

The ascending pathways from the spinal cord to brain include:
1. Posterior column tracts of Goll and Burdach
2. Spinothalamic tract (lateral or dorsal and ventral or anterior)
3. Spinocerebellar tract (Dorsal and ventral)
4. Spinotectal tract
5. Spino-olivary tract.

The first 3 tracts are very important clinically.

Posterior column tracts: The tract of Goll and Burdach are also known as Fasciculus gracilis and cuneatus. They are made of heavily myelinated fibers of the medical division of the posterior nerve roots of the same side. They convey epicritic tactile sensations, tacticle localization and discrimination and deep sensations—sense of position and movement (conscious proprioception) and vibration senses (deep pressure). Fibers enter the spinal cord through the medeal division of the posterior nerve root, enter the posterior white column.

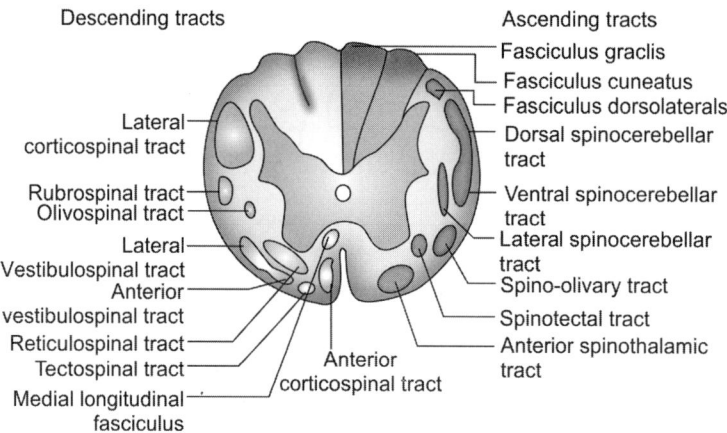

Fig. 17.12: Descending tracts and ascending tracts

Basis of Reffered Pain
Principle of Dermatomal rule. One segment of the spinal cord supplies a well-defined area of skin with somatic nerves (dermatome). But autonomic nerve from the same segment innervate a visceral area. The somatic and visceral areas innervated by one particular segment may be either close to each other or may be at a considerable distance from each other, causing the pair to be felt at a distance from diseased viscus.
For example:
1. Pain arising in heart may be substernal or is felt over the inner aspect of left arm.
2. Pain in the region of the diaphragm is felt over the tip of the shoulder. Previous experience also has a role for if pain from abdominal organ may be reffered to a previous surgical scar.

Mechanism of Referred Pain
1. *Convergence theory:* Both somatic and visceral afferents converge upon the same spinothalamic neurons. But the brain is accustomed to receiving somatic pain impulse much more frequently than visceral impulses brain is learnt, that impulses arriving along a certain pathway is from the somatic area.
2. *Facilitation theory:* Visceral and somatic pain afferents connect with separate but adjoining spinothalamic neurons and there may be some overlap of the neurons. Visceral afferents have collaterals connecting to the spinothalamic neurons receiving somatic pain afferents. Normally weak signals horn cells (chief sensory nucleus).

Second order neurons: Arise from horn, cross to the opposite side in the anterior commissure enter and ascend in the anterior white column. On entering the medulla moves medially, tranesss brain stem close to medial lemniscus, and in posteroventral nucleus of thalamus.

Third order neurons: Arise from thalamus some passes to the medical thalamic nuclei, other goes to sensory area of cerebral cortex.

Lateral Spinothalamic Tract

Carries sensations of pain, temperature and visceral and sexual sensations.

First order neurons enter the spinal cord via lateral division of posterior nerve root, and ascend or descend a short distance between the tip of the posterior horn and periphery of the cord before ending in the cells of substantia gelatinosa rolandis (SGR). This is tract of Lissonr.

Second order neurons which form the LST arise from SGR cross to opposite side in the anterior commissure to reach the lateral white funiculus, and ascend up to medulla. The fibers pass through medulla and close to VST in mid brain and pons called spinal leminiscus to pass to the posteroventral neurons of thalamus.

Third order neurons arise from posteroventral nucleus of thalamus and most of the fibers pass to medial nucleus of thalamus. Some fibers ascend to area 3, 1, 2 of cerebral cortex of the same side and ascend in the posterior columns. They enter the medulla and enter the corresponding N. cureatus and N. Gracilis. The fasciculus gracilis begins at the lowest level of the spinal cord (sacral segments) and carries fibers from lower limb. The arrangement of fibers from medical to lateral side are fibers from the sacral, lumbar, thoracic and cervical (SLTC) segments.

First order neurons—dorsal root ganglion up to medulla is N. Gracilis and cureatus.

Second order neurons—from N. Gracilis and N. cureatus fiber decussate with those coming from the opposite side forming sensory decussation and ascend as medial leiminiscus pass through medulla, pons and midbrain to terminate in posteroventral nucleus of thalamus.

Third order neurons—arise in the thalamus and ascend to the cortex lying in the posterior limb of internal capsule behind the corticospinal fibers diverges in the corona reliata and ends in the cerebral cortex area 3, 1, 2.

Spinothalamic Tract

Ventral spinothalamic conveys sensations of crude touch and some crude localization. First order neurons—enterspinal cord via the posterior nerve root and end in dorsal. Arrangement of fibers in the upper part from lateral to medial side are sacral, lumbar, thoracic and cervical (SLTC) opposite to that in posterior columns.

The Descending Pathways

They convey efferent impulses from various parts of brain to spinal cord. All the tracts end in anterior horn cells mostly through internuncial neurons while only a few connect directly with the anterior horn cells.
- Cortico spinal (Pyramidal) and corticobulbar tracts
- Extra pyramidal tracts
  - Vestibulospinal
  - Reticulospinal
  - Tectospinal
  - Rubrospinal
  - Olivospinal

Pyramidal Tract (Fig. 17.13)

The fibers arise from cerebral cortex. Thirty percent of the fibers come from primary motor area 30% from premotor and supplementary moter area and 40% from parietal lobe mainly from the sensory area in the post central gyrus, large chamiter fiber from Betz cells concerned with skilled movements.
- Fibers descend in the corona radiata and converge in the internal capsule. In the internal capsule they occupy the genn and anterior two-thirds of posterior limb.
- In the midbrain, fibers occupy the middle three-fifths of crus cerebri.
- The fibers descend in the pons and in the lower part of pons form a compact bundle descends in the ventral part of the medulla forming the prominent pyramids of the medulla (Its name is pyramidal tract).
- While passing down the brain stem, some of the fibers connect with the moter nuclei of cranial nerves of the opposite side. This part is called corticobulbar tract.
- At the lower part of medulla most of the fibers (80–85%) cross to the opposite

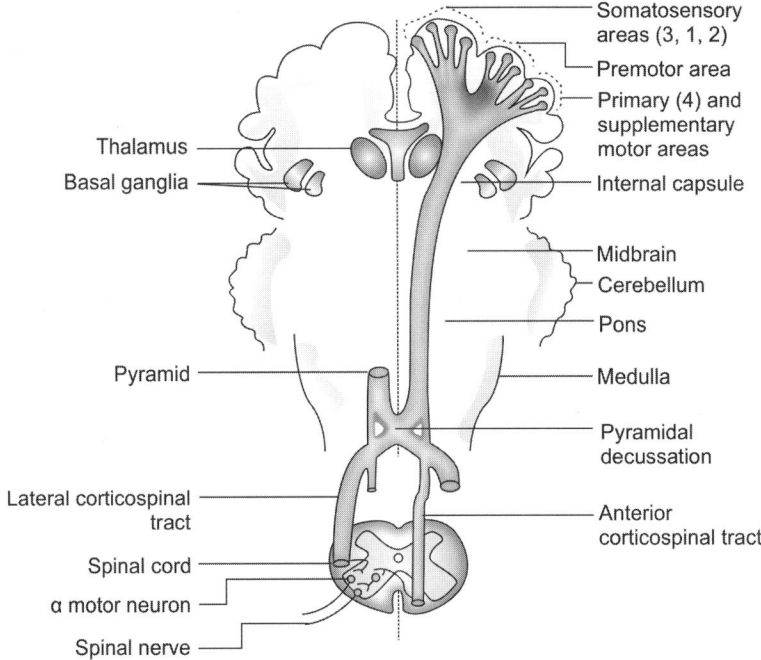

Fig. 17.13: Pyramidal tract

side in the pyramidal decussation, and descend in the leteral white column of spinal cord as lateral corticospinal or crossed pyramidal tract, and end in the anterior horn cells of spinal cord.
- The remaining uncrossed fibers (15–20%) descend in the anterior white column of the spinal cord of the same side, as the anterior or ventral corticospinal or direct pyramidal tract (Fig. 17.14).
- *Hemiplegia:* Paralysis of one half of the body.
  - *Contra lateral hemiplegia:* If the lesion is on left side of brain the paralysis is on right side of body.
  - *Crossed hemiplegia:* If the lesion is in the brain stem, cranial nerve of the same side of lesion and paralysis of opposite half of body occurs. This is crossed hemiplegia.
- *Paraplegia:* If the lesion is in the mid thoracic level of spinal cord, there is paralysis of both lower limbs. This is paraplegia.
- *Quadriplegia:* Paralysis of all four limbs occurs when the spinal cord lesion is at the upper cervical segments.
- *Muscle tone:* Tone in skeletal muscle is a state of slight partial, sustained contraction of the muscle. It consists of simultaneous contraction of a few muscle fibers at a time, replaced at regular intervals by contraction of other fibers. It is present mainly in the antigravity muscles and is concerned in the maintenance of posture. It is reflex in nature and hence intact nervous connections are essential.
- *Posture:* It is the position of the body in relation to the environment can be analysed as:
  - Head in relation to environment
  - Body in relation to head
  - Body in relation to environment
  - Tone of muscles especially limbs.

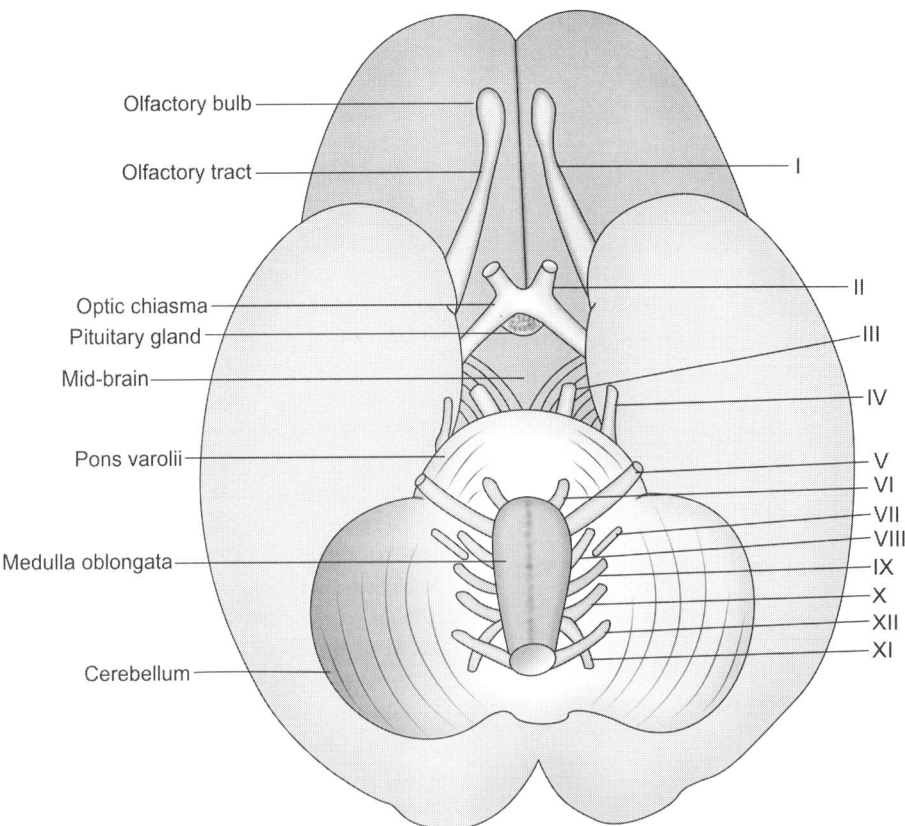

Fig. 17.14: Diagram illustrating the origin of cranial nerves from the base of the brain

Maintenance of posture is usually a reflex phenomenon which does not require a conscious effort, except in the adoption of complex postures as in yoga or other exercises or postures by circus artists. Tone of muscle is involved in the maintenance of posture. Muscle tone is due to low frequency asynchonous discharge of impulses from moter neurons (anterior horn cells). The distribution and degree of tone varies with the attitude adopted by the animal. The fundamental basis of muscle tone is the stretch reflex. Tone is also influenced by higher centers–cerebral cortex, basal ganglia midbrain, cerebellum and labyrinth.

■ THE BRAIN

The brain is that portion of the central nervous system which lies within the cavity of the skull. It consists of the following parts.

- The **forebrain**, consisting of the two cerebral hemispheres (the cerebrum) and the diencephalon or 'interbrain', which largely corresponds to the third ventricle and the structures bounding it.
- The **midbrain** or mesencephalon.
- The **hindbrain**, comprising
  - The pons
  - The medulla oblongata
  - The cerebellum.

The midbrain, pons and medulla oblongata together constitute the brainstem. When there is irreversible cessation of function of the brainstem, **brain death** is diagnosed. The heart may continue to beat but no spontaneous breathing occurs and respiration depends upon mechanical ventilation. Before the ventilator may be turned off, the diagnosis of brain death has to be substantiated, with due safeguards, by the repeated demonstration of **absence of all brainstem reflexes** by two doctors, one of whom has to be appropriately experienced and to have been registered for five years or more.

■ CEREBRUM

General consideration: Cerebral hemisphere comprises of cortical grey matter as outer surface and white matter beneath cortex. Each hemisphere contains the lateral ventricle. The cerebral cortex is folded into numerous gyri or convolutions separated by sulci or fissures. Till the third month of intrauterine life, the surface of brain is smooth. In the fourth month, lateral sulcus appears on the superolateral surface of cerebrum (Fig. 17.15). All sulci are formed by the end of 7th month. Sulci may be limiting, axial or operculated. Central sulcus may be an example of limiting sulcus. Lunate sulcus is an example of operculated sulcus and calcarine sulcus is an example of axial sulcus.

Gross anatomy of cerebral hemisphere: Cerebral hemispheres are separated by median longitudinal fissure. Each hemisphere has three surfaces, three borders and three poles.

Surfaces are: Superolateral, medial and inferior. The inferior surface is divided into an anterior (orbital) surface and posterior (tentorial) surface.

Borders are: Superomedial (between superolateral and medial surface), inferomedial (between medial and inferior surfaces) and inferolateral (between superolateral and inferior surface).

Poles are: Frontal pole, occipital pole, temporal pole. Each hemisphere is divided into four lobes—frontal, parietal, temporal, occipital. These lobes are separated by central sulcus, lateral sulcus, parieto-occipital sulcus.

Superolateral surface: This surface extends between superomedial border and inferolateral border. The sulci seen in this surface is central and posterior ramus of lateral sulci.

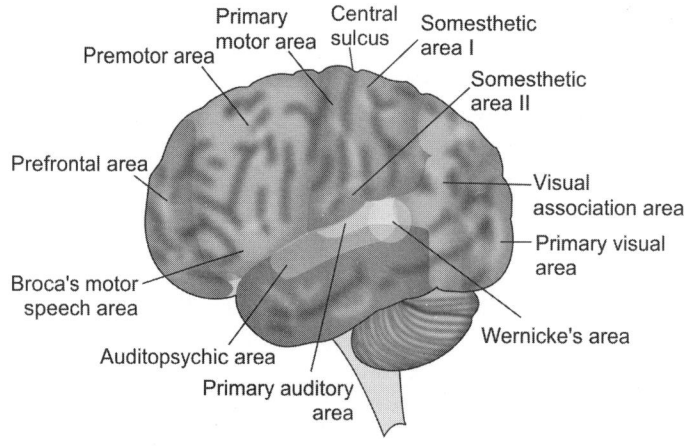

Fig. 17.15: Superolateral surface of cerebrum

Central sulcus of Rolando: Arises near the superomedial margin just behind the midpoint between frontal and occipital pole. The sulcul passes downwards on the superolateral surface towards posterior ramus of lateral sulcus and ends just above the lateral sulcus. Upper end of lateral sulcus appears partly on the medial surface.

Lateral sulcus (Sylvian fissure): It consists of stem and three rami. Stem is situated in the inferior surface and divide into three rami which spread on superolateral surface. The stem of the lateral sulcus lies between orbital and tentorial surface. The three rami are anterior horizontal, anterior ascending, and posterior. A pyramidal-shaped insula is situated at the bottom of the stem.

The parieto-occipital sulcus: It lies partly in medial surface and partly in superolateral surface. It lies in 5 cm in front of occipital pole.

Occipital notch: It lies 5 cm in front of occipital pole in the inferolateral border.

Frontal lobe: It lies in front of central sulcus and above lateral sulcus.

Parietal lobe: It is bounded in front by the central sulcus and behind by an imaginary line drawn from occipital notch to parieto-occipital sulcus.

Occipital lobe: It lies behind the parieto-occipital sulcus.

Temporal lobe: It lies in front of occipital lobe and below the posterior ramus of lateral sulcus.

Frontal lobe: It has four gyri and three sulci. Precentral sulcus lies in front of central sulcus and precentral gyrus lies between the two sulcus. Precentral gyrus is motor in function. Superior and inferior frontal sulcus lie in front of precentral gyrus and divides frontal lobe into superior, middle, inferior frontal gyrus.

Parietal lobe: Postcentral sulcus lies parallel to and behind the central sulcus. The postcentral gyrus is sensory in function. The intraparietal sulcus arises from the middle of postcentral sulcus and divides the parietal lobe to superior and inferior parietal lobule.

Occipital lobe: The sulci present in occipital lobe are transverse occipital, lateral occipital and lunate sulcus. The lateral occipital sulcus divides the occipital lobe into superior and inferior occipital gyri. Lunate sulcus lodges the primary visual area.

Temporal lobe: It has two sulci and three gyri. The two sulci are superior and inferior temporal sulci and three gyri are superior, middle, inferior temporal gyri. The upper surface of superior temporal gyri presents three or more transverse gyrus. The anterior most of them is the primary auditory area.

Medial surface: Medial surface is flat and presents an arched band of white matter the corpus callosum made of commissural fibers. Callosal sulcus lies above corpus callosum. Cingulate gyrus lies above cingulate sulcus. Above cingulate sulcus is medial frontal gyrus (anteriorly), paracentral lobule (in the middle), behind it is precuneus and posteriorly is cuneus and lingual gyrus.

Paracentral lobule is divided into motor and sensory area by central sulcus which extends to the medial surface.

Occipital lobe presents parieto-occipital sulcus which lies 5 cm in front of occipital pole. Calcarine sulcus meets parieto-occipital sulcus at an acute angle forming a triangular area in cortex called cuneus.

Lingual gyrus lies below cuneus.

Lingual gyrus, cuneus and calcarine sulcus together form primary visual area.

■ MOTOR SYSTEM

Cerebral Cortex

It is divided into two parts. Newer neocortex and older archi pallium (allocortex).

Neocortex contains pyramidal, granular spindle-shaped and other cells.

Layers from without Inwards

Outer molecular or plexiform layer—pear-shaped cells

Outer granular layer

Outer pyramidal layer

Internal granular layer—stellate cell layer

Internal pyramidal layer—small medium and large pyramidal cells called Betz cell.

The fusiform cell layer (spindle cell layer) consists of an outer layer of triangular cells and an inner layer of small spindle-shaped cells.

Types of Cortex

1. *Agranular:* Cortex is thicker. The pyramidal cells are very prominent. Granular cells are fewer and the Layers are thinner – seen in primary motor area with Betz cells. Other parts of the frontal cortex are also agranular but do not have Betz cells.
2. *Granular type:* Cortex is thinner. Granular cell layers are well-developed. Pyramidal cell layers are inconspicuous and poorly developed. The sensory areas are granular type → referred as Koniocortex.

The old cortex: It has only three or two layers inner granular and inner pyramidal (v) of the iso cortex.

Functions of Ceribral Cortex (Fig. 17.16)

- Motor functions in precentral gyrus (Area 4) somatic sensory functions in the postcentral gyrus. (Area 3, 1, 2) Visual functions in the occipital cortex (area 17)
- Right motor area in the left lower limb is represented in the upper part. The head and face in the lower part.

Lobes of the Cerebral Cortex

- Frontal lobe situated in front of the central sulcus or fissure of Roland.

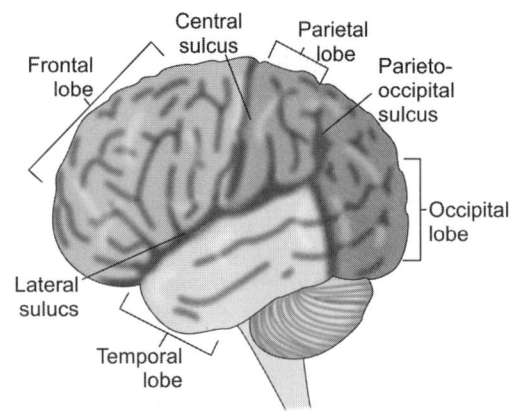

Fig. 17.16: Lobes of cerebral cortex

- Parietal lobe situated behind the frontal lobe, between the central sulcus and the parieto-occipital sulcus.
- Occipital cortex behind the parieto-occipital sulcus and is the most posterior part of the cortex.
- Temporal lobe below the lateral or sylvian fissure.

Frontal Lobe

The principal areas in the frontal lobe are:
- Brodmann's Area 4 in the precentral gyrus and is the primary motor area.
- Supplementary motor area on the medial aspect anterior to Areas 4 or 6.
- Premotor area (Area 6) in front of area 4.
- Area 4S of Hiner (The suppressor band between Areas 4 and 6 in the upper part.)
- Area 8 in front of the upper part of Area 6 in the posterior part of the second frontal convolution.
- Area 44 (Broca's or motor area for speech) in the posterior part of the frontal operculum in the dominant hemisphere. (left side in the right handed person).
- Prefrontal or orbitofrontal areas in the frontal lobe, in front of Areas 4, 6, 8 and 44 and include structures on the lateral medial and orbital surfaces. (Areas 9–14, 45–47).

Area 4 (Primary motor area, motor cortex): It is the highest center for voluntary movements. The muscles of the body are represented in the inverse sequence except for the face, which is not inverted.

Hands, fingers, thumb, lips and tongue which are extensively used have a greater area of representation than trunk which is much larger in size. The representation is called motor homunculus.

Supplementary motor area: Lies on the medical surface of the hemisphere in front of the Areas 4 and 6. In the medial frontal gyrus, representation is head to foot, anteroposteriorly. It projects to motor cortex.

Plasticity in motor area: The motor area shows a certain degree of plasticity.

Sensory Functions

The sensory tracts end in different parts of the sensory cerebral cortex. Somesthetic sensations are relayed to the postcentral cortex (areas 3, 1, 2) of parietal lobe.

Visual sensations end in occipital cortex (area 17) and the auditory sensations in superior temporal gyrus (area 41).

Functions → Somesthetic area: (Sensory area I)

- Perception and mediation of all epicritic and deep sensations.
- Discrimination and synthesis of sensation.
  - Recognition of spatial relationships
  - Recognition of relative intensities of stimuli
  - Recognition of similarities and differences
  - Stereognosis.

■ FUNCTIONAL AREAS OF CEREBRAL CORTEX

Cortical areas are divided into motor, sensory, and psychical areas.

Motor Areas

Motor areas are primary motor area, premotor area, supplementary motor area, prefrontal area.

Primary motor area (area 4): It includes precentral gyrus and extends to medial surface. It lies in the anterior part of paracentral lobule.

Functions

Primary motor cortex controls movements of the voluntary muscles of the opposite side of the body (contralateral side). Body is represented upside down (motor homunculus) in motor area with head represented in the lower part of gyrus and leg in the upper part. Motor area in the para-central lobule is the area for controling micturition and defecation reflux.

Effects of lesion: Lesion in motor cortex results in flaccid paresis of opposite side.

Premotor cortex: Area 6 lies immediately in front of area 4 and behind superior, middle and inferior frontal gyri. Area 8 lies in front of area 6. Both areas are motor in function.

Functions of area 6 is to perform voluntary movements like skilful acts. Upper part of area 6 is writing center and is concerned with coordinated movements of writing.

Broca's area (Motor speech area): The lower part of area 6 in the inferior frontal gyrus is Broca's speech area. It is motor speech center. It coordinates movement of lips, tongue, palate, larynx and pharynx. Area 8 lies in front of area 6 and is known as frontal eye field which regulates voluntary conjugate eye movements.

Prefrontal area (Area 9 to 12): The part of frontal lobe anterior to premotor area is prefrontal area 9, 10, 11, 12. This area is well-developed in human.

Functions of prefrontal area: This area is essential for abstract thinking, fair judgement, tactfulness, pleasure and displeasure. Lesion in this area results in a mental state which lacks sense of responsibility, vulgarity in speech, feelings of euphoria.

Sensory area: Sensory areas include primary sensory area, visual area, auditory area.

Primary sensory area: It is located in post-central gyrus and extends to the posterior part of para-central lobule on the medial surface (Area 3, 1, 2).

Function of sensory area: Cutaneous and proprioceptive senses are analysed in this area like touch, pressure, position and vibrating senses. Areas of sensations are represented upside down with head below and leg above (sensory homunculus). In the paracentral lobule sensations of distension of bladder and rectum appreciated. Lower end of post central gyrus acts as taste receptive area. Pain is appreciated most in the lower part of precentral and post-central gyrus.

Visual Area

Area 17: This area is situated in the walls of calcarine sulcus including cuneus and lingual gyrus. Visual cortex is thinner compared to other cerebral areas.

Functions: Visual area receives information from own half of each retina. Thrombosis of posterior cerebral artery produces partial blindness. Macular vision is spared because it has dual arterial supply.

Visual association area (area 18, 19): This area include area 18 and 19 which is surrounded by primary visual area. They connect with motor nuclei of extraocular muscles.

Functions: These areas include help in recognition of objects by relating with past visual experiences. These areas also produce conjugate movements of eye.

Higher visual association area (angular gyrus–area 39): This area helps identifying various objects and symbols by vision. Lesion in this area produce inability to recognize known objects by vision.

Primary auditory area (area 41): This area is present in the upper surface of superior temporal gyrus in the floor of posterior ramus of lateral sulcus. Fibers of auditory radiation terminate here. This area detects the change in frequency of sound and the place from where sound originated. Auditory area is bilaterally represented.

Auditory association area: It lies behind primary auditory area (area 42) in the upper surface of superior temporal gyrus. Rest of the superior temporal gyrus forms higher auditory association area (area 22). The association and higher association areas are connected by association fibers. Area 22 is called Wernicke's area. It analyses sound and is concerned with comprehension of spoken language.

In lesion of Wernicke's area, person is unable to understand words spoken by him itself. His speech will contain empty words (meaningless words).

Vestibular area: This area lies in front of auditory area. Stimulation of this area causes dizziness and vertigo.

Psychical cortex: It is the anterior part of temporal lobe and includes temporal pole. It is the area which recollects recent and past experiences. Irritation of this area causes epileptic seizures with auditory and visual hallucination and memory disturbances.

Speech function in brain: Speech requires muscles, vocal cords, visual senses, auditory senses. Dominant hemisphere and talking brain is left cerebral hemisphere. The four areas of speech are:

- *Area 22:* It is located in superior temporal gyrus. It helps to identify familiar sounds.
- *Area 39:* Angular gyrus—this area recognizes objects by sight.
- *Area 40:* Supramarginal gyrus—recognizes objects with help of touch. So, area 22, 39, 40 are sensory speech area. Information are processed by Wernicke's speech area and projected to Broca's speech area (Motor speech area).
- *Broca's speech area:* This area is located

in inferior frontal gyrus (area 44, 45). In lesion of Broca's speech area, person cannot speak properly and speech is very slow.

■ THALAMUS

Thalamus is a complex mass of grey matter around cavity of third ventricle. It lies above the hypothalamus separated by hypothalamic sulcus.

Thalamus has anterior and posterior ends and four surfaces like upper, lower, medial, lateral. Anterior end lies behind interventricular foramen. Posterior end presents medial and lateral geniculate body separated by pulvinar.

Upper surface forms floor of lateral ventricle covered by choroid plexus. Lower surface is related to hypothalamus. Medial surface is related to third ventricle. The medial surfaces of both thalami are linked by interthalamic adhesion. Lateral surface is related to posterior limb of internal capsule.

Thalamus is divided by Y-shaped internal medullary lamina and between the two limbs of 'Y' is anterior group of nuclei. Intralaminar nuclei lie within the internal medullary lamina.

Six groups of nuclear masses are present in thalamus.

These groups are:
1. Anterior
2. Medial or dorsomedia group
3. Intralaminar nuclei
4. Midline nuclei
5. Reticular nuclei
6. Lateral nuclei:
   - Ventral anterior, ventral lateral, ventral posterior
   - Lateral dorsal, lateral posterior, pulvinar.

Anterior group: It is connected to mammillary body via mammillothalamic tract – (Papez's circuit). Lesion leads to loss of recent memory.

Media group: It is connected to hypothalamus and prefrontal cortex.

This connection with prefrontal cortex controls emotional aspect of behavior.

Ventral anterior nucleus: It receives fibers from substantia nigra and globus pallidus. These fibers are projected to premotor cortex (area 6).

Ventral lateral nucleus: It receives major input from dentate nucleus of cerebellum. It is also connected to globus pallidus and substantia nigra. It is connected to area 4.

Function: Prime mover of motor pathway.

Ventral posterior nucleus: Ventral posteromedial (VPM)

Ventral postero lateral (VPL): Fibers of touch and vibration sense relay in this nucleus. Pain and temperature pathway also relay in this nuclei.

VPM nucleus: Taste fibers relay in medial part.
- Touch fibers relay in lateral part.
- Temperature fibers relay in intermediate part.
- Efferent fibers from the nucleus are projected to postcentral gyrus.

Functions of ventral posterior nucleus: Acts as the longest specific somatosensory relay nucleus of the thalamus.

Lateral dorsal nucleus: Receives input from mammillary body and output is projected to cingulate gyrus.

Lateral posterior nucleus: Receives inputs from medial geniculate body (MGB) and lateral geniculate body (LGB). Efferents are projected to area 5 and 7 (superior parietal lobule).

Pulvinar part of thalamus: Major input is from MGB and LGB, superior colliculus, VP nucleus of thalamus. Efferents are connected with parietal, temporal and occipital lobes.

Connections Between Cerebral Cortex and Thalamus

Thalamic radiations are divided into four peduncles—anterior, posterior, superior, inferior.

Anterior peduncle: Connects frontal lobe to anterior nucleus and passes through anterior limb of internal capsule.
Superior peduncle: Fibers passing from thalamus to frontal and parietal lobe constitute this peduncle. The fibers passes through genu and posterior limb of internal capsule.
Posterior peduncle: Fibers passing to occipital lobe from thalamus constitute this peduncle. They pass through retrolentiform part of internal capsule. Connects lateral geniculate body to visual cortex.
Inferior peduncle: Fibers from thalamus to temporal lobe constitute this peduncle. Fibers pass through sublentiform part of internal capsule. It connects medial geniculate body with auditory area (area 41, 42).
Functions of thalamus: Final relay station of all sensory pathway except olfaction. Thalamus is concerned with interpretation of pain and temperature. Thalamus regulates the activities of motor pathway.

HYPOTHALAMUS

Functions

- Control of autonomic nervous system.
- Centers for regulation of body temperature.
- Regulation of water balance of the body.
- Neurosecretory functions.
  - Posterior pituitary hormones
  - Releasing and inhibiting hormones.
- Control of sexual functions.
- Control of appetite, hunger and feeling.
- Emotional behavior, emotional exteriorization.
- Influences on sleep.
- Stressful stimuli cause the hypothalamus to discharge CRH which cause release of ACTH from anterior pituitary.
- Biological rhythms → such as sleep – wakefulness rhythm, etc.

INTERNAL CAPSULE

Afferent and efferent fibers from cerebrum traverse the internal capsule. Internal capsule is continuous above with corona radiata and below with crus cerebri.

The internal capsule is bounded medially by the head of caudate nucleus and thalamus and laterally by lentiform nucleus.
Parts of internal capsule are: Anterior limb, genu, posterior limb, retrolentiform part (behind lentiform nucleus) and sublentiform part (below lentiform part).
Anterior limb: This part of internal capsule lies between head of caudate nucleus medially and lentiform nucleus laterally.
Fibers traversing anterior limb are: fronto-pontine and anterior thalamic radiation.
Fibers traversing genu are: Corticonuclear fibers from motor area (area 4, 6, 8) and superior thalamic radiation.
Posterior limb: This part lies between thalamus and lentiform nucleus. Anterior 2/3 of posterior limb contain efferent fibers (corticospinal). Posterior 1/3 of posterior limb contain afferent fibers.

Fibers traversing posterior limb are:
- Corticospinal tract from area 4, 6 which control movements of opposite side of body.
- Corticorubral tract from area 4, 6 and are connected to red nucleus.

Sub-lentiform part: Auditory radiations pass through sub-lentiform part. Some fibers of optic radiation also pass through sub-lentiform part.
Retrolentiform part: Optic radiations pass through retrolentiform part and project to visual cortex (occipital lobe). Posterior thalamic radiation traverse retrolentiform part.

VENTRICLES

Lateral Ventricle (Fig. 17.17)

Each cerebral hemisphere contain lateral ventricle which is C-shaped filled with

The Nervous System 351

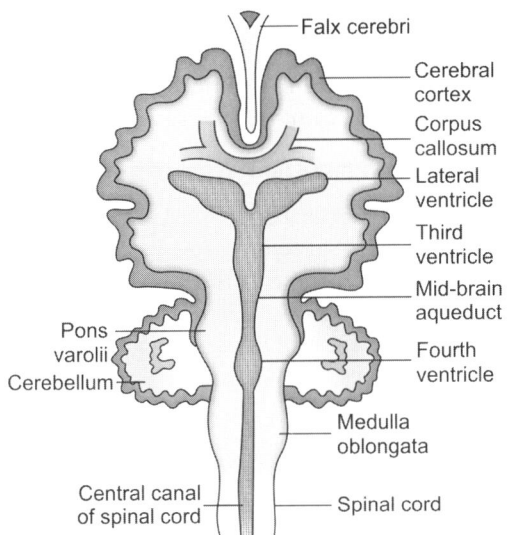

Fig. 17.17: Diagram of the ventricles of the brain (anterior view)

cerebrospinal fluid. The lateral ventricles are separated from each other by septum pellucidum. It communicates with third ventricle by the interventricular foramen of Monro.

Lateral ventricle has body or central part and three horns anterior, posterior and inferior.

Lateral ventricle is roofed by the under surface of corpus callosum.

Anterior horn: Extends in the frontal lobe.
Roof: It is formed by body of corpus callosum.
Floor: It is formed by rostrum of corpus callosum and head of caudate nucleus.
Anterior wall: It is formed by genu of corpus callosum.
Medial wall: It is formed by septum pellucidum.

Body of Lateral Ventricle

It extends from interventricular foramen to the splenium of corpus callosum.
Roof: It is formed by the body of corpus callosum

Floor: It is formed by rostrum of corpus callosum.
Anterior wall: It is formed by genu of corpus callosum.
Medial wall: It is formed by septum pellucidum.

Posterior Horn

It extends to the occipital lobe.
Roof and lateral wall: It is formed by tapetum of corpus callosum.
Medial wall and floor: It has two elevations:
1. *Bulb of posterior horn:* It is produced by forceps major.
2. *Calcar avis:* It is produced by projections of calcarine sulcus.

Inferior Horn

It begins at posterior end of central part. It runs downwards to temporal lobe. It has roof and floor.
Roof: It is formed by tail of caudate nucleus.
Floor: It is formed by hippocampus.

Third Ventricle (Fig. 17.18)

Third ventricle is a midline, slit like cavity formed on the medial surface of the anterior part of thalamus and the lower part is formed by the hypothalamus. Third ventricle is derived from fore-brain vesicle.
Lateral wall of ventricle: It is formed by medial surface of anterior 2/3 of thalamus and the lower part by hypothalamus.

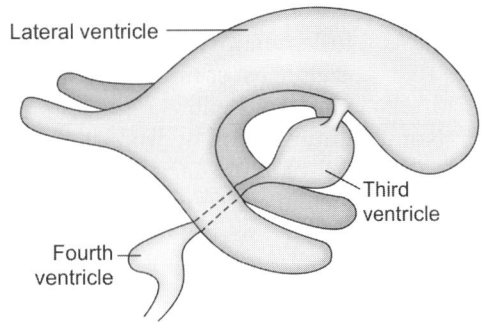

Fig. 17.18: Diagram of the ventricles of the brain (lateral view)

Lateral walls of the ventricle is joined by interthalamic adhesion (band of grey matter extending from one thalamus to the other.
Roof of the third ventricle: It is a thin ependymal layer. Above the roof is fornix.
Posterior boundary of ventricle: It is formed by supra pineal recess, pineal gland, pineal recess.
- The spinal cord level
- The lower brain level
- Higher brain or cortical level

The spinal cord of the human being retains many functions of the multi segmental animal. All the spinal cord motor responses are automatic and occur almost instantaneously nervously in response to the sensory signal. These occur in specific patterns of response called reflexes.

■ HYDROCEPHALUS

Pathological accumulation of CSF within brain spaces.

Types

- Communicating (or external) hydrocephalus is excess of fluid accumulation in subarachnoid space.
  Causes:
  - Increased formation of CSF: Overdevelopment of choroid plexus
  - Decreased absorptive capacity of arachnoid villi due to
    - Thrombosis of venous sinuses
    - Inflammatory changes in meninges casing occlusion of arachnoid villi
- Non-communicating hydrocephalus
  - Excess of fluid accumulation in ventricular system proximal to block. Common sites (1) foramen of Monro aqueduct of sylvius, foramen of Luschka and Magendie.
  - Diagnosis of the site of obstruction found out by injection of phenol sulfonephthalein into a lateral ventricle. Normally, it appears (1) in CSF obtained by lumbar puncture in 2–3 min. (2) in urine in 10–12 min.

■ BLOOD BRAIN BARRIER

Applies to barrier between blood and brain tissue. It exists at two places.
- Located at the choroid plexus and CSF interface. (Blood CSF barrier)
- Other is located between CSF and brain capillaries elsewhere than the choroid plexuses.

Both barriers are similar and blood brain barrier is the most common term used to refer to the net exchange of substances between blood and brain.

H^+ gradient between brain CSF and blood is (2) pH of brain is 7.33; whereas blood is 7.4 water soluble polar compounds cross slowly.

The blood brain barrier (BBB) is:
- Highly permeable to water, O_2, CO_2, sulfa drugs and erythromycin
- Slightly permeable to electrolytes H^+, Na^+, K^+, Mg^{++} Cl^-, HCO_3^-, and, glucoce and some drugs. e.g. penicillin, chloromycetin, tetracycline.
- *Almost impermeable to:* Arsenic, gold, sulfur, urea, catecholamine, proteins and bile salts.

Development of BBB

BBB develops during early years of life. At this time cerebral capillaries are much more permeable than adulthood. So, in severally jaundiced bile pigments penetrate into nervous system and in the presence of asphyxia damage the basal ganglia. (Kernicterus).

Functions of BBB

- BBB protects the sensitivity of the cortical neurons to ionic changes with fluid bathing them. This helps

to maintain constancy of internal environment, i.e. concentration of K^+, Ca^{++}, Mg^+, H^+ and other ions in the CNS.
- Protects brain from endogenous and exogenous toxins in the blood.
- It prevents the escape of neurotransmitters into the general circulation.

Clinical Importance of BBB
- Selection of drugs during management of meningitis sulfa and erythromycin are most commonly given to treat meningitis which can easily cross BBB.
- BBB breakdown in the areas of irradiation infection or tumors. Therefore, localization of pathological area is possible with dyes or radioactive iodine labeled with albumin.
- BBB also breaks down by sudden marked increase in BP or by IV administration of hypertonic fluids.

These are four small areas in or near brainstem outside the BBB. Substances in the circulating blood can act to trigger changes in brain function without penetrating BBB.
1. Postpituitary and ventral part of median eminence of hypothalamus secrete oxytocin and vasopressin.
2. The area postrema chemoreceptor zone that produce vomiting in response to chemical changes in the plasma
3. *Organum vasculosum of the lamina terminalis. (OVLT supraoptic crest):* Site of specialized osmoreceptors controlling thirst by ADH.
4. *Subfornical organ:* Circulating angiotensin II acts here and area 3 to increase water intake.

Learning: Conditional Reflexes
Ability to alter behavior on the basis of experience is called learning.

Conditional reflexes are an important type of learning.
- Inborn (unconditional)
- Acquired (conditioned).

Unconditioned: This reflex is present in all normal individuals such as superficial, deep and organic reflexes. For example:
- *Superficial reflex:* Plantain, abdominal reflex
- *Deep reflex:* Knee and biceps jerk
- *Organic reflex:* Deglutition's defecation, sucking, grasping and micturition reflex.

The Acquired or Conditional Reflex
Features
- It is a reflex response to a stimulus that did not previously produce the response, however it can be developed by respectively pairing the stimulus with another stimulus that normally does produce the response.
- It therefore peculiar to the individual and refers to certain conditions that must be present if this class of response is to develop.
- It occurs due to formation of new functional connections in the CNS. For example, Pavlov's dog experiment.
- The introduction of food (unconditional stimulus) into the month sets up reflex salivation in a dog. This is unconditional reflex.
- Application of a neutral stimulus like ringing of a bell alone produce no salivation.
- Application of ringing of a bell just before the unconditional stimulus (taking of food) produces salivation. If this procedure is repeated several times, the ringing of a bell alone produces salvation. The initial neutral stimulus acquires fresh properties, i.e. new connections in the CNS can now by itself produce salivation.

The flow of saliva in response to ringing of the bell (conditional stimulus) is referred to as conditional reflex.

Bio Feedback
A large number of somatic, visceral and other neural changes can be made to

occur as conditioned reflex responses. The conditioning of visceral responses is calls bio feedback. The changes that can be produced include alteration in bowel movements, heart rate and blood pressure. Conditioned decrease in BP has been used for the treatment of hypertension.

THE BRAINSTEM

This connects the forebrain and spinal cord. It consists of three parts, the midbrain and two portions of the hindbrain, namely the pons and the medulla oblongata.

The **midbrain** (mesencephalon), which is the shortest segment of the brainstem, joins the forebrain above to the pons and cerebellum below. For descriptive purposes the midbrain is divided into right and left **cerebral peduncles**. The two ventral portions of these are distinctly separate from each other and are called the **crura cerebri**. A layer of gray matter, called the substantia nigra, separates them from the dorsal part of the midbrain which is continuous across the midline and is known as the **tegmentum** (L. covering). The latter is traversed by the **cerebral aqueduct**, which connects the third and fourth ventricles. The part of the tegmentum dorsal to the aqueduct is called the tectum (L. roof) and it presents four rounded elevations known as the colliculi. The upper pair, the **superior colliculi**, are visual reflex centers and the lower pair, the **inferior colliculi**, are auditory reflex centers. There are connections between the superior and inferior colliculi which are involved in the integration of visual and auditory function.

The **pons** (L. bridge) is that part of the brainstem which lies between the midbrain and the medulla oblongata. On each side it is connected to the cerebellum by a middle cerebellar peduncle. The dorsal surface of the pons forms the upper part of the floor of the fourth ventricle. The white matter of the pons consists of nerve fibers passing up and down the brainstem and its gray matter comprises the nuclei of some of the cranial nerves.

The **medulla oblongata** also consists of white and gray matter. About 3 cm (1.2 in) in length, it is continuous above with the pons and below, through the foramen magnum, with the spinal cord. The upper portion of the posterior surface of the medulla forms the lower part of the floor of the fourth ventricle. Two inferior cerebellar peduncles connect the pons with the cerebellum.

The anterior surface of the medulla is characterized by two longitudinal swellings, one on each side of the midline fissure, caused by the pyramidal tracts and known as the **pyramids**. They contain the fibers which descend from the cerebral cortex to the spinal cord, namely the corticospinal fibers. In the lower part of the medulla most of these fibers cross the median plane, in what is known as the **decussation of the pyramids**, and pass down the opposite side of the spinal cord in the lateral corticospinal tract.

The medulla oblongata contains collections of gray matter known as the **vital centers**, because death usually follows damage to them. They integrate the complex reflexes which regulate heart rate, blood pressure and ventilation of the lungs; hence the terms cardiac center, vasomotor center and 'respiratory' center.

Other autonomic reflex responses which are integrated in the medulla are swallowing, gagging, vomiting, coughing and sneezing.

RETICULAR FORMATION

Reticular formation is made up of group of cells that extend from the upper cervical segments of the spinal cord through the medulla pons and midbrain up to the thalamus (Fig. 17.19).

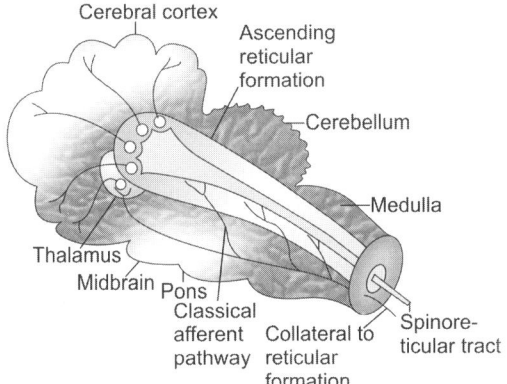

Fig. 17.19: Reticular formation

Nervous Connections

Afferent Connections

- Spinal cord via the spinoreticular tract and via collaterals from all ascending tracts.
- Brainstem afferents from the cranial nerves.
- *Tectum:* Tectumreticular conveying visual and auditory impulses.
- Cerebellum
- Basal ganglia
- Neocortex
- Limbic lobe including the amygdaloid, hippocampus.

Efferent Connections

- To the spinal cord
- To brainstem
- To the cerebellum
- To the red nucleus, substantia nigra and tectum in the midbrain.
- To the thalamus, subthalamic nuclei and hypothalamus.

Functions

- Reticular formation of the medulla contains respiratory and cardiovascular centers.
- The descending fibers exercise influence on
  - Motor control and stretch reflexes
  - Sensory modulation and autonomic ability.
- Ascending fibers controls the levels of cortical activity and electrical activity of the cortex.

Functions of the Descending Pathways

- Regulation of stretch reflexes and muscle tone
  - Stimulation of reticulospinal inhibitory pathway reduces muscle tone, reflex movements and the gamma efferent discharge.
  - Reticulospinal facilitatory pathway increase muscle tone and the gamma efferent discharge.
- Modulation of sensory input. Stimulation of the bulbar reticular formation inhibits transmission of the first synapse of the ascending sensory tracts.
- Influence on autonomic and visceral function.

Functions of the Ascending Reticular Fibers

Ascending reticular activating system which control the level of cortical activity wakefulness, alertness, sleep, etc.

■ CEREBELLUM

Cerebellum is divided into three parts:
1. Flocculonodular lobe
2. Spinocerebellum
3. Neoceribellum.

Histology

It has inner white matter and outer cortex.

Cortex has Three Layers

1. The molecular or plexiform layer
2. Purkinje cell layer
3. Inner granular layer.

There are two types of fibers reach cerebellar cortex from the white matter.
1. Mossy fibers
2. Fibers
3. Projection climbing fibers.

Cerebellar Nuclei

- Nucleus fastigial
- Nucleus globosus
- Nucleus emboliformis
- Nucleus dentatus.

Three types of fibers, white matter contains:
1. Commissural fibers
2. Association fibers
3. Projection fibers

Functions of the Cerebellum

- Role in the maintenance of body equilibrium
- Control of stretch reflexes and regulation
- Muscle tone and posture
- Coordination of voluntary movements.

Symptoms of Cerebellar Disease

- A synergia—finger nose test
- Adiadochokinesis
- Dysmetria
- Intention tremor
- Rebound phenomenon
- Decomposition of movement
- Asthenia—muscular weakness and slowness
- Hypotonia
- Pendular knee jerk
- Speech—slurring
- Wide-based staggering gait towards the side of lesion
- Vertigo
- Nystagmus
- Deviation of the eyes.

■ BASAL GANGLIA

- Corpus Striatum
- Substantia Nigra
- Subthalamic Nucleus.

Extra Pyramidal System (EPS)

Two important relay stations for the EPS.
1. Basali ganglia
2. Reticular formation.

Basal ganglia: A group of subcortical neurons in the forebrain. Accessory motor system. It control posture and movement.

In birds and lower animal basal ganglia (BG) is the highest motor area.

In human: Motor center take over the function called encephalization.

Physiological anatomy: Lateral to thalamus. No direct contact to spinal cord.

Importance: Role in background posture.

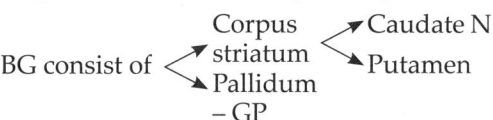

Lentiform nucleus → Putamen + GP.
Substantia Nigra and subthalamic N.
or
Body of Luys.
Red nucleus is also included in the BG.

Internal capsule passes bet. CN and putamen, these nuclei have got complex interconnections.

Major afferent part → Corpus striatum
Efferent part → Globes pallidus.

Afferent connections of striatum	Afferent connections of pallidum
- From different parts of cortex (Motor and Sensory)—Corpus striatum - From thalamus - Median Raphe of brainstem - From substantia nigra or pars compacta (other pars reticulata)	- From C. Stricutum - Sub thalamic N
Efferents from striatum	**Efferents**
- To thalamus - To substantia nigra - To globes pallidus - To pars reticulata	- Area lenticularis - Lenticular nucleus and join to form - Thalamic nucleus to enter the thalamus

Transmitters Released from BG

Corticostriate fiber release glutamate. It is excitatory.

Corpus Striatum ⟨ Cholinergic fibers (excitatory)
GABAergic fibers (inhibitory)

GABA project to globus pallidus.

Substantia nigra to striatum → Dopamine is the transmitter (inhibitory).

Median Raphe nucleus project to striatum. Transmitter is scrotonine.

Nigrostriatum → Dopamine (excitatory)

Caudate nucleus to substantia nigra → GABA (inhibitory)

Others:
- Norepinephrine
- Encephalin
- Substance P.

Functions of BG

- Role in muscle tone. → Inhibits muscle tone due to connect to
    Reticular formation, scandal part
    Disease of BG → increasing muscle tone.
    Modulation of muscle tone– connection to red neuclei and olivery nuclei.
- Role in voluntary motor activity →
    Globes pallidus subthalamic nucleus and brianstem nuclei control axial muscles.
- Role in background posture →
- Role in planning and programing, the motor activity, sequence of timing of movements. An abstract thought is connected to voluntary action.
- Along cerebral cortex and cerebellum initiate and regulate gross intentional movement.
- Along corticospinal tract BG control automatic execution of different complex pattern of motor activity.
- Important for control of associated movement that accompany normally subconcerned done, e.g. swinging of hand during walking along with laughing characteristic facial expression.
- **Reflex activity:** Because of connection of BG to red nucleus. It has role in postural reflexes.
- *Cognitive due to connection to cortex:* Dementia can occur. Thinking process may be lost.
- Role in infants and lower animal responsible for instinctive behavior like feeding.

Disorders in Basal Ganglia

Two basic types of diseases:

Dyskinesia ⟨ Akinesia, Bradykinesia
Hypokinesia
Hyperkinesia, e.g. choria (Hyperkinetic) Ballisum

- In muscle tone
- Rigidity, tremor

Causes
- Progressive degenerative disorders
- Genetic defects
- Vascular lesion.
    Metabolic disturbance result in loss or poverty of movement.
    Hence poverty of movement.

Release Phenomenon

Chorea: Degeneration of caudate nucleus characterized by rapid involuntary dancing movement. Normal movement cannot be changed.

Two types:
1. Sydenham's chorea
2. Huntington's chorea

Sydenham's chorea: Saint Vitus's dance seen in rheumatic fever.

Huntington's → Heriediraty autosomal dominant disorder. Gene is in short arm of chromosome. No : 4. Manifest in 3rd or 4th decade of life. It is due to degeneration of CN and Pulamen that secrete GABA. So no inhibition of GF and SN. Hence, spontaneous activity occurs continuously uncomfortable quick movements, dementia due to loss of ACh secreting neuron in BG and cortex. Hence, thinking process is also blocked.

Athetosis: Due to lesion of lentiform nucleus. Hence, interception of feedback circuit. The limbs, hand and fingers perform continuous, slow irregular, writhing movements. This is exaggerated by emotion when it also include jerky movement it is called Choreoathetosis.

Ballism: Degeneration of Subthalamic Nucleus. Here that is spont, violent or forceful involuntary movement involving muscle groups in limb, and trunk.

If half of body is affected due to involvement of Oppo. STN → Hemiballism.

Another disease → Parkinson's desease paralysis agitans → By James Parkinson.

Causes

- Idiopathic
- Atherosclerosis
- Late Complication of influenza
- Post-encephalitic Complication.

R_x with phenothiazine group of drug. In this condition dopamin deficiency and unbalanced action of ACh. Produce the manifestation.

- Rigidity
  - Isolated (Localized)
  - Widespread
- Tremor
- Akinesia
  - Increasing in tone both in agonists and antagonist due to activity of γ motor neurons. Mainly in the big muscle masses of the proximal part of limb. A plastic type of limb.
    - *Led pipe rigidity:* resistance throughout. Series of catches during passive movement
    - Cogwheel type rigidity.
  - Tremor
    - Seen in Rest. Resting tremor or involuntary tumor. It is

due to removal of inhibition of oscillation in feedback circuit.

Tremor disappears in voluntary activity due to motor signals of cortex over rides the signals.

L. Dopa → can cross BBB. Dopamine cannot cross BBB.

Carbidopa → Prevent peri. Decarboxilation of L. Dopa

- Stops in sleep
- Emotion ↑ the tremor.

- ***Akinesia (Bradykinesia):*** Slowness of movement. Progressive defect in initiating the movement.

It needs more concentration and effort even in the performance of simplest movement.

Weakness of muscles of speech.

Associated movements disappear: No swinging of movement of hand.

Peculiar gait: After initial slowness, slow short quick steps are taken, Bend forward while walking called festinating gait. When walking pushed forwards or backwards.

We cannot stop immediately move with a series of two steps.

- ***Disorders:***
  - Hypokinetic—Parkinsonism
  - Hyperkinetic—Chorea, Athetosis

Parkinsonism:
  Rigidity
  Mask like face
  Poverty of movement.

Tremor:
  Resting tremor
  Festinating gait
  Slurred speech.

Functions

- Planning and programing of voluntary movements
- Control of complex movements associated with corticospinal system
- Production of automatic associated movements

- Contributes to coordination of movements.

MOVEMENT AND THE MOTOR PATH (FIG. 17.20)

Movement may be voluntary or involuntary. Involuntary movement is considered in the section on reflex action.

Voluntary movement commences with an impulse sent out by the pyramidal cells of the motor cortex situated in front of the central sulcus (fissure of Rolando). The axons of these cells pass through the white matter of the brain and brainstem. In the medulla oblongata they cross to the opposite side and travel down in the lateral column of the spinal cord as the lateral corticospinal or pyramidal tract. At the appropriate level the fibers leave the pyramidal tract and end around the cells in the anterior horn of grey matter.

The pyramidal nerve cell in the motor cortex and its axon extending as far as the anterior horn cell is called the upper motor neuron.

The motor impulse is then relayed through the anterior horn cell whose fiber passes via the anterior nerve root to form, with the incoming fibers of the posterior root, the main nerve trunk. The motor nerve reaches its destination in muscle via the peripheral nerve.

The anterior horn cell and its axon passing in the peripheral nerve to the muscle is called lower motor neuron.

Because the upper motor neurons cross over in the medulla (at the decussation of the pyramids), one side of the brain controls the muscles on the opposite side of the body.

Autonomic Nervous System (ANS)

Innervations of all tissues other than skeletal muscle is by way of the ANS. It regulates the activity of smooth muscles, heart glands of GIT, sweat glands, adrenal gland and of certain endocrine organs. Its main aim is to maintain the optimal internal environment of the body. It governs the body functions which are carried out without conscious control or awakeness and is called vegetative or involuntary nervous system.

ANS is divided into sympathetic and parasympathetic division.

Sympathetic Division of ANS (Fig. 17.21)

- Also called thoracolumbar division sympathetic preganglionic fibers leave the spinal cord with the ventral roots of spinal nerves.
- Preganglionic fibers pass via the white rami communicantes to the par vertebral sympathetic ganglia which lies close to the spinal cord. These ganglia form the two chains of ganglia one on each side of the cord called sympathetic trunk. Most of the preganglionic fibers end on the cell bodies of the postganglionic neurons in the sympathetic chain.
- The sympathetic trunk extends the entire length of the spinal cord from the cervical levels high in the neck

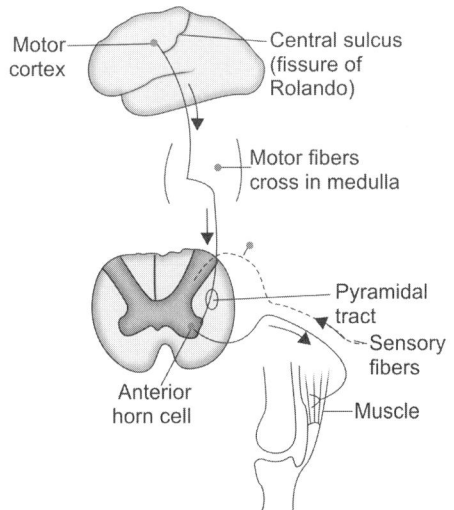

Fig. 17.20: The motor path

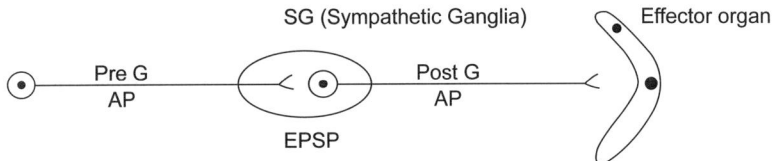

Pre G-Pregangionic neuron, Post G-Post ganglionic neuron, AP-action potential, EPSP–excitatory postsynaptic potential

Fig. 17.21: Sympathetic division of an effector cell

down to the sacral levels. The extra-ganglia in the sympathetic trunk receives preganglionic fibers from the thoracolumber regions because some of the preganglionic fibers turn to travel upward or downward for several segments before forming synapses with postganglionic neurons.

- The postganglionic fibers:
  - Pass to the viscera in the various sympathetic nerves.
  - Other re-enter the spinal nerves via grey rami communicantes from the chain ganglia and are distributed to the autonomic effectors in the area supplied by these spinal nerves, part, e.g. to the smooth muscles of blood vessels sweat gland and piloerector muscles of hair, etc.
- Some preganglionic fibers pass through the paravertebral ganglion chain (sympathetic trunk) and end on the postganglionic neurons located in the collateral ganglia (prevertebral ganglia) to the celiac, superior and inferior mesenteric ganglia. These ganglia lie far away from the spinal cord, closer to the innervated organs.
- In the sympathetic chain there is a ganglion for each segment except in the neck region, where several ganglia merge to form large ganglia, e.g. interior cervical ganglion fuse with T_1, ganglion to from stellate ganglion.
- Exceptions:
  - Myometrium of the returns is innervated by a special system of short adrenergic neurons, with cell bodies in the uterus and the preganglionic fibers to these post-ganglionic neurons go all the way to uterus.
  - In adrenal medulla, perganglionic fibers directly supply the adrenal medulla, where the postganglionic neurons have lost their axons and become specialized for secretion directly into the blood stream. It is really an endocrine gland whose secretion section is controlled by the sympathetic preganglionic nerve fibers.
- Sympathetic ganglia can act either as:
  - Automatic relay stations with practically no change in the information they transmit to the effector organ or
  - Important integrating centers capable of generating individualized responses. Sympathetic nervous system can act as a single unit.

Parasympathetic Division of ANS

- The nerve fibers of this division leave the CNS from the brain and the sacral portion of the spinal cord called craniosacral division. Here, the synapse between pre- and postganglionic neurons occur is the parasympathetic ganglia which are located within or near the effectors organs (except: Sphenopalatine and otic).
- ***Cranial outflow:*** It supplies the visceral structures in the lead via the

occulomotor facial (7th) nerves and glossopharyngeal (IX).
- *Sacral outflow:* It supplies the visceral via the pelvic branches of 2nd to 4th sacral spinal nerves.

Chemical Transmission at Autonomic Junctions

- In both sympathetic and parasympathetic division the major neurotransmitter released between pre- and postganglionic fibers in acetylcholin.
- In the parasympathetic division the main neurotransmitter between the postganglionic fibers and effectors cell is also acetylcholine.
- In the sympathetic division the main transmitter between the postganglionic fibers and effectors cells is non-epinephrine.
- On the basis of the chemical transmitter released the neurons in the entire nervous system are either cholinergic or adrenergic.
  - Cholinergic nerves:
    - All preganglionic autonomic (parasympathetic as well as sympathetic endings).
    - Postganglionic parasympathetic endings.
    - Postganglionic sympathetic endings which innervate sweat glands, skeletal muscle blood vessels, i.e. sympathetic vasodilator nerves.
    - Neuromuscular junction
    - Many parts of the brain (specially cerebral cortex, thalamus and forebrain nuclei).
    - Endings of some amacrine cells in the retina.
  - *Advantage:* Neurons which secrete NE or epinephrine at their nerve endings. For example:
    - Postganglioni sympathetic endings other than
      - Cerebral cortex
      - Hypothalamus
      - Cerebellum
      - Brainstem
      - Spinal cord
      - Adrenal medulla.
- Many of the drugs that stimulate or inhibit various components of the ANS effect receptors for ACh and NE. These are several types of receptors for each neurotransmitter.
  - ACh receptors on all autonomic (sympathetic and parasympathetic) postganglionic neuronal membranes respond to low doses of the drug nicotine and are called nicotine receptors.

■ SYNAPSE

The structure of synapse varies in the different parts of mammalian nervous system. The ends of the presynaptic fibers are generally enlarged to form terminal buttons (synaptic knobs). The axon or some other portion of one cell (the presynaptic cell terminates on the dendrites, soma, or axon of another neuron or a muscle or gland cell (the post synaptic cell).

Different Types of Synapses (Fig. 17.22)

Chemical Synapse

A synaptic cleft seperates the terminal of the presynaptic cell from the postsynaptic cell. An impulse in the presynaptic axon causes secretion of a chemical that diffuses across the synaptic cleft and binds to receptors on the surface of the postsynaptic cell. This triggers events that open or close channels in the membranes of postsynaptic cell.

Electrical Synapse

The membranes of the presynaptic and postsynaptic neurons come close together and gap junctions form between the cells. Like

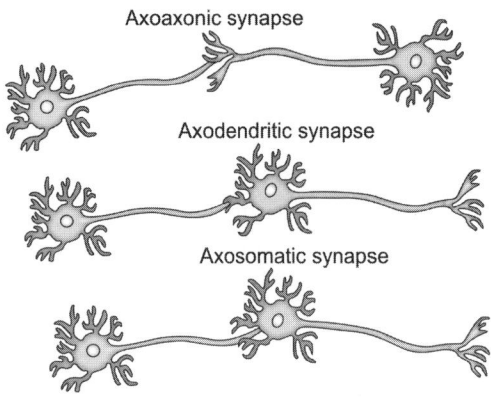

Fig. 17.22: Types of synapses

the intercellular junctions in other tissues, these junctions form low-resistance bridges through which ions pass with relative case.

Conjoint Synapses

The transmission is both electrical and chemical transmission is not a simple jumping of action potential from the presynaptic to synaptic cells. The effects of discharge can be excitatory or inhibitory.

When the postsynaptic cell is a neuron, the summation of all excitatory and inhibitory effects determines whether an action potential is generated.

In cerebral and cerebellar cortex endings, are located on dendrites and on dendritic spines (small knobs projecting from dendrites. Each neuron divides to form over 2000 synaptic endings and the human CNS has 10^{11} neurons and there are 2×10^{14} synapses. In cerebral cortex 98% of synapses are on dendrites and only 2% are on cell bodies. In the spinal cord the proportion of endings on dendrites is less. Eight thousands endings are on dendrites of a typical spinal neuron and about 2000 are on cell body.

The presynaptic terminal of a chemical synapse is separated from the postsynaptic structure by a synaptic cleft that is 20–40 nm wide. Across the synaptic cleft there are many neurotransmitter receptors in the postsynaptic membrane. In side the presynaptic terminal there are many mitochondria as well as many membrane enclosed vesicles, which contains neurotransmitters. The vesicles and the proteins in their walls are synthesized in the neuronal cell body and transported along the axon to the endings by fast axoplasmic transport. These vesicles are fused with the cell membrane and release transmitters through exocytosis and are then recovered by endocytosis to be refilled locally. In some instances they enter endosomes and budded off the endosome and refilled starting the cycle over again. The Ca^{++} that triggers exocytosis of transmitters enters the presynaptic neurons and transmitter release starts within 200/μs. Neurexins are proteins bound to the membranes of the postsynaptic neurons. The neurexins are not only hold synapse together but provide a mechanism for the production of synaptic specificity.

Vesicle budding, fusion and discharge of contents with subsequent retrieval of vesile membrane are fundamental processes occurring in most of cells. The exocytosis and endocytosis involves the v-SNARE protein synaptobrevin in the vesicle membrane locking with the t-SNARE protein syntaxin in the cell membrane.

Botulinum and Tetanus Toxins

Botulinum toxin C acts on syntaxin.
Tetanus toxin: Spastic paralysis by blocking presynaptic transmitter release in the CNS.

Botulinum: Clinical Application

Flaccid paralysis by blocking the release of ACh at N-M. Junction Botulinum toxin used in small doses into lower esophageal sphincter to release achalasia. Injection into facial muscles to remove wrinkles.

SYNAPTIC TRANSMISSION

The sequence of events that occur during synaptic transmission.
- The action potential (AP) travels along the presynaptic neuron and arrives at the synaptic knob.
- AP increases the permeability of the presynaptic membrane to Ca^{++} ions and causes Ca^{++} influx from extracellular fluid (ECF) into synaptic knob.
- Ca^{++} triggers the release of the chemical transmitter substance from synaptic vesicles. The transmitter traverses the synaptic cleft to reach the postsynaptic membrane.
- Transmitter combined with the receptor on the postsynaptic surface membrane alters the permeability of the membrane to ions.
- Na^+ influx produces a localized non-propagated depolarization immediately under the synaptic knob. This is excitatory postsynaptic potential (EPSP).
- When the EPSP reaches the threshold of about 10–15 mv it sets up a propagated AP in the postsynaptic neuron. During EPSP the excitability of neuron is increased and EPSP can be summated to produce AP. But AP cannot be summated. The all or none law is obeyed by AP. The initial segment is the Ist part of the neuron to fire and the nerve impulse passes down the axon. It also sweeps backwards toward the soma and dendrites. An impulse can be set up is the soma and dendrites only when EPSP reaches about 30 mv.

The resting membrane potential is – 65 milli-volt for the neuronal soma. Decreasing the voltage to a less negative value makes neuron more excitable. Increasing the voltage to a more negative value makes the neuron less excitable.

When an impulse reaches the presynaptic terminals an interval of at least 0.5 ms. The synaptic delay occur before a response is obtained in post-synaptic neuron.

Synaptic Transmission in CNS

- *The structural complexity:* Between the primary afferent neuron and the efferent neuron there are one or more internuncial neurons.
- An afferent fiber ending in a synapse may be either excitatory or inhibitory.
- There are several different chemical transmitters.

Synaptic transmission in autonomic ganglia: It is simple because:
- The structure is simple with preganglionic fiber synapsing with the post ganglionic neuron.
- If the incoming impulse is effective it is always excitatory. Inhibition does not occur at the ganglion. The inhibitory effects of autonomic nerve activity is only at the periphery at the post ganglionic nerve terminal.
- The chemical transmitter is always acetylcholine. The ACh is rapidly removed from the synapse so that repolarization may occur. Most of the ACh is hydrolyzed by acetyl cholinesterase, but some may be taken up by the presynaptic terminal by diffusion.

Excitatory transmission in central synapses is similar to that in autonomic ganglia, i.e. AP in the presynaptic neuron causes the release of a chemical transmitter at the synaptic knob. This sets up an EPSP in the postsynaptic neuron which causes a nerve impulse in the postsynaptic neuron. The transmitter released is different in different neurons.

Inhibition in Central Synapses

Inhibition is defined as the arrest or prevention of nerve action through a temporary operation of a process that involves no damage to the tissue. During inhibition there occurs an increase in the resting potential of the postsynaptic cell, i.e. hyperpolarization instead of depolarization. So, unlike in excitatory transmission, where there is a reduction in the resting potential, there is an increase in resting potential which prevents the discharge along the axon of the postsynaptic cell.

Different Types of Inhibitions

Direct or Postsynaptic Inhibition

This is mediated by an interneuron which connects an afferent neuron with the motor neuron. This is a short neuron with a thick axon and is called golgi bottle neuron. It acts by releasing the neurotransmitter glycine which causes a localized hyperpolarization called inhibitory postsynaptic potential (IPSP). The incoming AP via the interneuron releases the transmitter which acts on the postsynaptic surface and increases its permeability to Cl⁻ (Not Na⁺) ions and chloride. Conductance causing Cl⁻ influx into the cell. Hyperpolarization results due to larger number of negative ions inside the cell. This hyperpolarization reduces excitability as greater depolarization is necessary for reaching the firing level. The IPSP begins after 1 ms, peaks is about 2 ms and then declines (slow IPSP may also be produced by increase in K⁺ efflux or closing Na⁺ or Ca⁺⁺ channels.

Presynaptic Inhibition (Fig. 17.23)

This type of inhibition is medicated by an interneuron which ends on the synaptic knob of an excitatory neuron.

This is an axoaxonal synapse. The magnitude of action potential reaching the excitatory neuron is reduced by hyperpolarization due to increased Cl⁻ influx in the presynaptic neuron terminal. This reduces the Ca⁺⁺ entry into the ending in the excitatory neuron and decreases the

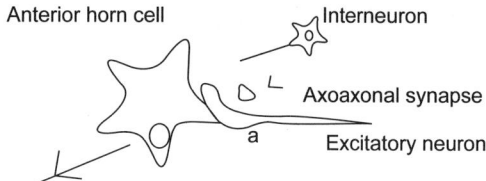

Fig. 17.23: Presynaptic inhibition

amount of transmitter substance released. Other contributing factors which contribute to inhibition are:
- Opening of K⁺ channels causing K⁺ efflux.
- A direct inhibitory effect on transmitter release
- The transmitter is GABA.

GABA is antagonized by the convulsant drug picrotoxin, but not strychnine.

Barbiturates increase presynaptic inhibition by facilitating Cl⁻ influx.

Recurrent Inhibition (Renshaw Cell Inhibition) (Fig. 17.24)

The spinal motor neuron gives off a collateral which connects with an inhibitory interneuron within the anterior horn. (The Renshaw cell and releases ACh). This in turn connects with the same motor neuron

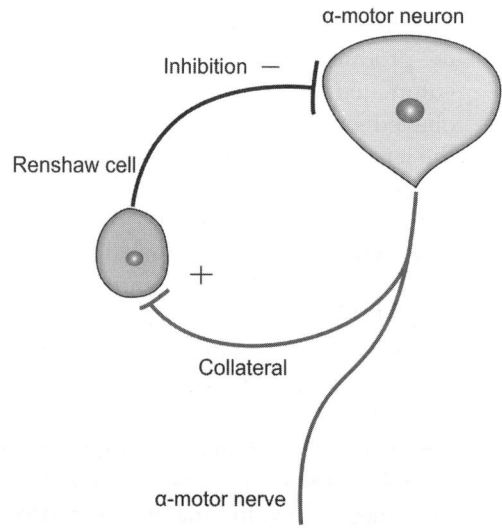

Fig. 17.24: Renshaw cell inhibition

and other motor neurons and inhibits its activity, and helps prevent excess discharge of impulse. Thus, the motor neuron regulates its own activity via an inhibitory collateral.

Similar mechanism is regulated in cerebral cortex and limbic system.

This is a negative feedback inhibition.

Pre and postsynaptic inhibitions are afferent inhibitions.

Properties of Synapses

- *One way conduction:* Conduction in a synapse is always in only one direction from the axon of the presynaptic neuron to the dendrites and cell body of the postsynaptic neuron and never in the opposite direction.
- *Delay in conduction:* A delay occurs in the synapse, which is at least 0.5 msec due to the events that occur in the synapse, i.e. time required for release of transmitter, diffusion across cleft, combining with receptor and set up AP.
- Susceptibility to fatigue, O_2 lack, anesthetics and some drugs. These factors tend to depress synaptic transmission. The synapse is more excitable in acidic and less excitable in an alkaline environment.
- Synapse permits modulation and grading of impulses modifications such as:
  - Summation
  - Facilitation
  - Inhibition
  - After discharge, etc.
    which occur at the synapses are necessary for appropriate neural activity in the body.

  For example, electrical synaptic transmission
  - Invertebrates
  - *Mammals:* Retinal neurons, or olfactory cells.

- *Synaptic Plasticity:* This refers to changes that occur in synaptic function offer repeated exposure to stimuli. The effects may be augmentation or inhibition of conduction and may be either of short duration or long duration. They are the effects of past experiences, and have a role in learning and memory. Some of the changes produced are:
- *Post-tetanic potentiation or facilitation:* If an excitatory presynaptic neuron is stimulated for a short-time by a tetanizing current then, after cessation of stimulus, the synapse become more excitable. This is a short-term effect lasting a few seconds or a minute. It is due to accumulation of Ca^{++} in the presynaptic endings caused by the tenanizing current. The Ca^{++} facilitates transmission by increasing transmitter release.
- *Long-term potentiation (LTP):* This is a prolonged increase in excitability tetanic stimulation of presynaptic neuron. It is more often due to Ca^{++}. Increase in the postsynaptic rather than presynaptic neurone. Glutamate released from presynaptic terminal facilitates entry of Ca^{++} and Na^+ into the postsynaptic neuron. It has also been suggested that retrograde signals sent from post to presynaptic neurons (probably via nitric oxide or arachidonate) favors long-term release of glutamate from presynaptic neurons. LTP is best seen in the hippocampus.
- *Habituation and sensitization:* Repeated application of a benign stimulus causes the response to disappear gradually. The synapse gets habituated to the stimulus. This habituation may be of short duration or may persist for long period depending upon the number of times the benign stimulus is repeated. This is brought about by gradual inactivation of Ca^{++}

channels and consequent reduction in intracellular Ca^{++}.

The benign, habituated stimulus is combined with a noxious stimulus (or a pleasurable stimulus) there is an increases in the postsynaptic response. This is called sensitization, as the synapse has become more sensitive to the stimulus. The sensitization is of short duration but can be prolonged, if the combination of the two stimuli are repeated. The transient sensitization is due to increased production of cAMP via Ca^{++} and adenylate cyclase. The long-term effects result from growth of presynaptic and postsynaptic neurons and increase in their connections, brought about by increased protein synthesis. Sensitization shows many features of short-term and long-term memory.

- *Inhibition or depression:* Short-term depression can occur with brief repetition of inhibitory afferent inputs.

Long-term depression (LTD) is the opposite of LTP described above. It occurs when afferent stimulation produces a partial depolarization not exceeding 20 mV. LTP is produced. When the depolarization is less than 20 mV, the Ca^{++} channels do not open up and Ca^{++} influx does not occur causing depressed conduction. This has been noted in hippocampus. It has also been found that afferent stimulation of climbing and parallel fibers in the cerebellum causes a long-term depression of conduction in the synapse between the parallel fibers and Purkinje cells. It is considered to be mediated by nitric oxide (NO) formed in the climbing fibers. It appears that NO causes LTD in the cerebellum whereas in the hippocampus it causes a potentiation. The mode of action of NO, and the details of the mechanism of LTP and LTD is uncertain.

The events that occur in the synapse constitute important physiological basis of learning and memory.

■ REFLEXES (FIG. 17.25)

The basic unit of integrated reflex activity is the reflex arc. These are consists of a sense organ, an afferent neuron, one or more synapses in the central integrating station or sympathetic ganglion, an efferent neuron and an effector. The afferent neurons enter via the dorsal roots or criminal nerves and have their cell bodies in the dorsal root ganglia or in the homologous ganglia on the cranial nerves. The principle that in the spinal cord the dorsal roots are sensory and the ventral roots are motor is known as Bell–Magendie law. The simplest reflex arc is one with a single synapse between the afferent and efferent neurons. Such arcs are monosynaptic and the reflexes occurring in them are monosynaptic reflexes. Reflex are in which one or more interneuron's are interposed between the afferent and efferent neurons are polysynaptic the no. of synapse varying between the afferent and efferent neurons are polysynaptic the number of synapses varying between two to many hundreds.

Monosynaptic Reflexes

When a skeletal muscle with an intact nerve supply is stretched it contracts. The response is called a stretch reflex. The stimulations that imitations the reflex is stretch of the muscle and the response is contraction of the muscle being stretched. The impulses originating in the spindle are conducted into CNS by fast sensory fibers that pass

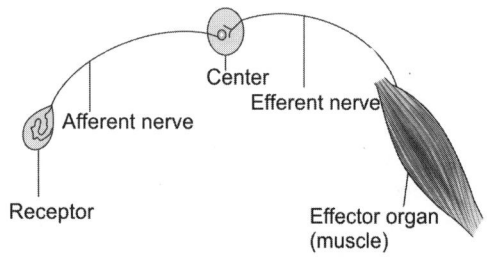

Fig. 17.25: Reflex action

directly to the motor neurons which supply the same muscle. The neurotransmitter at the central synapse is glutamate.

For example, tapping the patellar tendon elicits knee jerk a stretch reflex of the quadriceps muscle because the tap on the tendon stretches the muscle.

Structure of Muscle Spindles
Muscle Spindle (Fig. 17.26)

Each muscle spindle consists of up to about 10 muscle fibers enclosed in a connective tissue capsule. These are embryonal fibers and have less district striations than the rest of the fibers. They are called intrafusal fibers to distinguish it form the extrafused fibers, the regular contractile units of the muscle. The intrafusal fibers and in parallel with rest of the muscle fibers because the ends of the capsule of the spindle is attached to the tendons at either end of the muscle or to the sides of the extramural fibers. There are two types of intrafusal fibers in mammalian muscle spindle. The first type contains many nuclei in a dilated central area and is called a nuclear bag fiber.

There are two nuclear bag fiber per muscles spindle. Spindle fiber I and fiber II. The nuclear chain fiber is thinner and shorter and lack a definite bag. There are four or more of these fibers per spindle.

Their ends connect to the sides of the nuclear bag fibers. The ends of the intrafusal fibers are contractile whereas the central portions and not contractile.

There are two kinds of sensory ending in each spindle. The primary (annulospiral) ending are the terminations of rapidly conducting group Ia afferent fibers. One branch of the Ia fiber innervates nuclear beg fiber 1. Whereas another branch innervates nuclear bag fiber 2 and nuclear chain fibers. These sensory fibers wrap around the center of the nuclear bag and nuclear chain fibers. The secondary (flower spray) endings are terminations of Group II sensory fibers and as located nearer the ends of the intrafusal fibers but only on nuclear chain fibers.

The spindles have a motor nerve supply of their own. These nerves are 3–6 μm in diameter constitute about 30% of fibers in the ventral roots and belong to AR group. They go exclusively to the spindles. In addition larger β-motorneurons innervate both intrafusal and extrafusal fibers. γ efferents have plate endings on nuclear bag fiber and trail (network) endings on nuclear chain fibers.

The spindles produce two kinds of sensory nerves patterns dynamic and static and both γ and β motor axons produce two functional types of responses.

Central Connections of Afferent Fibers

Ia fibers from the primary endings and directly on motor neurons supplying the extrafusal fibers of the same muscle. The time between application of stimulus and response is the reaction time central delay is the time taken for the reflex activity to traverse the spiral cord. Minimal synaptic delay is 0.5 ms central delay for knee jerk is 0.6–0.9 ms. So far knee jerk only one synapse have been traversed.

Muscle spindle also make connections that cause muscle contractors via poly-

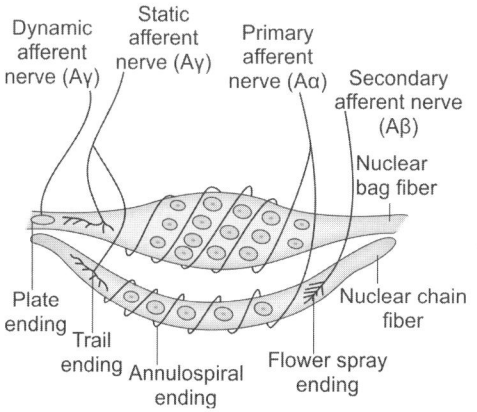

Fig. 17.26: Muscle spindle-structure

synaptic pathways and the afferents involved are those from the secondary ending.

Function of Muscle Spindles

When the muscle spindle is stretched its sensory ending are distorted and receptor potentials are generated. This set up AP in the sensory fibers at a frequency proportionate to the degree of stretching. The spindle is in parallel with the extrafusal fibers and when the muscle is passively stretched the spindles are also stretched. This initiate reflex contraction of the extrafusal fibers in the muscle. The spindle afferents characteristically stop firing when the muscle is made to contract by electrical stimulation of the nerve fibers to the extrafusal fibers because the muscle shortens while the spindle does not.

Thus spindle and its reflex connections constitute a feedback device that operates to maintain muscle length. If muscle is stretched, spindle discharge increase and reflex shortening is produced, whereas if the muscle is shortened without a change in γ efferent discharge, spindle discharge decreased and the muscle relaxes.

Primary endings on the nuclear bag fibers and nuclear chain fibers one both stimulated when the spindle is stretched, but the pattern of response differs. The nerves from the endings in the nuclear bag region show a dynamic response, i.e. they discharge most rapidly while the muscle is being stretched and less rapidly during sustained stretch. The nerves from the primary endings on the nuclear chain fibers show a static response, i.e. they discharge at an increased rate throughout the period. When a muscle is stretched. Thus, primary endings respond to both changes in length and changes in the rate of stretch. The response of the primary endings to the phasic as well as static events in the muscle is important because the prompt marked phasic response helps to dampen oscillations caused by conduction delays in the feedback loop regulating muscle length. There is normally a small oscillation in this feedback loop. This physiologic tremor has a frequency of approximately 10 Hz. However, the tremor will be worse if it were not for the sensitivity of the spindle to velocity of stretch.

Effects of Gamma Efferent Discharge

Stimulation of the γ efferent system does not lead directly to contraction of the muscle because the intrafusal fibers are not strong enough to cause shortening. But stimulation cause the contabile ends of the intrafusal fibers to shorten and therefore stretches the nuclear bag portion of the spindles deforming the annulospiral ending leading to reflex stimulation of the muscle. Thus, muscle can be made to contract by the stimulation of α motor neurons that innervate extrafusal fibers or the γ efferent neurons that initiate contraction by stretch reflex. When the rate of γ efferent discharge is increased the intrafusal fibers are shorter than the extrafusal fibers. Increased γ efferent discharge increases the sensitivity of the spindle to stretch. Increased γ efferent discharges along with the increased discharge of α motor neurons that initiate the two movements. Because of this α-γ linkage spindle shortens with the muscle and spindle discharge continue throughout the contraction.

There are dynamic and static γ and β efferent stimulation of dynamic efferent increases spindle sensitivity to the rate of change of stretch stimulation of static efferent increase spindle sensitivity to steady maintained stretch.

Control of Gamma Efferent Discharge

Anxiety causes increased 1st discharge, stimulation of the skin by noxious agents increase γ efferent discharge to ipsilateral

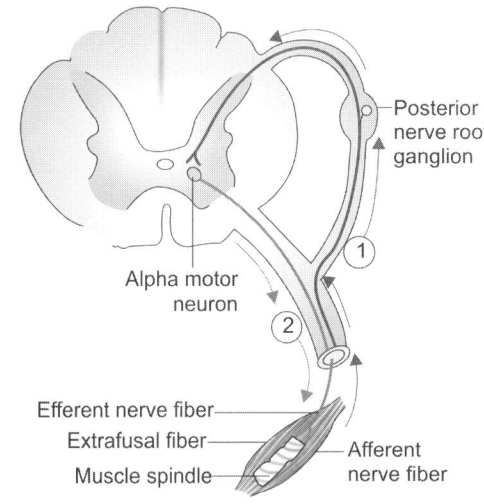

Fig. 17.27: Golgi tendon reflex

flexor muscle spindles decreasing that to extensors. Jendrassik's maneuver, i.e. trying to pull the hands a part when the flexed fingers are hooked together facilitates the knee jerk reflex. This is due to increased γ efferent discharge initiated by afferent impulses from the hand.

When a stretch reflex occurs the muscles that antagonize the action of the muscle involved relax. This is due to reciprocal innervations. Impulses in the Ia fibers from the muscle spindles of the protagonist muscle cause postsynaptic inhibition of motor neurons to the antagonists. The pathway mediating this effect is bisynaptic. A collateral from each Ia fiber passes in the spiral cord to an inhibitory interneuron (Golgi bottle neuron) that synapses directly on one of the motor neurons supplying the antagonist muscles (Fig. 17.27).

Inverse Stretch Reflex

Up to a point the harder a muscle is stretched the stronger is the reflex contraction. However when the tension becomes great enough contraction suddenly ceases and the muscle relax. This relaxation in response to a strong stretch is called the inheres stretch reflex or auto genic inhibition.

The receptor for the inverse stretch reflex is in the Golgi tendon organ. This organ consists of a net-like collection of knobby nerve endings among the fascicles of a tendon. The fibers from Golgi tendon organs makeup the Ib group of myelinated rapidly conducting sensing nerve fibers. Stimulation of these Ib fibers lead to the production of IPSP on the motor neurons that supply the muscle from which the fiber arises.

The Ib fibers end in the spinal cord inhibitory interneurons that in turn terminate directly on the motor neurons supplying antagonist to the muscle.

The Golgi tendon organ are in series with the muscle fibers and they are stimulated by both passive stretch and active contraction of the muscle. The thrash hold of the Golgi tendor organs are low. The degree of stimulation by passive stretch is not great because the more elastic muscle fibers take up much of the stretch and this is why it takes a strong stretch to produce relaxation. However, discharge is regularly produced by contraction of the muscle and the Golgi tendon organ function as a transducer in a feedback circuit that regulate muscle force in a fashion analogous to the spindle feedback circuit that regulator muscle length.

Muscle Tone

The resistance of a muscle to stretch is often referred to as its tone or tonus. If the motor nerve to a muscle is cut the muscle offers very little resistance and is said to be flaccid. A hypertonic (spastic) muscle is one in which the resistance to stretch is high because of hyperactive stretch reflexes. The muscles are generally hypotonic when the rate of referent discharge is low and hypertonic when it is high.

Clonus: This neurologic sign is the occurrence of regular rhythmic contractions of a muscle subjected to sudden maintained stretch. Ankle clonus is typical example. This is initiated by brisk maintained dorsiflexion of the foot and the response is rhythmic planter flexion at the ankle. The stretch reflex inverse stretch reflex sequence described above may contribute to this response.

Polysynaptic Reflex

The Withdrawal Reflex

Polysynaptic reflex paths branches in a complex fashion. The number of synapses in each of their branches is variable. The reverberating circuits that causes prolonged bombardment of the motor neurons from a single stimulus and consequently prolonged responses are responsible for withdrawal reflex.

When a strong stimulus is applied to a limb the response includes not only flexion and withdrawal of that limbs but also extension of the opposite limb. This crossed extensor response is a part of the withdrawal reflex. Flexor responses can be produced by stimulation of the skin or by stretch of the muscle. But strong flexor responses with withdrawal are initiated only by stimuli that are noxious are at least harmful to the animal. These stimuli and therefore called nociceptive stimuli.

General Properties of Reflects

- *Adequate stimulus:* A stimulus that triggers a reflex is generally very precise. The stimulus is called the adequate stimulus for the particular reflex. For example, scratch reflex in the dog. This spinal reflex is adequately stimulated by multiple linear touch estimate such as those produced by an insect crawling across the skin. The response is vigorous strutting of the area stimulated. It multiple touch stimuli are widely separated or not in a line, the adequate stimulus is not produced and no scratching occurs. Jumping of the fleas separate the touch stimuli so that an adequate stimulate for scratch reflex is not produced.

- *Final common path:* The motor neurons that supply the extrafusal fibers in skeletal muscles are the efferent side of many reflex arcs. All neural influences affecting muscular contraction ultimately funnel through them to the muscle and are called final common path. There are at least five inputs from the same spinal segment to a typical spinal motor neuron. In addition to this there are excitatory and inhibitory inputs relayed via interneurons from other levels of spinal cord and tracts from brain. All of these pathways coverage on and determine the activity in the final common paths.

- *Central excitatory and inhibitory state:* The spread up and down the spinal cord subliminal fringe effects from excitatory stimulation occurs in the spinal cord. Direct and presynaptic inhibitory effects can also be wide spread. The terms central excitatory state and central inhibitory state have been used to describe prolonged states in which excitatory influences over balances and vice versa.

- *Habituation and sensitization of reflex responses:* When a stimulus is benign and is repeated over and over the response gradually disappear. This is associated with decreased release of neurotransmitter from the presynaptic terminal because of deceased intracellular Ca^{++}. The decrease in the intracellular Ca^{++} is due to a gradual inactivation of Ca^{++} channels. Sensitization is the prolonged occurrence augmented postsynaptic responses after a stimulus to which an animal has become habituated is paired one or several times with a noxious stimulus.

- *A reflex action is capable to being summated:* Summation can either be temporal or spatial. Each inadequate stimulus produces a certain amount of excitatory state in the center which is incapable of sending a discharge through the motor nerve. But the state of excitation persists for a short while and can combine with the excitatory state produced by the next and succeeding stimuli. By such stimulation, the central excitatory state is raised to the threshold value and a discharge of impulse occurs. At an individual synapse the summation interval is equal to or smaller than the refractory period of the afferent nerve. So, temporal summation is only of academic value. Special summation is seen if subliminal stimuli are applied simultaneously to two afferent nerves which synapse on a common reflex center.
- *One way conduction:* Conduction is irreversible in a reflex arc. Centripetal in the afferent limbs and centrifugal in the efferent limb. This is called Bell-Magendie law.
- *Synaptic delay:* The cause of synaptic delay is due to the time taken to build up the threshold excitatory state. It is 5–6 milli sec.
- After discharge a single stimulus applied to the afferent nerve is followed by a series of impulses from the center. As a result of this repetitive discharge of impulse from the center, there is a time lag between the moment of cessation of the stimulus and termination of response from the effecter organ to center after cessation of the stimulus is called after discharge.
- *Recruitment:* The motor components of many reflexes gradually increase

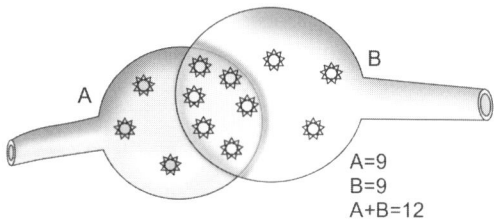

Fig. 17.28: Occlusion

to a maximum when a stimulus of unaltered intensity is merely prolonged due to progressive activation of a greater number of motor neurons.

- *Occlusion or Convergence (Fig. 17.28):* Simultaneous stimulation of two afferent nerves produces a response smaller than the maximum response expected by sum total of the effects of the two stimuli. Stimulation of 'a' produce response from four neurons, stimulation of 'b' produce response from four neurons. Simultaneous stimulation of a and b produce response from six neurons only. This is due to convergence of afferent nerves or central overlap of neurons.
- *Subliminal fringe:* The resulting response from concurrent stimulation of afferents will be greater when they are stimulated successively. So instead of a deficit, there is augmentation of muscular contraction. A stimulus applied to the afferent nerve builds up threshold excitatory state in certain neurons. Fringing on the effective excitatory field is a zone in which there are neurons, the excitatory state of which is raised, but is beneath the threshold level. This area is called subliminal fringe.
- *Fatigue:* A reflex action can easily be fatigued. Site of fatigue is synapse.
- *Susceptibility to O_2 lack:* Reflex conduction is susceptible to O_2 lack, shock and anesthesia due to presence of nerve cells in the conducting pathway.

- *Refractory period:* Nerve centers show absolute and relative refractory period and a phase of super normal excitability. The interval during which a reflex cannot be elicited by stimulating an afferent nerve is the absolute refractory period (ARP) and is followed by a relative refractory period (RRP).
- *Successive induction:* Two reflexes may exert their effects on each other if the 2nd immediately follows the 1st.
- *Rebound:* During elicitation of a reflex arc, if an inhibitory stimulus is applied to the afferent nerve augmentation of reflex response occurs when the inhibitory stimulus is withdrawn.
- *Irradiation:* When the strength of a stimulus over a receptive area is gradually increased the central excitatory state spreads to a greater number of neurons and additional groups of muscles take part in the reflex response. This is called irradiation.
- *Fractionation:* When a motor nerve is stimulated directly the response is greater than that produced by stimulation of the corresponding afferent nerve. It means fraction of the afferent impulses is lost in the CNS as the impulses make connections with other motor neurons supplying different groups of muscles.
- *Reciprocal innervation:* voluntary or reflex contraction of a muscle is accompanied by simultaneous relaxation of its antagonist.

RECEPTORS

Definition

Receptor is a specialized/modified sensory nerve ending which undergoes depolarization in response to a specific stimulus and in turn send information to CNS.

Functions: It acts as a transducer that converts various forms of energy in the environment into electric energy (i.e. action potential) in the neuron.

Different forms of energy converted by receptors include:
- Mechanical (touch pressure)
- Thermal (degrees of warmth)
- Electromagnetic (light)
- Chemical (smell, taste, O_2 and CO_2 content).

The receptor along with the surrounding non-neuronal cells is called a sense organ.

Classification of Receptors
According to Type of Stimulus

- *Mechanoreceptors:* Mechanical e.g. touch, pressure.
- *Chemoreceptors:* Chemical (change in chemical composition of the environment in which receptors are located), e.g. taste receptors and receptors of glucoreceptors.
- *Thermoreceptors:* Thermal (degree of warmth)
- *Nociceptors:* (Noxious stimuli → damaging), e.g. pain.
- *Photoreceptors:* (Electromagnetic) Light, e.g. rods and cones cells.

General or Anatomical Classification

- *Special Senses:* They are located at one (end in the head) very close to the CNS and are special for one type of sensory stimulation. Information from them is carried by cranial nerve, e.g. vision, hearing, smell, taste, rotational and linear acceleration.
- *Superficial or cutaneous senses:* Receptors are located in the skin. For example, touch, pain, pressure, the temperature sensation (cold/warmth).
- *Deep senses:* Carried by the muscular branches of the spinal or cranial nerves from deep body tissues. For example, sensation of joints, muscles and tendons.
- *Visceral senses:* These senses are concerned with perception of internal environment and carried by the automatic nervous system (ANS). For

example, pain from visceral structures, conc. of glucose in blood.

According to the Type of Receptors Sherrington's Classification

- *Tele receptors:* Sensory perception at a distance, e.g. hearing, vision, smell.
- *Exteroceptors:* Perception of external environment, e.g. touch, temperature, pain, pressure.
- *Interoceptors:* These receptors respond to changes within the body.
  - *Proprioceptors*, e.g.
    - Muscle spindle
    - Joint receptors
    - Golgi tendon organs
    - Vestibular receptors.
  - *Visceroceptors*, e.g. baroreceptor, osmoreceptors and glucoreceptors
  - *Chemoreceptors*.

Cutaneous Receptors

They respond to touch, pressure, pain and temperature. Most of the sensory nerve fibers in the skin are unmyelinated, few large myelinated sensory fibers.

Types of Receptors

Different types of receptors are also found that respond to touch, vibration and pressure. The temperature and pain sensations are conveyed by small myelinated (AS) fibers and unmyelinated 'C' fibers.

Mechanoreceptors

Concerned with sensations of touch and pressure. Consists of a lamellated connective tissue capsule which surrounds an unmyelinated axon. These include (Fig. 17.29):

- Merkel's discs and Meissner's corpuscles.
  - Concerned with perception of touch (tactile receptors).
  - They from expanded tips and encapsulated endings respectively on the sensory nerve terminals of A fibers (β and δ group)
  - They occur in groups in the cutaneous papillae with maximum

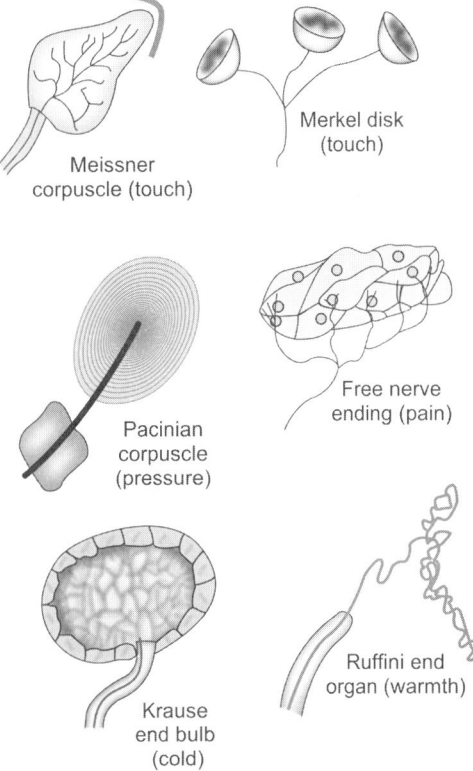

Fig. 17.29: Receptors structure

density in the skin of fingertips, lips, nipples, orifices of the body and around the base of hair follicles.
  - *They are rapidly adapting receptors:* This is why we do not feel our clothes once they are put.
- *Pacinian corpuscles:*
  - They are nerve terminals of Aβ fibers mainly and concerned with perception of pressure (or sustained touch)
  - They are large receptors, resemble an onion in shape and lamination.
  - They are found in large numbers in the skin subcutaneous tissues, mesentery and in the neighborhood of tendons and joints.
  - They respond to deformation caused by firm pressure and are quickly adapting. This is why we do not feel seat pressure when sitting.

- *Ruffini's end organs:*
  - They are encapsulated expanded endings myelinated Aδ or unmyelinated C group of fiber. They are concerned with perception of degree of warmth and also act as mechanoreceptors.
  - They are found in the dermis and supplied by large myelinated axons. They are slowly adapting receptors.
- *Krause's end bulbs:*
  - They are spherical mechanoreceptors and their afferent fibers belong to the Aδ group.
  - They occur in conjunctiva, papillae of the lips and tongue, in the skin of genitalia and in the sheath of nerves.
- *Naked nerve endings:*
  - These are the terminal branches of thin myelinated Aδ or unmyelinated C fibers.
  - They are concerned with perception of pain and injurious or (noxious) stimuli. They can also convey sensations of touch and temperature.

Thermoreceptors

They are terminal branches of thin myelinated. Aδ and unmyelinated 'C' fibers. These are found on the nose, nipples, anterior aspect of chest and on abdomen

There are 4–10 times more cold receptors than warm receptors. Differences:

Cold	Warm
Cold receptor fibers are mainly the thin myelinated Aδ fibers, 2.5 mm in diameter.	Warm receptor fibers are unmyelinated C. fibers 0.4–1.2 mm in diameter.
They fire with a steady discharge at any one tissue temperature between 10 and 35°C.	They fire with a fairly steady discharge at any one tissue temperature between 35 and 45°C.
The maximal frequency of the steady discharge is at a tissue temp of 25–30°C.	The maximal frequency of the steady discharge is at a tissue temperature of 38–43°C.

- Both the warm and cold receptors respond primarily to the temperature of the tissues which immediately surround them and not the gradient of temperature between the deep subcutaneous tissue and the surface. Therefore a stimulus of 35 °C will feel warm if the skin is at 30 °C and cool if the skin is at 40 °C. This explains why the cold metal objects feel colder than wooden objects of the same temperature because the metal conducts heat away from the skin more rapidly.
- If the tissue temp is raised beyond 45 °C the warm receptors do not respond but the cold receptors discharge at an increasing rate producing a mixed sensation of cold and pain. (Paradoxical cold fiber) Discharge is increased the 150 times. This is probably becauses above 45°C tissue damage occurs.

Pain Receptor

The pain receptors are called nociceptors. They are located at the ends of small C unmyelinated or myelinated Aδ afferent neurons.

Mechanism of Natural Excitation

(Generator Potential or Receptor Potential) It originates from the unmyelinated nerve endings and not from the capsule or from first node of Ranvier. It depolarizes the 1st node of Ranvier.

The magnitude of the generator potential is directly proportional to the intensity of stimulus.

Frequency of AP in a sensory nerve is also directly proportional to the magnitude of generator potential.

Frequency of AP – S.
Intensity of initiating stimulus – I
K, C – Contents.
According to Weber-Fechner law.
$S = K \log I + C$

Ionic basis of GP – Na^+ influx though unmyelinated terminal.

CHAPTER 18

The Sense Organs

The afferent or sensory nerves reaching the central nervous system have their beginnings (although these are sometimes referred to as nerve endings) in various peripheral structures such as the skin, muscles, joints and special organs such as the eye and ear.

Sensations are the conscious results of processes taking place in the brain following the arrival of impulses derived from the sensory nerves.

The structures concerned in the production of a sensation are:
- An end organ or sensory receptor, situated in the periphery to the terminations of the sensory nerves;
- The afferent nerve fibers in the peripheral nerve and spinal cord;
- The thalamus, which is a cell station relaying sensations to the cerebral cortex;
- The sensory reception areas in the brain which are connected with various psychic areas where the impulse is interpreted and may be stored as memory.

It is important to remember that, although the brain receives and appreciates the sensation, it projects it back to the site or end organ at which it was received and it is actually felt by the individual as being in the peripheral region

The end-organs for each sense are specially adapted in structure to respond to the particular stimulus for that sense. Thus, waves of light are described as being the *'adequate stimulus'* for the nerve endings in the retina of the eye. Sound waves are the adequate stimulus for the endings of the cochlear nerve in the ear, and have no effect on the eye, nose or skin.

Sensation may be classified in various ways. In describing the nervous system it was sufficient to make the simple subdivisions of (a) special senses, i.e. sight, hearing, taste and smell, (b) general sensations, including all the others. Numerous other classifications of the senses have been made, however, and the reader may encounter some of the terms used to describe the various receptors. These include:
- Telereceptors or 'distance receivers' (e.g. for sound and smell);
- Exteroceptors, concerned with elements of the immediate external environment (e.g. for taste);
- Interoceptors, concerned with the internal environment (e.g. hunger and thirst);
- Proprioceptors, concerned with the position of the body or its parts in space (e.g. receptors in the joints and semi-circular canals).

■ SENSATION IN THE SKIN

The sensations from the skin are those of pain, temperature (hot and cold) and light touch. Situated in the skin is a mosaic of minute sensory areas, which correspond with the nerve endings. Specific endings are present for each of the varieties of sensation. Further, the endings for one type of sensation may be more numerous in one area of skin than in another.

■ THE SENSE OF SMELL

The mechanism of smell is dependent on:
- The receptor or end-organ, i.e. the endings of the 1st cranial or olfactory nerve in the mucous membrane of the upper part of the nasal cavity;
- The olfactory bulb and tract which convey the impulses to the brain;
- The limbic lobe situated in the medial surface of the cerebral hemisphere.

The appropriate or adequate stimulus for the sense of smell must be either in the form of gas or minute particles which are soluble in the secretions of the nasal mucous membrane. These gases or particles are conveyed to the nasal cavities by the air and the quantity reaching the upeear part of the nasal cavities may be increased by the process of 'sniffing.'

Smell is a sense characterized by its extreme delicacy and the ease with which it becomes fatigued. This is shown by the fact that persons sitting in a closed room for some time may cease to be aware of an odor which is very apparent to someone entering from the fresh air.

The sense of smell is also diminished by inflammation or excess of secretion in the nasal mucous membrane which occurs in the common cold.

Odors are most simply classified into pleasant and unpleasant. It is important to remember that the sense of smell is closely associated with the sense of taste and that the majority of flavors are actually appreciated by the olfactory organ. This is clearly shown by the loss or change of taste which accompanies a severe head cold. Loss of the sense of smell is called anosmia.

■ THE SENSE OF TASTE

The true sense of taste is localized in the tongue. There are four basic tastes, namely

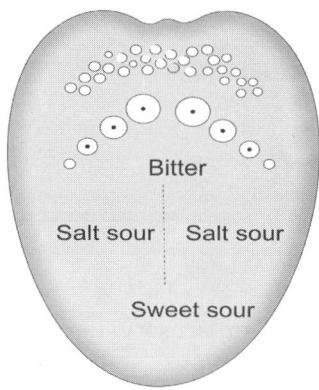

Fig. 18.1: Parts of the tongue in which the various sensations of taste are appreciated

bitter, sweet, sour and salt (Fig. 18.1). These only are appreciated by the tongue. All other flavors are appreciated by the sense of smell as already stated.

The tongue is a very mobile organ, consisting of muscles some of which arise from the hyoid bone and the lower jaw. It is covered by mucous membrane. The roughness of its upper surface is due to numerous minute elevations called papillae. The end-organs for the sense of taste are called taste buds, which are situated most densely at the tip, sides and base of the tongue. They consist of collections of receptor cells and supporting cells together with the sensory nerve endings which are wrapped intimately around the receptor cells. The taste bud has a pore which opens on to the epithelial surface of the tongue. A number of hairs projects from each receptor cell into this taste pore. The nerve fibers conveying impulses to the brain from the taste buds of the anterior two-thirds of the tongue travel in the facial nerves while those from the posterior third of the tongue travel in the gloss opharyngeal nerves (Fig. 18.2). The sensations of pain and touch are conveyed by the trigeminal nerves. There is no area of the cerebral cortex concerned solely with taste. This sense is represented in that portion of the postcentral gyrus which subserves cutaneous sensation from

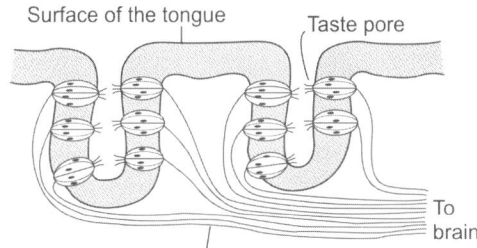

Fig. 18.2: Taste buds and their nerve supply. NB only one nerve fiber is shown for each taste bud

the face. The motor nerve to the tongue is the XIIth cranial or hypoglossal nerve.

The functions of the tongue are:
- *Motor:*
  - Mastication and the act of swallowing
  - Speech
- *Sensory:*
  - Taste (bitter, sweet, sour and salt)
  - Touch

As in the case of smell, in order that substances may have taste, they must be soluble in the watery secretion of the mouth and salivary glands.

■ THE SENSE OF HEARING (FIGS 18.3 AND 18.4)

The auditory apparatus consists of (1) the external ear, (2) the middle ear, (3) the cochlea of the internal ear, (4) the cochlear nerve and acoustic areas in the temporal lobe of the brain.

The External Ear

This consists of:
- The auricle or pinna
- The external acoustic meatus
  - Cartilaginous portion
  - Bony portion

The auricle or pinna (Fig. 18.5) is attached to the side of the head about midway between the forehead and the occiput. It has a deep shell-like cavity called the concha. Beneath the skin, the auricle is composed of yellow elastic cartilage, apart from the lobule or ear lobe, which is soft because it is composed of fibrous and adipose tissues.

The function of the auricle is to collect sound waves and conduct them to the

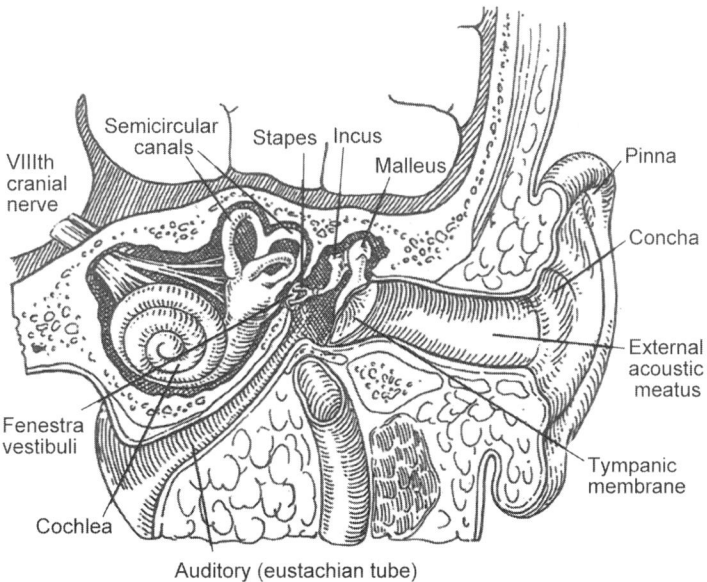

Fig. 18.3: The structure of the ear

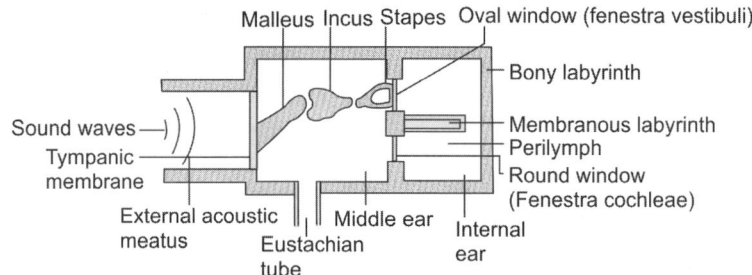

Fig. 18.4: Anatomy of the auditory apparatus

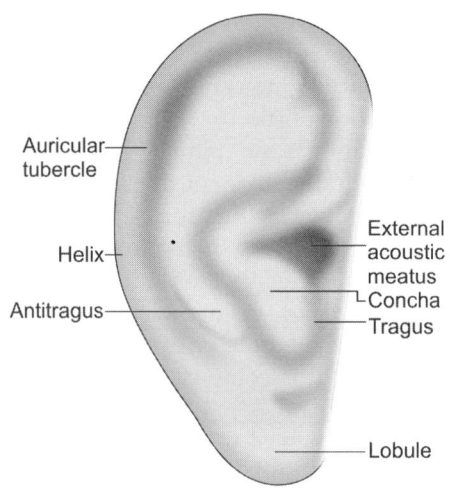

Fig. 18.5: The pinna

external acoustic meatus. This function is more marked in many animals than in man and in consequence their auricles are relatively larger and more mobile. Although there are several small muscles attached to the human ear, in only a few people is a limited amount of movement possible.

The external acoustic meatus leads from the pinna to the tympanic membrane or ear-drum. It is a tubular passage about 2.5 cm (1 in) long. Its course is not straight but shows a slight double or S-shaped bend, being directed at first medially, forwards, and slightly upwards, and then medially and slightly backwards. In order to bring the meatus into a straight line the pinna should be lifted upwards and backwards in adults, but in children owing to a slightly different course the pinna should be pulled downwards and backwards. This is of importance when it is desired to examine the tympanic membrane.

Structurally, the external acoustic meatus consists of two parts: The outer *cartilaginous* portion (lateral one-third) which is continuous with the cartilage of the pinna; and the inner *bony* part in the temporal bone.

The meatus is lined by skin which is continuous with that covering the pinna, but is characterized by special glands, the ceruminous glands, which secrete a yellow greasy substance called crewmen or wax. They are modified sweat glands and their secretion helps to prevent the entry into the meatus of foreign bodies, especially insects. A few hairs are present which also assist in this function. If there is excessive production or retention of wax, the meatus may become blocked and require syringing to dislodge and wash out the wax and restore normal hearing.

The Middle Ear

The middle ear or tympanic cavity is a small irregular cavity situated in the petrous portion of the temporal bone. It contains a chain of small bones or ossicles by which the sound waves are transmitted from the tympanic membrane to the internal ear. Roughly speaking, it is a narrow oblong box having anterior, posterior, medial and lateral walls with a roof and a floor.

Its walls are both bony and membranous in structure. The outer or lateral wall is formed by the tympanic membrane. Its medial wall, though mainly consisting of bone, has two openings which are covered by membrane, namely the fenestra vestibuli (f. ovalis) or oval window of the vestibule above, and the fenestra cochleae (f. rotunda) or round window of the cochlea below.

In addition to these membranous defects in its outer and inner walls, both the anterior and posterior walls have openings. Entering the middle ear in its anterior wall is the outer or lateral end of the auditory (Eustachian) tube which communicates with the nasopharynx. Posteriorly the middle ear communicates with the mastoid tantrum and the mastoid air cells which occupy the mastoid process of the temporal bone.

The whole of the cavity of the middle ear is lined by mucous membrane which, therefore, forms the inner lining of the tympanic membrane and is continuous with the mucous lining of the Eustachian tube and with that of the mastoid antrum and cells.

The auditory tube connects the nasopharynx with the middle ear and is less than 4 cm (1½ in) in length. There is thus a connection between the middle ear and the outer air so that the pressure of air on each side of the tympanic membrane is equalized.

The pharyngeal opening of the Eustachian tube is normally closed by the approximation of its walls, but is opened by the action of muscles in swallowing and yawning. In catarrhal conditions of the nasopharynx, as in a severe head cold, the opening of the tube may be defective and a degree of deafness is not uncommon from this cause.

The effect of atmospheric pressure is also demonstrated in going to the top of a high hill rapidly in a car, or going up in an aeroplane. Until air escapes from the middle ear by the Eustachian tube the atmospheric pressure on the outer surface of the tympanic membrane, being diminished by reason of the height, is less than the pressure on its inner side. An uncomfortable sensation in the ear and slight temporary deafness is produced but disappears with the adjustment of pressure, which is often accompanied by clicking sounds and is aided by the act of swallowing.

The main function of the Eustachian tube is, therefore, to equalize the pressure in the middle ear with the atmospheric pressure outside.

The Ossicles (Fig. 18.6)

The ossicles or small bones of the middle ear are three in number, the malleus, the incus and stapes. They stretch from the tympanic membrane to the fenestra vestibuli or oval window of the vestibule.

The malleus or hammer bone consists of a head which articulates with the incus and a handle which is attached to the tympanic membrane. The incus or anvil is the middle of the three bones and consists of a body

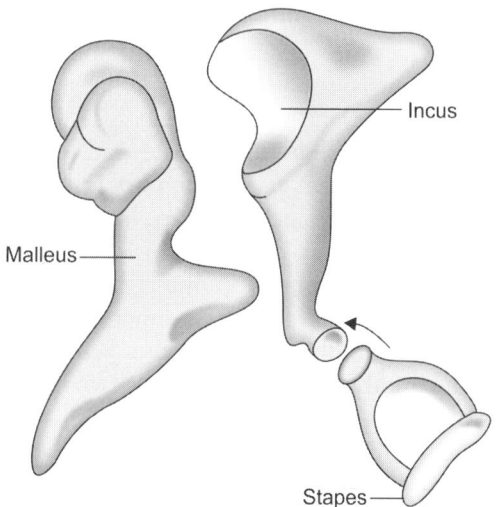

Fig. 18.6: The bones of the middle ear

and two short legs, one of which articulates with the roof of the middle ear, the other with the stapes. The stapes or stirrup bone is the smallest of the three. Its head articulates with the incus while its base or foot-plate is attached to the membrane covering the fenestra vestibuli.

These three bones act as a series of levers transmitting the movements or vibrations of the tympanic membrane, caused by sound waves impinging upon it, to the membrane covering the fenestra vestibuli. It will be seen later that from the fenestra vestibuli the vibrations are passed onto the internal ear.

The movements of the ossicles are controlled to some extent by two tiny muscles, the tensor tympani inserted into the handle of the malleus, and the stapedius muscle inserted into the neck of the stapes. These muscles act as dampers to prevent excessive movement of the ossicles in response to loud noise. They also attenuate low frequency components of sound so that weaker high frequency components are not masked. This improves the perception of sounds obscured by background noise.

The Tympanic Membrane

The tympanic membrane (tympanum, or ear-drum) is situated at the deepest part of the external acoustic meatus which it separates from the middle ear. It lies obliquely so that its upper part is nearer the exterior than its lower part. In structure, its outer surface consists of epithelium continuous with the skin lining the external acoustic meatus, while its inner lining is mucous membrane continuous with that of the middle ear. Between these two layers is a small amount of fibrous tissue. Firmly attached to its inner wall (and passing downwards and slightly backwards from its upper edge to a point just below and behind its center) is the handle of the malleus.

It appears as an almost circular structure tightly stretched between the walls of the bony meatus except for a small area in its upper part (known as the flaccid membrane of Shrapnell). It is easily seen with the aid of an auriscope and it appears red and sometimes bulging in patients with acute middle ear infections (acute otitis media). In some cases, it perforates and pus escapes through the perforation into the external acoustic meatus.

The Internal Ear (Fig. 18.7)

The internal ear or labyrinth consists of a series of irregular cavities situated in the petrous portion of the temporal bone. These cavities constitute the bony or osseous labyrinth. Within these bony walls is a membranous structure, which more or less follows the shape of the bony labyrinth and is called the membranous labyrinth.

Between the bony walls and the membranous part of the labyrinth is a clear fluid called **perilymph,** while the membranous labyrinth itself is a sac filled with a similar fluid called the **endolymph.**

The osseous labyrinth consists of the following parts:
- The vestibule or entrance which communicates with
- The cochlea (little shell) or organ of hearing in front and
- The semi-circular canals behind. These are concerned with equilibrium and the sense of position.

The vestibule is closely connected to the middle ear, from which it is separated by the membrane covering the fenestra vestibuli (the oval window of the vestibule) with the attached foot-plate of the stapes.

The cochlea or anterior portion of the labyrinth contains the organ of hearing. In some respects, it resembles the shell of a small snail and, in section, looks something like a spiral staircase with a central bony structure called the modiolus

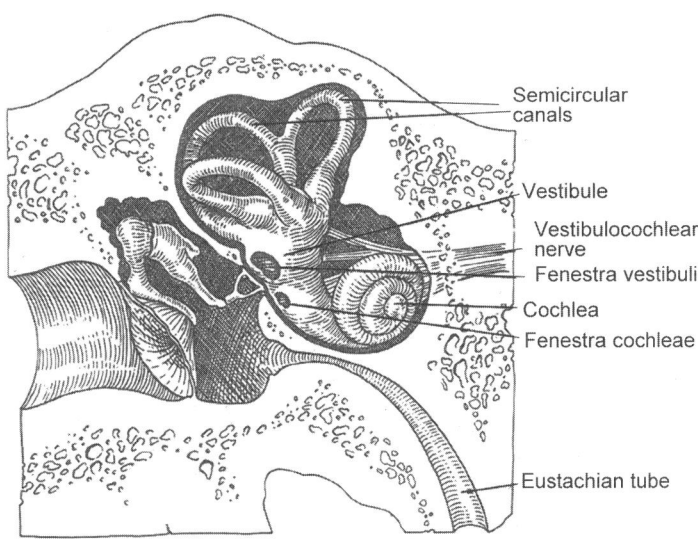

Fig. 18.7: Osseous labyrinth

from which ridges project to the outer wall. The membranous portion of the cochlea, called the duct of the cochlea, is contained within these bony walls and in it is the most important part of the structure, the organ of Corti, which is the true end-organ of hearing.

The organ of Corti, is a spiral structure contained in the membranous labyrinth, which follows the shape of the cochlea and is bathed in endolymph. It consists of special epithelial cells, called rods of Corti, on either side of which are layers of cells (hair cells) having hair-like processes on their free surface rather like ciliated epithelium in appearance. It is around these cells that the fibers of the cochlear or auditory division of the VIIIth cranial nerve commence. The nerve cell bodies are located in the spiral ganglion within the modulus.

Mechanism of Hearing

Sound is due to waves or vibrations in the air and has three main qualities.
1. Pitch, which depends on the frequency of the vibrations. The more rapid the frequency the higher the pitch of the note produced.
2. Intensity or loudness, which depends on the amplitude of the vibrations.
3. The quality, which is due to the combination of various vibrations. These may blend to produce harmony or music, or fail to unite giving rise to a discord or noise.

Sound waves in the air are collected by the pinna and directed along the external acoustic meatus to the tympanic membrane which they cause to vibrate. These vibrations are transmitted across the middle ear by the movements of the malleus, incus and stapes to the membrane covering the fenestra vestibuli. The inner surface of this membrane is in contact with the perilymph in the vestibule which picks up the vibrations and, in turn, passes them onto the end lymph by means of which they reach the organ of Corti.

The stimulus thus reaching the organ of Corti is conveyed by the cochlear portion of the VIIIth cranial or vestibulocochlear nerve, which leaves the petrous portion of the temporal bone by a foramen (the internal acoustic meatus) to reach the brainstem. The fibers are then carried to the acoustic areas of the brain situated in the temporal lobe of the opposite side.

Summary of the Sense of Hearing

Sound waves → pinna → external acoustic meatus → tympanic membrane → malleus → incus → stapes → fenestra vestibuli → vestibule → cochlea (perilymph → endolymph) → organ of Corti → VIIIth cranial nerve → temporal lobe of brain (of opposite side).

Hearing loss may be classified as conductive or sensorineural. In conductive deafness, sound is not transmitted to the cochlea because of a lesion affecting the external acoustic meatus or middle ear.

Sensorineural deafness may be of sensory type, resulting from a lesion within the cochlea, or neural due to a lesion affecting the VIIIth cranial nerve or any part of the pathway from the cochlea to the temporal lobe.

Audiometry, with an electronic audiometer, is used to measure hearing acuity and to localize the site of a lesion causing loss of hearing.

The Semicircular Canals

These are three canals situated in the posterior part of the bony labyrinth and set at right angles to each other. They are anterior (superior), posterior and lateral canals. Within the bony walls are the membranous canals or ducts surrounded by perilymph and containing endolymph. Each canal is enlarged at one end into an ampulla where the special nerve fibers end around cells which have fine hair-like processes projecting from them. Movements of the head and alteration in its position cause movement of the endolymph in the semicircular canals. This movement of fluid acts as a stimulus to the nerve endings in the ampullae and the impulses are conveyed to the brain (both the cerebrum and cerebellum) by the vestibular division of the VIIIth cranial nerve. Lesions of this portion of the nerve cause vertigo (dizziness).

The ampullae of the semicircular ducts open into a sac called the utricle. A thickened part of the floor and lateral wall of this sac is known as the macula or otolithic organ. It contains hair cells innervated by fibers which join those from the ampullae to form the vestibular nerve. Surmounting the hair cells and their supporting cells is a membrane containing the otoliths ('ear dust') which are crystals of calcium carbonate.

The semicircular canals provide the brain with information on head movement. The otolith organs give information on the position of the head.

It will be remembered that the sense of equilibrium and position is also dependent on impulses received from the eyes and from the muscles and joints which contain receptor organs described as proprioceptive.

■ THE SENSE OF SIGHT—VISION

The eye or organ of sight is situated in the orbital cavity of the skull and is well protected by its bony walls except on its anterior aspect.

In addition to the essential organs of the visual apparatus, namely, the eyeball, the optic nerve and the visual centers in the brain, there are certain accessory organs which are necessary for the protection and functioning of the eye. These include: (1) the eyelids; (2) the conjunctiva; (3) the lacrimal apparatus; and (4) the muscles of the eye.

Accessory Organs of the Eye

The Eyelids

These are two movable folds, upper and lower, which form the anterior protection for the eye. The upper is the larger and more mobile of the two and is provided with a muscle which elevates it. The eyelids are covered externally with skin and their inner lining consists of mucous membrane, the conjunctiva. Between these layers is a dense plate of fibrous tissue called the tarsus. Into the tarsal plate of the upper lid the muscle which raises it is inserted (levator palpebrae superioris). Surrounding both lids is a circular sphincter muscle (orbicularis oculi) which closes them and, when fully contracted, 'screws them up.'

The space between the two lids is the palpebral fissure. Its lateral angle is also called the lateral canthus and its medial angle the medial canthus.

The eyelids blink every few seconds. This movement keeps the front of the eye free from dust and helps to move the tears across the conjunctival sac. In addition to protecting the eyes from the entrance of foreign bodies, the eyelids also prevent the entry of excessive light.

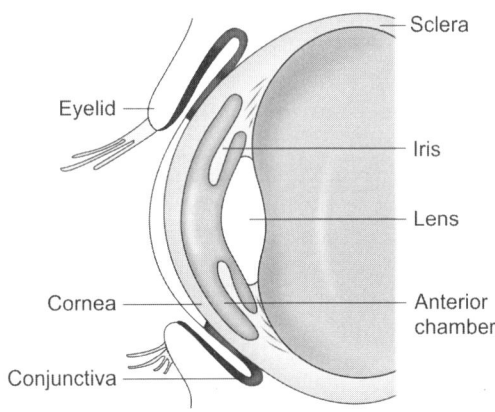

Fig. 18.8: The conjunctiva

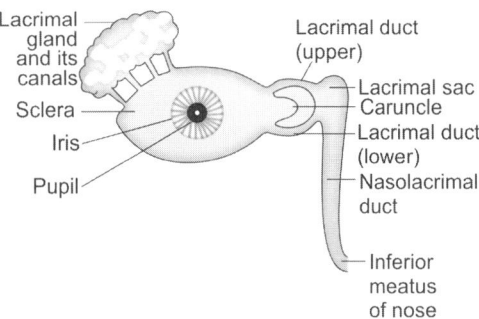

Fig. 18.9: The lacrimal apparatus

The Conjunctiva (Fig. 18.8)

This is a delicate mucous membrane which lines the inner surface of the eyelids and is then reflected onto the outer surface of the eyeball. The space between the two layers is called the conjunctival sac.

The Lacrimal Apparatus (Fig. 18.9)

This is concerned with the formation of tears and consists of the following structures: (1) the lacrimal glands; (2) the lacrimal canaliculi; and (3) the lacrimal sac and nasolacrimal duct.

The Lacrimal Glands

These are situated in the orbital cavity immediately above the lateral angle of the eye. Each is almond-shaped and lies in a depression in the orbital plate of the frontal bone. A number of small canals leads from it to the lateral angle of the conjunctival sac.

The Lacrimal Canaliculi

If the medial end of each eyelid is carefully examined the orifice of a minute duct can be seen. From this opening the lacrimal canaliculus passes inwards to enter the lacrimal sac.

The Lacrimal Sac and Nasolacrimal Duct

The lacrimal sac may be regarded as the upper expanded portion of the nasolacrimal duct which passes downwards inside the bony wall of the nasal cavity to open into the inferior meatus of the nose.

Tears are a slightly alkaline watery fluid containing a small amount of sodium chloride which give them a salty taste. Normally, there is a constant secretion from the lacrimal glands just sufficient to keep the interior of the conjunctival sac moist and free from dust. By the frequent movement of the eyelids the tears pass across the front of the eye from the lateral to the medial side, where they pass through the openings of the lacrimal canaliculi and are drained into the nose by the nasolacrimal duct to mix with the secretions of the nose.

Having observed the minute openings of the lacrimal canaliculi at the medial corners of the eyelids it is clear that any excess of tears must overflow from the conjunctival sac and run down the cheek. Some of the excess, however, does pass down the ducts and accounts for the excess of watery secretion from the nose after crying which, if severe, requires the use of a handkerchief, although in these circumstances its place is frequently taken by 'sniffing.'

The secretion of tears is increased by the presence of foreign bodies and inflammation caused by bacteria or irritating vapors. Irritation of the nasal mucous membrane and very bright light provoke reflex lacrimation, while emotional states and pain also result in the flowing of tears.

The functions of the tears may be summarized as:
- Keeping the eyes moist, thereby allowing free movement of the lids;
- Removal of dust and foreign bodies, including bacteria;
- Acting as a mild antiseptic;
- Expression of emotion or pain.

The Extraocular Muscles of the Eye (Figs 18.10 and 18.11)

Each eyeball is moved by muscles which arise from the posterior wall of the bony orbit close to the entrance of the optic nerve and are inserted into the outer fibrous coat (sclera) of the eye. There are four straight and two oblique muscles in addition to the muscle elevating the upper lid (levator palpebrae superioris).

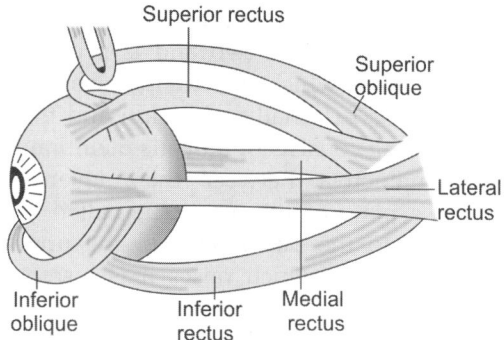

Fig. 18.10: Eye muscles. Left orbit (lateral aspect)

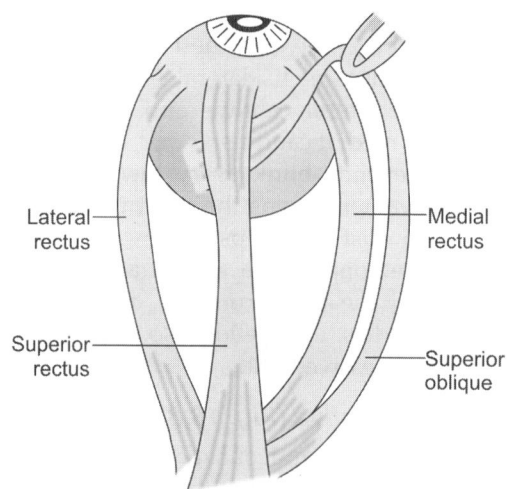

Fig. 18.11: Eye muscles. Left orbit (from above)

The straight muscles are the superior rectus, inferior rectus, medial rectus and lateral rectus. Their position in relation to the eyeball is indicated by their names. The action of these muscles is not too difficult to follow if two facts are remembered. (1) If one eye alone is considered, contraction of the superior rectus turning the eye upwards will be associated with relaxation of the inferior rectus, and vice versa. The medial and lateral recti move the eye to one side or the other respectively and work together in the same way. This action is similar to the opposing action of the flexor and extensor muscles of the forearm. When one set contracts the opposite set relaxes. (2) In normal vision both eyes move together (conjugate deviation). Therefore, if the eyes are turned upwards both right and left superior recti will contract and both inferior recti will relax. On the other hand, if both eyes are turned to the right it follows that the right lateral rectus and the left medial rectus will contract while the right medial rectus and left lateral rectus will relax. The converse is true if the eyes are turned to the left. This is quite simple, and with a little thought the individual can work it out for herself or himself.

Of the two oblique muscles, the superior oblique is so arranged as to direct the eye downwards and outwards. The inferior oblique muscle turns the eye upwards and outwards.

The muscles of the eyes are supplied by the cranial nerves (IIIrd, IVth and VIth). The lateral rectus is supplied by the VIth or abducens nerve. The superior oblique is supplied by the IVth or trochlear nerve. All the others (levator palpebrae superioris, medial rectus, inferior rectus, inferior oblique and superior rectus) are supplied by the IIIrd or oculomotor nerve. These extraocular muscles are sometimes referred to as the extrinsic muscles of the eye. The internal or intrinsic muscles are mentioned later.

The common condition of squint is usually due to imperfect balance between opposing muscles and may be treated by operations designed to shorten or lengthen the appropriate muscles.

The Eyeball or Bulb of the Eye

The eyeball is situated in the anterior part of the orbital cavity and is almost spherical in shape. It is surrounded by a pad of fat.

The structure of the eye may be considered in the following way.
- Three tunics or layers
  - Fibrous
    - Sclera
    - Cornea
  - Vascular
    - Choroid
    - Ciliary body
    - Iris
  - Nervous retina
- The light-transmitting mechanism
  - Aqueous humor
  - The lens
  - The vitreous body.

The Fibrous Coats

- The sclera (or sclerotic coat). The posterior five-sixths of the outer coat of the eyeball consists of strong, opaque fibrous tissue and is called the sclera. It is protective in function and helps to maintain the shape of the eyeball. When viewed from the front it is that portion which is referred to as 'the white of the eye' and, in this position, is covered by the conjunctiva. Posteriorly, the optic nerve passes through it to reach the retina inside the eye, and in the orbit the nerve is protected by a sheath of fibrous tissue continuous with the sclera.
- The cornea occupies the anterior one-sixth of the external surface of the eyeball and, being transparent, allows light to enter the interior of the eye. The cornea is sometimes described as the 'window of the eye' and its anterior surface can be seen to be slightly curved or convex. Over the cornea, the conjunctiva becomes very thin and is only represented by a few layers of epithelial cells. The cornea has no blood vessels but derives its nourishment from the aqueous humor.

The Vascular Coat

This is the middle layer of the eye. It contains many blood vessels and capillaries, which are derived from the ophthalmic branch of the internal carotid artery, and is pigmented. The choroid, ciliary body and iris together form the uveal tract. Hence, the term uveitis for inflammation of the iris (iritis) and the structures in continuity with it.

- *The choroid:* This is a thin pigmented membrane, dark brown in color, which lines the posterior compartment of the eye. It is situated between the inner surface of the sclera and the retina.
- *The ciliary body:* This is a circular structure, continuous with the anterior part of the choroid, which surrounds the periphery of the iris immediately behind the outer margin of the cornea where it joins the sclera (Fig. 18.12). It contains muscle fibers (the ciliary muscle) and to it is attached the ligament which helps to suspend the lens in position.
- *The iris:* This is the pigmented membrane which surrounds the pupil of the eye. It arises from the margin of the ciliary body and forms a diaphragm with a black central opening (the pupil) immediately in front of the lens. The color of the eye is dependent on the pigment in the iris. In dark eyes the pigment is plentiful, but in blue eyes it is scanty.

The iris contains two sets of muscle fibers. Those comprising the sphincter pupillae encircle the pupil. The fibers of the other muscle, the dilator pupillae, pass in a radial direction from the outer margin of the iris to the edge of the pupil. It will be clear that the circular muscle acting as a sphincter will reduce the size of the pupil when it contracts. Contraction of the radial fibers, on the other hand, increase its size and they are, therefore, dilators. These, with the ciliary muscle, are the intrinsic muscles of the eye.

The function of the iris is to regulate the amount of light entering the posterior part of the eye. Thus, when a bright light shines on the retina the pupil contracts.

The iris is under the control of the autonomic nervous system, the effect of sympathetic stimulation being pupillary dilatation (mydriasis) and that of parasympathetic stimulation being pupillary constriction (miosis). Parasympathetic blockade with anticholinergic drugs such as atropine therefore dilates the pupils. Drugs which dilate the pupils are called mydriatics and one which is frequently used as a topical solution (drops) for this purpose is the anticholinergic agent cyclopentolate. Drugs which act like or prolong the action of acetylcholine (parasympathomimetic drugs) constrict the pupil. An example is physostigmine (Eserine) which blocks the enzyme cholinesterase, which normally terminates the action of acetylcholine. Physostigmine is therefore an example of an anticholinesterase.

The Retina (Fig. 18.13)

The retina is the innermost coat of the eye. It lines the posterior chamber and

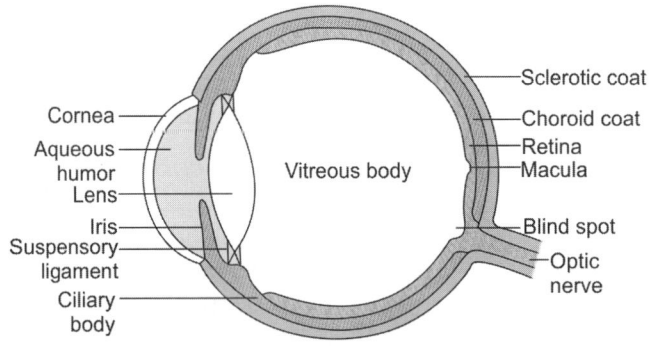

Fig. 18.12: Section through eyeball viewed from above

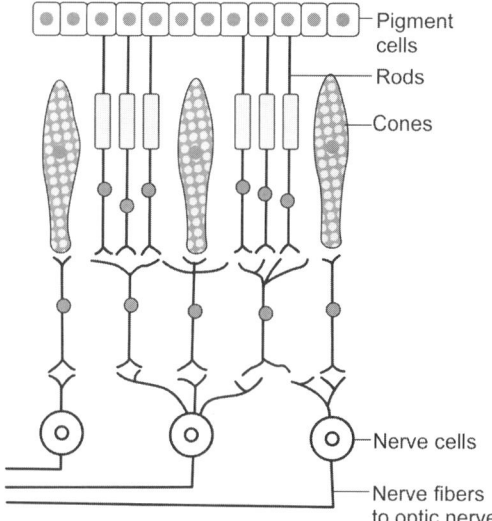

Fig. 18.13: Layers of the retina

ends anteriorly at the margin of the ciliary body. It is a delicate membrane consisting of neurons, that is, nerve cells and nerve fibers, together with a layer of special structures called rods and cones. These are situated on the outer or choroidal surface of the retina, while the nerve fibers are on the inner surface facing the chamber of the eye. The rods and cones are the actual receptors of sight and light reaching them sets up the impulses which are transmitted to the nerve. The impulses are generated by the action of light on photosensitive pigments in the rods and cones. In the rods, the pigment is known as visual purple or rhodopsin. The cones are responsible for color vision. The rods give only monochromatic (black and white) vision but their much greater sensitivity enables us to see in very poor lighting conditions.

The retina is the nervous portion of the eye and is therefore the true end-organ of vision. The fibers of the optic nerve commence in the cells of the retina and are collected together at a point just medial to the most posterior part of the eyeball where they pierce the choroid and sclera and pass backwards as the optic nerve through the orbit to the optic chiasma and brain.

The point at which the optic nerve fibers all converge contains no nerve cells and no rods and cones. It is, therefore, insensitive to light and is called the blind spot.

The retina is supplied with blood by a branch of the ophthalmic artery which enters the eye with the optic nerve and is called the central artery of the retina.

The macula is situated just to the lateral side of the exit of the optic nerve, i.e. at the very center of the posterior part of the eye. It is a small area of the retina of great sensitivity on which the images seen by direct or near vision are focused. No rods are present in this area hut cones are especially numerous.

The retina may become partially detached from the choroid, particularly in people with severe myopia (short sightedness).

The Light-transmitting Mechanism
The Aqueous Humor

Situated between the cornea in front and the iris and ciliary body behind is the anterior chamber of the eye which contains a clear watery fluid called the aqueous humor.

The Lens

This is a firm transparent structure, convex in shape, which is suspended in its capsule by a ligament attached to the ciliary body. It is placed immediately behind the iris and pupil of the eye, its function is to focus rays of light entering the eye through the pupil onto the retina.

The Vitreous Body

This is a colorless, transparent jelly-like substance which fills the posterior four-fifths of the eye. It helps to preserve the spherical shape of the eyeball and to support the retina.

The presence of fluid and semi-fluid material or gel in the interior of the eye maintains its shape by keeping up a constant pressure on its walls. This is referred to as the intraocular tension.

In certain conditions drainage of the fluid may be impaired and there will be a consequent increase in the intraocular tension, a serious effect which may disturb the nutrition of the retina and lead to blindness. This is known as glaucoma. It may be treated medically and surgically:

- By instilling drops which cause the pupil to contract (miotics, e.g. physostigmine), thereby helping to open up the canals situated at the point of attachment of the iris to the ciliary body where the excess of fluid is normally drained off into the circulation;
- By making a small hole (trephine) through the sclera into the anterior chamber of the eye so that fluid can drain under the conjunctiva and so relieve the tension within the eyeball.

Diminution in intraocular tension is seen in cases of severe shock and marked fluid loss from the body. Complete loss of tension is observed after death.

The Mechanism of Sight

From a structural point of view the eye may be compared with a camera (Fig. 18.14). The eyelids act as a shutter and there is an entrance window for light—the cornea; a diaphragm to regulate the aperture and therefore the amount of light entering—the iris; a lens to focus the image; a darkened interior formed by the choroid, and a light-sensitive plate which receives the image—the retina.

The optic nerve and its connections convey the details of the image to the occipital region of the cerebral cortex where they are processed before reaching consciousness.

In order to understand the mechanism of vision, it is necessary to know something about light and the action of lenses. Light consists of electromagnetic waves which

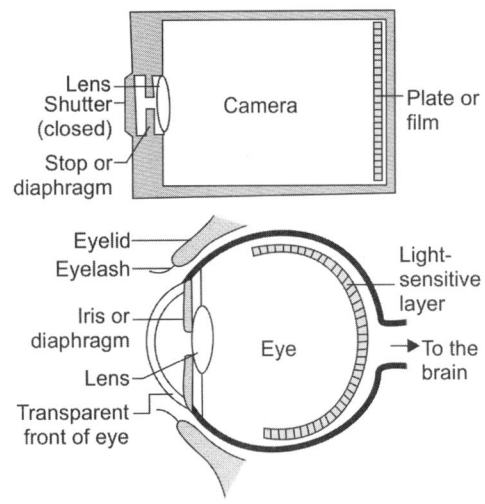

Fig. 18.14: The eye compared with a camera

travel faster than anything else known in the universe, at the rate of 186000 miles per second.

Some objects, such as the sun, electric light or candle, emit light rays and are self-luminous sources of light. Other objects, such as the things we normally see, merely reflect light received from other sources; If there is no source of light, complete darkness exists and no object can be seen.

Rays of light ordinarily travel in straight lines. A lens, which may be roughly defined as a curved transparent structure, has the power of bending or refracting rays of light. A lens which is thicker at the center than at the periphery is described as convex. One, which is thinner in the middle is called concave.

A convex lens has the power of bending rays of light so that they converge and meet at a point of focus behind the lens. The stronger the lens, i.e. the greater the degree of curvature of its surfaces, the nearer is the focal point. A concave lens, on the other hand, bends the light rays so that they diverge and do not focus behind the lens. The lens of the eye is convex and focuses the rays of light passing through it onto the retina.

Actually the image reaching the retina is inverted but this is turned the right way up by the visual cortex in the brain.

Accommodation

Rays of light from distant objects are for all practical purposes parallel and therefore strike the vertical axis of the lens at right angles. The eye is so adjusted that such rays are bent by the lens to focus exactly on the retina, forming a sharp image. Rays of light from a near object (say 25 cm or 10 in) are divergent and strike the lens obliquely. In order that such rays may be accurately focused on the retina the lens must be made more powerful (of greater focusing power) by increasing its curvature, i.e. making it more convex. This is accomplished by the action of the ciliary muscles. At the same time the clearness of the image is increased by cutting down the number of rays entering the eye by contraction of the iris. The process of altering the shape of the lens is called accommodation and operates every time a near object is looked at. The nearest point at which an object can be brought clearly into focus by accommodation is called the near point. For a normal child of 10 years it is about 9 cm (3.5 in) but it recedes throughout life and by the age of about 45 may become so distant that reading is difficult without spectacles. This defect of accommodation with advancing age is due to decreasing elasticity of the lens and is called presbyopia.

When an object is placed near the eyes, in order to obtain a clearly focused picture on both retinae the eyes turn slightly inwards towards each other. This is called convergence. The extreme of convergence is illustrated by 'squinting down the end of the nose'. The triple response of accommodation, convergence and pupillary constriction is called the near response.

It is of interest at this point to note some of the common defects of vision requiring

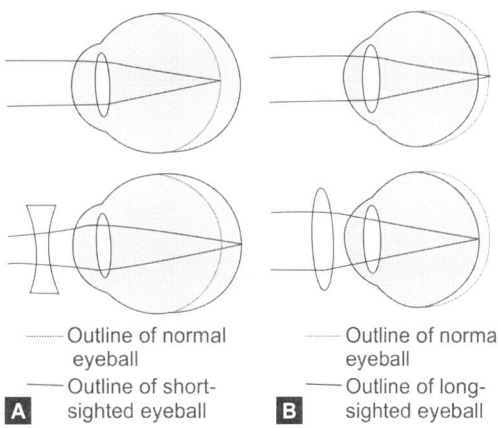

Figs 18.15A and B: A. Myopia (short sight) and its correction; **B.** Hypermetropia (long sight) and its correction

the use of spectacles. Whereas, the normal eye is practically spherical, in some people it tends to be slightly elongated and in others flattened. In other words, in the former case the distance from the lens to the retina is increased and in the latter it is decreased. It follows, therefore, that the lens will not naturally focus the image accurately on the retina in these conditions. In the former, elongated or myopic eye (short sighted), the image will tend to fall in front of the retina, while in the shortened or hypermetropic eye (long sighted) it will fall behind the retina (Figs 18.15A and B). In both instances the objects seen will be blurred and out of focus.

These defects can be compensated by using additional lenses in the form of spectacles. By placing a concave glass lens in front of a myopic eye the rays of light will become divergent before reaching the lens, so that its point of focus is shifted back on to the retina. A convex lens in front of a hypermetropic eye will bring the image nearer the front of the eye by increasing the convergence of the rays so that they are focused on the retina.

Astigmatism is due to unequal curvature of the surfaces of the cornea, i.e. it may be curved more vertically than horizontally.

This also may require correction with spectacles (cylindrical lenses).

Vision

Rays of light reflected from visible objects fall on the retina and, in near vision, are focused on the macula. The light falling on the retina produces certain chemical changes there, which stimulate the endings of the optic nerve. These stimuli are conveyed by the optic nerve to the optic chiasma where some of the fibers cross and are then carried back to the cortex of the occipital lobe to be interpreted into consciousness.

Binocular Vision

In considering the sense of sight it must be remembered that although we can see with each eye separately, normal stereoscopic vision is obtained by the simultaneous use of both eyes.

Rays of light strike the retina from all directions. Those coming from the left-hand side of the body will fall on the nasal side of the retina of the left eye and the temporal side of the retina of the right eye. These images produced by objects on the left side of the body are eventually received by the occipital lobe on the right side of the brain. This explains the crossing of certain fibers of the optic nerve in the optic chiasma and is part of the principle that one side of the body is controlled by the cerebral hemisphere of the opposite side. These facts are easily appreciated from Fig. 18.16.

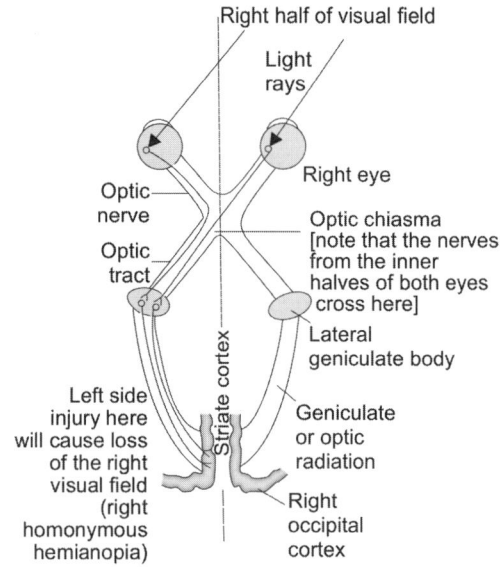

Fig. 18.16: The visual pathways

Summary of the Sense of Sight

Light waves → cornea → aqueous humor → lens → vitreous body → retina → optic nerve → optic chiasma → occipital lobe of brain.

CHAPTER 19

Reproductive System

Introduction: Sex organs, genetic basis of sex, sex chromatin, role of hormones in sexual differentiation during fetal life. Aberrations of sexual development chromosomal and hormonal.

■ SEX ORGANS

Development of the Gonads

On each side of the embryo a primitive gonad arises from genital ridge a condensation of tissue near the adrenal gland. The gonad develops a cortex and medulla. Until the 6th week of the development these structures are identical in both sexes. In genetic males, the medulla develops during the 7th and 8th weeks into a testis and the cortex regresses. Leydig's and Sertoli cells appear and testosterone and mullerian inhibiting substance (MIS) are secreted. In genetic females, the cortex develops into an ovary and medulla regresses. The embryonic ovary does not secrete hormones.

In the 7th week of gestation the embryo has both male and female primordial genital ducts. In a normal female fetus, the Mullerian duct system then develops into uterine tube and a uterus. In the male fetus the Wolffian duct system on each side develops into the epidedimis and vas deference.

External genitalia are similarly bi-potential until the 8th week. Thereafter, the urogenital slit disappears and male genitalia forms or alternatively it remain open and female genetialia form.

When there are functional testes in the embryo male internal and external genitalia develops. The Laydig's cells of the fetal testis secrete testosterone and the sertoli cells secrete MIS. MIS is a 536 AA homodimer that is the member of the TGFB super family of growth factor which includes... inhibins and activins. In their effects on the internal and external genetalia MIS and testosterone act unilaterally. MIS causes regression of Mullerian duct by apoptosis on the same side on which it is secreted. Testosterone causes the development of the vas deference and related structures from the Wolffian ducts. The testosterone metabolite DHT induces the formation of male external genitalia and male secondary sex characteristics.

MIS continues to be secreted by the Sertoli cells, and it reaches mean values of 48 ng/ml in plasma in 1–2 year old boys. Then it declines to low levels by the time of puberty, but persists at low but detectable levels throughout life. In girls MIS is produced by granulosa cells in small follicles in the ovaries but low undetectable levels until puberty. Thereafter MIS is about the same as in adult men, i.e. about 2 ng/mL. The functions of MIS after early embryonic life are unsettled, but are involved in germ cell maturation in both sexes and in control of testicular descent in boys.

Affected by androgens in early life. In rats a brief exposure to androgens during the first few days of life causes the male pattern of sexual behavior and male pattern of hypothalamic control of gonadotropin secretion to develop after puberty. In the absence of androgens female pattern develop. In monkeys similar effects on sexual behavior produced by exposure to androgens in utero. But the pattern of gonadotropin secretion remains cyclic. Early exposure of female human fetuses to androgens also causes subtle but significant masculinizing effects on behavior. Women with adrenogenital syndrome due to congenital adrenocortical enzyme deficiency develop normal menstrual cycles when treated with cortisol.

■ MALE REPRODUCTIVE SYSTEM (FIG. 19.1)

The Scrotum

The scrotum is a pouch of pigmented skin situated below the root of the penis, and is continued with the skin of perineum and groin. It is divided into two by a midline fibrous septum, which is marked on the surface by a ridge, the scrotal raphe. Each half of the scrotum contains a testis, an epididymis and the lower end of the spermatic cord.

The subcutaneous tissue of the scrotum contains smooth muscle fibers, constituting the dartos muscle. This muscle contracts in response to cold or exercise to hold the testes closer to the body, causing the scrotum to become smaller and wrinkled. The muscle relaxes in response to warmth and thus helps to maintain an optimal temperature for spermatogenesis.

The Testes

The testes (singular: testis) are small ovoid glands suspended in the scrotum. They are the reproductive glands, or gonads of the male.

In the embryo the testes develop within the upper abdominal cavity and during the seventh month of fetal life they migrate down the posterior abdominal wall and leave the abdominal cavity by passing through the inguinal canals into the scrotum, drawing with them the blood vessels and ducts which form the spermatic cords. As it passes into the scrotum, each testis carries with it a coat of peritoneum which normally becomes separated from the rest of the abdominal peritoneum. If this separation does not take place a channel remains between the abdominal cavity and the scrotum, and thus abdominal viscera may protrude into the scrotum, giving rise to a hernia or rupture.

Structure of the Testis (Fig. 19.2)

The separated coat of peritoneum forms the serous outer covering of the testis, the tunica vaginalis. The testis and the tunica vaginalis are attached to the lower part of the scrotum by fibrous tissue.

Each testis is surrounded by a dense white fibrous capsule, the tunica albuginea, which projects into the substance of the testis to divide it into 200 or more cone-shaped lobules. Lining the tunica albuginea is a delicate layer of connective tissue which supports a network of blood capillaries called the tunica vasculosa.

The lobules of the testis contain the seminiferous tubules. Each seminiferous tubule is highly convoluted, and if unravelled would measure about 70 cm (27.5 in) in length. The tubules are coiled in such a way that both ends join a series of

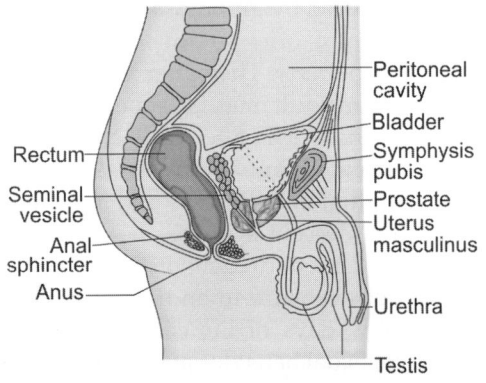

Fig. 19.1: Section through the male pelvis

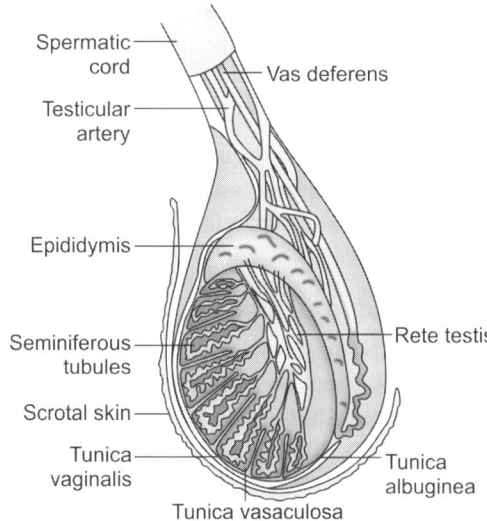

Fig. 19.2: Testis and epididymis

straight tubules which converge to form a network called rete testis.

The seminiferous tubules are lined by germinal epithelial cells (spermatogonia) resting on a basement membrane. The germinal epithelial cells form the *spermatozoa*. Lying between the germinal cells of the tubule and the sustenacular cells (of Sterol). Immature spermatocytes become attached to these cells and appear to be nourished by them at an early stage of their development.

The seminiferous tubules are embedded in loose connective tissue containing blood vessels, nerves and groups of interstitial cells (the cells of Leydig), which secrete the male hormones.

The rete testis is continued with a series of efferent ductules which drain into the epididymis.

Functions of the Testes

Spermatogenesis

Spermatogenesis is the process by which primitive male gametes (spermatogonia) become mature sperm.

The spermatogonia are the germinal epithelial cells lining the seminiferous tubules; they are present at birth but do not produce spermatozoa until puberty. At puberty, spermatogonia begin to actively divide under the influence of follicle stimulating hormone (FSH) from the anterior pituitary gland; and will continue to do so throughout life, although there may be a decrease in the numbers of spermatozoa produced in the later years due to a decrease in testosterone secretion.

Some of the spermatogonia begin to enlarge and undergo mitotic division to form primary spermatocytes, each containing 44 somatic and 2 sex chromosomes (XY). The primary spermatocytes move away from the basement membrane and undergo their first meiotic division, to produce a pair of secondary spermatocytes each containing 22 autosomes and one sex chromosome, either X or Y. Thus, half the spermatozoa contain the Y chromosome and become male spermatozoa, while the other half contain the X chromosome and become female spermatozoa.

Each of the secondary spermatocytes rapidly divides again by mitosis to form a pair of spermatids (each containing 23 chromosomes). The spermatids become attached to the Sterol cells and elongate to develop a head and a tail. The head contains the pronucleus, and is covered by the acrosome which is thought to contain proteolytic enzymes (Fig. 19.3). The tail, comprising the neck, middle piece, main piece and end piece, is the organ of motility. The neck contains the centriole and the middle piece contains mitochondria,

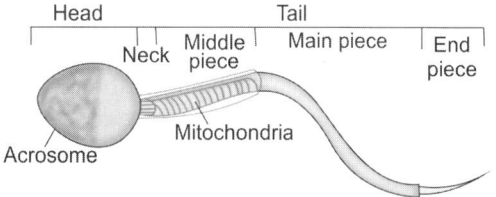

Fig. 19.3: Spermatozoon. The head is almost entirely composed by the nucleus

arranged around an axial sheath, which provide energy for motility. The axial sheath extends into the main piece which is covered by a tough fibrous coat that terminates at the end piece. The end piece consists of the exposed axial sheath which forms a fine filament.

The spermatozoa pass from the seminiferous tubules of the testis into the epididymis. They are non-motile and are transported by contraction the smooth muscle of the epididymis. It is here that the spermatozoa become mature and capable of fertilizing an ovum. The secretion of testosterone is necessary for the complete maturation of the spermatozoa.

Secretion of Hormones

Testosterone

The interstitial cells of Leydig, which lie in compact groups in the connective tissue surrounding the seminiferous tubules, secrete the male sex hormones collectively known as androgens. Testosterone, a steroid compound, is the principal hormone secreted; dehydroepiandrosterone and androstenedione are produced in lesser amounts.

Very little testosterone is secreted in childhood, but at puberty the secretion of luteinizing hormone (LH) by the anterior pituitary gland stimulates the interstitial cells to produce testosterone. (In the male LH is often referred to as interstitial cell-stimulating hormone or ICSH).

Testosterone secretion promotes maturation of the male reproductive organs and causes the appearance of secondary sexual characteristics. It causes growth of hair over the chest, abdomen and pubis; and on the face. It causes enlargement of the larynx which results in the voice 'breaking' and gradually changing to the deeper base voice of the adult male.

Although FSH initiates spermatogenesis, testosterone must be secreted simultaneously for development of the spermatozoa beyond the primary spermatocyte stage. Testosterone also has a powerful anabolic action, stimulating protein synthesis and growth of bones.

Estrogen

The testes secrete small amounts of estrogen, but its exact function in the male is unknown.

The Epididymis and Vas Deferens

The epididymis is a tightly coiled tubule surrounded by connective tissue. It is described as having a head which is connected to the testes by the efferent ductules, a body and a tail which is continued with the vas deferens. The convoluted tubule is lined with pseudo stratified columnar epithelium. The epithelial cells have long cellular processes on their surfaces through which cellular secretions enter the lumen of the duct. The secretions contain hormones, enzymes and nutrients and may be important in the maturation of spermatozoa. The duct is surrounded by a circular layer of smooth muscle fibers which contract to aid the passage of spermatozoa along the duct.

At its termination, the duct of the epididymis straightens and becomes continuous with the vas deferens. This is a thick-walled fibromuscular tube approximately 45 cm (17.7 in) long which passes upwards behind the testis and through the spermatic cord and inguinal canal to enter the pelvic cavity. It passes backwards to the base of the bladder and joins the seminal vesicle on its own side to form the ejaculatory duct. At its termination the vas deferens becomes dilated and tortuous to form an ampulla. The thick muscular walls of the duct move spermatozoa along the lumen by peristaltic contraction towards the ampulla. The pseudo stratified epithelial lining of the duct is thrown into longitudinal folds. The walls of the ampulla are thinner and the lining is folded to form pocket like recesses.

Mature spermatozoa are stored in the vas deferens and the ampulla. Vasectomy is the surgical interruption of the vas deferens via an incision through the scrotum. It renders a man sterile since it prevents spermatozoa leaving the epididymis.

The Spermatic Cord

The spermatic cords extend through the inguinal canals and then pass in front of the pubis to reach the scrotum and testes. Each spermatic cord contains the testicular artery, the pampiniform plexus of veins, lymphatic vessels, nerves and the vas deferens.

Blood Supply

The testicular artery arises from the aorta immediately below the renal artery. It passes downwards through the spermatic cord, supplying branches to the vas deferens and the epididymis before reaching the testis.

Veins emerge from the posterior surface of the testis to form the pampiniform plexus, which passes upwards through the inguinal canal in the spermatic cord to form the testicular vein. The right testicular vein drains into the inferior vena cava, while the left vein drains into the left renal vein.

Lymphatic Drainage

The lymphatic vessels of the testis and epididymis accompany the veins and drain into the lateral and preaortic nodes.

Nerve Supply

The testis receives its nerve supply from the 10th and 11th thoracic nerve segments of the spinal cord.

Seminal Vesicles (Fig. 19.4)

The seminal vesicles are two small convoluted pouches situated behind the bladder and above the prostate gland. Each vesicle is about 5 cin (2 in) long and consists of three coats.

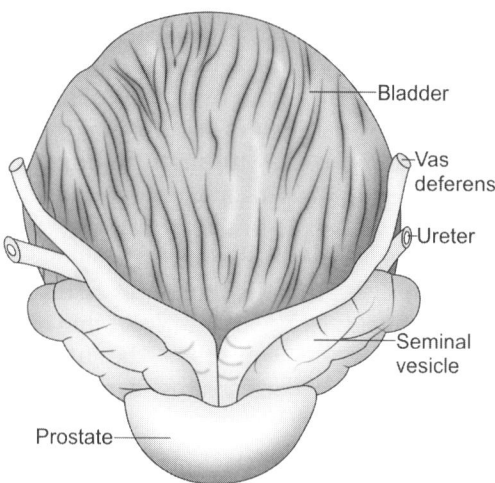

Fig. 19.4: Base of the bladder (from behind)

1. An outer coat of connective tissue containing elastic fibers.
2. A middle coat of smooth muscle fibers consisting of an outer layer of longitudinal fibers and an inner layer of circular fibers.
3. An inner coat of secretory columnar epithelium which is folded to form numerous pockets. Under the influence of testosterone the epithelium secretes a viscid liquid containing fructose and other nutrients, which is stored within the seminal vesicles until ejaculation occurs. Just prior to ejaculation, the seminal vesicles empty their contents into the ejaculatory ducts to join the spermatozoa from the vas deferens.

Blood Supply

The seminal vesicles are supplied with arterial blood by the inferior vesical and middle rectal arteries.

The veins drain into the vesicoprostatic venous plexus.

Nerve Supply

The seminal vesicles are innervated by nerve fibers from the pelvic plexuses.

The Ejaculatory Ducts

Each ejaculatory duct is formed by the union of the vas deferens with the duct of the seminal vesicle. It is about 2 cm (0.8 in) in length and passes through the prostate gland to enter the prostatic urethra.

The Prostate Gland

The prostate gland is about the size of a chestnut and is situated below the base of the bladder surrounding the urethra. The prostate is enclosed by a sheath of fibroelastic tissue which is called false capsule. It contains an extensive plexus of veins, the vesicoprostatic plexus. Beneath this lies the true capsule consisting of dense fibrous tissue.

The glandular tissue of the prostate is formed by secretory alveoli and tubules of very irregular size and shape, composed of columnar epithelial cells. These are surrounded by a fibroelastic stroma containing smooth muscle fibers. The prostate secretes a thin, milky, slightly alkaline fluid which contains calcium, acid phosphate and citric acid. During emission the prostatic capsule contracts and expels the fluid into the urethra through numerous small ducts.

Blood Supply

The arterial blood supply of the prostate gland is from the inferior vesical, middle rectal and internal pudendal arteries.

The veins form a plexus around the gland (which also receives venous blood from the deep dorsal vein of the penis) and drain into the internal iliac veins.

Nerve Supply

The prostate receives both sympathetic and parasympathetic nerve fibers from the inferior hypogastric (pelvic) plexus.

In many elderly men the prostate gland may become enlarged and by pressing on the urethra can obstruct the flow of urine from the bladder, thus causing retention of urine. Surgical removal of the gland (prostatectomy) is usually required.

Bulbourethral Glands

The bulbourethral glands (of Cowper) lie, one on each side, in the connective tissue behind the membranous urethra just below the prostate gland. Each gland is about the size of a pea and consists of compound tubuloalveolar tissue and has a duct which enters the penile portion of the urethra. The bulbourethral glands produce a clear, viscid alkaline secretion.

The Penis (Fig. 19.5)

The penis is composed mainly of three cylindrical columns of erectile tissue (i.e. tissue which becomes firm and rigid when congested with blood). The two larger dorsal columns are the corpora cavernosa penis, and the single inferior column is the corpus spongiosum. Numerous trabeculae divide each column of tissue into cavernous spaces (sinuses) giving the entire structure a spongy appearance.

The penis has a fixed root arising from the perineum and a free shaft. The corpora cavernosa originate separately but unite beneath the pubic arch and run forward together. Each corpus cavernosum is surrounded by a thick fibrous sheath. Between the two columns lies a fibrous septum through which the cavernous spaces of both sides communicate (Fig. 19.6).

The corpus spongiosum is surrounded by a thin fibrous sheath containing elastic and smooth muscle fibers. It encloses the penile portion of the urethra. The corpus spongiosum arises at the root of the penis and passes forwards inferiorly in the deep groove formed between the corpora cavernosa. Its tip is expanded to form a cap, the glans penis, overlapping the terminal ends of the corpora cavernosa.

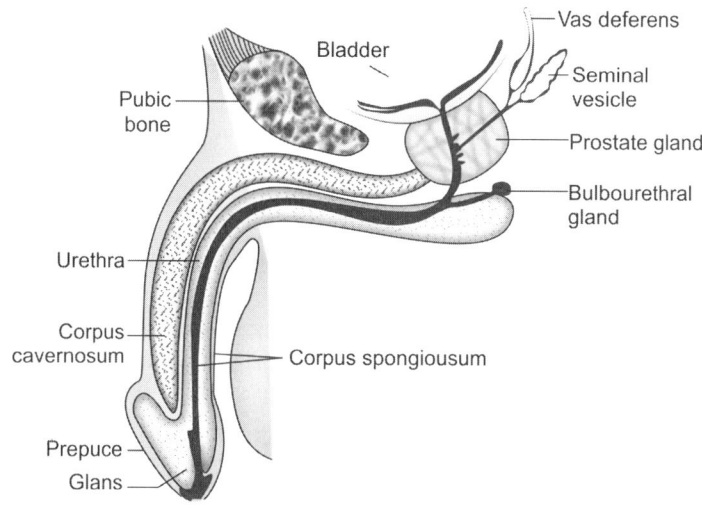

Fig. 19.5: Penis and related organs

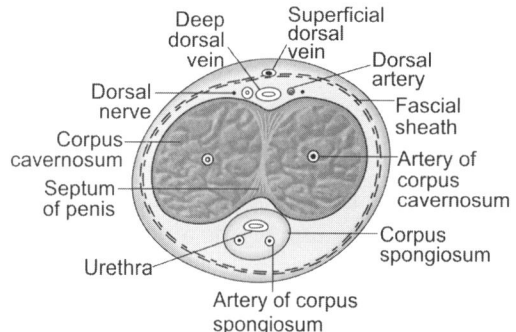

Fig. 19.6: Transverse section through the body of the penis

The three columns of erectile tissue are surrounded by a small amount of subcutaneous tissue containing numerous smooth muscle fibers; this is covered by thin delicate skin, which forms a double fold over the glans penis called prepuce (foreskin).

The urethra serves as a common outlet for urine and for semen.

If the prepuce covers the glans penis too tightly a condition known as phimosis is caused which results in difficulty in micturition. This is not uncommon in young children and may require circumcision.

Blood Supply

Arterial blood is supplied to the penis by branches of the internal and external pudendal arteries. The deep arteries of the penis and branches of the dorsal arteries of the penis supply the cavernous spaces, some branches dividing to form convoluted vessels opening directly into the sinuses of the erectile tissue.

The veins draining the cavernous spaces converge on the dorsum of the penis to form the deep dorsal vein which empties into the prostatic venous plexus.

Nerve Supply

The penis is innervated by the 2nd, 3rd and 4th sacral spinal nerves through the pudendal nerve and pelvic plexuses.

Semen

Semen (seminal fluid) is a mucoid, milky white fluid consisting of the spermatozoa suspended in the mixed secretions from the vas deferens, seminal vesicles, prostate gland and bulbourethral glands. The average pH of the semen is approximately 7.5.

Functions of the Male Reproductive System

The male reproductive system is concerned with spermatogenesis and the introduction of spermatozoa into the female vagina during sexual intercourse (coitus).

Erection of the penis is necessary for penetration of the vagina. Parasympathetic stimulation causes dilation of the penile arterioles and constriction of the veins, this results in engorgement of the erectile tissue, and the penis becomes elongated and rigid.

Emission is the reflex movement of spermatozoa and secretions from the epididymis, vas deferens and seminal vesicles into the urethra.

Ejaculation is caused by rhythmic contractions of the prostate and the bulbocavernosus muscles which result in wave-like increases in pressure on the erectile tissue causing propulsion (ejaculation) of the semen out of the urethra.

■ FEMALE REPRODUCTIVE SYSTEM

- *Primary sex organs or ovaries:* Function is to produce ova and to secrete female sex hormones.
- *Accessory sex organs:* Divided into two major sex organ:
  - Internal genital organs
  - External genital organs

Internal Genital Organs

- Uterus
- Body
- Fundus
- Isthmus
- *Cervix:* Cylindrical lower part

The Uterus

The uterus is a hollow, pear-shaped organ situated in the pelvic cavity. It has thick muscular walls and a small central cavity. In the adult, it measures about 7.5 cm (3 in) in length, 5 cm (2 in) in width and 2.5 cm (1 in) in thickness.

It consists of the *fundus*, the *body* and the *cervix*. The fundus is the upper part of the uterus situated between the two uterine tubes.

The body or corpus forms the greater part of the organ and gradually tapers downwards towards the cervix. The cervix or neck is the lowest portion, part of which projects like an inverted cone into the vault of the vagina. It is traversed by a canal opening above into the cavity of the uterus by an orifice called the *internal os*, and below into the vagina by the *external os*.

The cavity of the uterus is a mere slit when viewed from the side, but is flat and triangular when seen from the front. The uterine tubes open into the cavity at the upper outer angles of the fundus. The area of insertion of each tube is called the *cornu*.

The *walls of the uterus* consist of three layers.
1. The *perimetrium*, an outer coat of peritoneum which covers the uterus except at the sides and is closely adherent to the underlying muscle layer. The peritoneum on the anterior surface of the uterus is reflected forwards on to the superior surface of the bladder forming a shallow uterovesical pouch. The peritoneum covering the posterior surface continues downwards to cover the upper part of the vagina before being reflected on to the rectum. This space between the uterus and the rectum is called the *rectouterine pouch (of Douglas)*.

    The peritoneum passing laterally from the uterus extends to the side walls of the pelvis being continuous with the folds of the broad ligament.
2. The *myometrium* is a thick middle coat of smooth muscle fibers arranged in three layers, an inner layer of circular fibres, a middle layer of oblique fibers and an outer layer of longitudinal fibers. The bundles of muscle fibers are interlaced with elastic and fibrous tissue.

3. The *endometrium* is a specialized form of mucous membrane which varies in thickness according to the phase of the menstrual cycle. It is covered by a layer of partially ciliated columnar epithelium which contains glands that dip down into the basal layer.

Position of the Uterus (Figs 19.7A and B)

Normally the uterus is bent forwards on itself in a position of *anteflexion* so that the fundus rests on the bladder. When a woman is standing the uterus lies in a position which is almost horizontal with the cervix inclined forwards at an angle of 90° with the long axis of the vagina. This position is called *anteversion*.

In some women the uterus is angled backwards in a position of *retroversion*.

The uterus is held in place by *four pairs of supporting ligaments* and indirectly by the muscles of the pelvic floor.

The broad ligaments: Each broad ligament consists of a double fold of peritoneum continuous with the perimetrium and extending from the uterus to the side walls of the pelvis. The uterine tube is enclosed within the upper margin.

The *round ligaments* are fibromuscular cords extending from the cornua of the uterus through the inguinal canals to be inserted in the labia majora. They help to maintain the uterus in a position of anteversion and anteflexion.

The transverse cervical ligaments (cardinal ligaments). The lower border of each broad ligament is thickened and strengthened by fibrous tissue, fascia and some smooth muscle to form the transverse cervical ligament. These fan out from the cervix and upper vagina to the side walls of the pelvis. They are important in preventing the uterus from prolapsing into the vagina.

The *uterosacral ligaments* are continuous with the transverse cervical ligaments and extend backwards around the rectum to the sacrum. By pulling the cervix backwards they help to maintain the uterus in a position of anteversion.

The *pelvic floor* consists of muscles, fascia and connective tissue which fills the irregular shape of the pelvic outlet.

Blood Supply

The uterus receives arterial blood from the uterine arteries which are branches of the internal iliac arteries. Each uterine artery passes forwards in the base of the broad ligament and reaches the uterus at the level of the cervix. It divides into branches which supply the cervix and upper vagina, then turns upwards in a tortuous fashion to supply the body of the uterus.

In addition, branches of the ovarian artery pass from the ovary and uterine tube to supply the fundus of the uterus and anastomose with the uterine artery.

Venous drainage is by the uterine and ovarian veins which accompany the arteries.

Lymphatic Drainage

The uterus has a wide distribution of lymphatic vessels; those of the fundus drain with the ovarian vessels into the aortic nodes, while those of the lower part of the body and of the cervix drain into the inguinal, external and internal iliac nodes.

Nerve Supply

The uterus receives sympathetic and parasympathetic fibers from the autonomic nervous system.

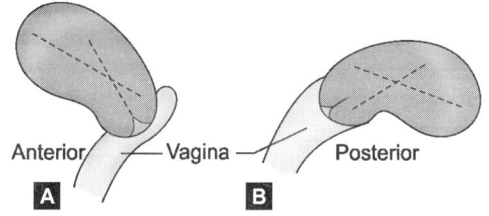

Figs 19.7: Position of the uterus. **A.** Normal position of anteflexion and anteversion; **B.** Retroversion

Functions of the Uterus

During the reproductive years the female experiences regular cyclical changes (the menstrual cycle). Each cycle prepares the uterus to receive the fertilized ovum, and to retain and nourish the developing fetus throughout the duration of pregnancy. At the end of pregnancy the muscular walls of the uterus contract to expel the fetus.

Fallopian Tubes

10 cm in length 8 mm diameter medial uterine end attached to and opens into the uterus and lateral end opens into peritoneal cavity.
- Uterine or interstitial part
- Isthmus
- Ampulla
- Infundibulum.

Functions: The uterine tubes convey ova, shed by the ovaries to the uterus. Ova enter the tube at its fimbriated end.

The sperms enter the uterine tube at its medial end after traversing the vagina and uterine cavity. Secretions present in the tube provide nutrition, oxygen and other requirements for ova and spermatozoa passing through the tube. Fertilization takes place in the ampulla and the fertilized ovum travels towards the uterus through the tube. The ciliated epithelial cells lining the tube help to move ova towards the uterus.

The Ovary (Fig. 19.8)

The two ovaries are small ovoid structures, measuring 3–4 cm (1.2–1.6 in) in length, 2 cm (0.8 in) in width and 1 cm (0.4 in) in thickness, lying one on either side of the uterus. They are attached to the posterior surface of the broad ligament by the mesovarium, a fold of peritoneum. Blood vessels, lymphatics and nerves enter the ovary through the mesovarium at the hilum of the ovary. Each ovary is suspended from below the cornu of the uterus by an ovarian ligament.

Structure

The ovary consists of a medulla and a cortex which merge together and are not clearly defined.

The medulla is composed of loose connective tissue containing numerous blood vessels, lymphatics and nerves. Close to the hilum and mesovarium it contains small groups of hilus cells which are thought to be homologous to the interstitial cells of the testis.

The cortex consists of a compact connective tissue stromal containing ovarian follicles in all stages of development. Surrounding the cortex is a layer of dense connective tissue called tunica albuginea. The outer surface of the ovary is covered by a single layer of simple cuboidal epithelium called germinal epithelium.

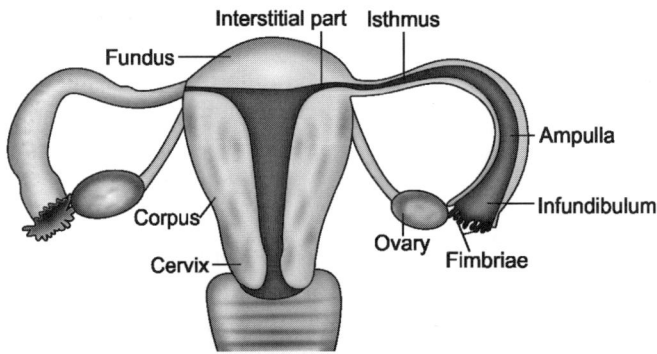

Fig. 19.8: Uterus, uterine tubes and ovary

Functions of the Ovaries

Oogenesis

Oogenesis is the process by which primitive female gametes become mature ova.

Before birth, primitive female sex cells (oogonia) reproduce in the ovaries by mitosis to form primary oocytes (immature ova). At birth the ovaries contain about 2 million primordial follicles, each containing a primary oocyte surrounded by epithelial cells. During childhood many of these follicles degenerate, so that at puberty only about 400 000 remain. During the reproductive years, some 500 of the follicles will mature and expel their ova; the remainder degenerate and by the end of the reproductive period (menopause) only a few primordial follicles are left.

Very little development takes place in the ovaries between childhood and the onset of puberty. During puberty the internal organs of the reproductive system reach maturity, become active and menstruation begins (menarche).

The mature ovary has a cycle of activity which occupies approximately 28 days (although it may be as short as 21 days or as long as 35 days).

The ovarian cycle begins on the first day of menstruation. The secretion of follicle stimulating hormone (FSH) by the anterior pituitary gland stimulates several primordial follicles, which begin to grow and develop, although only one will reach maturity (Fig. 19.9).

The primary oocyte within the follicle enlarges and the epithelial cells of the follicle (membrana granulosa) proliferate and becomes separated from the oocyte by a membrane called zona pellucida. The stromal cells of the ovary form a capsule around the follicle. The capsule consists of two layers, an inner vascular layer, the theca interna, and theca externa, an outer fibrous layer. The granulosa cells begin

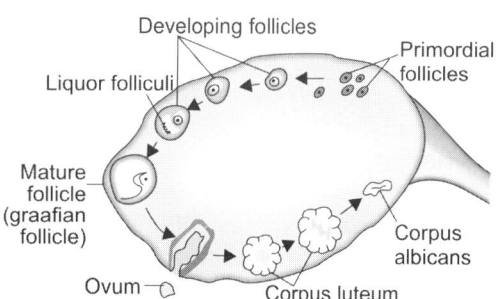

Fig. 19.9: Ovary showing stages in development of an ovum from primordial follicle to corpus albicans

to secrete fluid, the liquor folliculi which causes the ovum to be displaced to one side of the follicle, where it becomes surrounded by a mass of granulosa cells called cumulus oophorus. By the time ovulation occurs the oocyte undergoes the first phase of meiosis.

During development the follicle is known as Graafian follicle, and as it ripens the follicle secretes the hormone estrogen in increasing amounts until production reaches a peak just before ovulation.

Ovulation

During development of the follicle the anterior pituitary also secretes luteinizing hormone (LH), which assists FSH to promote final follicular growth and ovulation. A few hours after estrogen production reaches a maximum there is a marked increase in the secretion of LH. The follicle swells with fluid and ruptures through the surface of the ovary, expelling the ovum into the peritoneal cavity. About the time of ovulation the outer end of the uterine tube moves closer to the ovary to facilitate the entry of the ovum into the tube.

After ovulation the follicle collapses and the granulosa cells enlarge and proliferate. This process is called luteinization, and is controlled by LH.

The resulting glandular structure is called the corpus luteum (yellow body). The corpus luteum grows for about 7–8 days, secreting increasing amounts of progesterone and estrogen, which initiate a feedback mechanism to cause a decrease in the production of FSH and LH by the anterior pituitary.

If the ovum is not fertilized the corpus luteum begins to degenerate and its production of hormones ceases. Connective tissue invades the corpus luteum and it is gradually transformed into a white scar, the corpus albicans.

The anterior pituitary, which is no longer inhibited by the secretion of progesterone and estrogen, begins to secrete increasing amounts of FSH. Menstruation occurs and a new ovarian cycle begins.

If the ovum is fertilized and implants in the uterus the corpus luteum continues to grow and produces large amounts of estrogen and progesterone during the early months of pregnancy.

Ovulation occurs approximately 14 days before the next ovarian cycle commences; thus in a 28 day cycle ovulation occurs about day 14. However in cycles of different lengths the preovulatory phase is variable; for example in a 21 day cycle ovulation would occur about day 7.

Although normally only a single ovum is released from the ovaries in each cycle, multiple ovulation sometimes occurs.

Secretion of Hormones

Ovarian endocrine activity is mainly concerned with the secretion of estrogen and progesterone, but in addition the ovaries synthesize androgens.

Estrogen is a collective name for a group of steroid compounds (Estradiol, estriol and estrone) which are of similar structure. Estrogen is responsible for the development of secondary sexual characteristics at puberty, and for the growth and development of the female reproductive tract and mammary glands.

Progesterone is a steroid compound which can only affect tissues that have already been influenced by estrogen. Its principal function is to initiate secretory changes in the endometrium in preparation for pregnancy. It also acts in conjunction with estrogen to promote the proliferation and enlargement of the alveolar cells of the breast.

Androgens are secreted in small amounts by the ovaries, and are thought to be synthesized by the stromal cells and hilus cells of the ovarian medulla.

Control of Ovarian Functions (Fig. 19.10)

The production of ovarian hormones, and thus the ovarian cycle, are controlled by the *gonadotrophic hormones* released by the pituitary gland.

Puberty and the Menarche

Puberty means being functionally capable of procreation and is characterized by sexual maturation. It is the beginning of adolescence, during which mental and emotional maturation occurs and physical growth becomes complete. The menarche is the onset of menstruation.

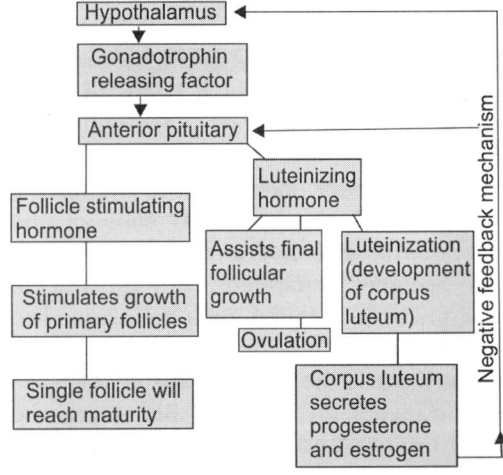

Fig. 19.10: Hormonal control of the ovarian cycle

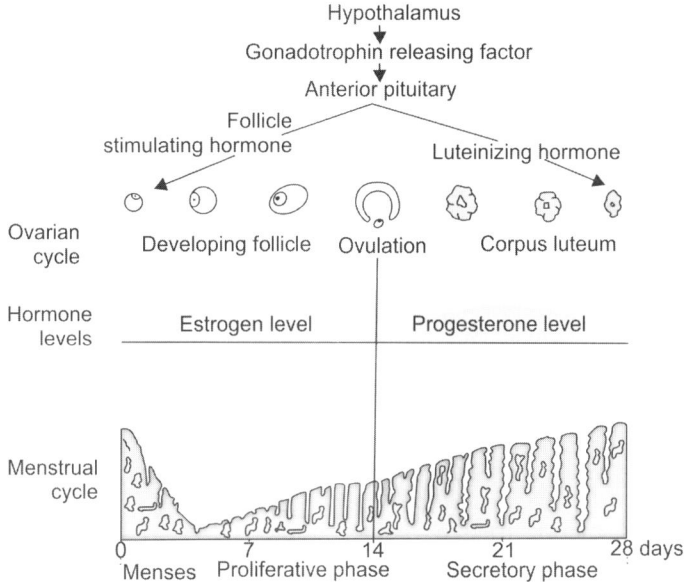

Fig. 19.11: Relationship of ovarian and menstrual cycles

Menstruation

Throughout the reproductive years, from the menarche until the menopause, the endometrium undergoes cyclical changes. The endometrial or menstrual cycle is closely related to the ovarian cycle and takes place over approximately 28 days. It can be described in three phases, each phase passing gradually into the next (Fig. 19.11).

The Proliferative Phase

During menstruation most of the endometrial lining of the uterus is shed, leaving only a thin basal layer of the endometrium. The proliferative phase begins at the end of menstruation. Estrogen, secreted in increasing quantities by the ovaries during the first part of the ovarian cycle, causes rapid proliferation of the epithelium. The endometrial blood vessels and glands grow longer and more coiled. By the end of the proliferative phase, (about 14 days from the onset of menstruation) the endometrium is from 2–3 mm in thickness.

This phase ends when ovulation occurs.

The Secretory Phase

Following ovulation the endometrium continues to hypertrophy under the influence of *progesterone* secreted by the corpus luteum. The endometrial glands become larger and more tortuous, store large amounts of glycogen, and begin secretory activity. The epithelium becomes increasingly vascular and edematous.

Towards the end of this phase, which lasts approximately 14 days, the endomefrium has a thickness of 4–6 mm. This thick, soft vascular surface is ready to receive a fertilized ovum. If implantation of a fertilized ovum takes place the endometrium continues to grow and becomes the decidua of pregnancy. In this case the next phase of the menstrual cycle does not occur.

The Menstrual Phase

If the ovum is not fertilized, the corpus luteum degenerates and the secretion of estrogen and progesterone decreases rapidly. The endometrium is infiltrated by leucocytes and the blood vessels constrict causing shrinking and ischemia. The necrotic surface layers of the endometrium are shed as the menstrual flow. The average duration of the menses is about 5 days, although 1 to 10 days may be considered with in the normal range.

Normally the blood loss during menstruation causes a slight fall in the hemoglobin level; hence women need a greater intake of iron in their diets.

■ THE FEMALE CLIMACTERIC AND MENOPAUSE

The female climacteric is a transitional phase which occurs at the end of the reproductive years. Over a period of one to five years ovarian function gradually declines as the supply of ova becomes exhausted. The resulting fall in estrogen secretion causes many physiological changes. The menstrual cycle and menstruation become irregular and infrequent. Complete cessation of menstruation is known as menopause. Vasomotor instability occurs, resulting in a tendency to sudden flushing (hot flushes), night sweats and palpitations. These effects are often precipitated by anxiety, warm environments and alcohol. The severity of these symptoms varies greatly in each individual. The breasts and the organs of the genital tract atrophy. Psychological symptoms may occur such as anxiety, irritability, fatigue and loss of concentration.

The climacteric may be induced by surgical removal of the ovaries, or by pelvic irradiation in a woman of any age.

■ THE BREASTS (MAMMARY GLANDS) (FIG. 19.12)

The breasts are accessory glands of the female reproductive system. In childhood and in the male they are present in a rudimentary form only. In the female the breasts begin to develop at puberty due to the influence of the ovarian hormones.

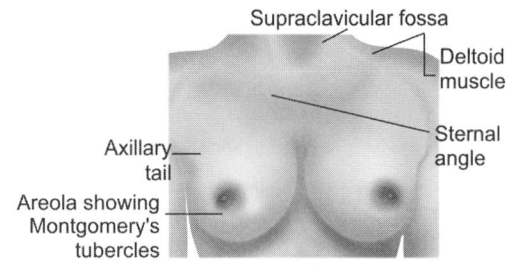

Fig. 19.12: The breasts of a girl aged eighteen years

Estrogen stimulates growth of the ducts, while progesterone stimulates development of the alveoli.

Following puberty the breasts continue to enlarge due to deposition of fat and connective tissue. However, the breasts remain incompletely developed until pregnancy occurs, when there is further growth of both ducts and alveoli.

Each breast lies over the pectoralis muscles, extending from the second rib downwards to the sixth rib, and horizontally from the margin of the sternum to the mid-axillary line.

The size and shape of the breasts of mature women vary considerably.

Structure (Fig. 19.13)

The breast consists of 15 to 20 lobes separated by fibrous tissue, which also acts as a supporting framework by forming suspensory ligaments. Each lobe is divided into numerous lobules by delicate connective tissue containing fat cells. Embedded in the lobules are clusters of alveoli, the secretory cells of the gland. The alveoli are drained by minute ducts, which unite to form one lactiferous duct for each lobe. The lactiferous ducts pass towards the nipple, and close to their termination widen to form ampullae or lactiferous sinuses.

The nipple is composed of erectile tissue covered by pigmented epithelium containing smooth muscle fibers, which when contracted harden and elevate the

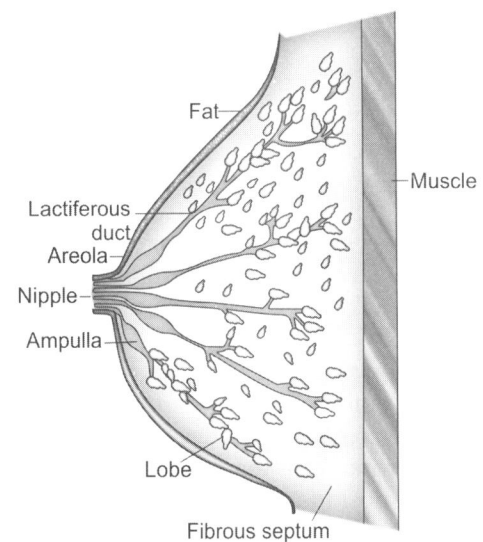

Fig. 19.13: Section of the breast

nipple. The lactiferous ducts open onto the surface of the nipple.

Surrounding the nipple is a pigmented area of skin, the areola, which contains a number of specialized sebaceous glands (the glands of Montgomery).

Blood Supply

Arterial blood is supplied by branches of the thoracic arteries and the anterior intercostal arteries.

The veins of the breast drain into a venous plexus encircling the nipple, which in turn drains into the axillary, internal thoracic and intercostal veins.

Lymph Drainage

The mammary glands are drained by superficial and deep lymphatic vessels.

The superficial vessels drain the skin and subcutaneous tissues of the breast, and converge to form a diffuse lymphatic plexus with the lymphatic vessels draining the nipple and areola. The deep lymphatic vessels are found within the lobes of the breast draining the alveoli and ducts.

The lymphatic plexuses of the superficial vessels join the deep lymphatics. Over 85% of the lymph from the breasts drains into the axillary nodes; the remainder drains into the lymph nodes accompanying the internal thoracic artery. In addition there are communicating channels between the lymphatic plexuses of the two breasts.

The extensive lymphatic drainage of the breasts provides an important route for the rapid spread of cancerous cells throughout the body.

Nerve Supply

The breast receives sympathetic nerve fibers from branches of the second to sixth thoracic nerves, which are accompanied by sensory nerve fibers. The breast tissue contains numerous free and encapsulated nerve endings, particularly around the nipple.

■ FUNCTIONS OF THE BREAST

The mammary glands are inactive until stimulated by pregnancy to secrete milk to nourish a newborn infant.

Profound changes occur in the breast during pregnancy in preparation for lactation. After conception there is a general enlargement and hardening of the breasts; the veins on the surface become dilated and dark brown pigment is deposited in the areola. These changes are initially due to the increased production of ovarian hormones, but later are due to placental hormones. Estrogen stimulates growth of the intralobular ducts, and progesterone, acting on the estrogen-primed tissues, stimulates growth of the alveoli and development of the secretory cells. Other hormones, including growth hormone, prolactin, thyroxin and adrenocorticoids, are also important in the development of the mammary glands.

Towards the end of pregnancy, and for a few days after delivery, a watery fluid called colostrum is secreted by the breast. After childbirth there is a fall in the blood levels of estrogen, which stimulates the anterior pituitary to release prolactin. Prolactin stimulates the process of lactation. Milk production commences 3–4 days after childbirth. The posterior pituitary hormone oxytocin causes the expulsion of milk from the alveoli to the ducts. The secretion of oxytocin is stimulated by the infant suckling at the breast. Regular suckling if the infant is necessary to maintain lactation.

■ PREGNANCY

Following expulsion of the ovum from the ovary it enters one of the uterine tubes. The ovum remains viable for approximately 12 to 24 hours and is still surrounded by a mass of granulosa cells, the cumulus oophorus, which radiates out from the oocyte and is known as the corona radiata. During sexual intercourse sperm enter the female vagina with each ejaculation of semen. Passage of the sperm to the uterine tubes is accomplished partly by sperm motility and partly by contractions of the uterus. Fertilization usually takes place in the uterine tube. Only one sperm is required for fertilization of the ovum. The head of the sperm enters the ovum by penetrating the corona radiata and the underlying zona pellucida. Penetration of the sperm into the ovum is facilitated by proteolytic enzymes. Changes occur in the zona pellucida which prevent penetration of the ovum by other sperm.

When the sperm enters the ovum it loses its tail and body, and the head of the sperm begins to swell forming a male pronuclear. The pronucleus of the ovum and the male pronucleus do not merge but form a new nucleus, each contributing 23 chromosomes to produce a total of 46.

The fertilized ovum begins a series of cell divisions by mitosis, and by the time it has reached the uterine cavity 3–4 days later it forms a mass of cells called morule. During the next few days the morula develops a central fluid filled cavity and is now known as blastocyst. The cells of the blastocyst become differentiated into a double layered wall called trophoblast and an inner cell mass from which the fetus will be formed.

Following fertilization of the ovum, the endometrial lining of the uterus continues to develop under the influence of progesterone from the corpus luteum, and is called decidua. The trophoblast secretes proteolytic enzymes which digest the cells of the decidua to obtain nourishment; and to embed the blastocyst into the deeper layers of the endometrium. The trophoblast develops projections which invade the endometrium and which will become the placental villi.

As the cells of the inner cell mass continue to divide, two cavities appear; one is the amniotic cavity and the other forms the yolk sac. The two cavities are separated by a double layer of cells, the embryonic plate. The cells of the embryonic plate are destined to become the embryo; the layer lining the amniotic cavity is the ectoderm and that lining the yolk sac is the endoderm. A third layer of cells, the mesoderm develops between these two, and grows out to form the umbilical cord through which the embryonic circulation will extend into the placenta. Blood capillaries grow into the villi of the trophoblast through the umbilical cord from the vascular system of the embryo, and maternal blood sinuses form in the endometrium surrounding the villi. Oxygen and nutrients pass from the maternal blood sinuses to the blood capillaries of the embryo by diffusion, while waste product from the embryo diffuse in

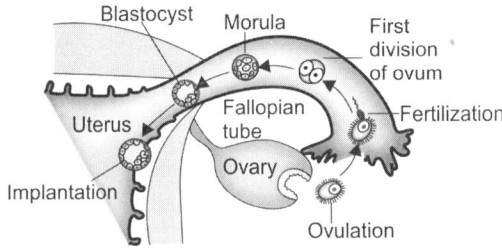

Fig. 19.14: From ovulation to implantation

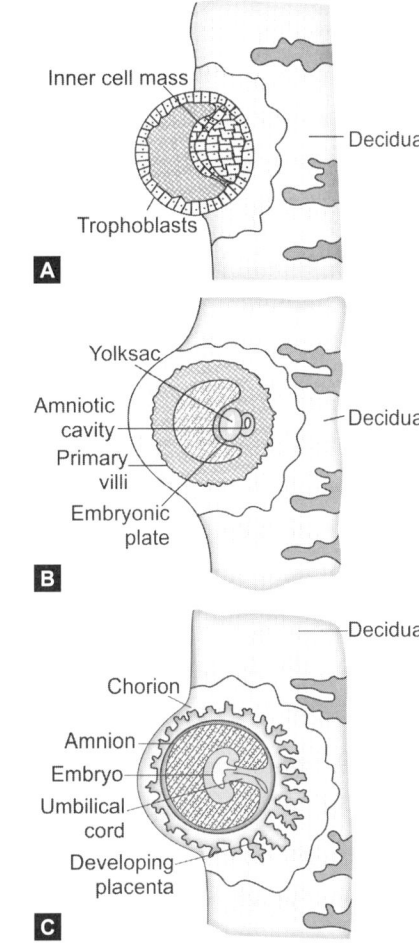

Figs 19.15A to C: Development of the embryo and placenta: **A.** At implantation; **B.** Differentiation of inner cell mass; **C.** Development of the umbilical cord and placenta

the opposite direction to the mother for excretion. At no time during pregnancy do the two circulations come into direct contact, the exchange of nutrients taking place across a membrane called chorion.

As the blastocyst increases in size it bulges into the uterine cavity and the villi on the exposed surface atrophy. The remaining villi become restricted to one area and form the placenta. From the time of implantation (Fig. 19.14) the trophoblast begins to secrete small amounts of human chorionic gonadotropin (hCG); this prevents the corpus luteum from degenerating and causes it to continue to secrete progesterone and estrogen, which maintain the decidual endometrium to provide for the early development of the placenta and embryo (Figs 19.15A to C).

The corpus luteum reaches its peak activity during the first eight weeks of pregnancy, and then begins to wane. By the sixteenth week it has ceased to be active and the placenta becomes totally responsible for the secretion of estrogen and progesterone. The placenta continues to produce HCG in increasing amounts until about the eighth week; from this time the HCG production falls to a low constant level for the remainder of the pregnancy. The presence of HCG forms the basis of pregnancy tests, since it is excreted in the maternal urine soon after the first missed menstrual period.

In addition, from the fifth week of pregnancy the placenta begins to secrete a hormone called human placental lactogen (HPL) which has actions similar to those of growth hormone, and probably plays an important role in the growth and development of the fetus.

By the sixth week of pregnancy the ectoderm, mesoderm and endoderm will have formed all the essential structures of the body, and by the eighth week the embryo is recognizable as human baby. It now becomes known as fetus. By the sixteenth week it is possible to determine the sex of the fetus and further development is mainly growth (Fig. 19.16).

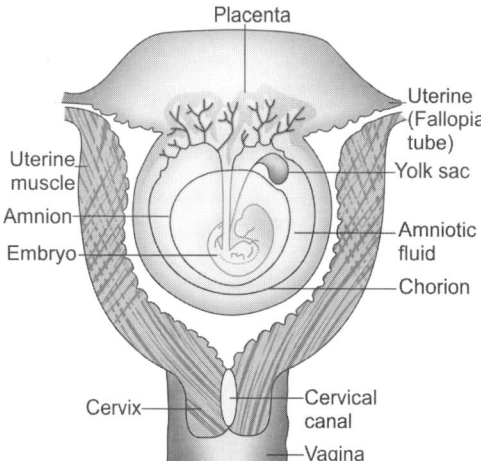

Fig. 19.16: Uterus and embryo in early pregnancy

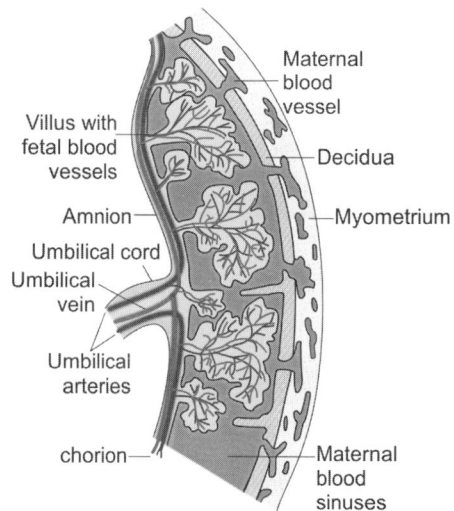

Fig. 19.17: Fully developed placenta

During the development of the embryo the trophoblasts produce an inner layer of cells which form a membrane called chorion; this covers the fetal surface of the placenta and umbilical cord (Fig. 19.17). The amniotic cavity grows rapidly until it fills the original blastocyst and its cells come into close contact with the chorionic. This membrane is the amnion; it lines the chorion and covers the umbilical cord, being continuous with the skin of the fetus at the umbilicus. The amnion produces a fluid, liquor amnii, in which the fetus is suspended.

The chorion and amnion form the fetal sac, which encloses and protects the fetus until it ruptures during labor and allows expulsion of the baby (Fig. 19.18).

Changes in Maternal Physiology in Pregnancy

During pregnancy there are widespread physiological changes in the mother, involving most of the systems of the body, which result in alteration of metabolic, chemical and endocrine balance.

- The uterus gradually enlarges, mainly due to hypertrophy of individual muscle fibers and partly by the formation of new fibers. The uterine growth rate is usually regular and provides a means of estimating the period of gestation by measurement of the fundal height (Fig. 19.19).

  The cervix becomes softer and the cervical glands secrete a tenacious mucus which forms a plug that fills the cervical canal. Expulsion of this mucoid plug as the 'show' frequently occurs a few hours before the onset of labor.

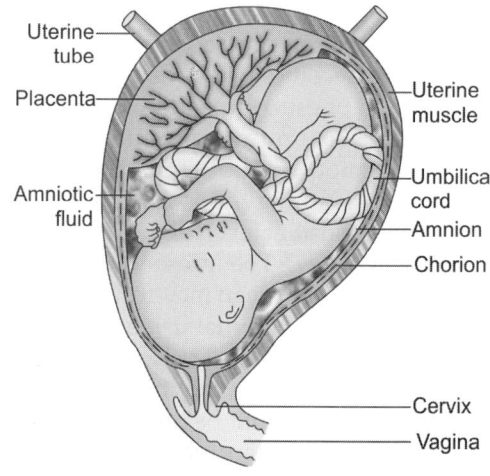

Fig. 19.18: Full-term pregnancy

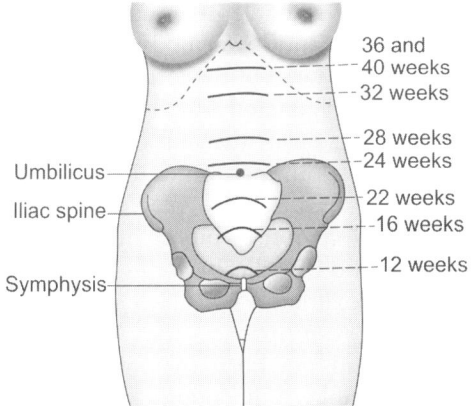

Fig. 19.19: Height of the fundus of the uterus during weeks of pregnancy

- The breasts begin to enlarge early in pregnancy with increased brown pigmentation of the areola. The sebaceous glands of the areola become raised, appearing as small nodules, and are known as Montgomery's tubercles. A small amount of fluid (colostrum) can be expressed from the nipples. In mid-pregnancy, patchy pigmentation develops around the areola and forms the secondary areola.
- The skin of the abdominal wall becomes stretched and pink striations sometimes develop (striae gravidarum). Increased pigmentation of the skin may also occur on the forehead and cheeks (known as the chloasma or mask of pregnancy), and a dark line (the linea nigra) may be seen extending from the umbilicus to the pubis.
- *Metabolism:* In addition to placental hormone production in pregnancy, there is increased secretion of many hormones including thyroxine, adrenocorticoids and sex hormones. Carbohydrate metabolism is altered, and there may be a lowered renal threshold for glucose resulting in glycosuria. As a result of the increased endocrine functions the basal metabolic rate rises by 15–20% during the latter part of pregnancy.
- *Weight gain:* In the entire pregnancy averages about 24 lbs (11 kg). The fetus, placenta and liquor amnii account for approximately 10 lbs (4.5 kg). The increase in uterine and breast size accounts for about 4 lbs (1.8 kg). The remainder is due to increased blood volume, fat deposition and fluid retention.
- *Nutrition:* Early in pregnancy nausea and vomiting commonly occurs ('morning sickness') and is thought to be due to hormonal changes, but usually disappears after the first three months.

  During pregnancy the mother's diet must supply the energy requirements for the additional maternal tissues and the growing fetus as well as for her own health. If the diet is inadequate, the fetus will obtain its nourishment at the expense of the mother's tissues. The mother's diet therefore should contain adequate quantities of protein, carbohydrate and fat as well as vitamins, calcium and iron.
- *The Cardiovascular System:* The volume of the circulating plasma is increased by approximately 30%, mainly during the second half of pregnancy. There is also a small increase in red cells, but the total hemoglobin concentration falls to about 12 g/100 mL of blood. This must not be interpreted as anemia, although this may occur if the dietary intake of iron and folate is inadequate for the combined needs of the mother and fetus.

  As a result of the increased blood volume and the rise in general metabolic demands the cardiac output increases by 25–30%.
- Respiration increases in depth rather than rate, to supply the extra oxygen

- **Fetal circulation:** The placenta is the fetal lung. Its maternal portion is in effect a large blood sinus. In this lake project the villi of the fetal portion containing the small branches the fetal umbilical arteries and vein. O_2 is taken up by fetal blood and CO_2 is charged into the maternal circulation across the walls of the villi in a fashion analogous to O_2 and CO_2 exchange in the lungs. The cellular layers covering the villi are thicker and less permeable than the alveolar membranes in the lungs and exchange is less efficient. The placenta is also the route by which all nutritive materials enter to the fetus and by which fetal waste are discharged to the maternal blood.

  Fifty-five percent of the fetal cardiac output goes through the placenta. The blood in the umbilical vein in human is 80% saturated with O_2. In adult arterial circulation is 98% saturated. The ductus venosus divert some of this blood directly to the IVC and the remainder mixes with the portal blood of the fetus. The portal and systemic venous blood of the fetus is only 26% saturated and saturation of the mixed blood in the IVC is approximately 67%. Most of the blood entering the heart through the IVC is diverted directly to the left atrium via the patent foramen ovale. Most of the blood from the SVC enters the right ventricle and is expelled into pulmonary artery. The resistance of the collapsed lungs is high and the pressure in pulmonary artery is several mm Hg higher than it is in the aorta, so that most of the blood in the pulmonary artery passes through ductus arteriosus to the aorta. In this fashion the relatively unsaturated blood from the right ventricle is diverted to the trunk and lower body of the fetus, while the head of the fetus receives the better oxygenated blood from the left ventricle. From the aorta some of the blood is pumped into the umbilical arteries and back to placenta. The O_2 saturation of the blood in the lower aorta and umbilical arteries of the fetus is approximately 60%.

- **Fetal respiration:** The tissues of fetal and newborn mammals have a remarkable but poorly understood resistance to hypoxia. The O_2 saturation of the maternal blood in the placenta is so low that the fetus might suffer hypoxic damage if the fetal red cells did not have a greater O_2 affinity than adult red cells. The fetal red cells contain fetal Hb (HbF) whereas adult cells contains adult Hb (HbA). The cause of the difference in O_2 affinity between the two is that HbF binds 2,3,OPG less effectively than HbA. does.Decrease in O_2 affinity due to the binding of 2,3, OPG is responsible for this.

  Some HbA is present in blood during fetal life. After birth no more HbF is normally formed and by the age of 4 months 90% of the circulating Hb is HbA.

- **Changes in fetal circulation and respiration at birth:** Because of the patent ductus arteriosus (PDA) and foramen ovale the left heart and right heart pump is parallel in the fetus than in series as they do in adult. At birth the placental circulation is cut off and the peripheral resistance suddenly rises. The pressure in aorta rises until that it exceeds that in pulmonary artery. By that time placental circulation has been cut off the infant become increasingly asphyxial. Finally infant gasps several times, lung expand, and the markedly negative intrathoracic pressure

(–30—50) during the gasps contribute to the expansion of the lungs. The sucking action of the first breath plus constriction of umbilical vein squeezes as much as 100 ml of blood from the placenta (the placental transfusion).

Once the lungs are expanded the pulmonary vascular resistance falls to less than 20% of the *in vitro* value and pulmonary blood flow increases markedly. Blood returning from the lungs raises the pressure in the left atrium closing the foramen ovale by pushing the valve that guards it against the inter arterial septum. The ductus arteriosus constricts within a few hours after birth producing functional closure and permanent anatomic closure follows in the next 24–48 hours due to extensive intimal thickening.

The mechanism producing the initial constriction is not completely understood but the increasing arterial O_2 tension plays an important role relatively high concentration of vasodilators are present in the ductus in utero—especially PG2å and synthesis of these PG is inhibited, by the inhibition of cyclooxygenase (COX) at birth.

In many premature infants, the ductus fail to close spontaneously but closure can be produced by infusion of drugs that inhibits COX. Better results have been obtained with drugs that inhibit COX1 and COX2.

- *Chorionic Villus Sampling:* Chorionic villus sampling can be for the antenatal diagnosis of certain genetic diseases such as Down syndrome, spina bifida, hemophilia, Tay-Sach's diseases, sickle cell anemia and certain muscular dystrophies. Chorionic villus sampling can be preferred as early as 8th week of gestation which permits and earlier decision on whether or not to continue the pregnancy. The procedure does not require penetration of abdomen, uterus and amniotic cavity. There is 1–2% chance of spontaneous abortion after the test. A catheter is placed through the vagina and cervix of the uterus and advanced to chorionic villi under ultra sound guidance. About 30 mg of tissue are suctioned out and prepared for chromosomal analysis. Chorion cells and fetal cells contain identical genetic information.
- *Infertility:* In 30% of cases problem is in the man and in 45% in the woman, in 20% there is problem in both partners and in 5% no cause can be found.

Diagnosis of the Cause

- In the male semen collected after abstinence for 5 days is analyzed after 30 minutes but within 2 hours for volume sperm count, motility, etc.
- The female is tested to determine if ovulation is occurring by different tests of ovulation.
- Patency of fallopian tubes determined by insufflation of tubes with air or CO_2 via cervix or by hysterosalpingography.

In Vitro Fertilization

On July 12, 1978 first recorded case of *in vitro* fertilization (IVF) (fertilization in laboratory dish) was done. In this procedure for IVF, the mother is to be given follicle stimulating hormone soon after menstruation so that several secondary oocytes are produced. Administration of LH ensure the maturation of the secondary oocytes. Next a small incision is made near umbilical and secondary oocytes are aspirated from the follicles and then transferred to a solution of the male's sperm.

Once fertilization has taken place the fertilized ovum is put in another medium and observed for cleavage. When fertilized ovum reaches the 8 cell or 16 cell stages it is introduced into the uterus for implantation and further growth.

Embryo transfer: It is a type of IVF in which a husband's semen is used to artificially inseminate a fertile secondary oocyte donor and after fertilization, the morula or blastocyst is transferred from the donor to the infertile wife who carries it to term.

Indication: Infertile female carriers of serious genetic disorder who do not want to pass their own genes to progeny.

GIFT: In this, the normal process of conception by uniting sperm and secondary oocyte on the prospective mother's uterine tubes is mimicked. The female is given FSH and LH to stimulate the production of several secondary oocytes. The secondary oocytes are aspirated with a laparoscope fitted with suction device, mixed with solution of male's sperm outside the body and then immediately inserted into the uterine tubes.

Hyper prolactinemia: Up to 70% patients with chromophobe adenomas of anterior pituitary have elevated plasma prolactin levels. It produce galactorrhea. Fifteen to twenty percent of women with secondary amenorrhea have elevated prolactin levels and when prolactin secretion is reduced normal menstrual cycles and fertility return. Prolactin produces amenorrhea by blocking the action of gonadotrophins on the ovaries.

There are two principle types of estrogen receptors (ER) are as follows:

One on chromosome 6, second on chromosome 14. After binding estrogen they form homodimers, bind to DNA altering its transcription.

Estrogen receptor 1 found in uterus, kidneys, liver and heart, estrogen receptor 2 found in ovaries, prostate, lungs, GIT, hematopoietic system and CNS. Most of the effects of estrogen are genomic due to actions of the nucleus. Neuronal discharge in brain and feedback effects on gonadotropin secretion are very rapid. They produced their effects by intracellular nitrogen activated protein kinase pathways.

Synthetic and environmental estrogens: Ethinyl derivative of estradiol is a potent estrogen, and is active when given by mouth because it is resistant to hepatic metabolism. Other naturally occurring estrogen are having relatively low activity when they are administered by mouth (due to portal venous drainage of intestine which carry them to the liver where they are inactivated).

Dioxins: Found in environment has both estrogenic and antiestrogenic effects.

Tamoxifen: Not stimulate breast.

Raloxifene: Not stimulate breast or uterus.

Selective estrogen receptor modulators (SERM): The effects of SERM brought about is related to the complexity of estrogen receptors and hence to differences in the way Receptor-Ligand complexes they form bind to DNA.

CHAPTER 20

Ageing

Ageing is not something that happens suddenly after 40, 50, 60 or some other determinate number of years. Old age (senescence) is, with certain exceptions, the culmination of many years of slowly declining function and degenerating structure. All physiological functions decline as ageing increases and ageing results in increased susceptibility to stress and disease. Disease and trauma may accelerate the effects of ageing. Healing and recovery are much slower in the elderly. Normal elderly people have a physiology that is adequate for resting conditions but, compared to young people, they show slower adjustment to environmental change and a diminished reserve capacity.

It is therefore particularly important for doctors, nurses and others to know what changes ageing causes, as these must be taken into account in the treatment of disease.

■ CHANGES DUE TO AGEING

The Skin

With ageing the skin becomes wrinkled because there is a loss of subcutaneous fat and the dermis shrinks, losing its elasticity. With less support from the dermis and subcutaneous tissues the epidermis develops folds or wrinkles. Blood flow to the skin is reduced, the epidermis becomes thinner and surface blood capillaries become more fragile. There is an overall decrease in the number of functioning melanocytes, resulting in grey hair and changes in skin color. However, some melanocytes increase in size producing brown 'age spots'.

Sebaceous glands atrophy, skin and hair become dry and brittle and, because it breaks easily, the skin is more susceptible to infection. Sweat glands also atrophy, a fact which contributes to the reduced ability of the elderly to adjust to increased environmental temperatures.

Axillary and pubic hair decrease and nails thicken.

The Musculoskeletal System

Body stature diminishes with age. While the length of the long bones remains constant there is thinning of the intervertebral disks resulting in decreased height. Bone mass is reduced as the bones tend to lose calcium and become thinner and more brittle with ageing. The risk of injury resulting in fractures, especially of the femur, are greater.

Joint capsules and cartilage becomes calcified resulting in stiff joints which limit the elderly person's mobility.

Muscle fibers atrophy and are replaced by fibrous tissue, resulting in decrease in muscle power.

The Cardiovascular System

Myocardial function diminishes and cardiac output falls gradually with age. The older heart has a reduced myocardial reserve and is unable to respond to a demand for an increased cardiac output as efficiently as a young heart, and cardiac failure is more easily induced (e.g. by over-zealous intravenous therapy).

With ageing, arteries become less elastic because the muscle fibers of the tunica media are replaced by collagen fibers. The gradual development of arteriosclerosis may cause a further decrease in the distensibility of the arteries. These changes cause an increase in peripheral resistance which results in an increase in blood pressure, especially the systolic pressure.

The Respiratory System

Chest movement diminishes because of increasing rigidity of the thoracic cage, and vital capacity is reduced. Alveoli become less elastic and enlarge as the alveolar walls become weakened. Bronchioles and alveolar ducts also lose their elasticity and become dilated. A decrease in ciliary action combined with the structural changes increases the susceptibility of the elderly to respiratory infection. Ageing also results in less efficient diffusion and tissue utilization of oxygen. It is not surprising that elderly people more easily become short of breath than do young people.

The Urinary System

In the ageing kidney the number of functioning nephrons is reduced and the kidneys become smaller. The basement membrane of Bowman's capsule becomes thicker leading to a diminished permeability of the membrane. These changes result in a reduction in the glomerular filtration rate. Additionally, the excretory and reabsorptive capacities of the renal tubules decrease as age increases. Therefore, the kidneys do not concentrate urine as efficiently in the elderly, although under normal circumstances renal function, remains adequate.

Bladder capacity diminishes, especially in the female, and can result in an immediate, urgent need to urinate. It often becomes necessary for the older person to void urine during the night.

The Digestive System

Some characteristic changes occur in the anatomy and physiology of the digestive system with ageing.

Teeth become darker with age and the permeability of the enamel decreases. The enamel at the contact points of teeth is gradually reduced and the grinding surfaces of the molars wear down. Changes in the formation of dentine result in a gradual reduction in the size of the pulp cavity. Gum margins tend to recede leading to exposure of the roots.

Dryness of the mouth may be noted due to a reduction in mucus secretion. Since mucus secretion is necessary for the retention of complete dentures an elderly person may experience considerable difficulty in keeping their dentures in place, especially when dentures are new.

A reduction in the flow of saliva, diminishes the moisture added to food in the mouth and may affect an individual's enjoyment of particular foods.

Atrophy and diminished enzyme secretion mean that the digestion of food takes longer and its absorption may be impaired. The reduced gastrointestinal movement may lead to constipation, which is exacerbated by a reduction in mucous secretion by the mucosal cells lining the large intestine due to atrophy.

The Endocrine System

The secretion of sex hormones declines sharply in women at the menopause while in men there is a slower progressive decrease. Thyroxine secretion and hence basal metabolic rate (BMR) gradually diminishes with age. Glucose tolerance also diminishes.

The Reproductive System

In the male, changes in the reproductive system occur gradually. The testes continue to produce spermatozoa well into advanced old age, although there is a decrease in the number of viable spermatozoa. Testosterone secretion tends to diminish with increasing age. Sexual arousal is slower with ageing, the number and volume of ejaculations is reduced but feelings of stimulation and satisfaction remain. The prostate gland usually increases in size and may cause urinary difficulties.

Following the menopause, the female is no longer able to reproduce because of atrophy of the ovaries. The uterus and cervix shrink. The walls of the vagina become less elastic and the mucosal rugae flatten. Vaginal secretions diminish and become less acid. There is a loss of subcutaneous fat in the external genitalia; pubic and vulval hair becomes thinner. Due to lack of ovarian hormones there is atrophy of the glandular tissue of the breasts. However, despite the changes occurring in the genital tract there is no loss of female libido.

The Nervous System

The Brain

Each day approximately 1000 neurons are lost from the brain. Fortunately there is a large reserve and many elderly people never show obvious senile mental changes. The velocity of transmission of nerve impulses is reduced and reaction time is slower in the elderly.

The Autonomic Nervous System

Vasomotor control is often impaired in elderly people. Diminished blood supply to the brain may cause unsteadiness, faintness and falling after sudden assumption of the erect posture. Nurses have to remember this when getting elderly patients out of bed, and may have to proceed very slowly.

■ THE SPECIAL SENSES

Eyes

The lens capsule of the eye becomes less elastic and is unable to accommodate to a shape sufficiently convex to focus on near objects. The 'long sight' resulting from this ageing process is known as presbyopia. Sometimes the lens becomes opaque and prevents light entering the eye (cataract). There is loss of peripheral vision, and it takes longer to adapt to light changes.

Ears

Hearing impairment increases with ageing, and is associated with increased deposition of wax in the external auditory meatus, rigidity of the ossicles and degeneration of the vestibulocochlear nerve (VIIIth cranial nerve).

Taste

The number of taste buds on the tongue is reduced with ageing. There appears to be a decreased sensitivity to sweet and salty substances, while there is an increased sensitivity to bitter substances. These changes may result in a preference for very sweet foods.

■ TEMPERATURE REGULATION

With ageing the ability of the temperature-regulating system to maintain core temperature in extreme environmental temperatures appears to be impaired. There is impairment of the mechanisms for heat production and preservation. Some people feel the cold more as they age whilst others are uncomplaining in a cold home environment which their younger relatives, accustomed to efficient modern heating, would not tolerate.

Old people commonly fail to produce a pyrexia when suffering from infections such as pneumonia.

■ THIRST

The sensation of thirst may be diminished in elderly people, who become dehydrated more easily, especially when they are ill.

■ PAIN

Pain is sometimes less keenly appreciated by elderly people. A myocardial infarction or 'acute abdomen' may be painless (silent).

■ RESISTANCE TO INFECTION

There is increased susceptibility to infection in old age because of a diminished antibody response and reduced serum immunoglobulin concentrations.

■ THE RELEVANCE OF AGEING TO CLINICAL MEDICINE

Nurses, physiotherapists and other professional people will realize that, because of impaired vasomotor control, elderly people often cannot be got out of their beds hurriedly without making them feel faint and unsteady.

Doctors avoid misguided attempts at treatment of a raised blood pressure by relating the degree of elevation to the patient's age. For example, a blood pressure of 180/95 mm Hg in a patient aged 70 years would not call for any treatment. Indeed, effective treatment would be likely to induce disabling postural hypotension.

Drug treatment of any condition may be fraught with special problems in old age. The absorption, metabolism and excretion of a drug may all be slowed. Therefore, it is often necessary to reduce the standard dosage of some drugs. Failure to do this may result in digitalis intoxication in elderly patients.

Weights and Measures

1 ounce (oz) = 28.35 gram (g)
1 pound (lb) = 16 ounces = 0.45 kilogram (kg)
1 stone = 14 lb = 6.3 kg

1 fluid ounce = 28.41 milliliter (mL)
1 pint = 560 mL

1 yard = 36 inches (in) = 0.91 meters (m)
1 foot = 30.48 centimeters (cm)
1 inch = 2.54 centimeters

1 kilogram = 2.2 pounds = 35.27 ounces

1 liter = 1.75 pints = 35 fluid ounces (fl oz) = 0.22 gallon
1 mL = 15 minims

1 meter = 1.09 yards = 39.37 inches = 3.28 feet

To convert:
grams to ounces multiply by 0.03
ounces to gram multiply by 28.0
minims to milliliter multiply by 0.06
pints to liters multiply by 0.57

Fahrenheit to Centigrade or Celsius, subtract 32 and multiply by $\frac{5}{9}$

Centigrade or Celsius to Fahrenheit, multiply by $\frac{9}{5}$ and add 32

SI Units

The International System of Units (Systeme International, SI) is the system used in British Medicine for weights and measures. It is based on seven fundamental units: the meter (m); kilogram (kg); second (s); ampere (A); kelvin (K); candela (cd); and mole (mol). Other units such as those of pressure, the pascal (Pa) and energy, the joule (J), are derived from the basic units. Prefixes are used to indicate fractions or multiples of all these units. The prefixes are as given in the following table:

Prefixes for SI units

Factor by which unit is multiplied	Prefix	Symbol of prefix
10^{12}	tera	T
10^{9}	giga	G
10^{6}*	mega	M
10^{3}*	kilo	k
10^{2}	hecto	h
10^{1}	deca	da
10^{-1}*	deci	d
10^{-2}*	centi	c
10^{-3}*	milli	m
10^{-6}*	micro	m
10^{-9}*	nano	n
10^{-12}*	pico	p
10^{-15}	femto	f
10^{-18}	atto	a

*These are the factors which the nurse is likely to encounter in clinical practice

Index

Page numbers followed by *f* refer to figure and *t* refer to table, respectively

A

Abdominal cavity 35
   boundaries of 35
Abdominal wall 210
   anterior 104
   posterior 105
Abdominothoracic in males 123
Abducent nerve 335
Abductor pollicis brevis 48
Absolute refractory period 372
Accoucher's hand 274
Acetabular
   articular surface 83
   fossa 83
Acetabulum, formation of 50
Acetyl coenzyime A 241, 242
Acid base balance 139
Acid citrate dextrose 164
Acid phosphatase myeloperoxidase 151
Acid secretion 226
Acidophilic
   cosin stain 148
   hemoglobin 148
Acidosis 196
Acinar cells 221
Acromegaly 260
ACTH *See* adrenocorticotropic hormone
Actin 90
Actin-based molecular motors 13
Action potential 26
   different types of 27
      biphasic 27
      compound 27
      monophasic 27
      plateau type 27
      rhythmic type 27
      spike potential 27
   functions of neuroglia 27
   in neuron 26*f*
   ionic basis of 27
Activate cellular genes 29
Active transport 15
   primary active transport 15
   secondary active transport 16
Adductor magnus muscle 53
Adenohypophysis 253
Adenoid 112
Adenoidectomy 112
Adenoids 204
Adenosine 121
   diphosphate 238
   monophosphate 238
   triphosphate 238
Adequate stimulus 375
ADHD *See* attention deficit hyperactivity disorder
Adherens junctions 14
Adhesion molecules of IgG subfamily 14
Adipose tissue 19*f*
ADP *See* adenosine diphosphate
Adrenal
   cortex 278
   medullary secretion, regulation of 283
   medullary tumor 194
Adrenalin 193, 187
Adrenergic receptors 281*t*
Adrenocorticotropic hormone 252-254
Adrenogenital syndrome 392
Adrenomedullin 283
Afibrinogenemia 142
Ageing 413
   cardiovascular system 413
   changes due to 413
   digestive system 414
   endocrine system 414

musculoskeletal system 413
nervous system 415
pain 416
reproductive system 415
resistance to infection 416
respiratory system 414
skin 413
special senses 415
temperature regulation 415
thirst 416
urinary system 414
Agglutinogen 161
Aglutinins 138
Agranulocytes 151, 153
Agranulocytosis 154
    clinical features 154
    severe cases 154
Agregation 155
Akinesia 358
Aldosterone 193
    causes 278
    secretion 277
Alkaline phosphatase 139
Alkaline urine 134
Alpha cells 284
Alveolar
    epithelium 121
    fluid 121
    stability 120
Alveoli, collapse of 120
Ameboid movement 151
Amine precursor uptake and decarboxylation 121
Amino acid 139, 149
    absorption of 236
    deamination of 218
    essential and non-essential 243*t*
    gamma aminobutyric acid
    level in blood 288
    reabsorption of 309
Amniotic cavity 408
AMP *See* adenosine monophosphate
Anabolic hormones 244
Anabolism 238
Anaphylactic shock 165
Anastomotic fibers 23
Androgens *in utero* 392
Anemia 140, 144
    break down of Hb 145
    classification of 145
    polycythemia 145
Aneuploidy 11

Angiotensinogen 138
Angiotensin 122
Angstrom, symbol of 12
Animal cell, anatomy of 7*f*
Anisocytosis 140
Ankle bones 42
Ankle joint 88*f*
Annulospiral 367
ANS *See* autonomic nervous system
Anterior pituitary hormones, functions of 253
Anti-allergic effects 280
Anticholinergic agent, cyclopentolate 386
Anticholinesterase enzyme 97
Anticoagulants 158
Anticoagulated blood 138
Antidiuretic hormone 193, 195, 261
Antigen 30, 161
Antithyroid drugs 269
    iodides 269
    propylthiouracil 269
Aorta 167
Aortic
    body 131
    impedance 187
    resistance 186
    valve stenosis 194
Apex 168
Apnea deglutition 133
Apneustic center 131
Apocrine glands 292
Aponeurosis 106
Appendicitis, acute 211
Appendicular skeleton 69
Appendix 204
Appetite 250
APUD *See* amine precursor uptake and
    decarboxylation
Aquaporins 311
Aqueous humor 385
Areolar connective tissue 19*f*
Arginine vasopressin 263
Arm 42
Arneth count 151
Arterial pulse genesis and characters of
    normal pulse 173
Arterioles 188
Arthroscopy of knee 87
Articular, surface 79, 80, 87
Articulations 79
Aryepiglottic folds 114
Arytenoid cartilage 114

Asphyxia 134
    carbon monoxide poisoning 134
    cyanosis 134
Asterocytes 24, 27
Atherosclerosis 169
Atherosclerotic lesions 196
Athetosis 358
Atlanto-axial joint 72
Atonic bladder 319
ATP *See* adenosine triphosphate
Atrial
    depolarization 177
    fibrillation 180
    flutter 180
    natriuretic peptide 193
    systole 186
Atrioventricular 167
    groove (coronary) 168
Attention deficient hyperactivity disorder 268
Auditory apparatus, anatomy of 378
Auerbach's plexus 222
Auricle 377
Autocrine hormones 252
Automatic bladder 319
Automatic nervous system 372
Automobile exhaust 134
Autonomic junctions, chemical transmission 361
Autonomic nervous system 212, 359
    parasympathetic division of 360
    sympathetic division of 359
Autoregulation 196, 197
Axillary nerve 45, 46
Axoaxonal synapse 364
Axon reflex 199

B

Ball and socket joint 45, 80
Ballism 358
Baroreceptor mechanism 187
Baroreceptors 193
Barr body 152
Basal ganglia 356
    disorders 357
    functions of 357
    release phenomenon 357
Basal lamina 96
Basal metabolic rate 239, 414
Basopenia 154
Basophil 152
Basophilic normoblast 148
BCOP *See* blood colloidal osmotic pressure

Becker's muscular dystrophy 94
Bellini 300
Bell-Magendie law 366
Betz cells 341
Biceps femoris 107
Bicondylar joints 80
Bile 220, 230
    canaliculi 218
    composition of 230
    functions of 231
    pigments 220, 231
    salts 220
    secretion of 218
Biliary tract 219
    common bile duct 219
    cystic duct 219
    hepatic duct 219
Bilirubin albumin complex 146
Biliverdin 213
Binocular vision 390
Biot's breathing 135
Bitemporal hemianopia 334
Blast cells, develop to RBC 147
Blastemal stage 37
Blood 137
Blood arterial 128
Blood brain barrier 352
    acquired or conditional reflex 353
    clinical importance of 353
    conditional reflexes 353
    development of 352
    functions of 352
Blood cells and lymphatic organs, effects on 280
Blood coagulation 156
Blood colloidal osmotic pressure 303
Blood composition and functions of
    albumin 138
    difference between serum and plasma 138
    different types of globulins 138
    hypoproteinemia: causes 138
    physical properties 138
    plasma and formed elements 137
    plasma proteins 139
    specific gravity 138
Blood flow
    factors affecting 189
    in various chambers and vessels of heart 170f
Blood group 161
    ABO systems 161
        agglutinins in plasma 162
        chemistry of blood group antigen 161

determination of blood group 162
inheritance of blood group
substances 162
    Landsteiner's law 161
  blood transfusion 164
  complications of blood transfusion 164
  immediate signs and symptoms 165
  importance of 163
  indication 164
  other hazards 165
  Rh blood group 162
    inheritance of Rh system 163
    prevention 164
    treatment 163
Blood pressure 190
  control, factors influencing 192
  measurement of 191
  regulation of 192
Blood venous 128
Blood vessels 38, 201, 291
Blood volume 186
  regulation of 193
BMR *See* basal metabolic rate
Body
  as whole 33
  fluids distribution of total body water 16
  lies 221
  systems of 36
    cardiovascular system 36
    of digestive system 36
    endocrine system 36
    hemopoietic system 36
    locomotor system 36
    nervous system 36
    reproductive system 36
    respiratory system 36
    skin and organs 36
    urinary system 36
    urogenital system 36
  temperature, regulation of
    control of temperature 296
    heat loss 295
    heat loss conduction 295
    heat loss convection 295
    heat loss evaporation 295
    heat loss radiation 295
    heat production 295
    hyperpyrexia 297
    hypothermia 297
    pyrexia 296
Bohr effect 127

Bone 21
  cells 39
  cranium 42
  development of 39
  forearm 46
  growth 39, 261
  lining cells 22
  lower limb 52
    femur 52
    fibula 55
    foot 55
    knee-cap 53
    patella 53
    shin bone 54
    thigh bone 52
    tibia 54
  macroscopic, structure of 21
  matrix microscopy of 22
  microscopic, organization of 22
  microscopy of cells 22
  middle ear 379
  pelvic girdle 49
  right foot, medial view 55
  shoulder girdle 43
  structure of 41
  wrist and hand 48
  types of 40
    articulation 41
    border 41
    condyle 41
    crest 41
    epicondyle 41
    facet 41
    flat bone 41
    foramen 41
    fossa 41
    irregular bones 41
    long bones 40
    of sesamoid bones 41
    process 42
    short bones 41
  upper limb 43
Bony labyrynth 382
Botulinum
  clinical application 362
  tetanus toxins 362
Bowman's capsule 304
Brachial plexus 328
Brachialis 101
Bradykinesia 358

Brain 343
  bridge reflex 187
  death 344
  forebrain 343
  gut peptides 252
  hindbrain 343
  metabolism and oxygen requirements 198
  midbrain 343
Brainstem 354
  cerebral aqueduct 354
  cerebral peduncles 354
  crura cerebri 354
  decussation of the pyramids 354
  inferior colliculi 354
  medulla oblongata 354
  midbrain 354
  pons 354
  pyramids 354
  reflexes 344
  superior colliculi 354
  tegmentum 354
  vital centers 354
Breasts 404
  blood supply 405
  functions of 405
  lymph drainage 405
  nerve supply 405
  section of 405f
  structure 404
Breathing, types of 123
  intrapleural pressure changes 123
  intrapulmonary pressure 123
  pressure changes during respiratory cycle 123
Bregma 59
Broca's 198
Broca's area 347
Brodmann's area 346
Bronchial carcinoma 78
Bronchiectasis 78
Bronchoconstriction, factors producing 121
Bronchodilation, factors producing 121
Bronchopulmonary, segments of 116t
  left lung 116t
  right lung 116t
Bulbourethral glands 396
Burst promoting activity 149

C

Cadherins 14
Calcaneus articulates 56
Calcific nodules 61
Calcitonin 38, 274
  inhibits bone 38
Calcitriol 275
Calcium metabolism 271
  applied aspect 272
  body calcium 272
  deposition and resorption of bone 271
  functions of ionic calcium in the body 272
  main features of 244f
  physiology of bone 271
Callosal sulcus lies 345
Calorigenic effect 282
CAM *See* cell adhesion molecules
Cancellous bone 21, 38, 44, 62
Capillaries 188
Capillary endothelium 121
Capsular hydrostatic pressure 302
Carbamino compounds 128
Carbohydrate metabolism 240, 266, 282
Carbon dioxide (CO_2) 6, 36, 130, 166
  diffusion
    from tissues 126
    to alveolus 126
  dissociation curve 128
  in arterial blood 129
  narcosis 132
  transport 128
    in blood 126
    the form of bicarbonate 128
Carbon monoxide poisoning 134
Carbonic anhydrase inhibitors 309
Cardiac
  branches
    inferior 337
    superior 337
  cycle 180
    aortic pressure changes 183
    events of 181
    isometric relaxation phase 183
    mechanical changes 182
    pathologically 183
    proto diastole 182
    rapid ejection phase 183
    ventricular diastole 181, 182
    ventricular systole 181
  damage 196
  disorders 133
  external features 168
  failure, causes of 194
    decreased myocardial contractility 194
    increase in after load 194
    increase preload 194

impulse, spread of 177
investigations 190
muscle 23, 94
    Ca^{++} binding 94
    Ca^{++} channel 94
    Ca^{++} ions 94
    contraction 95f
output 184
    distribution of 185
    effect of end diastolic volume on 186
    methods of measurement 184
    regulation of 186
    variations of 185
shape 168
size 168
veins 169
Cardiomyopathy 194
Cardiovascular, physiology 170
Cardiovascular system 409
Carotid bodies, mechanism of stimulation 132
Carpus 42
Carrying angle 82
Cartilage 20
    cells 20
    growth of 21
    matrix 20
    structure of 20
    varieties of 20
Cartilaginous joint 79
    primary 79
    secondary 79
Catabolism of
    fats 241
    glucose 240
Catecholamines, actions of 282
Cauda equina 73
Cecum 211
Cell 7
Cell adhesion molecules 14
Cell
    body 24
    mediated 30
    membrane 11, 154
        arrangements of carbohydrates 13
        functions of 13, 14, 140
        structure 12f
    physiology 11
    surface projections 9
    types and hormones 253
        anterior pituitary 253
        posterior pituitary 253

Cellular immunity 205
Cellular organization 7
Celsius 417
Centigrade 417
Centrosome 13
Cephalic phase, control in 229
Cephalometry 51
Cerebellum 37, 355
    functions of 356
    histology 355
    layers 355
    symptoms of cerebellar disease 356
Cereberal 197
    circulation factors, determining the flow 197
    cortex, functional areas of 347
        motor areas 347
        visual area 348
Cerebrospinal fluid 322
    absorption 324
    clinical aspects 324
    composition 323
    formation of 324
    functions of 324
    measurement of 324
Cerebrum 344
Ceribral cortex
    functions of 346
    lobes of 346
Ceruminous glands 292
Cervical
    plexus 327
    vertebra 71f
Chelating agents 158
Chemical regulation 131
    aim of 132
    central chemoreceptors 131
    peripheral chemoreceptors 131
Chemoreceptors 129, 193
    primary response 193
    secondary response 193
Chest in section 117f
Cheyne-Stokes breathing 135
Chloride reabsorption 309
Chloride shift 128
Cholecystokinin 220
Cholesterol 242
Cholesterol esterase 236
Chorea 357
Chorionic villi 411
Chorionic villus sampling 411
Choroid 386

Choroid plexuses 321
Choroidal surface 387
CHP See capsular hydrostatic pressure
Christmas disease 160
Chromosomal abnormalities 11
Chromosomes 10
    analysis 11
    banding 11
    morphology of 11f
    structure of 10f
Chylomicron 237
Chymotrypsin carboxypeptidase 236
Cilia and flagella 10f
Ciliary body 385, 386
Ciliated columnar epithelium 18, 19f
Cingulate gyrus lies 345
Circulation 167f
Circulatory
    shock 133
    system 166
Circumvalate papilla 207
Cisterna chyli 202
Cisterna magna 321, 324
Cisternae 8
Citric acid cycle 241f
Clavicle 42, 44
Clinoid process, anterior 61
Clonus 370
Clot retractions 157
Clotting factors, production of 219
Coagulation
    mechanism of 156
    proteins 138
Coarctation of aorta 194
Coccygeal 42
Cochlear nerve 336
Collagen deseases 141
Collagen underneath endothelium 155
Colles' fracture 48
Colloid of the follicular spaces 266
Colon
    ascending 211
    descending 211
    pelvic 211
    sigmoid 211
    transverse 211
Columnar epithelium 18
Complement system 31
Conduction 25
Condyloid joint 57
Congenital adrenocortical enzyme deficiency 392
Congestive cardiac failure 133
Conjugate deviation 385
Conjunctiva 383
Conn's syndrome 194
Connective tissue 14, 19
    adipose tissue 19
    dense irregular connective tissue 19
    irregular connective tissue 19
    loose (areolar) connective tissue 19
    mucoid tissue 20
    regular connective tissue 20
Conus arteriosus 168
Conus medullaris 322
Conventional kinesins 13
Convergence theory 340
Convex lens 388
Coracoclavicular ligament 43
Coracoid process 43
Corium 290
Coronary
    artery 168
    circulation 196
    disease 169
    distribution 169
    mechanical 196
    metabolic factors 197
    neural factor 197
    sinus 170
Coronoid fossa 46
Corpus
    albicans 402
    luteum 402, 406
Cortex, types of 346
    agranular 346
    granular type 346
Corti 381
Cortical nephron 304
Corticobulbar tracts 132
Corticospinal tracts 132
Corticotropin-releasing
    factor 254
    hormone 256, 260
Cough 117
Counter current mechanism 315
Coupling 266
Cranial fossa, posterior 62, 64
Cranial nerves 333
    abducent 334
    accessory nerve 338
    facial nerve 335
    glossopharyngeal nerve 336

hypoglossal nerve 338
oculomotor 334
olfactory nerves 333
optic nerve 334
trigeminal nerve 335
trochlear 334
vagus nerve 337
vestibulocochlear nerve 336
Cretinism 240, 270
CRF *See* corticotropin-releasing factor
Cribriform plate 66
Cricoid cartilage 114
Crista galli 61
Crista terminalis 168
Cruciate ligaments 86
Cryoprecipitates 160
Cushing's syndrome 194, 260, 277
Cutaneous circulation 198
    special functions 198
    triple response 198
        flare 199
        red reaction 198
        wheal 199
Cutaneous senses 372
Cyanosis 135
Cyclooxygenase 411
Cyclooxygenase pathway 155
Cylindrical lenses 390
Cytokins 121
Cytoplasm 8, 154
    cytoplasmic inclusions 13
    cytoskeleton 13
    organelles 13
Cytoskeleton 9

D

DCT *See* distal convoluted tubule
Deamination 218
Deep cervical fascia 208
Deep muscles 101
Deep senses 372
Defecation 213, 234
Deglutition 207, 224
Degranulation 151
Dense irregular connective tissue 19f
Dent disease 307
Deoxygenated 166
Deoxygenated hemoglobin binds 128
Dermis 290
Desmopressin 263
Detoxification 219

Diabetes mellitus 286
    classical features 286
    classification of 287
    complications 286
    cut off level for hyperglycemia 286
Diabetic ketoacidosis 135, 287
Dialysis 317
    indications 317
    types of
        hemodialysis 317
        peritoneal dialysis 317
Diameter, anteroposterior 51
Diaphragm 103
Diaphragmatic (inferior) surface 168
Diaphragmatic
    movements 122
    surface 204
Diaphysis 40
Diffusing capacity 118
Diffusion 15
    facilitated diffusion 15
    K^+ ions through membrane 25
    Na^+ through nerve membrane 25
    types of channels 15
Digestion and absorption of
    fat 236
    food 235
    proteins 235
    lipids 236
Digestive
    function
        gastric lipase 227
        pepsin 227
        rennin 227
    organs 34
    peristalsis 232
    system 207
Digits 42
Dioxins 412
Dipalmitoylphosphatidylcholine 120
Dipeptidases 236
Diploe 60
Diplopia 335
Disorders of respiration 135
Disseminated intravascular coagulation 161
Distal convoluted tubule 305
Distal tubule and collecting ducts in excreting a concentrate urine 315
Diuretics 317
DNA, structure of 10

Dopamine 193
   effects of 283
   estrogen 275
   metabolism steps 282
   moderate rate 283
Dorsal 42
   and ventral 339
   nucleus of vagus 187
   surface of left scapula 43f
Dorsum sellae 65
Down syndrome 11
DPPC *See* dipalmitoylphosphatidylcholine
Ductless glands 36
Duodenum 210
   first (superior) part 210
   fourth part 210
   second (descending) part 210
   third (horizontal) part 210
   vascular supply 210
Dwarfism 258
Dwarfism pituitary 259
Dyneins 13
Dystrophin 91

E

Ear structure of 377f
ECF *See* extracellular fluid
ECG
   bipolar leads 175
   calibration of time and voltage on 177
   normal 177
   recording of 175
   unipolar leads 176
   unipolar limb leads 176
   uses of 179
   waves of 178
      P wave 178
      T wave 178
      U wave 178
Echocardiography 1
Edentulous atrophied 68
EDV *See* end diastolic volume
Einthoven's law 178
Ejaculatory ducts 396
Elastic cartilage 21f
Electrocardiograph 176
Electroencephalogram 2
Ellipsoid joint 80
Embryo
   development of 407f
   transfer, indication of 412

End diastolic volume 185
Endemic colloid goiter 271
Endocardium 172
Endocrine 252
   cells 226
   function 122
   glands action on 282
   pancreas 284
   system 251
Endocytic system 9
Endocytosis 15, 16
Endolymph 380, 382
Endoplasmic reticulum 8, 24
Endosome, system of vesicles 9
Endothelial cells 155
Endothelial factor 157
Enteric nervous system, physiological anatomy 222
Enterochromaffine cells 226
Enterogastric reflex 233
Enterohepatic, circulation of bile salts 231
   cholagogue 231
   choleretic effect 231
Entrapment neuropathy 48
Enzyme
   anticholinesterase 96
   tyrosinase 289
Eosinophil 152, 153
Eosinophilic
   cationic proteins 152
   peroxidase 152
Epicondyle
   lateral 45
   medial 45
Epidermis 289
Epidermolysis bullosa 9f
Epididymis 394
Epiglottis 113
Epinephrine 281
Epiphyseal cartilage 261
Epithelial cells 14, 18, 265
Erector spinae 106
Erythroblastosis fetalis 146, 163
Erythrocyte sedimentation rate, factors affecting 141
   plasma factors 141
   variations 141
Erythropoiesis 146
   development of blood cells 147
   factors influencing and regulating 149
   origin of blood cells 147
   site of synthesis 146
   stages of 147

Erythropoietin
    deficiency of 150
    secretion 133, 134
Eserine 386
ESR *See* erythrocyte sedimentation rate
Ethmoidal air cells 66
Eukaryotic cells 13
Excess volume transfusion 165
Excessive CO_2 132
Excitability 25
Excitation contraction coupling 92
Excretory system 298
Exocrine 221
Exocytosis 15, 16
Extensor digitorum communis 102
External acoustic meatus 377
Extracellular fluid 137, 277
Extrafusal fibers 368
Extrahepatic biliary tract 219
Extraocular muscles 384
Extrapyramidal nuclei 37
Extrapyramidal system 356
Extrinsic pathway 157
Eye
    accessory organs of 382
    bulb of 385
    muscles 384
    sockets 58
Eyeball 385
Eyelids 382
Eye-sockets 58

F

Facilitated diffusion 15f
Facilitation theory 340
Factors maintaining stability 81
Fahrenheit 417
Fair-skinned people 290
Fallopian tubes 215, 400
    function of 400
False localizing sign 335
False pelvis 50
Falx cerebri 61, 321
Fasciculus gracilis 339
Fat
    catabolism 242f
    metabolism 241
Fate of
    CO_2 in blood 126
    Na^+ 308
Fatiguability, abnormal 206

Fatigue 371
    causes of 94
Feces 213
Female climacteric and menopause 404
Female human fetuses 392
Female pelvis 52
    sagittal section 52f
Female reproductive system 398
    accessory sex organs 398
    ovary
        functions of 401
        structure 400
    primary sex organs 398
Femur 42
Fenestra vestibuli 379, 380, 381
Fetal
    circulation 410
    respiration 410
    testis secrete testosterone 391
Fetuin 138
Fetus ultrasound image 2f
FF *See* filtration fraction
FGFR 3 *See* fibroblast growth factor receptor 3
Fiber 248
    traversing anterior limb 350
    traversing genu 350
Fibrinogen 138, 141
Fibrinolytic
    enzyme 158
    inhibitors 160
    system 122
Fibroblast growth factor receptor 3 258
Fibrocartilage 21f
Fibrocartilaginous rim 83
Fibrocellular membrane 37
Fibrous 385
    areolar tissue 97
    band 48
    capsule 79, 81
    coats 385
    joint 79
Fibula 42
Fibular group 109
Filiform 207
Filopodia 20
Filtration fraction 305
Filum terminale 322
Flail chest 58
Flat foot 56
Flexor carpi radialis 102
Flexor digitorum longus 54, 108

Flexor digitorum sublimus 101
Fluid mosaic, model of membrane structure 12
Follicle stimulating hormone 253, 255, 393, 401
Follicular cells 265, 266
Food
    control of 249
    mixing of food 232
Foot 42
Foramen ovale 65
Forearm 42
Formed elements 139
Fluid therapy 16, 17
Fossa ovalis 168
FRC *See* functional residual capacity
Fresh frozen plasma 160
Fructose 235
FSH *See* follicle stimulating hormone
Fucose transferase 161
Fungiform 207
Funny bone 45, 329

G

GABA *See* amino acid gamma aminobutyric acid
Gactin 90
GAG *See* glycosaminoglycan
Galactose 235
Gallbladder 219, 231
    functions of 220
    structure of 220
Gallstones 232
Gamma efferent discharge control of 368
Gap junction 14
Gas
    content of inspired and expired air 118*t*
    transfer factor 118
Gastric
    branches 337
    curvatures 209
        greater curvature 209
        lesser curvature 209
    emptying 233
    hormonal mechanism 228
    motility 232
    orifices 209
        Barrett's esophagus 209
        cardiac orifice 209
        gastroesophageal junction 209
        internal appearance 209
        nerve supply 210
        pyloric orifice 209
        small intestine 210
        vascular supply 210
        veins 210
    phase, regulation in 230
    secretion, functions of 227
    secretion, phases of 228
        cephalic phase 228
        of gastric phase 228
        intestinal phase 229
    secretion, regulation of 227
    surfaces
        antero-superior surface 209
        postero-inferior surface 209
Gastrin, actions of 228
Gastroileal reflex 234
Gastrointestinal tract, organization of the wall 222
Gastrostomy 210
Genesis of expiration 131
Genetic sex 152
Genioglossus 207
Genitalia 391
GFR *See* glomerular filtration rate
GH *See* growth hormone
Ghost cells 142
Ghrelin 258
Giemsa 11
Gigantism 259
Girdle muscular dystrophy 94
Glandular epithelium 18*f*
Glenohumeral abduction 81
Glenoid cavity 44, 45, 46, 101
Glenoid labrum 81
Glisson's capsule 218
Globulin 138, 141
Glomerular
    blood hydrostatic pressure 302
    filtration rate 302
        factors affecting 303
        factors influencing 302
        regulation of 303
    ultrafiltration coefficient 303
Glomerulus 304
Glossopharyngeal 204
Glossopharyngeal nerve fibers 129
Glottis 118*f*
Glucagon 221, 287
Glucagon
    control of glucagon secretion 287
    effects on hepatocytes 287
    functions of 287
Glucocorticoids 276
    actions of 279
    anti-inflammatory effects of 280

Gluconeogenesis 240, 266
Glucose reabsorption, mechanism of 307
Glutathione peroxidase 139
Gluteus
    medius 50, 106
    minimus 50
Glycocalyx 13
Glycogen, storage of 218
Glycogenolysis 222
Glycogenosis 283
Glycolipids 12, 13, 139
Glycolysis 240, 241f
Glycophorin 139
Glycoproteins 12, 13, 138
Glycosaminoglycan 20
Glycosphingolipid 161
Glycosuria 284
GnRH *See* gonadotropin-releasing hormone
Golgi apparatus 8, 9f, 24
Golgi bottle neuron 369
Golgi complex 20
Golgi tendon organ 369
Gomphoses 79
Gonadotropin-releasing hormone 255, 256, 260
Gonads 275
Granular endoplasmic reticulum 8
Granular preumocyte secrete 120
Granulocytes 150
Grave's disease 270
Great vessels 167
Greater omentum 211
Growth hormone 253, 254, 256
    metabolic effects of 256
    secretion, abnormalities of 258
    secretion, factors affecting 257t
    secretion, regulation of 257

H

Hair 292
Hair follicle 292f
Hair layers
    cortex 292
    cuticle 292
    medulla 292
Haldane effect 128
Hand 42
Hand supinated 47
Haustral contractions 234
Haustral shuttling 234
Haversian canal 22, 38, 39
Haversian system 22

Hearing loss 382
Heart 167, 170
    block
        complete 180
        first degree 180
        second degree 180
        third degree 180
    conducting system of 171f
    contractile unit of 172
    layers of wall
        inner endocardium 171
        middle myocardium 171
        outer pericardium 171
    muscle fibers forming
        conductive system 172
        pacemakers 172
    pacemaker and conducting tissue 172
    rate factors influencing 187
    sound 172, 183
        first heart sound 173, 174
        fourth sound 173
        second heart sound 173, 174, 184
        third and fourth sounds 173, 184
Helper T cells mechanism of action of 32f
Hemalytic jaundice 144
Hematopoietic growth factors 149
Hemiplegia 342
Hemoglobin 142
    breakdown 143
    derivatives of 142
    estimation of 142
    functions of 143
    structure, synthesis 143
    synthesize 143
Hemolysis 29
Hemolytic
    disease of newborn 163
    jaundice 145
        causes 146
    transfusion reactions 165
Hemophilia A and hemophilia B 159
    clinical features 159
    diagnosis 159, 160
    treatment 160
Hemopoiesis 205
Hemopoietic
    function 228
    system 137
Hemorrhagic fever 259
Hemorrhoidal plexus 212

Hemostasis 156
    abnormalities of 159
    tests of
        bleeding time 158
        capillary tube method 159
        clotting time 158
        Dukes method 158
        Ivy methods 158
        prothrombin time 159
Heparin 157
Hepatic ducts 218
Hering-Breuer
    deflation reflex 133
    inflation reflex 132
Heterometric autoregulation 185
Hiccough 117
Hinge joint 80
Hirchsprung's disease 234
Histochemical techniques 333
Hodgkins disease 154
Homometric regulation 185
Homonymous hemianopia 334
Hormonal mechanism 193
Hormones adrenal medulla 281
    applied physiology 281
    biosynthesis 281
Hormones
    classification of 252
    influence of 187
    producing cell 264
    secretion of 394, 402
        estrogen 394
        testosterone 394
HPA *See* hypothalamic pituitary-adrenal
HPL *See* human placental lactogen
Human chromosome 10f
Human placental lactogen 407
Human plasminogen 157
Human skeleton 42
Humeroradial articulations 81
Humerus 42, 45
    articulates 44
Humoral 30
Huntington's chorea 357
Hyaline
    articular cartilage 45, 52
    cartilage 20, 39, 79
    membrane disease 121
Hydrocephalus 352
    types of 352
Hydrogen ion concentration in the body 5f

Hydrop's fetalis 163
Hyoglossus 207
Hyoid bone 376
Hyperapnea 193
Hypercapnea, effects 134
Hyperkalemia 131
Hyperparathyroidism 274
Hyperplastic thyroid gland 271
Hyperprolactinemia 412
Hypersecretion 251
Hypertension
    endocrine 194
    primary 194
    renal 194
    secondary 194
    treatment of 194
Hyperthyroidism 270
    diagnosis of 270
    physiology of treatment 270
Hypoglycemia 288
Hypokalemia 312
Hypoparathyroidism, abnormalities 274
Hypophyseal fossa 61, 65
Hypophysis cerebri 61, 65
Hypothalamic pituitary-adrenal axis 276
Hypothalamic releasing and inhibitory hormones
    control anterior pituitary secretion 260
    secreted into the median eminence 260
Hypothalamus, functions of 350
Hypothermia 297
Hypothyroidism, features of 269
Hypoxia
    anemic 135
    clinical features 133
Hypoxia histotoxic 135
Hypoxia oxygen
    therapy 134
    toxicity 134
Hypoxia, types of
    anemic hypoxia 133
    histotoxic hypoxia 133
    hypoxic hypoxia 133
    stagnant hypoxia 133

I

Icterus gravis neonatorum 163
Idiopathic non-toxic colloid goiter 271
Ileum 210
    Meckel's diverticulum 211
    superior mesenteric artery 211
    vascular supply 211
    veins 211

Iliac bones 50
Iliofemoral ligament 84
Iliotibial tract 106
Ilium, innominate bone 49
Immovable joints 57
Immune response 30, 205
Immune system development of 31
Immunity 28
    acquired 30
    active 30
        artificial 30
        natural 30
        passive 30
    cellular 31
    disorders of 154
    humoral 31
    natural (innate) 30
Immunoglobulin, molecule 31f
Immunoglobulins 205
In vitro fertilization 411
Infertility 411
Infraspinatus muscle 43
Infraspinous fossa 43
Infundibulum 168
Ingestion of food 222
Innate immunity 28
Innominate bone 49
Inorganic compounds 139
Inspiration 122
Inspiratory reserve 117
Insulin 221, 284
    action of 285
    applied physiology 286
    control of secretion 285
    effects of
        adipocytes 285
        liver 285
        skeletal muscle 285
    glucose entry 285
    hormonal control 286
    like growth factors 257
    mechanism of 285
    neural control 286
    substrate control 285
Integral proteins 13
Integrins 14
Intense phagocytic activity 205
Intercellular
    junctions 13, 14
    matrix 20

Intercondylar
    area 54
    fossa 53
Intercostal
    muscles 103
    space 78
Interdigestive phase 229
Interlobular veins 217
Intermediary metablolism 279
Internal capsule 350
Interneuron 364
Interosseous border 54
Interosseous membrane 46, 54, 55
Interstitial space 121
Intertrochanteric crest 53
Intertubercular sulcus 45
Interventricular septum 170, 171
Intervertebral discs 69
Intestinal
    mucosal cell 237
    phase regulation in 230
Intracartilaginous 37
Intracellular
    bacteria 31
    enzymes 29
Intrafusal fibers 367
Intralobujar ductules 218
Intramembranous 37
Intrapericardial pressure 186
Intrapulmonary pressure 123
Intrinsic
    pathway 156
    proteins 13
    vascular mechanism 193
Inverse stretch reflex 369
Iodide, oxidation of 266
Iodine deficiency 266, 270
Ionized 5
Iris 386
Iron
    balance 138
    metabolism 144
    sources and requirements of 144
    storage of 219
Irreversible shock 196
Ischiopubic ligament 84
Ischium 49, 50

J

Jaundice 232
    hemolytic (prehepatic) 232
    hepatic 232
    obstructive (posthepatic) 232

Jejunum 210
    jejunal feeding 210
Jendrassik's maneuver 369
Joint capsules 413
Joints of 79
    pelvic girdle and lower limb 83
        articular surfaces 83
        fibrous capsule 83
        hip joint 83
        ligament of head of femur 84
        ligaments of hip joint 84
        relations 84
    upper limb
        articulating surfaces 81
        carrying angle 82
        distal radioulnar joint 83
        elbow joint 81
        fibrous capsule 81
        glenohumeral joint 80
        ligaments 82
        radiocarpal joint 83
        radioulnar joints 82
        shoulder joint 80
        synovial membrane 82
        wrist joint 83
Jugular venous pressure 174
    wave form of 174
Jugulodigastric group 204
Juxtaglomerular apparatus 305
Juxtaglomerular cells secrete 301
Juxtamedullary nephrons 304
Juxtapulmonary capillary receptors 133
JVP *See* jugular venous pressure

K

Kala-azar 154
Karyotype 11
Keratohyalin 289
Kernicterus 163
Kidneys 278
Kidneys 298
    blood supply 301
    CT scan at the level of 2f
    functions of 301
    functions of
        composition of urine 302
        factors favoring filtration 302
        factors influencing 302
        glomerular filtration 302
        maintenance of homeostasis 301
        mechanism of urine formation 302
        net filtration pressure 302

    position of 299f
    relations 298
    renal corpuscle 299
    renal tubule 300
    structure 299
Kinin 301
Knee joint 55
    arthroscopy of 88f
Koniocortex 346
Krause's end bulbs 374
Krebs cycle 241f
Kupffer cells 232
Kussmaul's breathing 135
Kyphosis 70

L

Lacrimal
    apparatus 383f
    canaliculi 383, 384
    glands 383
    sac 383
Lambdoid suture 59, 63, 69
Lamellar bone 22
Landsteiner's law 161
Langerhans islets of 221
Large intestine
    functions of 212
    motility of 234
    movements of 213
    structure of 212
Laryngeal cavity, middle part of 114
Laryngeal
    stridor 274
    vestibule 114
Laryngopharynx 113
    constrictor muscles 113
    longitudinal muscles 113
    muscles of pharynx 113
    piriform fossa 113
Larynx 58, 113
    ventricle of 114
Lateral epicondyles 45
Lateral geniculate body 349
Laydig's cells 391
Led pipe rigidity 358
Left atrium 168
Left brachiocephalic vein 202
Left cerebral hemisphere 323f
Left clavicle 44f
Left humerus, anterior and posterior aspects of 45f
Left scapula, costal surface of 43f

Left ventricle 168
    general and external features 169
    internal features 169
Left ventricular outflow tract 167
Leg bones 42
Leishman stain 150
Lens 387
Leucocytes 137
Leukemia 154
    electron microscopic structure 154
    platelets 154
Leukopenia 154
Leukotriens 151
Levator palpebrae superioris 385
LH *See* luteinizing hormone
Ligaments of shoulder joint 81
Ligamentum flava 74
Ligamentum patella 86
Ligamentum teres 52
Linea
    aspera 53, 107
    nigra 409
Lingual gyrus 345
Lining thoracic wall 115
Lipases in pancreatic juice 236
    cholesterol esterase 236
    pancreatic lipase 236
    phospholipase a_1 and a_2 236
Lipid
    bilayer 12f
    metabolism 267, 282
Lipolysis 283
Lipoproteins 12, 138
Liquor folliculi 401
Liver 215
    blood supply 216, 217f
    disease 160
    functions of 218
    inferior surface of 217
    lobes 216
    lobule 218
    structure of 216
    surfaces of 216
        anterior surface 216
        inferior surface 216
        posterior surface 216
Lobectomy 78
Lobes 115
Lobulated mass lying 208
Loop of Henle 300, 305
    characteristics of 315

Lower limb 42
Lumbar lordosis 70
Lumbar plexus 329
Lumbosacral 73
Lunate bones 46
Lung 115
    apex 115
    base 115
    capacities 123
    changes occurring 128
    costal surface 115
    coverings of 121
    diffusion, capacity of 126
    factors affecting diffusion capacity of 127
    functions of 122
    left (2 lobes) 116
    medial surface 115
    pulmonary surface features 115
    right (3 lobes) 116
    ventilation of 118
    volumes 123
Luteinizing hormone 253, 255
Lymph nodes 201f, 202
    major groups of 203t
Lymphangitis 201
Lymphatic
    circulation 166
    vessels 291
Lymphocytosis 154
Lymphoid systems 200
Lymphoid tissue elsewhere 203
Lymphopenia 154
Lysosomes 8, 9, 13
Lysozyme 28

M

Malaria 146
Male reproductive system 392
    functions of 398
    scrotum 392
    testes 392
        functions of 393
        structure of 392
Malleolus, lateral 55
Malpighian bodies 204, 299
MALT *See* mucosa-associated lymphoid tissue
Mammalian cells shapes of 7
Mammary glands 404
Mandibular
    angle 208
    division 335

Manubrium 76
Marey's reflex 187
Mass peristalsis 234
Mast cells secrete heparin 122
Mastoiditis 64
Maxilla 58
Maxillary division 335
Maxillofacial injuries 58
Medial geniculate body 349
Medullary and pontine centers 131
Megakaryoblast 155
Megakaryocytes 7, 155
Meibomian glands 293
Meissner inner 222
Meissner's plexus 222
Melanin 289
Membrane potential, measurement of 26
Memeory cell 32
Menarche 401, 402
Meninges 321
Menstruation 403
    menstrual phase 403
    proliferative phase 403
    secretory phase 403
Mesangial cells 304
Mesenteric artery 212
    inferior 212
    superior 212
Metabolic acidosis 135
Metabolic functions
    carbohydrate metabolism 232
    destruction of blood cells 232
    detoxification 232
    excretory 232
    fat metabolism 232
    protein metabolism 232
    storage 232
    synthetic 232
Metabolism 238
    factors influencing 239
    of fats 218
Metacarpals 42
Metalloproteinases 152
Metamorphosis: metabolism 266
Metatarsalgia, anterior 56
Metatarsals 42
Micelles 236
Microbiocidal, effect 28
Microfilaments 9
Microflora 28
Microglia 24, 27

Microtubule based molecular motors 13
Microtubules 9
Microvilli 9
Micturite, urinary bladder 318
Micturition reflex 318
    abnormalities of bladder function 319
    higher control of micturition reflex 318
    reflex mechanism of voluntary micturition 318
Milk
    let down 263
    synthesis of 263
Mineral 267
Mineral metabolism 244, 282
    calcium 244
    fluorine 245
    iron 245
    magnesium 245
    phosphorus 245
    potassium 245
    sodium 245
    zinc 246
Mineralocorticoids 276
Mineralocorticosteroids 278
Miosis 386
Miotics 388
MIS *See* mullerian inhibiting substance
Mismatched blood transfusion 146
Mitochondria 9, 24
Mitochondrial matrix 9
Molecular motors 13
Molecules in cell membrane 12
Monocytes 29, 153
Monocytic leukemia 154
Monoglyceride 236
Mononuclear phagocytic
    cells 29
    system 29
Monosomy 11
Monosynaptic reflexes 366
Monro-Kellie doctrine 197m 324
Motor
    path 359
    system 345
        cerebral cortex 345
        layers from without inwards 346
    unit 93
Movement 359
Mucin secreted 213
Mucoid plug 408
Mucoid tissue 20f
Mucosa 222, 223

Mucus, functions of 228
Müllerian duct 391
    system 391
Müllerian inhibiting substance 391
Multifiber summation 93
Multinucleated fiber 23
Murmurs 184
Muscle 14
    abdomen 104
    actions of 98
    attachments of 98
    back of 106
    back of leg 108f
    back of the thigh 107
    buttock 106
    contraction, mechanism of 92
    contraction, physiology of 89
    expiration 122
    fatigue 93
    female pelvic floor 106
    fibers 17, 413
    forearm 101
    front of the leg 108f
    front of the thorax 105f
    hand and fingers 103
    head and neck 99
    leg 107
    lower extremity 106
    pelvis 106
    principal groups of 99
    producing movements of 81
    right upper limb: posterior aspect of 102
    shoulder girdle 101
    spindles, function of 368
    spindles, structure of 367
    superficial 100
    thigh 106
    thoracic wall 103
    tone 342, 369
    tongue 207
    trunk 103
    upper limb 101
Muscular dystrophy, types of 94
    Duchene's muscular dystrophy 94
    limb 94
    milder form 94
Muscular pump 166
Muscular ridges 168
Muscular tissue 23
Muscularis 222
Musculi pectinati 168

Myasthenia gravis 97
Mydriasis 386
Mydriatics 386
Myelin 24, 25
Myeloid stems cells 147
Myenteric
    plexus 222
    reflex 228
Mylohyoid muscle 207
Myocardial contractility 187
Myocardium 172
Myoepithelial cells 24
Myofibril 89
Myoglobin 128
Myosin 91
    light chain phosphates 95
    molecule 91
Myxedema 154, 240, 269

N

Nails 293
Naked nerve endings 374
Nasal cavity 110
    cartilagenous septum 110
    floor 110
    lateral wall 110
    medial wall 110
    nerve supply of 112
    roof 110
Nasal septum 110f
    arterial supply of 111
Nasolacrimal duct 383, 384
Nasopharyngeal tissues 204
Nasopharynx 64, 112
Natural antibiotics 29
Navicular bone 56
Neck 59
Neoplasmic lesion 263
Nephritic syndrome 194
Nephrogenic diabetes insipidus 311
Nephron, functional anatomy 304
Nerve 24
    functions of myelin 25
    morphology 24
    sensory information 291
    supply 121
Nervi irigentes 318
Nervous control of the
    blood vessels 192
    heartbeat 189

Nervous system 320
    effects on 280
    function major levels of
        higher brain or cortical level 322
        lower brain level 322
        spinal cord 322
    organization of 320
Neurexins 362
Neurilemma 24
Neurocrine hormones 252
Neurofibrils 24
Neurohypophysis 253, 255
Neuromuscular
    junction 96, 206
    transmission 96
Neuronal cell bodies 261
Neurons
    cluster of 250
    properties of 25
    types of
        bipolar 24
        multipolar 24
        unipolar 24
Neurotransmitters 332
Neurovascular bundle 78
Neutropenia 154
Neutrophil 150-152
    granules 152
Neutrophilia 153
Nigro striatum 357
Nissl bodies 24
Nitric oxide 253, 366
Nocturnal enuresis 319
Nonadrenalin 193
Normoblast
    early 148
    late 148
Nuchal lines, superior 59
Nucleus 13, 148
    consists 3
    nuclear membrane 13
    nucleolus 13
    nucleoplasm 13
Nutrition 248

O

Obesity 250
Obligatory urine volume 314
Obstetric gland 274
Obturator
    externus muscle 53
    foramen 50
    membrane 50
    muscles 85
Occipital bone, outer surface of 63f
Odontoid process 72
Olecranon
    fossa 47
    process 46, 47
Olegodentroglia 27
Olfactory mucosa 111
Oligo dendrocytes 24
Oligosaccharides 161
Omenta 214
Oogenesis 401
Oogonia 401
Ophthalmic division 335
Opioid peptides 281
Opsonization 151
Opsonizing antibody 30
Optic
    chiasma 334
    neuritis 334
Oral (presulcal) part 207
Orbits 58
Organification 266
Oropharynx 113
    boundaries 113
    palatine tonsil 113
    palatoglossal 113
    palatopharyngeal arches 113
Osmosis 15
Osmotic
    fragility 142
    pressure 138
    stimuli 262
Osseous labyrinth 381
Ossicles 379
Osteoblasts 22, 38
Osteoclasts 22
Osteon 23f
Osteoprogenitor cells 22
Ovarian, functions control of 402
Ovaries 36, 400
Ovulalion 401
Oxalated blood 159
Oxaloacetic acid 242
Oxidative metabolism 266

Oxygen (O$_2$)
    affinity of Hb 143
    content and partial pressure 127t
    diffusion from
        alveolus 125
        capillaries to tissues 126
    Hb dissociation curve 127
    in arterial blood 129
    transport in blood 126
Oxytocin 256, 262
    function of milk ejection 263

P

Pacemaker 172
Pacinian corpuscles 373
PAF *See* platelet, activating factor
Pain 338
    receptor 374
    reffered pain 338
    stimuli for visceral pain 338
    visceral pain 338
Palatoglossal arch 207
Palmar surface 48
Pancreas 221, 283
    functions of 221
    structure of 221
Pancreatic
    juice 229
    polypeptide 288
    secretion, regulation of 229
        composition 229
        inorganic substances 229
        lipolytic enzymes 229
        proteoytic 229
        regulation of 229
Panhypopituitarism in the adult 259
    causes 259
    effects 259
    treatment 259
Papilloedema 334
Paracrine hormones 252
Paraesthesias tingling sensations 274
Parafollicular cells 265
Paraplegia 342
Parasitic infestation 154
Parasympathomimetic drugs 386
Parathyroid
    glands 273
    hormone 38
Parieto-occipital sulcus 345
Parkinsonism 358

Parotid capsule 208
Parotid gland 208, 223
    anteromedial surface 208
    innervations of 224
    parotid capsule 208
    parotid duct 208
    posteromedial surface 208
    superficial surface 208
    vascular supply 208
Pars intermedia 253
Patellar ligament 85
Patent ductus arteriosus 410
PDA *See* patent ductus arteriosus
Pectoralis
    major 103
    minor 103
Peculiar gait 358
Pelvic
    aperture superior 51
    axis 51
    cavity 51
        boundaries of 36
        contents of 36
    floor 399
    girdle 42
    inlet 51
    peritoneum 215
Pelvimetry 51
Pelvis 51f
    false 50
    true 51
Pendular contractions 233
Penis 396
    blood supply 397
    nerve supply 397
Peptidases 229
    amylase 229
    lipase 229
    nucleases 229
    phospholipases 229
    procarboxy peptidase 229
    trypsin and chymotrypsin 229
Peptide bonds 243
Peptides 236
Perfusion pressure 197
Pericardium 172
    parietal layer 214
    visceral layer 214
Perilymph 380, 381, 382
Periodic breathing, types of 135
    Biot's breathing 135
    Cheyne-Stokes breathing 135

Periosteum 39
Peripheral chemoreceptors 129
Peripheral protein 13
Peristaltic contractions 233
Peritoneal
	dialysis 215
	ligaments 214
Peritoneum 214
	functions of 215
Peritubular capillaries 315
Peroneal nerve 55
Peroxisomes 9, 13
Pes planus 56
Petromastoid part 64
Petrous portion 64
Peyer's patches 204
pH See hydrogen ion concentration
Phagocytes 29
Phagocytic cells 29
Phagocytosis 30, 151, 205
Phalanges 42, 49
Pharyngeal (post-sulcal) part 207
Pharynx 112
Phenylbutazone 309
Pheochromocytoma 283
Phospholipids 12, 242
Phosphorus, metabolism
	action on
		bone 273
		intestine 273
		kidney 273
	functions of 272
	mechanism of 274
Physostigmine 388
Pia mater 321
PIF See prolactin inhibiting factor
Pineal gland 275
Pinna 377, 378
Pisiform 48
Pituitary
	gland 253
	growth hormone 40
	hyperfunction 259
	insufficiency in humans, features 259
Pivot joint 80
Placenta, developed 408f
Plane joint 80
Plasma proteins
	production of 219
	prothrombin 243

Plasma thromboplastin 160
Plasmin lyses fibrin 157
Plasticity 96
Platelet 155
	activating factor 155
	activation 155
	adhesion 155
	plug formation 156
	properties and functions of 155
Pleura 115
	cervical 115
	costovertebral 115
	diaphragmatic 115
	parietal 121
	vascular supply of 115
	visceral 115, 121
Pleural
	effusion 203
	recess 115
Pneumotaxic center 129, 131
Poikilocytosis 140
Poiseuille's law 188
Polyarthritis nodosa 141
Polychromatophilic normoblast 148
Polycythemia 140, 142
Polymorphnuclear
	neutrophils 30
	leukocytes 28, 29, 200
Polypeptides 29
Polyphyletic 147
Polysynaptic reflex 370
Popliteal
	fossa 54
	surface 53
Popliteus 54
Porta hepatis 216
Postcentral gyrus 376
Postganglionic
	fibers 360, 361
	neurons 95, 360
Postsynaptic, membrane effect of ach on 96
Potts' fracture 55
pouch of Douglas 215, 398
Power stroke 92
Precapillary sphincter 188
Preganglionic fibers 359, 360
Pregnancy 406
	changes in maternal, physiology of 408
	diagnosis of the cause 411
	full-term 408f
Pregnant, uterus effect on 263

Presynaptic
    membrane 363
    neuron 363, 364
PRL *See* prolactin
Proenzymes 29
Proerythroblast 148
Progenitor cell 147
Prolactin 253, 255
    inhibiting factor 255
    inhibitory hormone 260
Prolongation of PR interval 179
Pronormoblast 148
Proprioceptors 373
Proprionobacterium acnes 28
Prostate gland 396
    blood supply 396
    nerve supply 396
Prostatic obstruction 28
Protective function 228
Protein and polypeptides 252
Protein C 157
Protein 91
    cell membrane 12, 13
    contractile elements 90
    metabolism 243, 267
        main features of 243f
    synthesis 243
Proteosomes 9
Prothrombin conversion of 156
Protruberances 45
Proximal convoluted tubule 305
Psoas muscle 53
Pterygoid processes 65
Pterygopalatine ganglion 204
Ptosis 335
Ptyalin 223
Puberty 402
Pubic rami 51, 52
Pubic symphysis 49, 50, 51
Pubis 49, 50
Pubofemoral ligament 84
Pulmonary
    artery 183
        atrial pressure changes 183
        isometric contraction 183
        jugular venous pressure 183
        volume changes in the ventricle 183
    edema 134
    fissures 115
    gas exchange 125
    ligaments 115
    veins 194
    ventilation, measurement of 123
Pulse 191
Pulvinar part of thalamus 349
Pyramidal decussation 342
Pyramidal tract 341
Pyrexia 296
Pyruvic acid molecules of 240

Q

QRS complex 179
Quadrates lumborum muscles 299
Quadriceps
    extensor 107
    muscle 53
    tendon 53
Quadriplegia 342
Queckenstedt's sign 324
Q wave 179

R

Radiation induced tissue injury 134
Radioulnar joint 48, 82f
Radius 42, 46, 47
Raloxifene 412
Rami 50
Ramus superior 50
Ramus terminates 67
Rathke's pouch 259
RBC *See* Red blood cells
RBM *See* red bone marrow
Receptors 372
    classification of 372
    exteroceptors 373, 375
    interoceptors 375
    proprioceptors 375
    telereceptors 375
    types of 373
Reciprocal innervation 372
Rectum and anal canal 212
Rectus
    abdominis muscle 76
    femoris 107
Red blood cells 200
    functions of 140
    life span of 142
    membrane, major proteins of 139
    properties of 140
    structure of 139

variations
   shape 140
   size 140
   structure of 140
Red bone marrow 31
Red cell storage 206
Reflexes 366
Regional
   circulations 196
   variation of supply 196
Reinke's edema 114
Relative refractory period 372
Relax mesangial cell 309
Relaxing protein 92
Renal
   blood flow
      measurement of 303
      special features of 304
   hypertension 194
   mechanisms for excreting a dilute urine 313f
   medullary interstitium hyperosmotic 315
   plasma flow 305
   tubule 300f
Renin
   angiotensin aldosterone 303
   angiotensin mechanism 193
      capillary fluid shift 193
      stress relaxation 193
Renshaw cell inhibition 364
Repolarization 27
Reproductive system 391
Residual volume 117
Resistance to stress 280
Respiration
   artificial
      mechanical methods of 136
      methods of 135
      procedure 136
   physiology of 119
   regulation of
      automatic control of respiration 130
      chemical control 129
      expiratory center 130
      inspiratory center 130
      nervous control 129
      pneumotaxic center stimulates 130
      pontine centers 130
Respiratory
   centers factors, affecting 132t
   membrane, structure of 121
   movements 116, 117

   system 110
   tract, movement of air 117
   volumes 117t
Resting membrane potential 25, 91
   origin of 25
Reticular formation 354, 356
   functions of the
      ascending reticular fibers 355
      descending pathways 355
   nervous connections
      afferent connections 355
      efferent connections 355
Reticulocyte 148
Retina 386
   layers of 387
Retinaculum bridges 48
Retro-mandibular vein 208
Rh blood group 162
Rheumatic
   fever 141
   arthritis 141
Rhodopsin 387
Rhythmical segmental contractions 233
Rib 42, 76
   movements of 116
Ribonucleic acid 321
Ribosomes 8f, 13, 24
Right atrium 168
Right heart failure 194
   backward failure 195
   forward failure 194
Right ventricle 168
Rima glottidis 114
RMP *See* resting membrane potential
RNA *See* ribonucleic acid
Rolando central sulcus of 345
Romanosky stain 150
Rough ischial tuberosity 50
Rouleaux formation 139, 140, 141f
RPF *See* renal plasma flow
Ruffini's end organs 374
Ryanodine receptor 94

S

Sacral outflow 361
Sacral plexus 330
Saddle joint 80
Saliva secretion of 223
Salivary ducts 223
Salivary glands 208, 223, 224f
Saphenous vein 54

Sarcoglycans 94
Sarcolemma 90
Sarcomere 23, 89, 95
Sarcoplasmic reticulum: functions 90
Scalp 59
Scapula 42, 43
Schindylesis 79
Schwann cells 24
Sciatica 331
Sclerotic coat 385
Sebaceous glands 293
Sebum 293
Segmental peristalsis 233
Selective estrogen receptor modulators 412
Selective vagotomy 337
Sella turcica 61, 62, 65
Semen 397
Semicircular canals 382
Semimembranosus 107
Seminal vesicles 395
    blood supply 395
    nerve supply 395
Semitendinosus 107
Sensation 331
    deep 331
    in the skin 375
    superficial 331
Sense of hearing 377
    external ear 377
    internal ear 380
    mechanism of hearing 381
    middle ear 378
    semicircular canals 382
    smell 376
    taste 376
    vision 382, 390
Sensorineural deafness 382
Sensory
    nerves 197
    path 331
Septal
    cartilage 66
    wall 168
SERM *See* selective estrogen receptor modulators
Serosa 222
Sertoli cells, secrete 391
Sesamoid bone 53, 107
Sex
    chromatin 391
    chromosomes 393
    glands 275
    hormones 40, 276
    organs, development of the gonads 391
Sexual growth 267
Sheehan's syndrome 259
Shock 195
    causes of
        cardiogenic shock 195
        hypovolemia 195
        septicemic shock 195
    compensatory mechanism 195
        conservation of body water 195
        tissue fluid shift 195
        vasoconstriction 195
    dangers of 195
Shoulder
    girdle 43
    joint 80f
        ligaments of 81
        movements of 81
Sickle cell
    anemia 142
    Hb 144
Sighs 117
Sight, mechanism of 388
Sigmoid
    flexure 211
    mesacolon 211
Sinoatrial node 170
Sinus 114
Sinusoids 217
Skeletal muscle 23, 89, 97
    contraction, mechanics of 93
    fasciae 97
    pump 185
    tone 93
Skeleton 37, 40
    main functions of 40
    larynx of 113
    thorax of 75f
Skin 289
    functions of
        absorption 294
        formation of vitamin d 294
        protection 294
        secretion 294
        sensation 294
        storage 294
    regulation of body temperature 289
    section through 290f
    systemic disease 294

Skull 34
  bones of
    anterior cranial fossa 61
    interior of the skull 60
    middle cranial fossa 61
    norma
      basalis 60
      frontalis 58
      occipitalis 59
      verticalis 59
    posterior cranial fossa 62
  ethmoid bone 66
  fontanelles 68
  frontal bone 62
  interior of 61f
  lacrimal bones 67
  lateral view 59f
  mandible jaw 67
  maxilla 66
  nasal bones 67
  occipital bone 63
  outline of 60f
  palatine bones 67
  parietal bone 63
  sphenoid bone 64
  temporal bone 64
  vomer 67
  zygomatic bone 67
Sliding filament theory 92
Small intestinal motility 233
Smooth endoplasmic reticulum 8
Smooth muscle 23, 24f, 95
SMR *See* submucous resection
Sodium glucose cotransport 16f
Soleus 54
Somatomedins 257
Somatostatin 288
Somatotropin 254
Spastic neurogenic bladder 319
Special senses 372
Spectrin 139
Speech 119
  consonants 119
  vowels 119
Spermatic cord 395
  blood supply 395
  lymphatic drainage 395
  nerve supply 395
Spermatogenesis 393
Spermatogonia 393
Spermatozoon 393
Sphenoid bones 58

Spherocytosis 140, 142
Spinal column 42
Spinal cord 324
  structure of 326
    grey matter 326
    of white matter 326
Spinal nerves 327, 328f
Spinocerebellar tract 339
Spinothalamic tract 341
Spinous process 71, 74
Spiral structure 381
Spirogram 124
  importance of FEV_1 125
  inspiratory capacity 125
  inspiratory reserve volume 124
  lung capacities 124
  pathological variations 124
  residual volume 124
  significance of residual volume 124
  tidal volume 124
  variations in vital capacity 124
Spleen 204
  functions 205
  medial or visceral aspect of 205
  structure of 204
Splenectomy 205
Splenic flexure 211
Spongy bone 21
Squamous
  epithelium 120, 289
  part 64
Starling's forces 309
Starvation 250
Stellate cells 304
Stercobilin 213
Sternocostal surface, anterior 168
Sternum 42
  during respiration 116
Steroid hormones 252
Stimulate parietal cells, agents 228
  ACh 228
  enterogastrone 228
  gastrin 228
  histamine 228
Stimulation 131
Stimulus 25
Stokes-Adams syndrome 180
Stomach 208
  motor functions of 226
  movements of 232
  parts of 208
  receptive relaxation of 226

secretions of 226
structure of 209f
Stratified squamous epithelium 18
Stratum
　　corneum 289
　　granulosum 289
　　lucidum 289
Striae gravidarum 409
Styloid process 46, 47, 56
Subarachnoid space 321
Subendocardial region of myocardium 196
Subliminal fringe 371
Sublingual glands 223
Submadibular gland 223
　　innervations of 224
Submandibular salivary gland 208
　　secretomotor supply 208
　　submandibular duct 208
　　superficial part 208
Submucosa 222
Submucous resection 66
Sulci 168
Summation 93
Suprapatellar bursa 53
Suprapubic arch 52
Suprarenal
　　cortex, functions of 276
　　glands 275
　　medulla, functions of 277
Suprascapular nerve 44
Suprasellar cysts 259
Supraspinous fossa 43
Surfactant 120
　　approximate, composition of 120
Suture 79
Swallowing, stages of 224
　　esophageal 226
　　nervous control of pharyngeal 225
　　pharyngeal 225
　　voluntary 225
Sweat glands 278, 291
　　apocrine gland 291
　　eccrine glands 291
Sydenham's chorea 357
Sylvian fissure 345
Symphysis menti 79
Synapse
　　different types of 24, 361
　　　　chemical synapse 361
　　　　conjoint synapses 362
　　　　electrical synapse 361
　　properties of 365

Synaptic transmission 363
Synarthroses 79
Syncope 189
Syndesmoses 79
Synovial
　　fluid 80
　　joint, classification of 80
　　membrane 80, 81

T

Tabetic bladder 319
Tachycardia 268
Taenia coli 212
Tailbone 73
Talocrural joint 87
Tamoxifen 412
Tank respirators 136
Tarsus 42
Taste buds 377f
T cell
　　cytotoxic 32
　　helper 31
　　suppressor 31
Tectum 355
Tele receptors 373
Temperature regulation 122, 267
Temporal summation 93
Tentorium cerebelli 61, 321
Terminal bronchioles histology of 120
Tetanus 93
Tetrahydrobiopterine deficiency 281
Thalamic radiations: anterior, posterior,
　　superior, inferior 349
Thalamus 349
Thalassemia 144
Thermoreceptors 374
Thiazides 309
Thick filament 91
Thoracic 42
　　nerves 329
　　vertebrae with ligaments 77f
Thoracoabdominal 123
Thoracolumbar division 189
Thoracotomy 78
Thorax 34
　　bones of
　　　　costal cartilages 77
　　　　intercostal spaces 78
　　　　ribs 76
　　　　sternum 75

boundaries of 34
contents of 35
section of 35f
Thromboasthenic purpura platelet 156
Thrombocytes 137
Thrombocytopenia 156
Thrombocytosis 156
Thromboembolic disorder 160
Thromboembolism 133
Thrombopoiesis 155
Thymus 206
Thyroid 265
   adenoma 270
   biosynthesis 265
   cartilage 114
   effect on
      CNS 268
      CVS 268
   functions 266
   gland 38, 264
   hormone 40, 239
   mechanism of action 268
   stimulating hormone 253, 254, 264
   storm 271
Thyrotoxic crisis 271
Thyrotoxicosis 240
Thyrotrophin-releasing hormone 254, 256, 260, 265
Tibia 42
Tibial
   collateral ligament 85, 86
   condyles 54
   tuberosity 54
Tibialis anterior muscle 54
Tissue
   anoxia 196
   thromboplastin activate prothrombin 159
Titin 91
TLC *See* total lung capacity
Toes 42
Tongue 207
   innervation of 207
   parts of 376f
Tonsils 204
Total knee replacement 88f
Total lung capacity 117
Tourniquet test 159
Toxemia 196
Trabecular 38
Transitional epithelium 18
Transmembrane proteins 13
Transmission of depolarization 179
Transport across cell membranes 15
Tremor 358
TRH *See* thyrotrophin-releasing hormone
Tricuspid valve 167, 168, 170, 174, 184
Trigeminal
   ganglion 335
   nerves 376
Triglycerides 236
Triiodothyronine 264
Tripeptidases 236
Trochanteric fossa 53
Trochlear
   nerve 335, 385
   notch 46, 47
Tropomyosin 90, 91
Troponin complex 90
Trousseau's sign 274
Truncal vagotomy 337
Trypsin 236
   inhibitor 229
TSH *See* thyroid stimulating hormone
Tubular
   fluid in distal 314
   function
      filtered load 305
      glucose reabsorption 306
      renal tubular transport maximum 305
   secretion 302, 311
   system 154
Tunica
   adventitia 188
   intima 188
   media 188
Tympanic membrane 380
Tympanic part 64

U

Ulna 47
Ulnar nerve 46
Ulnar nerve passes 45
Uniaxial joint 81
Unipolar
   chest leads 179
   recording 178
      active (exploring) electrode 178
      indifferent electrode 178
Upper limb 102
Upper motor neurones 37
Urea
   absorption 310
   role of 316

Urinary bladder 317
    afferent nerve supply 317
    function 318
Urine
    acidification of 316
    concentration and dilution 313
    volume decrease 262
Uterus 398
    blood supply 399
    cervix 398
    cornu 398
    external os 398
    functions of 400
    fundus 398
    internal os 398
    lymphatic drainage 399
    nerve supply 399
    position of 399
        anteflexion 399
        anteversion 399
        broad ligaments 399
        retroversion 399
        transverse cervical ligaments 399
    uterosacral ligaments 399
    walls of 398
        endometrium 399
        myometrium 398
        perimetrium 398
Uxtamedullary nephrons 305

V

Vagal trunks
    anterior 337
    posterior 337
Vagus
    nerves 222
    respiration role of 133
Vas deferens 394
Vascular
    coat 385
    constriction 156
    mural cells 195
    reactivity: 279
    spasm 156
    stasis 131
    supply 169, 208
        coronary arterial supply 169
        left coronary artery 169
        right coronary artery 169
    system, parts of systemic circulation 188
    trabecular bone 75

Vasoactive intestinal peptide 252
Vasoconstrictor nerves 192
Vasodilator nerves 192
Vasopressin 255, 261
Vasopressure action 262
Vasovagal reflex 228
Vastus medialis 107
Veins 188
Venous sinuses 321
Ventilators
    types of 136
        pressure ventilator pumps 136
        volume ventilator pumps 136
    response to
        CO_2 132
        H^+ 132
Ventral posterolateral 349
Ventricles 350
    body of lateral ventricle 351
    inferior horn 351
    lateral ventricle 350
    posterior horn 351
    third ventricle 351
Ventricular
    conduction 177
    fibrillation 180
    systole 181
        isometric contraction phase 181
        reduced ejection phase 181
Vermiform appendix 211
Vertebrae 42
Vertebral column 69, 70f
    cervical vertebrae
        atlas 71
        axis 72
    coccyx 73
    ligaments of the vertebral column 74
    lumbar vertebrae 73
    movements of the spinal column 75
    sacrum 73
    spine whole 70
    thoracic vertebrae 72
    vertebrae 70
Vessels and nerves 84
    ankle joint 87
    articular surfaces 85
    bursa around knee joint 87
    knee joint 85
    ligaments of knee 86
    ligaments of the joint 85
    menisci 86
    muscles producing movement 84, 87, 88

Vessels pressure change 188
Vestibular
    ganglion 336
    nerve 336
Vicious cycle 196
Villi movement 233
VIP *See* vasoactive intestinal peptide
Visceral senses 372
Visceroceptors 373
Viscosity 138
Vision 390
Visual pathways 390
Vital capacity 117
Vitamins 246
    B 213
    B complex 247
    folate 149
    storage of 219
    types of
        fat soluble
            A (retinol) 246
            D 38, 246, 247
            E (tocopherols) 246
            K 213, 246, 247
        water soluble
            B_1 (thiamine) 246, 247
            B_{12} (cyanocobalamin) 149, 246, 247
            B_2 (riboflavin) 246, 247
            B_3 (nicotinamide) 246, 247
            B_6 (pyridoxine) 246, 247
            C (ascorbic acid) 149, 248, 246
            folic acid 246, 248
            pantothenic acid 246, 248
Vitreous body 387
VMC ischemic 196
Vocal
    cords 114
    folds 114
Vocalization 122
Voice production 118
    loudness 118
    pitch 118
    quality 119
Volition 37
Voluntary
    control of respiration 133
    hyperventilation 133
von Willebrand 158
    factor 154, 155
    disease 156, 158

W

Waldeyer's ring 113
Warm antibody 162
Water 248
    balance 17, 122
    intoxication 311
    metabolism 259
        effects on 280
    reabsorption 310
WBC, lifespan of 153
Wernicke's area 198
Westergren's pipette 141
Whispering 119
White fibrocartilage 20, 21
Windkessel
    effect 188
    vessels 188
Window of the eye 385
Winslow 214*f*
Withdrawal reflex 370
Wolffian duct system 391
Wrist 42
    drop 329

X

Xanthine oxidase 309
X descend, tricuspid valve ring 174
X linked fatal 94
XO chromosomal pattern 258
XX in females 11
XY in males 11

Y

Yawns 117
Y chromosomes 11
Y descend, tricuspid valve opened 174
Yellow elastic cartilage 20, 21
Young
    cartilages 79
    cells 20, 151

Z

Zn 149
Zona pellucida 401, 406
Zygomatic
    arch 208
    bone 58, 60, 63, 67
    process 63